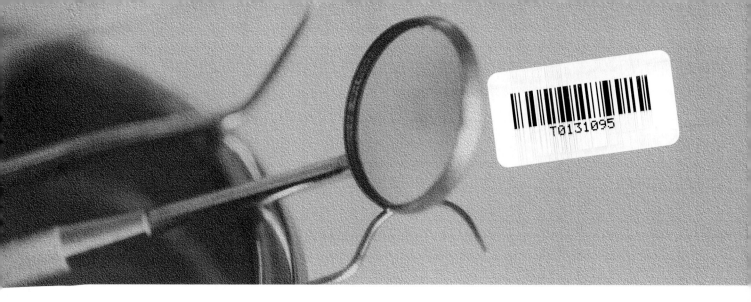

Mosby's
Review for the NBDE

Part Two

SECOND EDITION

edited by

FRANK DOWD, DDS, PhD
Professor Emeritus
Department of Pharmacology
School of Medicine
School of Dentistry
Creighton University
Omaha, Nebraska

ELSEVIER
MOSBY

3251 Riverport Lane
St. Louis, Missouri 63043

Notices

Knowledge and best practice in this field are constantly changing. As new research and experience broaden our understanding, changes in research methods, professional practices, or medical treatment may become necessary.

Practitioners and researchers must always rely on their own experience and knowledge in evaluating and using any information, methods, compounds, or experiments described herein. In using such information or methods they should be mindful of their own safety and the safety of others, including parties for whom they have a professional responsibility.

With respect to any drug or pharmaceutical products identified, readers are advised to check the most current information provided (i) on procedures featured or (ii) by the manufacturer of each product to be administered, to verify the recommended dose or formula, the method and duration of administration, and contraindications. It is the responsibility of practitioners, relying on their own experience and knowledge of their patients, to make diagnoses, to determine dosages and the best treatment for each individual patient, and to take all appropriate safety precautions.

To the fullest extent of the law, neither the Publisher nor the authors, contributors, or editors, assume any liability for any injury and/or damage to persons or property as a matter of products liability, negligence or otherwise, or from any use or operation of any methods, products, instructions, or ideas contained in the material herein.

Executive Content Strategist: Kathy Falk
Senior Content Development Specialist: Brian Loehr
Publishing Services Manager: Julie Eddy
Senior Project Manager: Marquita Parker
Design Direction: Brian Salisbury

Printed in the United States of America

Last digit is the print number: 9 8 7

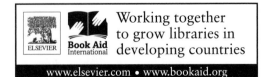

Section Editors

Myron Allukian, Jr., DDS, MPH
Oral Health Consultant
Boston, Massachusetts

Nikola Angelov, DDS, MS, PhD
Professor and Chair
Department of Periodontics
School of Dentistry
University of Texas Health Sciences Center
Houston, Texas

Oscar Arevalo, DDS, SCD, MBA, MS
Private Practice
Miami Children's Hospital
Pediatric Dentistry
Doral, Florida

Larry L. Cunningham, Jr., DDS, MD, FACS
Professor and Chief
Division of Oral and Maxillofacial Surgery
University of Kentucky
Lexington, Kentucky

Frank Dowd, DDS, PhD
Professor Emeritis
Department of Pharmacology
School of Medicine
School of Dentistry
Creighton University
Omaha, Nebraska

Jarshen Lin, DDS
Director, Predoctoral Endodontics
Department of Restorative Dentistry and Biomaterials
    Science
Harvard School of Dental Medicine
Boston, Massachusetts

Steven J. Lindauer, DMD, MDSc
Professor and Chair, Department of Orthodontics
Virginia Commonwealth University
School of Dentistry
Richmond, Virginia

Sanjay Mallya, BDS, MDS, PhD
Assistant Professor
Diagnostic and Surgical Sciences
School of Dentistry
University of California
Los Angeles, California

Karen Novak, DDS, MS, PhD
Professor
Department of Periodontics
School of Dentistry
University of Texas Health Sciences Center
Houston, Texas

Alejandro Peregrina, DDS, MS
Clinical Associate Professor
Restorative and Prosthetic Dentistry
College of Dentistry
The Ohio State University
Columbus, Ohio

Kenneth L. Reed, DMD, FADSA, NDBA
Private Practice
Tucson, Arizona

André V. Ritter, DDS, MS
Professor and Graduate Program Director
Department of Operative Dentistry
School of Dentistry
University of North Carolina
Chapel Hill, North Carolina

Jeffrey C.B. Stewart, DDS, MS
Associate Professor
Department of Pathology and Radiology
Oregon Health and Science University
Portland, Oregon

Mark Taylor, DDS, FACD
Chair, Department of Pediatric Dentistry
School of Dentistry
Creighton University
Omaha, Nebraska

Contributors

Marla W. Deibler, Psy.D.
Director, The Center for Emotional Health of Greater
   Philadelphia
Cherry Hill, New Jersey

Florence Kwo, DMD
Section of Endodontics
Division of Associated Clinical Sciences
School of Dentistry
University of Southern California
Los Angeles, California

Philip Lin, DDS
Resident
Division of Oral and Maxillofacial Surgery
University of Kentucky

Tom C. Pagonis, DDS, MS
Assistant Clinical Professor
Department of Restorative Dentistry and Biomaterials
   Science
Harvard School of Dental Medicine
Boston, Massachusetts

Catherine Frankl Sarkis, JD, MBA
Assistant Professor, Department of Health Policy &
   Health Services Research
Boston University
Henry M. Goldman School of Dental Medicine
Boston, Massachusetts

Bhavna Shroff, DDS, MDentSc, MPA
Professor, Department of Orthodontics
Virginia Commonwealth University
School of Dentistry
Richmond, Virginia

Eser Tufekci, DDS, MS, PhD
Associate Professor, Department of Orthodontics
Virginia Commonwealth University
School of Dentistry
Richmond, Virginia

Preface

How to Use This Text

This review book is the compiled work by experts in each of the relevant disciplines represented on the National Board Dental Exam (NBDE). This second edition includes recent updates and important changes from the first edition for each NBDE subject. This text is a tool to help prepare students for taking the NBDE and to help identify strengths and weaknesses so students can better utilize their study time. This text is not meant to replace years of professional training nor to simply provide questions so that students may pass the exams if they memorize the answers. Instead, this book will help direct students to the topic areas they may need to further review and will strengthen students' knowledge and exam-taking skills.

Dental schools generally do well in preparing their students for practice and for board exams. Usually, there is a good correlation between students who do well in their dental courses and those who score well on their board exams. Therefore to best prepare for board exams, students should focus on doing well in their course work. It is in the students' best interest to focus more board exam study time on the areas in which they have not performed as well in their dental coursework. Most students are aware of their areas of weakness and therefore will have the opportunity to focus more resources on these areas when studying for boards.

Helpful Hints for Preparing to Take Your Board Examinations

1. Pace yourself and make a study schedule. As when taking a course, it is always better to give yourself sufficient assimilation time rather than "cramming" over a short period of time, and if you start studying early enough, you should not have to make major changes in your daily schedule.
2. Study in a quiet environment similar to that in which the test is given. Stick to your schedule and minimize distractions to avoid last minute panic and the urge to "cram."
3. Know your weaknesses and focus more of your resources on strengthening these areas. Look back at your grades from the courses that relate to the exam topics. These will indicate areas that need more attention. Also, use this book as a trial run to help point to content areas that may need more review.
4. Many find practice exams useful. You can employ practice exams in several ways: study with others by asking each other questions; test yourself with flashcards or notes that are partially covered from view; or answer questions from this text. In each case, be sure to check your answer to find out whether you achieved the correct answer. Each section of this review book has practice exam questions. There is also a sample exam with questions from each discipline. This book also contains explanations as to why an answer is a correct answer and why the distracters are not. See if these explanations agree with the reasons for making your selections. The questions are written in the formats used on the National Boards including the new formats of matching, ordering and multiple correct/multiple responses.
5. Block off time for practice examinations, such as the review questions and sample exam in this text. Time yourself and practice your test speed; then compare your time to the estimated time needed to complete each section of the NBDE.
6. If your school offers board reviews, we highly recommend taking them. These may assist you with building your confidence with what material you have already mastered and may help you focus on material that you need to spend more time studying.
7. Stay positive about the board exam. If you prepare well, you should do well on the exam. Besides, think of all the people who have preceded you and have passed the exam. What has been done can be done. Consider making a study group composed of people who will be good study partners and who are able to help the other members in the group review and build confidence in taking the exam.
8. Exams are administered by the Joint National Commission on Dental Education (JNCDE) contracting with Prometric, Inc. (Prometric.com) at various testing centers. Exams are taken electronically. Students seeking to take the National Board Exam must be approved by their Dean, who recommends eligibility for the exam to JNCDE. More information on the exam is available at the American Dental Association (ADA) website.

Helpful Hints During the Taking of Examinations

1. It is important to note that questions that are considered "good" questions by examination standards will have incorrect choices in their answer bank that are very close to the correct answer. These wrong choices are called "distracters;" they are meant to determine

those who have the best knowledge of the subject. The present NBDE review questions should be used to help the test taker better discriminate similar choices, as an impetus to review a subject more intensively. (Distractors in questions on the actual board exam help determine which students have the best knowledge of the subject.) Most test takers do better by reading the question and trying to determine the answer before looking at the answer bank. Therefore consider trying to answer questions without looking at the answer bank.

2. Eliminate answers that are obviously wrong. This will allow a better chance of picking the correct answer and reduce distraction from the wrong answers.

3. Only go back and change an answer if you are absolutely certain you were wrong with your previous choice, or if a different question in the same exam provides you with the correct answer.

4. Read questions carefully. Note carefully any negative words in questions, such as "except," "not," and "false." If these words are missed when reading the question, it is nearly impossible to get the correct answer; noting these key words will make sure you do not miss them.

5. If you are stuck on one question, consider treating the answer bank like a series of true/false items relevant to the question. Most people consider true/false questions easier than multiple choice. At least if you can eliminate a few choices, you will have a better chance at selecting the correct answer from whatever is left.

6. Never leave blanks, unless the specific exam has a penalty for wrong answers. It is better to choose incorrectly than leave an item blank. Check with those giving the examination to find out whether there are penalties for marking the wrong answer.

7. Some people do better on exams by going through the exam and answering known questions first, and then returning to the more difficult questions later. This helps to build confidence during the exam. This also helps the test taker avoid spending too much time on a few questions and running out of time on less difficult questions that may be at the end. In addition, you may find additional insight to the correct answer in other exam questions later in the exam.

8. Pace yourself during the exam. Determine ahead of time how much time each question will take to answer. Do not rush, but do not spend too much time on one question. Sometimes it is better to move to the next question and come back to the difficult ones later, since a fresh look is sometimes helpful.

9. Bring appropriate supplies to the exam, such as reading glasses, appropriate for a computer screen. If you get distracted by noise, consider bringing ear plugs. It is inevitable that someone will take the exam next to the person in the squeaky chair, or the one with the sniffling runny nose. Most exams will provide you with instructions as to what you may or may not bring

to the exam. Be sure to read these instructions in advance.

10. Make sure that once you have completed the exam all questions are appropriately answered. Review before you submit your answers electronically.

11. Before coming to the exam, read over the checklist provided on the ADA website under "National Boards". Presently, the part II exam is constructed as follows:

Day 1

Description	# of Items	Time
Optional Tutorial	NA	15 minutes
Discipline-based, multiple-choice test items	~200	3.5 hours
Optional scheduled break	NA	One hour max.
Discipline-based, multiple-choice test items	~200	3.5 hours

Day 2

Description	# of Items	Time
Optional tutorial	NA	15 minutes
Patient case problems with multiple-choice questions	100	3.5 hours
Optional Post-exam Survey	NA	15 minutes

Helpful Hints for the Post-Examination Period

It may be a good idea to think about what you will be doing after the exam.

1. Most people are exhausted after taking board exams. Some reasons for this exhaustion may be the number of hours, the mental focus, and the anxiety that exams cause some people. Be aware that you may be tired, so avoid planning anything that one should not do when exhausted, such as driving across the country, operating heavy machinery or power tools, or studying for final exams. Instead, plan a day or two to recuperate before you tackle any heavier physical or mental tasks.

2. Consider a debriefing or "detoxification" meeting with your positive study partners after the exam. Talking about the exam afterwards may help reduce stress. However, remember that the feelings one has after an exam may not always match the exam score (e.g., students who feel they did poorly may have done well, or students who feel they did well may not have.)

3. Consider doing something nice for yourself. After all, you will have just completed a major exam. It is important to celebrate this accomplishment.

We wish you the very best with taking your exams and trust that this text will provide you with an excellent training tool for your preparations.

Additional Resources

This review text is intended to aid the study and retention of dental sciences in preparation for the National Board Dental Examination. It is not intended to be a substitute for a complete dental education curriculum. For a truly comprehensive understanding of the basic dental sciences, please consult these supplemental texts.

Biomechanics and Esthetic Strategies in Clinical Orthodontics
Ravindra Nanda

Carranza's Clinical Periodontology, Twelfth Edition
Michael G. Newman, Henry Takei, Perry R. Klokkevold, Fermin A. Carranza

Color Atlas of Dental Implant Surgery, Third Edition
Michael S. Block

Contemporary Fixed Prosthodontics, Fifth Edition
Stephen F. Rosenstiel, Martin F. Land, Junhei Fujimoto

Little and Falace's Dental Management of the Medically Compromised Patient, Eighth Edition
James W. Little, Donald Falace, Craig Miller, Nelson L. Rhodus

Dentistry, Dental Practice, and the Community, Sixth Edition
Brian A. Burt, Stephen A. Eklund

Functional Occlusion: From TMJ to Smile Design
Peter E. Dawson

Handbook of Local Anesthesia, Sixth Edition
Stanley F. Malamed

Jong's Community Dental Health, Fifth edition
George M. Gluck, Warren M. Morganstein

Management of Pain & Anxiety in the Dental Office, Fifth Edition
Raymond A. Dionne, James C. Phero, Daniel E. Becker

Management of Temporomandibular Disorders and Occlusion, Seventh Edition
Jeffrey P. Okeson

Medical Emergencies in the Dental Office, Sixth Edition
Stanley F. Malamed

Oral Radiology: Principles and Interpretation, Seventh Edition
Stuart C. White, Michael J. Pharoah

Orthodontics: Current Principles & Techniques, Fifth Edition
Thomas M. Graber, Robert L. Vanarsdall, Jr., Katherine W. L. Vig

Cohen's Pathways of the Pulp, Tenth Edition
Stephen Cohen, Kenneth M. Hargreaves

Periodontics: Medicine, Surgery, and Implants
Louis F. Rose, Brian L. Mealey, Robert J. Genco, Walter Cohen

Pharmacology and Therapeutics for Dentistry, Sixth Edition
John A. Yagiela, Frank J. Dowd, Barton S. Johnson, Angelo J. Mariotti, Enid A. Neidle

Endodontics: Principles and Practice, Fifth Edition
Mahmoud Torabinejad, Richard E. Walton, Ashraf Fouad

Sturdevant's Art & Science of Operative Dentistry, Sixth Edition
Theodore M. Roberson, Harald O. Heymann, Edward J. Swift, Jr.

Wong's Essentials of Pediatric Nursing, Ninth Edition
Marilyn Hockenberry-Eaton

A special thank you to Dr. Michael J. Hoover, Dr. W. Thomas Cavel, Dr. Steven J. Hess, and the Creighton University School of Dentistry, Department of Diagnostics Sciences, for their immeasurable help in preparing some of the cases.

Contents

SECTION 7
Periodontics   251

SECTION 8
Pharmacology   290

SECTION 9
Prosthodontics   343

Endodontics

JARSHEN LIN
FLORENCE KWO
TOM C. PAGONIS

OUTLINE

The word *endodontic* comes from two Greek words meaning "inside" and "tooth." *Endodontics* is the science of diagnosing and treating pulpal and apical disease. Endodontics is the branch of dentistry that is concerned with the morphology, physiology, and pathology of the human dental pulp and apical tissues. The study and practice of endodontics encompass the basic and clinical sciences, including the biology of the normal pulp and the etiology, diagnosis, prevention, and treatment of diseases and injuries of the pulp and associated apical conditions.*

This review outline is similar to the outline of the textbooks *Principles and Practice of Endodontics* (4th edition, 2009), *Problem Solving in Endodontics* (5th edition, 2011), and *Pathways of the Pulp* (10th edition, 2010). Some contents in this review have been taken from these texts. This review is not meant to be a comprehensive review of endodontics but rather a guide to study in preparing for the endodontic section of Part II of the National Board Dental Examination (NBDE). Students are referred to other sources including the aforementioned texts for a more complete discussion in each area of endodontics. This review is intended to help organize and integrate knowledge of concepts and facts. It also can help students to identify areas requiring more concentrated study.

The section editors acknowledge Dr. Meghan T. Cooper, Dr. Doreen Toskos, Dr. Louis Lin, Dr. Peggy Leong and Dr. Brooke Blicher for their contributions.

*Council on Dental Education and Licensure, American Dental Association.

Outline of Review

A practice analysis was conducted using the 63 *Competencies of the New Dentist*, developed by the American Dental Education Association.† For NBDE Part II, the findings of the dental practice survey were used to make changes in the content specifications. There are 31 endodontic questions on the examination, divided into the following six subjects:

1. Clinical diagnosis, case selection, treatment planning, and patient management (19)
2. Basic endodontic treatment procedures (7)
3. Procedural complications (1)
4. Traumatic injuries (1)
5. Adjunctive endodontic therapy (1)
6. Posttreatment evaluation (2)

The American Association of Endodontists Glossary of Endodontic Terms is used in reference to endodontic pathoses. In 2013, the endodontics diagnostic terminology adopted by the American Association of Endodontists as described in the December 2009 issue of *Journal of Endodontics* (Volume 35, Number 12, p. 1634) was incorporated in the NBDE Part II.

1.0 Clinical Diagnosis, Case Selection, Treatment Planning, and Patient Management

Outline of Review

1.1 Pulpal Diseases
1.2 Apical Diseases
1.3 Endodontic Diagnosis
1.4 Endodontic Examination and Testing
1.5 Cracked Tooth Syndrome

†Council on Dental Education and Licensure, American Dental Association.

1.1 Pulpal Diseases

A. The pulp.
  1. The pulp contains nerves, blood vessels, and connective tissue.
  2. Several factors make it unique and alter its ability to respond to irritation.
      a. The pulp is almost completely surrounded by hard tissue (dentin), which limits the available room for expansion and restricts the pulp's ability to tolerate edema.
      b. The pulp lacks collateral circulation, which severely limits its ability to cope with bacteria, necrotic tissue, and inflammation.
      c. The pulp possesses unique, hard tissue–secreting cells, or odontoblasts, as well as mesenchymal cells that can differentiate into osteoblasts that form more dentin in an attempt to protect the pulp from injury.
B. Physiology of pulpal pain.
  1. The sensibility of the dental pulp is controlled by A-delta and C afferent nerve fibers.
  2. Dentinal pain.
      a. A-delta fibers are large myelinated nerves that enter the root canal and divide into smaller branches, coursing coronally through the pulp.
      b. A-delta fiber pain is immediately perceived as a quick, sharp, momentary pain, which dissipates quickly on removal of the inciting stimulus (cold liquids or biting on an unyielding object).
      c. The intimate association of A-delta fibers with the odontoblastic cell layer and dentin is referred to as the *pulpodentinal complex.*
  3. Pulpitis pain.
      a. In pulpal inflammation, the response is exaggerated and disproportionate to the challenging stimulus (*hyperalgesia*). This response is induced by the effects of inflammatory mediators that are released in the inflamed pulp.
      b. Progression of pulpal inflammation can change the quality of the pain response. As the exaggerated A-delta fiber pain subsides, pain seemingly remains and is perceived as a dull, throbbing ache. This second pain symptom is from C nerve fibers.
      c. C fibers are small, unmyelinated nerves that course centrally in the pulp stroma.
      d. In contrast to A-delta fibers, C fibers are not directly involved with the pulpodentinal complex and are not easily provoked.
      e. C fiber pain surfaces with tissue injury and is mediated by inflammatory mediators, vascular changes in blood volume and blood flow, and increases in tissue pressure.
      f. When C fiber pain dominates, it signifies irreversible local tissue damage.
      g. With increasing inflammation of pulp tissues, C fiber pain becomes the only pain feature.
      h. Hot liquids or foods can increase intrapulpal pressure to levels that excite C fibers.
      i. The pain is diffuse and can be referred to a distant site or to other teeth.
      j. The sustained inflammatory cycle is detrimental to pulpal recovery, finally terminating in tissue necrosis.
C. Clinical classification of pulpal diseases.
  1. Normal pulp.
      a. A normal pulp is asymptomatic.
      b. A normal pulp produces a mild to moderate transient response to thermal and electrical stimuli that subsides almost immediately when the stimulus is removed.
      c. The tooth does not cause a painful response when percussed or palpated.
  2. Reversible pulpitis.
      a. In reversible pulpitis, thermal stimuli (usually cold) cause a quick, sharp, hypersensitive response that subsides as soon as the stimulus is removed.
      b. Any irritant that can affect the pulp may cause reversible pulpitis.
        (1) Early caries or recurrent decay.
        (2) Periodontal scaling or root planing.
        (3) Deep restorations without a base.
      c. Reversible pulpitis is not a disease; it is a symptom.
        (1) If the irritant is removed, the pulp reverts to an uninflamed state.
        (2) If the irritant remains, the symptoms may lead to irreversible pulpitis.
      d. Reversible pulpitis can be clinically distinguished from a symptomatic irreversible pulpitis in two ways.
        (1) Reversible pulpitis causes a momentary painful response to thermal change that subsides as soon as the stimulus (usually cold) is removed. However, symptomatic irreversible pulpitis causes a painful response to thermal change that lingers after the stimulus is removed.
        (2) Reversible pulpitis does not involve a complaint of spontaneous (unprovoked) pain.
      e. Frank penetration of bacteria into the pulp frequently is the crossover point to irreversible pulpitis.
  3. Symptomatic irreversible pulpitis.
      a. By definition, the pulp has been damaged beyond repair, and even with removal of the irritant, it will not heal.
      b. Microscopic findings.
        (1) Microabscesses of the pulp begin as tiny zones of necrosis within dense acute inflammatory cells.

(2) Histologically intact myelinated and unmyelinated nerves may be observed in areas with dense inflammation and cellular degeneration.

c. Following irreversible pulpitis, pulp death may occur quickly or may require years; it may be painful or, more frequently, asymptomatic. The end result is necrosis of the pulp.

d. Characterized by spontaneous, unprovoked, intermittent or continuous pain.

e. Sudden temperature changes (often to cold) elicit prolonged episodes of pain that linger after the thermal stimulus is removed.

f. Occasionally, patients may report that a postural change, such as lying down or bending over, induces pain.

g. Radiographs are generally insufficient for diagnosing irreversible pulpitis.

   (1) Radiographs can be helpful in identifying suspect teeth only.

   (2) Thickening of the apical portion of the periodontal ligament (PDL) may become evident on radiographs in the advanced stage.

h. Electrical pulp test is of little value in the diagnosis of symptomatic irreversible pulpitis.

4. Asymptomatic irreversible pulpitis.

a. Microscopically similar to symptomatic irreversible pulpitis.

   (1) Microabscesses of the pulp begin as tiny zones of necrosis within dense acute inflammatory cells.

   (2) Histologically intact myelinated and unmyelinated nerves may be observed in areas with dense inflammation and cellular degeneration.

b. There are no clinical symptoms, but inflammation produced by caries, caries excavation, or trauma occurs.

5. Pulp necrosis.

a. Death of the pulp, resulting from the following.

   (1) Untreated irreversible pulpitis.

   (2) Traumatic injury.

   (3) Any event that causes long-term interruption of the blood supply to the pulp.

b. Pulpal necrosis may be partial or total.

   (1) Partial necrosis may manifest with some of the symptoms associated with irreversible pulpitis. For example, a tooth with two canals could have an inflamed pulp in one canal and a necrotic pulp in the other.

   (2) Total necrosis is asymptomatic before it affects the PDL, and there is no response to thermal or electrical pulp tests.

c. In anterior teeth, some crown discoloration may accompany pulp necrosis.

d. Protein breakdown products and bacteria and their toxins eventually spread beyond the apical foramen; this leads to thickening of the PDL and manifests as tenderness to percussion and chewing.

e. Microscopic findings.

   (1) As inflammation progresses, tissue continues to disintegrate in the center to form an increasing region of liquefaction necrosis.

   (2) Because of the lack of collateral circulation and the unyielding walls of dentin, there is insufficient drainage of inflammatory fluids.

   (3) The result is localized increases in tissue pressure, causing the destruction to progress unchecked until the entire pulp is necrotic.

   (4) Bacteria are able to penetrate and invade into dentinal tubules. (It is necessary to remove the superficial layers of dentin during cleaning and shaping.)

6. Previously treated pulp.

a. Clinical diagnostic category indicating that the tooth has been endodontically treated and the canals are obturated with various filling materials other than intracanal medicaments.

7. Previously initiated therapy.

a. Clinical diagnostic category indicating that the tooth has been previously treated by partial endodontic therapy (e.g., pulpotomy, pulpectomy).

8. Other.

a. Hyperplastic pulpitis—reddish, cauliflower-like growth of pulp tissue through and around a carious exposure. The proliferative nature of this type of pulp is attributed to low-grade, chronic irritation of the pulp and the generous vascular supply characteristically found in young people.

b. Internal resorption.

   (1) Most commonly identified during routine radiographic examination. If undetected, internal resorption eventually perforates the root.

   (2) Histologic appearance.

      (a) Chronic pulpitis.

         (i) Chronic inflammatory cells.

         (ii) Multinucleated giant cells adjacent to granulation tissue.

         (iii) Necrotic pulp coronal to resorptive defect.

   (3) Only prompt endodontic therapy can stop the process and prevent further tooth destruction.

   (4) Partial pulp vitality is necessary for active internal resorption.

1.2 Apical Diseases

A. Definition of apical disease.

1. Apical lesions of pulpal origin are inflammatory responses to irritants from the root canal system.

2. Patient symptoms may range from an asymptomatic response to various symptoms.

a. Slight sensitivity to chewing.

b. Sensation of tooth elongation.

c. Intense pain.

d. Swelling.

e. Fever.

f. Malaise.

3. The sign most indicative of an apical inflammatory lesion is radiographic bone resorption, but this is unpredictable. Apical lesions are frequently not visible on radiographs.

4. Apical lesions do not occur as individual entities; there are clinical and histologic crossovers in terminology regarding apical lesions because the terminology is based both on clinical signs and symptoms and on radiographic findings. There is *no correlation* between histologic findings and clinical signs, symptoms, and duration of the lesion. The terms *acute* and *chronic* apply only to clinical symptoms.

B. Classification of apical diseases.

1. Symptomatic apical periodontitis.

a. Symptomatic apical periodontitis refers to painful inflammation around the apex (localized inflammation of the PDL in the apical region). It can result from the following.

(1) Extension of pulpal disease into the apical tissue.

(2) Canal overinstrumentation or overfill.

(3) Occlusal trauma such as bruxism.

b. Because symptomatic apical periodontitis may occur around vital and nonvital teeth, conducting pulp tests is the only way to confirm the need for endodontic treatment.

c. Even when present, the apical PDL may radiographically appear within normal limits or only slightly widened.

d. The tooth may be painful during percussion tests.

e. If the tooth is vital, a simple occlusal adjustment can often relieve the pain. If the pulp is necrotic and remains untreated, additional symptoms may appear as the disease advances to the next stage, acute apical abscess.

f. Because there is little room for expansion of the PDL, increased pressure can also cause physical pressure on the nerve endings, which subsequently causes intense, throbbing apical pain.

g. Histopathologic examination reveals a localized inflammatory infiltrate within the PDL.

2. Asymptomatic apical periodontitis.

a. Asymptomatic apical periodontitis is a long-standing, asymptomatic or mildly symptomatic lesion.

b. It is usually accompanied by radiographically visible apical bone resorption.

c. Bacteria and their endotoxins cascading out into the apical region from a necrotic pulp cause extensive demineralization of cancellous and cortical bone.

d. Occasionally, there may be slight tenderness to percussion or palpation testing.

e. The diagnosis of asymptomatic apical periodontitis is confirmed by the following.

(1) General absence of symptoms.

(2) Radiographic presence of an apical radiolucency.

(3) Confirmation of pulpal necrosis.

f. A totally necrotic pulp provides a safe harbor for the primarily anaerobic microorganisms—if there is no vascularity, there are no defense cells.

g. Asymptomatic apical periodontitis traditionally has been classified histologically as apical granuloma or apical cyst. The only accurate way to distinguish them is by histopathologic examination.

3. Acute apical abscess.

a. An acute apical abscess is painful, with purulent exudate around the apex.

b. It is a result of exacerbation of symptomatic apical periodontitis from a necrotic pulp.

c. The PDL may radiographically appear within normal limits or only slightly thickened.

d. The periapical radiograph reveals a relatively normal or slightly thickened lamina dura (because the infection has rapidly spread beyond the confines of the cortical plate before demineralization can be detected radiographically).

e. Only swelling is manifest.

f. Lesions can also result from infection and rapid tissue destruction arising from within asymptomatic apical periodontitis.

g. Histopathologic findings.

(1) Central area of liquefaction necrosis containing disintegrating neutrophils and other cellular debris.

(2) Surrounded by viable macrophages and occasional lymphocytes and plasma cells.

(3) Bacteria are not always found in the apical tissues or within the abscess cavity.

h. Presenting signs and symptoms of acute apical abscess.

(1) Rapid onset of swelling.

(2) Moderate to severe pain.

(3) Pain with percussion and palpation.

(4) Slight increase in tooth mobility.

(5) Extent and distribution of swelling are determined by the location of the apex and the muscle attachments and the thickness of the cortical plate.

(6) Usually the swelling remains localized. However, it also may become diffuse and spread widely (cellulitis).

i. An acute apical abscess can be differentiated from lateral periodontal abscess with pulp vitality testing and sometimes with periodontal probing.

4. Chronic apical abscess.
   a. Associated with either a continuously or an intermittently draining sinus tract without discomfort.
   b. The exudate can also drain through the gingival sulcus, mimicking a periodontal lesion with a "pocket."
   c. Pulp tests are negative because of the presence of necrotic pulp.
   d. Radiographic examination shows the presence of bone loss at the apical area.
   e. Treatment—these sinus tracts resolve spontaneously with nonsurgical endodontic treatment.
5. Condensing osteitis.
   a. Excessive bone mineralization around the apex of an asymptomatic vital tooth.
   b. Radiopacity may be caused by low-grade pulp irritation.
   c. This process is asymptomatic and benign. It does not require endodontic therapy.

1.3 Endodontic Diagnosis

A. Triage of patient with pain.
   1. Orofacial pain can be the clinical manifestation of various diseases involving the head and neck region.
   2. The cause must be differentiated between odontogenic and nonodontogenic.
      a. Numerous orofacial diseases mimic endodontic pain (may produce sensory misperception as a result of overlapping between the sensory fibers of the trigeminal nerve).
      b. Characteristics of nonodontogenic involvement (not all apply to all cases).
         (1) Episodic pain with pain-free remissions.
         (2) Trigger points.
         (3) Pain travels and crosses the midline of the face.
         (4) Pain that surfaces with increasing mental stress.
         (5) Pain that is seasonal or cyclic.
         (6) Paresthesia.
B. Medical history (developing data).
   1. Endodontic treatment is not contraindicated with most medical conditions. The only systemic contraindications to endodontic therapy are uncontrolled diabetes or a recent myocardial infarction (MI) (within the past 6 months).
   2. The patient's medical history enables the clinician to determine the need for a medical consultation or premedication of the patient.
C. Dental history.
   1. Chief complaint.
      a. "Can you tell me about your problem?"—as expressed in the patient's words.
      b. The dentist should paraphrase the patient's responses to verify them.

2. Location.
   a. The site or sites where symptoms are perceived.
   b. "Could you point to the tooth that hurts or swells?"—the patient is asked to indicate the location by pointing to it directly with one finger.
   c. The accuracy of the patient's description of pain depends on whether the inflammatory state is limited to the pulp tissue only.
      (1) If the inflammation has not reached the PDL, it may be difficult for the patient to localize the pain because the pulp contains sensory fibers that transmit only pain, not location.
      (2) The PDL contains proprioceptive sensory fibers. When the inflammatory process extends beyond the apex, it is easier for the patient to identify the source of the pain. (Percussion test can be used.)
   d. Referred pain.
      (1) Pain can also be referred to the adjacent teeth or in the opposing quadrant.
      (2) It is rare for odontogenic pain to cross the midline of the head.
      (3) Referred pain may also be ipsilaterally referred to the preauricular area, down the neck, or up to the temple, especially for the posterior teeth.
      (4) In posterior molars, pain can often be referred to the opposing quadrant or to other teeth in the same quadrant.
      (5) Maxillary molars often refer pain to the zygomatic, parietal, and occipital regions of the head, whereas lower molars frequently refer pain to the ear, angle of the jaw, or posterior regions of the neck.
3. Chronology.
   a. "When did you first notice this?"—inception.
   b. The patient may be aware of the history of dental procedures or trauma, clinical course, and temporal pattern of the symptoms.
      (1) Mode—is the onset of symptoms spontaneous or provoked (i.e., sudden or gradual)? If symptoms can be stimulated, are they immediate or delayed?
      (2) Periodicity—do the symptoms have a temporal pattern (i.e., sporadic or occasional)?
      (3) Frequency—have the symptoms persisted since they began, or are they intermittent? "How often does this pain occur?"
      (4) Duration—how long do symptoms last when they occur (i.e., momentary or lingering)?
4. Quality of pain.
   a. How the patient describes the complaint.
      (1) Bony origin—dull, gnawing, or aching.
      (2) Vascular response to tissue inflammation—throbbing, pounding, or pulsating.
      (3) Pathosis of nerve root complexes, sensory ganglia, or peripheral innervation (irreversible

pulpitis or trigeminal neuralgia)—sharp, electrical, recurrent, or stabbing.

(4) Pulpal and apical pathoses—aching, pulsing, throbbing, dull, gnawing, radiating, flashing, stabbing, or jolting pain.

5. Intensity and severity of symptoms.

   a. Quantify pain by assigning the pain a degree of 0 (none) to 10 (most severe).

6. Affecting factors—stimulated or spontaneous.

   a. "Does the pain ever occur without provocation?"

   b. Provoking factors.

   (1) "Does heat, cold, biting, or chewing cause pain?"

   (2) The dental pain may be exacerbated by lying down or by bending over. This change increases blood pressure to the head, which increases pressure on the inflamed, confined pulp.

   c. Attenuating factors.

   (1) "Does anything relieve the pain?"

   (2) "Does drinking warm or cold liquids relieve pain?"

   (3) "Does lying down or sitting up relieve pain?"

7. Disposition.

   a. How has the pain changed since it started—worse, dissipated, eliminated.

8. Supplemental history.

   a. Past facts and current symptoms characterizing the difficult diagnosis.

   (1) It might be necessary to wait a while for vague symptoms to localize.

   (2) This conservative approach is often necessary in pulpal pathosis confined to the root canal space, which can refer pain to other teeth or to nondental sites.

1.4 Endodontic Examination and Testing

Extraoral Examination

A. Examination should begin while the clinician is taking the patient's history.

B. Facial asymmetry might indicate swelling of odontogenic origin.

C. Occasionally, facial lesions (e.g., a sinus tract) can be traced to a tooth as the source. All sinus tracts should be traced with a gutta-percha point by radiograph (Figure 1-1).

Intraoral Endodontic Examination

A. Intraoral diagnostic tests (Tables 1-1 and 1-2).

1. Help define the pain by evoking reproducible symptoms that characterize the chief complaint.

2. Help provide an assessment of normal responses for comparison with abnormal responses.

3. The dentist should include adequate controls for test procedures. Several adjacent, opposing, and contralateral teeth should be tested before the tooth in

question to establish the patient's normal range of response.

B. Palpation.

1. When apical inflammation develops after pulp necrosis, the inflammatory process may burrow its way through the facial cortical bone and begin to affect the overlying mucoperiosteum.

2. Before incipient swelling becomes clinically evident, it may feel tender during shaving or applying makeup.

C. Percussion.

1. Although the percussion test does not indicate the health of the pulp, the sensitivity of the proprioceptive fibers reveals inflammation of the apical PDL.

2. A positive response to percussion indicates not only the presence of inflammation of the PDL but also the extent of the inflammatory process. The degree of response correlates with the degree of inflammation.

3. Other factors may also inflame the PDL and yield a positive percussion test result.

   a. Rapid orthodontic movement of teeth.

   b. A recently placed restoration in hyperocclusion.

   c. A lateral periodontal abscess.

4. The first percussion test should be performed with the clinician's finger on a nonsuspect tooth. If the patient is unable to discern, the blunt handle of a mouth mirror should be used.

5. Having the patient chew on a cotton roll, a cotton swab, or the reverse end of a low-speed suction straw may help.

D. Thermal tests (see Tables 1-1 and 1-2)—thermal testing is especially valuable when the patient describes the pain as diffuse. Thermal testing of vital pulps often helps to pinpoint the source. However, the sensory response of the teeth is refractory to repeated thermal stimulation. To avoid misinterpretation of a response, the dentist should wait an appropriate amount of time for tested teeth to respond and recover.

1. Cold test—cold testing can be done with cold water baths, sticks of ice, ethyl chloride ($-5°C$), dichlorodifluoromethane (Endo-Ice) ($-30°C$, $-21°F$), and carbon dioxide ice sticks ($-77.7°C$, $-108°F$).

   a. In the ethyl chloride or Endo-Ice method, ethyl chloride is sprayed liberally onto a cotton pellet.

   b. The chilled pellet is applied immediately to the middle third of the facial surface of the crown.

   c. The pellet is kept in contact for 5 seconds or until the patient begins to feel pain.

2. Heat test—these include warm sticks of temporary stopping, rotating a dry prophy cup to create frictional heat, and a hot water bath. The hot water bath yields the most accurate patient response.

3. Responses to thermal tests—the sensory fibers of the pulp transmit only pain, whether the pulp has been cooled or heated. There are four possible responses.

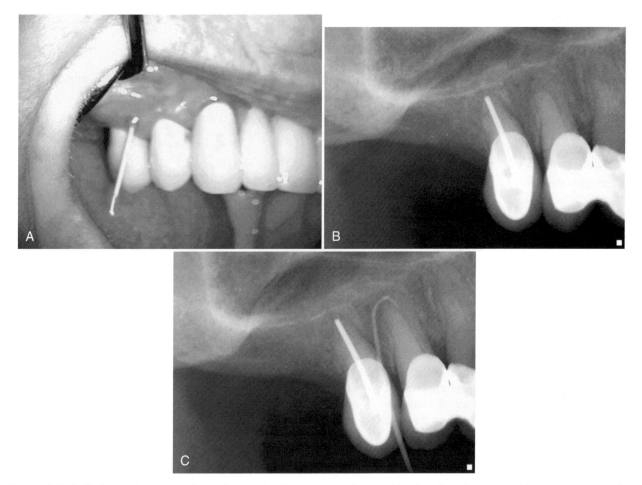

Figure 1-1 A, To locate the source of an infection, the sinus tract can be traced by threading the stoma with a gutta-percha point. **B,** Radiograph of the area shows an old root canal in tooth #4 and a questionable radiolucent area associated with tooth #5, with no indication as to the etiology of the sinus tract. **C,** After tracing the sinus tract, gutta-percha is seen to be directed to the source of pathosis, the apex of tooth #5. *(From Cohen S, Hargreaves KM:* Pathways of the Pulp, *ed 10. St Louis, Mosby, 2011.)*

Table 1-1

Pulpal Diagnosis

PULPAL DIAGNOSIS	CHIEF COMPLAINT OR HISTORY	RADIOGRAPHIC FINDINGS	EPT	THERMAL TESTING
Normal pulp	—	Normal	+	+
Reversible pulpitis	Cold sensitivity	Normal or widened PDL	+	++
Symptomatic irreversible pulpitis	Hot or cold sensitivity with lingering pain	Normal, widened PDL, or PRL	+	++ with lingering pain
Asymptomatic irreversible pulpitis	No clinical symptoms	Widened PDL or PRL	+	
Pulp necrosis	Variable	Normal, widened PDL, or PRL	–	–
Previously treated pulp	Tooth has been endodontically treated and canals obturated	Canals obturated	–	–
Previously initiated therapy	Tooth has been treated by partial endodontic therapy	Pulpotomy or pulpectomy	–	–

EPT, Electrical pulp test; *PDL,* periodontal ligament; *PRL,* periradicular (apical) radiolucency.

Table 1-2

Apical Diagnosis

APICAL DIAGNOSIS	CHIEF COMPLAINT OR HISTORY	RADIOGRAPHIC FINDINGS	EPT	THERMAL TESTING	PERCUSSION
Normal apical tissues	—	Normal			−
Symptomatic apical periodontitis	Biting sensitivity	Normal or widened PDL	+/−	+/−	+
Asymptomatic apical periodontitis	—	PRL	−	−	−
Acute apical abscess	Pain with swelling	Normal, widened PDL, or PRL	−	−	+
Chronic apical abscess	"Bump in the gum"	PRL	−	−	−
Condensing osteitis	Asymptomatic (usually) or variable pulpal symptoms	Increased radiopacity (increased apical bone density)	+/−	+/−	−/+

EPT, Electrical pulp test; *PDL,* periodontal ligament; *PRL,* periradicular (apical) radiolucency.

---

a. No response—a nonvital pulp is indicated; it can also indicate a false-negative response because of excessive calcification or recent trauma.

b. Mild to moderate degree of awareness of slight pain that subsides within 1 to 2 seconds—within normal limits.

c. Strong, momentary painful response that subsides within 1 to 2 seconds—reversible pulpitis.

d. Moderate to strong painful response that lingers for several seconds or longer after the stimulus has been removed—irreversible pulpitis.

E. Electrical pulp tests (see Tables 1-1 and 1-2).

1. Electrical pulp test does *not* suggest the health or integrity of the pulp; it simply indicates that there are vital sensory fibers present within the pulp.

2. Electrical pulp test does *not* provide any information about the vascular supply to the pulp, which is the true determinant of pulp vitality.

3. Electrical pulp test readings do not correlate with the relative histologic health or disease status of the pulp.

4. Several conditions can cause false responses to electrical pulp testing—it is essential that thermal tests be performed before a final diagnosis is made.

5. Electrical pulp testing technique.

a. The teeth must be isolated and dried.

b. The electrode of the pulp tester should be coated with a viscous conductor (e.g., toothpaste).

c. The electrode should be applied to the dry enamel on the middle third of the facial surface of the crown.

d. The current flow should be adjusted to increase slowly.

e. The electrode should not be applied to any restorations (false reading).

f. Thicker enamel yields a more delayed response; thinner enamel of anterior teeth yields a quicker response.

g. If the patient's medical history reveals that a cardiac pacemaker has been implanted, the use of an electrical pulp tester is contraindicated.

6. Causes of false readings.

a. False-positive response.

(1) Electrode or conductor contact with a metal restoration or the gingiva.

(2) Patient anxiety.

(3) Liquefaction necrosis may conduct current to the attachment apparatus.

(4) Failure to isolate and dry the teeth before testing.

b. False-negative response.

(1) The patient has been heavily premedicated with analgesics, narcotics, alcohol, or tranquilizers.

(2) Inadequate contact between the electrode or conductor and the enamel.

(3) A recently traumatized tooth.

(4) Excessive calcification of the canal.

(5) Recently erupted tooth with an immature apex.

(6) Partial necrosis.

F. Periodontal examination.

1. If a significant isolated pocket is discovered in the absence of periodontal disease, it increases the probability of a vertical root fracture.

2. To distinguish disease of periodontal origin from disease of pulpal origin, pulp vitality tests along with periodontal probing are essential.

G. Mobility.

1. Tooth mobility is directly proportional to the integrity of the attachment apparatus or to the extent of inflammation of the PDL.

2. The clinician should use two mouth mirror handles to apply alternating lateral forces in a faciolingual direction.
3. The pressure exerted by the purulent exudate of an acute apical abscess may cause transient mobility of a tooth.
4. Other causes of tooth mobility.
   a. Horizontal root fracture in the coronal half of the tooth.
   b. Very recent trauma.
   c. Chronic bruxism.
   d. Overzealous orthodontic treatment.
H. Selective anesthesia test—this test can be used when the clinician has not determined through prior testing which tooth is the source of pain. Because diffusion of the local anesthetic is not limited to a single tooth, the clinician cannot make a conclusive diagnosis on the basis of pain relief.
I. Test cavity—this test is done only in cases where pulp necrosis is strongly suspected and corroborated by other tests and radiographic findings, but a definitive test is required.
J. Radiographic examination.
   1. Findings on radiographic examination.
      a. A radiolucency does not begin to manifest until demineralization extends into the cortical plate of the bone. Clinicians should not rely exclusively on radiographs to arrive at a diagnosis.
      b. Because a radiograph is a two-dimensional image only, radiographic strategy should involve the exposure of two films at the same vertical angulation but with a 10- to 15-degree change in horizontal angulation (Figure 1-2).
      c. The status of the health and integrity of the pulp cannot be determined by radiographic images alone.
   2. Radiographic interpretation.
      a. A single root canal should appear tapering from crown to apex.
      b. A sudden change in appearance of the canal from dark to light indicates that the canal has bifurcated or trifurcated.
      c. A necrotic pulp does not cause radiographic changes until demineralization of the cortical plate. Significant medullary bone destruction may occur before any radiographic signs start to appear.
      d. The attending dentist should be cautious in accepting prior diagnostic radiographs from the patient or another dentist, no matter how recently they were made. Prior iatrogenic mishaps such as ledge formation, perforation, or instrument separation are critical for a newly treating dentist to uncover.
   3. Buccal object rule (SLOB rule—same lingual, opposite buccal).
      a. Principle—the object closest to the buccal surface appears to move in the direction opposite the

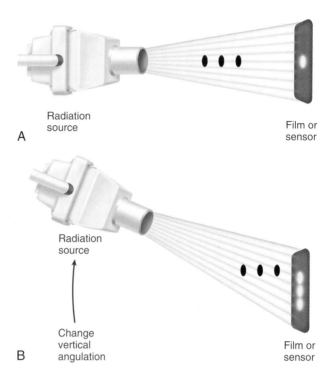

Radiation source

Film or sensor

A

Radiation source

Change vertical angulation

Film or sensor

B

Figure 1-2 Radiographic images are only two-dimensional, and it is often difficult to discriminate the relative location of overlapping objects. **A,** When the source of the radiation is directly perpendicular to overlapping objects, the image is captured without much separation of the objects. However, when the radiation source is at an angle to offset the overlapping objects, the image is captured with the objects being viewed as separated. **B,** The object that is closest to the film (or sensor) moves the least, with the object closest to the radiation source appearing farthest away. *(From Cohen S, Hargreaves KM:* Pathways of the Pulp, *ed 10. St Louis, Mosby, 2011.)*

movement of the tube head or cone when compared with a second radiograph. Objects closest to the lingual surface appear to move in the same direction of the cone.
      b. Proper application of this technique allows the dentist to do the following.
         (1) Locate additional canals or roots.
         (2) Distinguish between superimposed objects.
         (3) Differentiate various types of resorption.
         (4) Determine buccal-lingual positions of fractures and perforative defects.
         (5) Locate foreign bodies.
         (6) Locate anatomic landmarks in relation to the root apex.
   4. Radiographic differential diagnosis of apical radiolucencies.
      a. Vertical root fracture.
         (1) A long-standing vertical root fracture may be viewed as a variant of apical periodontitis.
      b. Lateral periodontal cyst.
         (1) Tracing of the lamina dura and normal responses to pulp vitality testing establish the diagnosis.

c. Osteomyelitis.
  (1) A highly variable radiographic appearance with sclerotic and osteolytic processes occurs sometimes in the same patient.
d. Developmental cysts.
  (1) An incisive canal cyst (nasopalatine duct cyst) may exhibit radiographic features similar to apical periodontitis. Tooth vitality responses become particularly important in differential diagnosis.
e. Traumatic bone cyst.
  (1) Cyst usually reveals a smoothly outlined radiolucent area of variable size sometimes with a sclerotic border.
  (2) Pulp vitality testing is within normal limits in most cases.
f. Ameloblastoma.
  (1) Occurs primarily in the fourth and fifth decade.
  (2) Aggressive lesions occur as multilocular radiolucencies.
  (3) Frequently causes extensive resorption of roots in the area.
g. Cemental dysplasia.
  (1) Lesion varies in radiographic expression from radiolucent initially to more radiopaque later.
  (2) It is more commonly associated with *vital* mandibular anterior teeth.
h. Cementoblastoma.
  (1) Radiographically appears as a well-circumscribed dense radiopaque mass often surrounded by a thin, uniform radiolucent outline.
  (2) Severe hypercementosis or chronic focal sclerosing osteomyelitis (condensing osteitis) has similar radiographic appearance.
i. Central giant cell granuloma.
  (1) Lesion produces a radiolucent area with either a relatively smooth or a ragged border showing faint trabeculae.
  (2) Associated teeth are usually vital.
j. Systemic disease.
  (1) *Giant cell lesion of primary hyperparathyroidism* gives rise to a generally radiolucent appearance of bone and later may give rise to well-defined oval or round radiolucencies.
k. Other nonanatomic radiolucency.
  (1) Odontogenic lesions—dental papilla (apical), dentigerous cyst, odontogenic keratocyst, residual (apical) cyst, odontoma (early stage).
  (2) Nonodontogenic lesions—fibro-osseous lesions, osteoblastoma, cementifying fibroma, ossifying fibroma, malignant tumor, multiple myeloma.
l. Anatomic radiolucencies.
  (1) Mandible—mental foramen, mandibular canal, submandibular fossa, mental fossa.
  (2) Maxilla—maxillary sinus, incisive foramen, greater (major) palatine foramen, nasal cavity.
  (3) Both jaws—marrow spaces, nutrient canal.
5. Cone-beam computed tomography (CBCT)—although valuable in endodontic diagnosis and treatment, current intraoral radiographs have limitations because they display a two-dimensional view, which could lead to diagnostic inaccuracies. CBCT acquires three-dimensional views, and its increased use should improve diagnostic capabilities.

1.5 Cracked Tooth Syndrome

A. Clinical features.
  1. Sustained pain during biting pressures.
  2. Pain only on release of biting pressures.
  3. Occasional, momentary, sharp, poorly localized pain during mastication that is very difficult to reproduce.
  4. Sensitivity to thermal changes.
  5. Sensitivity to mild stimuli, such as sweet or acidic foods.
B. Radiographic evidence—a mesiodistal crack is impossible to demonstrate on radiographs because the line of fracture is not in the plane of the radiograph.
C. Incidence—primarily mandibular molars, with a slight preference for the first over the second molar.
D. Diagnosis.
  1. Transillumination.
  2. Use of a "tooth slooth" or a cotton-tipped applicator. Noting which cusps occlude when the pain occurs aids in the location of the fracture site.
  3. Stain.
E. Treatment.
  1. Healthy pulp or reversible pulpitis.
    a. Splint with an orthodontic band and observe or prepare for crown (place sound temporary crown and observe before placing permanent crown).
  2. Irreversible pulpitis (symptomatic and asymptomatic) or necrosis with acute apical periodontitis (symptomatic and asymptomatic).
    a. Endodontic treatment.
      (1) Minimizing the removal of tooth structure.
      (2) Minimizing condensation force.
    b. Restoration.
      (1) If sufficient tooth structure remains, place a glass-ionomer or acid-etched, dentin-bonded core without post and restore with permanent crown. Core material can be placed 2 to 3 mm into the canal orifices.
      (2) If insufficient tooth structure remains, consider a passively placed post along with an acid-etched, dentin-bonded core and permanent crown with margins of 2 mm or more of sound tooth structure. Crown lengthening or extrusion or both may be necessary.

F. Prognosis.
   1. Presence and extent of an isolated probing—guarded prognosis.
   2. Extension of the crack to the floor of the pulp chamber—guarded prognosis.
   3. Fracture traceable all the way from mesial to distal—poor prognosis.

1.6 Vertical Root Fracture

A. Clinical findings.
   1. Vertical root fracture starts apically and progresses coronally.
   2. It is usually in the buccal-lingual plane of the root.
   3. There is an isolated probing defect at the site of the fracture in most cases.
   4. Important diagnostic signs include a radiolucency from the apical region to the middle of the root ("J" shape or "teardrop" shape) (Figure 1-3).
   5. May mimic other entities such as periodontal disease or failed root canal treatment.
B. Etiologies—predisposing factors are a weakening of the root structure by the following.
   1. Extensive enlargement of the canal.
   2. Mechanical stress from obturation.
   3. Unfavorable placement of posts.
C. Diagnosis—a vertical root fracture is confirmed by visualizing the fracture with an exploratory surgical flap.
D. Treatment—goal of treatment is to eliminate the fracture space.
   1. Single-rooted teeth—extraction.
   2. Multirooted teeth.
      a. Hemisection or root resection with removal of only the affected root.
      b. Extraction.
E. Prognosis—hopeless prognosis.

1.7 Endodontic-Periodontal Relationships

A. Communication of the pulp and periodontium.
   1. By way of the following.
      a. Dentinal tubules.
      b. Lateral or accessory canals.
      c. Furcation canals.
      d. Apical foramen.
   2. Endodontic pathosis can cause periodontal disease, but periodontal disease usually does not cause endodontic problems (unless periodontal disease involves the apex of the tooth).
   3. Periodontal treatment can affect pulpal health because periodontal treatment (i.e., root planing) can result in bacterial penetration into exposed dentinal tubules, which can cause thermal sensitivity and subsequent pulpitis.
B. Types of endodontic or periodontal lesions.
   1. Primary endodontic lesions.
      a. Clinical presentation.
         (1) Inflammatory processes may or may not be localized at the apex—may appear along the lateral aspects of the root or in the furcation or may have a sinus tract along the PDL space appearing like a "narrow deep pocket."
         (2) Tooth tests nonvital.
      b. Treatment—endodontic therapy only because the primary lesion is of endodontic origin that has merely manifested through the PDL.
   2. Primary periodontal lesions.
      a. Clinical presentation.
         (1) Periodontal disease is progressive—it starts in the sulcus and migrates to the apex as deposits of plaque and calculus produce inflammation that cause loss of surrounding alveolar bone and soft tissues.

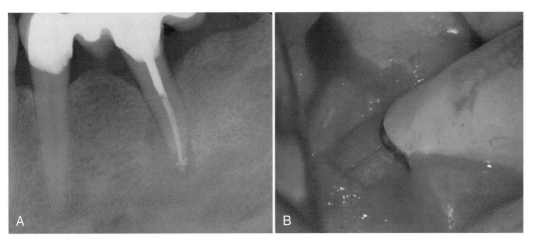

Figure 1-3 A, J-shaped radiolucency possibly indicating root fracture. **B,** Exploratory surgery confirms the presence of a vertical root fracture. *(From Cohen S, Hargreaves KM:* Pathways of the Pulp, *ed 10. St Louis, Mosby, 2011.)*

(2) Manifestation of a periodontal abscess during acute phase of inflammation.

(3) Broad-based pocket formation.

(4) Teeth are vital.

b. Treatment—periodontal therapy.

3. Primary periodontal lesions with secondary endodontic involvement.

a. Clinical presentation.

(1) Deep pocketing with history of extensive periodontal disease.

(2) Possibly past treatment history.

b. Treatment—endodontic therapy followed by periodontal treatment.

4. True combined lesions.

a. Clinical presentation—when endodontic and periodontal lesions coalesce, they may be clinically indistinguishable.

b. Treatment.

(1) Both the endodontic and the periodontal problem require treatment.

(2) Prognosis depends on how much of the periodontal component actually caused the destruction.

2.0 Basic Endodontic Treatment Procedures

Outline of Review

2.1 Nonsurgical Endodontics

2.2 Surgical Endodontics

2.3 Endodontic Emergencies

2.4 Sterilization and Asepsis

2.5 Radiographic Techniques

2.6 Microbiology of Endodontics

2.1 Nonsurgical Endodontics

A. Objectives.

1. To alleviate and prevent future adverse clinical symptoms.

2. To débride and shape the root canal.

3. To create the radiographic appearance of a well-obturated root canal system where the root canal filling extends as closely as possible to the apical constriction.

4. To maintain health or promote healing and repair of apical tissues.

B. Access preparation.

1. Most important phase of the technical aspects of root canal treatment.

2. Proper access preparation maximizes cleaning, shaping, and obturation.

3. Objectives.

a. Straight-line access.

(1) Improved instrument control, with less zipping, transportation, or ledging.

(2) Improved obturation.

(3) Decreased procedural errors, such as ledges or perforations.

(4) Requires adequate tooth structure removal.

b. Conservation of tooth structure.

(1) Minimal weakening of the tooth.

(2) Prevention of accidents.

c. Unroofing of the chamber to expose orifices and pulp horns.

(1) Maximum visibility.

(2) Prerequisite in locating orifices of canals.

(3) Improved straight-line access.

(4) Exposure of pulp horns.

C. Instruments for cleaning and shaping.

1. Gates-Gliddon—long thin shaft with parallel walls and short cutting head, side cutting with safety tips.

a. Used to preenlarge coronal canal areas; cut dentin as they are withdrawn from canal.

2. K-files—twisted square or triangular metal blanks along their long axis; partly horizontal cutting blades.

a. Can be used with the watch winding or balanced forces technique.

3. Hedstrom files—spiraling flutes cut into the shaft of round, tapered, stainless steel wire; very positive rake angle.

a. Cut in one direction only—retraction.

4. Barbed broaches—sharp, coronally angulated barbs in metal wire blanks.

a. Used to remove vital pulp from root canals, sever pulp at constriction level, and remove materials from canals.

5. Nickel-titanium rotary instruments—designs vary in tip sizing, taper, cross section, helix angle, and pitch.

a. Important properties—superelasticity and high resistance to cyclic fatigue, which allow continuously rotating instruments to be used in curved root canals.

b. Nickel-titanium instruments have reduced incidence of blocks, ledges, transportation, and perforation but are believed to fracture more easily than hand instruments.

c. Examples—EndoSequence, Lightspeed, ProFile, ProTaper, EndoSequence.

D. Working length determination.

1. Reference point selection.

a. Select a point that is stable and easily visualized.

2. Techniques for determining working length.

a. Estimate working length with a diagnostic film taken using a paralleling technique with a No. 10 or 15 K-file.

b. If necessary, correct the working length by measuring the discrepancy between the radiographic apex and tip of file. Adjust to 1 mm short of the radiographic apex.

c. Use an apex locator—an electronic instrument used to assist in determining the root canal working length or perforation; operates on the principles of resistance, frequency, or impedance.

d. Feel for the apical constriction; however, in many instances, this may be unreliable.

E. Cleaning and shaping.

1. Best indicator of clean walls is the level of smoothness obtained.

2. In shaping, it is best to precurve inflexible files because essentially all canals are curved.

3. Taper of canal permits débridement of apical canal, reduces overinstrumentation of the foramen, and improves ability to obturate.

4. Techniques.

a. Crown-down—clinician passively inserts a large instrument into the canal up to a depth that allows easy progress. The next smaller instrument is used to progress deeper into the canal; the third instrument follows, and this continues until the apex is reached. Hand and rotary instruments may be used in this technique.

b. Step-back—working lengths decrease in stepwise manner with increasing instrument size.

c. Hybrid technique—above-listed basic techniques may be combined into a hybrid technique to achieve the best outcome.

F. Apical preparation.

1. Apical stops help confine instruments, materials, and chemicals to the canal space and create a barrier against which gutta-percha can be condensed.

G. File dimensions.

1. D1—file size at the tip of the file (e.g., 0.08 mm for a size 8 file; 0.15 mm for a size 15 file).

2. The diameter of the file where the cutting flutes end (16 mm) is known as D2 or D16.

a. It is the diameter at the tip plus 0.32 mm (e.g., for 0.02 taper No. 8 file, it is 0.08 mm + [16 mm × 0.02] = 0.40 mm).

H. Irrigation and medicaments.

1. Sodium hypochlorite (NaOCl).

a. Indications.

(1) Disinfection of root canals—hypochlorite anion (ClO^-).

(2) Dissolving organic matter—proteolytic material.

(3) Does not remove smear layer.

(4) Concentrations vary from 0.5% to 6%.

b. NaOCl accident.

(1) Signs and symptoms.

(a) Instant extreme pain.

(b) Excessive bleeding from the tooth.

(c) Rapid swelling.

(d) Rapid spread of erythema.

(e) Later—bruising and sensory and motor nerve deficits.

(2) Treatment.

(a) Long-lasting local anesthetic.

(b) Encourage drainage.

(c) Steroids.

(d) Cold compresses.

(e) Antibiotics.

(f) Analgesics.

(g) Daily follow-up.

2. Ethylenediamine tetraacetic acid (EDTA).

a. Principal ingredient—aqueous solution of 17% EDTA.

b. Indications.

(1) Removes inorganic material.

(2) Removes smear layer.

3. Chlorhexidine—synthetic cationic hydrophobic and lipophilic molecule that interacts with phospholipids and lipopolysaccharides on the cell membrane of bacteria and enters the cell by changing osmotic equilibrium and is effective at a concentration of 2%. The combination of chlorhexidine and NaOCl forms an undesirable precipitate, para-chloroaniline, which is believed to affect the seal of root canal filling.

4. Calcium hydroxide.

a. Best intracanal medicament available.

b. Its high pH causes an antibacterial effect (pH 12.5).

c. It inactivates lipopolysaccharide.

d. It has tissue-dissolving capacity.

I. Obturation of the root canal.

1. Obturation purposes.

a. To eliminate all avenues of leakage from the oral cavity or the apical tissues into the root canal system.

b. To seal within the system any irritants that cannot be fully removed during canal cleaning and shaping procedures.

2. Gutta-percha.

a. Advantages.

(1) Plasticity—adapts with compaction to irregularities.

(2) Easy to manage.

(3) Little toxicity.

(4) Easy to remove.

(5) Self-sterilizing (does not support bacterial growth).

b. Disadvantages.

(1) Gutta-percha without sealer does not seal.

(2) Lack of adhesion to dentin.

(3) Elasticity causes rebound to dentin.

(4) Shrinkage after cooling.

2.2 Surgical Endodontics

A. Incision and drainage and trephination.

1. Objectives are to evacuate exudates and purulence and toxic irritants. Removal speeds healing and reduces discomfort from irritants and pressure. The best treatment for swelling from acute apical abscess

is to establish drainage and to clean and shape the canal.

2. Indications for incision and drainage of soft tissues.
   a. If a pathway is needed in soft tissue with localized fluctuant swelling that can provide necessary drainage.
   b. When pain is caused by accumulation of exudates in tissues.
   c. When necessary to obtain samples for bacteriologic analysis.

3. Indications for trephination of hard tissues.
   a. If a pathway is needed from hard tissue to obtain necessary drainage.
   b. When pain is caused by accumulation of exudate within the alveolar bone.
   c. To obtain samples for bacteriologic analysis.

4. Procedure.
   a. Incision and drainage is a surgical opening created in soft tissue for the purpose of releasing exudates or decompressing an area of swelling.
   b. Trephination refers to surgical perforation of the alveolar cortical bone to release accumulated tissue exudates.
   c. Profound anesthesia is difficult to achieve in the presence of infection because of the acidic pH of the abscess and hyperalgesia.
   d. The incision should be made firmly through periosteum to bone. Vertical incisions are parallel with major blood vessels and nerves and leave very little scarring.
   e. These procedures may include the placement and subsequent timely removal of a drain.
   f. Antibiotics may be indicated in patients with diffuse swelling (cellulitis), patients with systemic symptoms, or patients who are immunocompromised.

B. Root end resection (apical surgery or apicoectomy).
   1. Indications.
      a. Persistent or enlarging apical pathosis after nonsurgical endodontic treatment.
      b. Nonsurgical endodontics is not feasible.
         (1) Marked overextension of obturating materials interfering with healing.
         (2) Biopsy is necessary.
         (3) Access for root-end preparation and root-end filling is necessary.
         (4) The apical portion of the root canal system with apical pathosis cannot be cleaned, shaped, and obturated.
   2. Contraindications.
      a. Anatomic factors—such as a thick external oblique ridge or proximity of the neurovascular bundle.
      b. Medical or systemic complications.
      c. Nonrestorability.
      d. Poor root/crown ratio.

3. Procedure.
   a. Root end resection is the preparation of a flat surface by the excision of the apical portion of the root and any subsequent removal of attached soft tissues.
   b. Flap design.
      (1) Submarginal curved flap (semilunar flap).
         (a) Disadvantages.
            (i) Restricted access with limited visibility.
            (ii) Leaving the incision directly over the lesion.
            (iii) Often healing with scarring.
      (2) Submarginal triangular and rectangular flaps.
      (3) Full mucoperiosteal flap.
   c. A mucoperiosteal flap is elevated, and, when necessary, bone is removed to allow direct visualization of and access to the affected area.
   d. Root end resection.
      (1) Resect 3 mm of diseased root tip.
      (2) The traditional 45-degree bevel has been replaced with lesser bevel (0 to 10 degrees).
      (3) Leave 3 mm for root end cavity preparation and root end filling.
      (4) Prepare 3 mm of the root end with ultrasonic instrumentation.
      (5) Increasing the depth of root end filling significantly decreases apical leakage.
      (6) Increasing the bevel increases leakage.
   e. Root end filling (retrofilling).
      (1) A biologically acceptable filling material, such as mineral trioxide aggregate (MTA), is placed into the 3-mm root end preparation to seal the root canal system.
   f. Primary closure of the surgical site is desired.

C. Hemisection.
   1. Surgical division (in approximately equal halves) of a multirooted tooth (e.g., mandibular molars). A vertical cut is made through the crown into the furcation. The defective half of the tooth is extracted.
   2. Indications.
      a. Class III or IV periodontal furcation defect.
      b. Infrabony defect of one root of a multirooted tooth that cannot be successfully treated periodontally.
      c. Coronal fracture extending into the furcation.
      d. Vertical root fracture confined to the root to be separated and removed.
      e. Carious, resorptive root or perforation defects that are inoperable or cannot be corrected without root removal.
      f. Persistent apical pathosis in which nonsurgical treatment or apical surgery is impossible and the problem is confined to one root.
   3. Procedure.
      a. Often performed in mandibular molars.
      b. Hemisection requires root canal treatment on all retained root segments.

c. When possible, it is preferable to complete the root canal treatment and place a permanent restoration into the canal orifices before the hemisection.

D. Bicuspidization.

1. A surgical division (as in hemisection, usually a mandibular molar), but the crown and root of both halves are retained.

2. The procedure results in complete separation of the roots and creation of two separate crowns.

E. Root resection (root amputation).

1. Removal of one or more roots of a multirooted tooth.

2. Indications for root resection.

a. Class III or IV periodontal furcation defect.

b. Infrabony defect of one root of a multirooted tooth that cannot be successfully treated periodontally.

c. Existing fixed prosthesis.

d. Vertical root fracture confined to the root to be resected.

e. Carious, resorptive root or perforation defects that are inoperable or cannot be corrected without root removal.

f. Persistent apical pathosis in which nonsurgical root canal treatment or apical surgery is impossible.

g. At least one root is structurally sound.

3. Procedure.

a. Amputation is the surgical removal of an entire root leaving the crown of the tooth intact.

b. Root resection requires root canal treatment on all retained root segments.

c. When possible, it is preferable to complete root canal treatment and place a permanent restoration into the canal orifices.

F. Intentional reimplantation.

1. Indications.

a. Persistent apical pathosis after endodontic treatment.

b. Nonsurgical retreatment is impossible or has an unfavorable prognosis.

c. Apical surgery is impossible or involves a high degree of risk to anatomic structures.

d. The tooth presents a reasonable opportunity for removal without fracture.

e. The tooth has an acceptable periodontal status before the reimplantation procedure.

2. Procedure.

a. Intentional reimplantation is the insertion of a tooth into its alveolus after the tooth has been extracted for the purpose of accomplishing a root end filling procedure.

b. Stabilization of the reimplanted tooth may or may not be needed.

c. When possible, root canal therapy is performed before the reimplantation.

G. Surgical removal of the apical segment of a fractured root.

1. Indicated when a root fracture occurs in the apical portion and pulpal necrosis results.

2. The fractured segment may be removed surgically after or in conjunction with nonsurgical root canal treatment.

3. Surgical removal of the apical segment of a fractured root is indicated in the following clinical situations.

a. Root fracture in the apical portion of the root.

b. Pulpal necrosis in the apical segment as indicated by an apical lesion or clinical signs or symptoms.

c. Coronal tooth segment is restorable and functional.

4. Procedure.

a. A mucoperiosteal flap is surgically elevated, and, when necessary, bone is removed to allow direct visualization and access to the affected site.

b. The apical portion of the affected root and all of the targeted tissue are removed.

2.3 Endodontic Emergencies

A. Definition.

1. Endodontic emergencies are usually associated with pain or swelling or both and require immediate diagnosis and treatment.

2. Emergencies are usually caused by pathoses in the pulp or periapical tissues.

3. Emergencies include luxation, avulsion, or fractures of the hard tissues.

B. Categories.

1. Pretreatment.

a. Patient usually presents with pain or swelling or both.

b. Challenge in this case is the diagnosis and treatment of the offending tooth.

2. Emergencies occurring between appointments or after obturation.

a. Also referred to as "flare-up."

b. Easier to manage because the offending tooth has been identified and diagnosed.

3. Diagnosis.

a. A rule of a true emergency is that only one tooth is the source of pain, so avoid overtreatment.

b. Obtain a complete medical and dental history.

c. Obtain a subjective examination relating to the history, location, severity, duration, character, and eliciting stimuli of the pain.

d. Obtain an objective examination including extraoral and intraoral examinations.

(1) Observe for swelling, discolored crowns, recurrent caries, and fractures.

(2) Apical tests include palpation, mobility, percussion, and biting tests.

(3) Pulp vitality tests are most useful to reproduce reported pain.

(4) Probing examination helps differentiate endodontic from periodontal disease.

(5) Radiographic examination is helpful but has limitations because periapical radiolucencies may not be present in acute periapical periodontitis.

4. Treatment.
   a. Reducing the irritant, through reduction of pressure or removal of the inflamed pulp or apical tissue, is the immediate goal.
   b. Pressure release is more effective than pulp or tissue removal in producing pain relief.
   c. Obtaining profound anesthesia of the inflamed area is a challenge.
   d. Management of painful irreversible pulpitis.
      (1) Complete cleaning and shaping of the root canals is the preferred treatment.
      (2) Pulpectomy provides the greatest pain relief, but pulpotomy is usually effective in the absence of percussion sensitivity.
      (3) Chemical medicaments sealed in chambers do not help control or prevent additional pain.
      (4) Antibiotics are generally not indicated.
      (5) Reducing occlusion has been shown to aid in the relief of symptoms if symptomatic apical periodontitis exists.
   e. Management of pulpal necrosis with apical pathosis.
      (1) Treatment is twofold.
         (a) Remove or reduce pulpal irritants.
         (b) Relieve apical fluid pressure when possible.
      (2) When no swelling exists, complete canal débridement is the treatment of choice.
      (3) When localized swelling exists, the abscess has invaded soft tissues.
         (a) Complete débridement.
         (b) Drainage to relieve pressure and purulence—drainage can occur through the tooth or mucosa (via incision and drainage).
         (c) Patients with localized swelling seldom have elevated temperatures or systemic signs, so systemic antibiotics are unnecessary.
      (4) When diffuse swelling exists, the swelling has dissected into fascial spaces.
         (a) Most important is the removal of the irritant via canal débridement or extraction of the offending tooth.
         (b) Swelling may be incised and drained followed by drain insertion for 1 to 2 days.
         (c) Systemic antibiotics are indicated for diffuse, rapid swelling.

5. "Flare-ups."
   a. This is a true emergency and is so severe that an unscheduled visit and treatment is required.
   b. A history of preoperative pain or swelling is the best predictor of "flare-up" emergencies.
   c. No relationship exists between flare-ups and treatment procedures (i.e., single or multiple visits).
   d. Treatment generally involves complete cleaning and shaping of canals, placement of intracanal medicament, and prescription of analgesic.
      (1) Antibiotics are generally not indicated except in the instance of systemic symptoms and cellulitis.

2.4 Sterilization and Asepsis

A. Rationale for sterilization.
   1. Endodontic instruments are contaminated with blood, soft and hard tissue remnants, bacteria, and bacterial by-products.
   2. Instruments must be cleaned often and disinfected during the procedure and sterilized afterward.
   3. Because instruments may be contaminated when new, they must be sterilized before initial use.
B. Types of sterilization.
   1. Glutaraldehyde.
      a. Cold or heat labile instruments such as rubber dam frames may be immersed for a sufficient period of time in solutions such as glutaraldehyde.
      b. Generally 24 hours are required to achieve cold sterilization.
      c. Immersion may be effective for disinfection, but it fails to kill all organisms.
      d. Because this method is not presently verifiable with biologic indicators, it is least desirable in the office and should be reserved for instruments that cannot withstand heat.
   2. Pressure sterilization.
      a. Instruments should be wrapped and autoclaved for 20 minutes at 121° C and 15 psi.
      b. All bacteria, spores, and viruses are killed.
      c. Either steam or chemicals can be used.
         (1) Pressure sterilizers using chemicals rather than water have the advantage of causing less rusting.
      d. Both steam and chemical autoclaving dull the edges of all cutting instruments owing to expansion with heat and contraction with cooling, resulting in permanent edge deformation.
   3. Dry heat sterilization.
      a. Dry heat is superior for sterilizing sharp-edged instruments such as scissors for best preservation of cutting edges.
      b. The cycle time for dry heat sterilization is temperature dependent.
         (1) After the temperature reaches 160° C, the instruments should be left undisturbed for 60 minutes.
         (2) If the temperature decreases to less than 161° C, the full 60-minute heat cycle must be repeated.
      c. The disadvantage to this method is the substantial time required both for sterilization and for cooling.

C. Disinfection.
1. Surface disinfection during canal débridement is accomplished by using a sponge soaked in 70% isopropyl alcohol or proprietary quaternary ammonium solutions.
2. Files can be thrust briskly in and out of this sponge to dislodge debris and contact the disinfectant.
3. This procedure cleans but does not disinfect instruments.

2.5 Radiographic Techniques

A. Diagnostic radiographs.
1. Angulation.
   a. Paralleling technique—the most accurate radiographs are made using a paralleling technique.
      (1) With paralleling, there is less distortion, more clarity, and reproducibility of the film and cone placement with preliminary and subsequent radiographs.
   b. If a paralleling technique cannot be used because of low palatal vault, maxillary tori, or long roots, the next best choice is the modified paralleling technique. The film is not parallel to the tooth, but the central beam is oriented at right angles to the film surface.
   c. The least accurate technique is the bisecting angle.
B. Working films.
1. Working length image.
2. Master cone image.
3. Check image.
   a. Taken of the master cone with accessory cones, before searing off the excess gutta-percha during cold lateral obturation.
C. Exposure considerations.
1. Proper x-ray machine settings and careful film processing are important for maximal quality radiographs.
   a. The optimal setting for maximal contrast between radiopaque and radiolucent structures is 70 kV.
D. Cone image shifting.
1. The cone image shift reveals the third dimension of the structures.
2. Indications and advantages.
   a. Separation and identification of superimposed canals.
      (1) This is necessary in all teeth that may contain two canals in a faciolingual plane.
   b. Movement and identification of superimposed structures.
      (1) Occasionally, radiopaque structures may overlie a root, as in the case of the zygoma.
   c. Determination of working length.
   d. Determination of curvatures.
      (1) Buccal object rule (SLOB rule) applies—the object closest to the buccal surface appears to move in the direction opposite the movement of the tube head or cone when compared with a second radiograph. Objects closest to the lingual surface appear to move in the same direction of the cone. The fulfillment of this principle requires two radiographs: the original image and the second "shifted" image.
      (2) Depending on the direction of curvature relative to the cone, it can be determined if the curvature is facial or lingual.
   e. Determination of faciolingual location.
   f. Identification of undiscovered canals.
      (1) An anatomic axiom is that if a root contains only a single canal, that canal will be positioned close to the center of the root.
   g. Radiographs must be taken at either a mesial or a distal angulation to see if another canal is present.
   h. If the instrument is skewed considerably off center, another canal must be present.
   i. Location of "calcified" canals.
      (1) A root always contains a canal, however tiny or impossible to negotiate.
      (2) Canals are frequently not visible on radiographs.
   j. While searching for an elusive canal, two working radiographs must be made: one from a straight view and the other from a mesial or distal view. The direction of the bur is adjusted accordingly.
3. Disadvantages of cone-image shifting.
   a. Decreased clarity.
      (1) The clearest radiograph with the most definition is the parallel projection.
   b. Superimposition of structures.
E. Endodontic radiographic anatomy (Fig. 1-4).
1. Limitations.
   a. A considerable amount of bone must be resorbed before a lesion becomes visible radiographically.
   b. Periapical lesions become more evident if cortical bone is resorbed.
2. Differential diagnosis of endodontic pathosis.
   a. Characteristics of radiolucent lesions.
      (1) Apical lamina dura is absent.
      (2) Most often, radiolucency is seen to be circular about the apex, but lesions may have various appearances.
      (3) The radiolucency stays at the apex regardless of cone angulation.
      (4) A cause of pulpal necrosis is usually evident.
   b. Characteristics of radiopaque lesions.
      (1) These lesions are better known as focal sclerosing osteomyelitis (condensing osteitis).
      (2) Such lesions have an opaque diffuse appearance.
      (3) Histologically, they represent an increase in trabecular bone.
      (4) The radiographic appearance is one of diffuse borders and a roughly concentric arrangement around the apex.

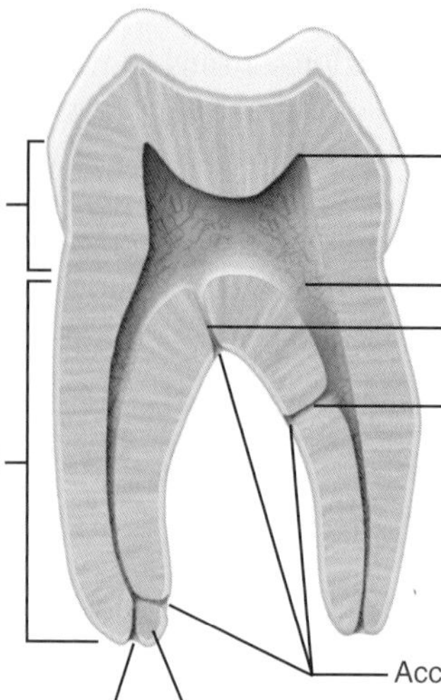

Figure 1-4 Major anatomic components of the root canal system. *(From Cohen S, Hargreaves KM: Pathways of the Pulp, ed 10. St Louis, Mosby, 2011.)*

(5) Condensing osteitis and apical periodontitis frequently manifest together.

(6) The pulp is often vital and inflamed.

2.6 Microbiology of Endodontics

A. Portals of entry of bacteria into the pulp.
  1. Caries.
  2. Permeable tubules.
    a. Cavity preparation.
    b. Exposure of dentin.
    c. Leaking restorations.
    d. Neither dentinal fluid nor odontoblastic processes are present in necrotic pulps.
  3. Cracks or trauma.
  4. Pulp exposure.
B. Nature and dynamics of root canal infection.
  1. Polymicrobial.
  2. Positive correlation between the number of bacteria in an infected root canal and the size of apical radiolucency.
  3. Difference between primary infection and unsuccessful root canal therapy.
    a. Primary endodontic infection.
      (1) Strict anaerobes predominate.
      (2) Gram-negative anaerobic—black pigmented *Bacteroides* (e.g., *Prevotella nigrescens*, *Porphyromonas*) most common in endodontic infections.
      (3) Gram-positive anaerobic—*Actinomyces* (root caries).
    b. Unsuccessful root canal therapy (retreatment needed because of persistent infection).
      (1) *Enterococcus faecalis* (rarely found in infected but untreated root canal).
      (2) High incidence of facultative anaerobes.
  4. Lipopolysaccharides.
    a. Lipopolysaccharides are found on the surface of gram-negative bacteria.
    b. When released from the cell wall, lipopolysaccharides are known as endotoxins.
      (1) Endotoxin is capable of diffusing across dentin.
      (2) A relationship has been established between the presence of endotoxins and apical inflammation.
C. Antibiotics used in endodontics.
  1. Penicillin V or amoxicillin are the first choice.
    a. They are effective against the following.
      (1) Most strict anaerobes (*Prevotella*, *Porphyromonas*, *Peptostreptococcus*, *Fusobacterium*, and *Actinomyces*).
      (2) Gram-positive facultative anaerobes (streptococci and enterococci) in polymicrobial endodontic infections.
  2. Clindamycin is effective against many gram-negative and gram-positive organisms, including strict and facultative anaerobes.
  3. Metronidazole is effective against strict anaerobes; since it is ineffective against facultative anaerobes and aerobes it must always be used in combination with another antibiotic, such as amoxicillin.

3.0 Procedural Complications

Outline of Review

3.1 Ledge Formation
3.2 Instrument Separation
3.3 Perforation
3.4 Vertical Root Fracture

3.1 Ledge Formation

A. Definition of a ledge.
  1. Artificial irregularity created on the surface of the root canal wall that impedes the placement of instruments to the apex.

2. Working length can no longer be ascertained.

3. Radiographic findings.

a. Instrument or obturation material is short of the apex.

b. Instrument or obturation material no longer follows the true curvature of the root canal.

B. Why ledges occur.

1. Lack of straight line access.

a. Can be caused by improper access preparation.

b. Can compromise the negotiation of the apical third of a canal through improper coronal flaring.

2. Anatomy of canal.

a. Length.

(1) Longer canals have a greater potential for ledge formation.

(2) With longer canals, recapitulate to confirm patency.

b. Canal diameter.

(1) Smaller diameter canals have greater potential for ledge formation.

c. Degree of curvature.

(1) As degree of curvature of the root canal system increases, the potential for ledge formation directly increases.

(2) Given buccal radiographic exposure, the degree of the buccolingual curvature of the root canal system may not be appreciated.

3. Inadequate irrigation or lubrication.

a. NaOCl is a good irrigant for disinfection and removal of debris, but an additional lubricant is necessary.

b. Lubricants allow for ease of file insertion, decrease of stress on instruments, and ease of debris removal.

4. Excessive enlargement of curved canal with files.

a. Instruments used to negotiate the root canal system have the tendency to cut straight ahead and straighten out.

(1) The files cut dentin toward the outside of the curvature at the apical portion of the root, a process called *transportation*.

b. The transported tip of the file may gouge into the dentin and create a ledge or perforation outside the original curvature of the canal.

c. Each successive file size should be used before a greater sized file is attempted (i.e., do not jump a file size).

d. Flexible files reduce ledge formation.

5. Obstruction or the packing of debris in the apical portion of the canal.

C. Correction of ledge formation.

1. The canal first must be relocated and renegotiated.

2. One technique is to use a precurved (1 to 2 mm apically) small file to reestablish correct working length.

a. Use plenty of lubrication.

b. Use a picking motion.

(1) If the true canal is located, use a reaming motion and occasionally an up-and-down movement to maintain the space and débride the canal.

c. Flaring the access may help improve access to the apical third of the canal.

3. Despite all effort, correction of a ledge is difficult because instruments and obturating materials tend to be directed into the ledge.

4. If unable to bypass ledge, clean and shape at the "new" working length.

D. Prognosis of the ledge.

1. Successful treatment after ledge creation depends on the extent of debris remaining in the region past the ledge.

a. The amount of debris depends on *when* the ledge formation occurred in the cleaning and shaping process.

b. Short and cleaned apical ledges have better prognoses.

2. Inform the patient of the prognosis, and instill the importance of recall and the signs that would indicate failure.

3.2 Instrument Separation

A. Definition.

1. A separated instrument is the breakage of an instrument within the confines of a canal.

B. How instruments separate.

1. Separation occurs because of limited flexibility and strength of the instrument.

2. Improper use.

a. May be overuse.

b. May be excessive force.

3. Manufacturing defects of instruments causing breakage are rare.

C. How to avoid separating instruments.

1. Recognize the stress limitations of the instruments being used.

2. Continual lubrication of the instrument within the canal.

a. Use irrigants.

b. Use lubricants.

3. Examine the instruments to be placed into the canal.

a. Before separation, steel instruments often exhibit fluting distortions, highlighting unwound or twisted regions of the file (signs of file fatigue).

b. Nickel-titanium files do not show the same visual signs of fatigue. These should be discarded before visual signs occur.

4. Replace files often.

5. Do not proceed to larger files until the smaller ones fit loosely within the canal.

D. Treating canals with separated instruments.

1. Bypass the instrument.

a. Use the same principles as bypassing a ledge.

2. Remove the instrument—this approach is usually unsuccessful, and referral to endodontist is necessary.
3. Prepare and obturate the canal to the point of instrument separation.
    a. Clean to the "new" working length, which corresponds to the coronal-most aspect of the separated instrument.
E. Prognosis of separated instrument.
    1. Successful treatment depends on the extent of debris remaining in the region below the separated instrument.
    2. Prognosis improves if instrument separation occurred during the later stages of cleaning and shaping, after much of the canal has been débrided to working length.
    3. Prognosis is poor for teeth where smaller instruments have been separated. Separating a No. 40 file at the working length is better than a No. 15 file, presumably because débridement to the working length would have been performed at least partially.
    4. Must inform patient and document history of the separated instrument.
    5. Overall, as long as the instrument separation is managed properly, the prognosis is favorable.
    6. If the patient has residual symptoms, the tooth is best treated surgically (root end resection).

3.3 Perforation

A. Definition—iatrogenic communication of the tooth with the outside environment.
B. Different kinds of perforations.
    1. Coronal perforation.
        a. Cause—failure to direct the bur toward the long axis of the tooth during access.
        b. During access preparation, visualize the long axis of the tooth periodically.
            (1) Magnification—use of loupes or a microscope aids.
            (2) Transillumination—the fiberoptic light illuminates the pulp chamber floor. The canal orifice appears as a dark spot.
            (3) Radiographs—use radiographs from different angles to provide information about the size and extent of the pulp chamber.
        c. In cases of rotated or tilted teeth, misoriented cast cores, or calcified chambers, follow the long axis of the roots carefully.
    2. Furcal perforation.
        a. Usually occurs during the search for canal orifices.
        b. Should be repaired *immediately*.
    3. Strip perforations.
        a. Involves the furcation side of the coronal root surface.
        b. Sequela of excessive flaring with instruments.

4. Root perforations.
    a. Apical perforation.
        (1) Can be a result of canal transportation, resulting in a perforated new canal.
    b. Midroot perforation.
        (1) Usually occurs after ledge formation, when a file is misdirected and creates an artificial canal.
C. Recognition of a perforation.
    1. Hemorrhage.
        a. Perforation into PDL or bone *may* cause immediate hemorrhage (bone, being relatively avascular, may cause little hemorrhage).
    2. Sudden pain.
        a. Occurs usually during evaluation of the working length.
        b. Usually the anesthetic used was adequate for access but not working length determination.
        c. Burning pain or bad taste with NaOCl use.
    3. Radiographic evidence.
        a. Files are malpositioned in reference to the canal.
        b. Take multiple x-rays from different horizontal angles to assess file.
    4. Apex locator readings—readings are far short of the initial file entry's working length.
    5. Deviation of a file from its previous course.
    6. Unusually severe postoperative pain.
D. Prognosis of a perforation.
    1. Perforation into the PDL results in a questionable prognosis, and the patient must be informed of this.
    2. Location.
        a. If located at or above the alveolar bone, the prognosis for repair is favorable.
            (1) Can be easily repaired with restorative materials (similar to a class V lesion).
            (2) May require flap surgery.
        b. If below the crestal bone or at the coronal third of the root, the prognosis is poor.
            (1) Attachment often recedes, usually to the extent of the defect.
            (2) Permanent periodontal pocket forms.
    3. Size of defect.
        a. Smaller perforations (<1 mm) are more amenable to repair.
        b. Cause less tissue destruction when smaller.
    4. Timing of perforation.
        a. Perforations occurring later in treatment, after complete or partial débridement of the canal, have a better prognosis.
    5. Timing of repair.
        a. The sooner the perforation is repaired, the better the prognosis.
        b. Minimizes the damage to the periodontal tissues by bacteria, files, and irrigants.

c. Immediate sealing of defect reduces periodontal breakdown.
6. Isolation—if tooth was well isolated at the time of repair, the prognosis is more favorable.
7. Accessibility of the repair.
8. Sealing ability of the restorative material.
9. Patient oral hygiene.
10. Capabilities of dentist performing the repair.
11. Treatment of perforations.
    a. Coronal perforation—refer case to an endodontist to locate the canals.
    b. Furcal perforation.
       (1) Usually accessible and able to be repaired nonsurgically.
       (2) Usually good prognosis if repaired (sealed) immediately.
    c. Strip perforation.
       (1) Rarely accessible.
       (2) Usual sequelae are inflammation followed by periodontal pocket.
    d. Root perforation.
       (1) Prognosis depends on the size and shape of perforation.
       (2) An open apex is difficult to seal and allows for extrusion of sealing materials.
       (3) Surgical treatment may be necessary.
12. Follow-up.
    a. Perforations should be monitored.
       (1) Assess symptoms.
       (2) Evaluate radiographs.
       (3) Periodontal probing to evaluate periodontal status.
E. Treatment—the ultimate goal is to clean, shape, and obturate as much of canal as is accessible. Avoid using high concentrations of NaOCl because it may inflame the periodontal tissues.
1. Surgical repair.
   a. Try to position the apical portion of the defect above the crestal bone.
      (1) Orthodontic extrusion.
      (2) Flap surgery and crown lengthening—used when the esthetic result is not compromised or if adjacent teeth require periodontal therapy.
      (3) Hemisection.
      (4) Root amputation.
      (5) Intentional reimplantation—indicated when the defect is inaccessible or when multiple problems exist (as with perforation and separated instrument).
   b. Prognosis is guarded because of increased technical difficulty of procedures. The remaining roots are often prone to caries, periodontal disease, and vertical root fracture.
2. Nonsurgical internal repair with MTA—studies have shown MTA is very biocompatible and promotes the deposition of cementumlike material.

3.4 Vertical Root Fracture

A. Vertical root fracture has a poor prognosis.
B. Definition of vertical root fracture (see Figure 1-3).
   1. Occurs along the long axis of the tooth.
   2. Often associated with a severe periodontal pocket in an otherwise periodontally sound dentition.
   3. Can be associated with a sinus tract.
   4. Can be associated with a lateral radiolucency extending to the apical portion of the root fracture.
   5. A fracture can be identified only with visualization, and surgery is often necessary to confirm the fracture.
C. How vertical fractures occur.
   1. Can occur after the cementation of a post.
   2. Can be the sequela of excessive condensation forces during obturation of an underprepared or overprepared canal.
      a. Prevent fracture via appropriate canal preparation.
      b. Prevent fracture via balanced pressure of condensation forces during obturation.
D. Treatment of vertical root fractures.
   1. Removal of the involved root in multirooted teeth or extraction.
   2. Results in extraction of single-rooted teeth.

4.0 Traumatic Injuries

Outline of Review

4.1 Examinations of Traumatic Injuries to Teeth
4.2 Types of Injuries
4.3 Avulsion
4.4 Biologic Consequences of Traumatic Injuries to Teeth
4.5 Inflammatory Root Resorption versus Replacement Root Resorption

4.1 Examinations of Traumatic Injuries to Teeth

A. Apical injuries.
   1. Injury may result in swelling and bleeding that involves the PDL.
   2. Teeth are sensitive to percussion.
   3. Apical displacement with injury to vessels entering the apical foramen may lead to pulp necrosis.
B. Pulp vitality testing.
   1. Test vitality of all teeth in the area.
   2. Testing immediately after the injury frequently yields a false-negative response.
   3. These data serve as a baseline for future reference. The test results may be unreliable for 6 to 12 months.
   4. False-negative test results.
      a. All the current pulp testing methods detect only the responsiveness and not the vitality of the pulp.

The vitality of the pulp is determined by the integrity of its blood supply. In reality, sensitivity tests for nerve function do not indicate the presence or absence of blood circulation within the pulp.

   b. In traumatic injury, the neural response from the pulpal sensory nerves may be disrupted, but the vascular supply may be intact.

5. These tests should be repeated at 3 weeks, 3 months, 6 months, and 12 months and yearly intervals thereafter. The purpose of the tests is to establish a trend as to the physiologic status of the pulps.

4.2 Types of Injuries

Fracture Injuries

A. Uncomplicated fractures (without pulp involvement).
   1. Infraction.
      a. Definition—incomplete crack of enamel without the loss of tooth structure.
   2. Enamel fracture (Ellis class I).
      a. Definition—involves enamel only (enamel chipping and incomplete fractures or cracks).
      b. Treatment—grinding and smoothing the rough edges or restoring lost structure.
      c. Prognosis—good.
   3. Crown fracture without pulp involvement (Ellis class II).
      a. Definition—uncomplicated fracture involving enamel and dentin only.
      b. Treatment—restoration with a bonded resin technique.
      c. Prognosis—good unless accompanied by a luxation injury.

B. Complicated fractures (Figure 1-5).
   1. Crown fracture with pulp involvement (Ellis class III).
      a. Definition—a complicated fracture involving enamel, dentin, and exposure of the pulp.
      b. Treatment—vital pulp therapy versus root canal therapy depends on the following factors.
         (1) Stage of development of the tooth—in an immature tooth, vital pulp therapy should always be attempted if feasible because of the tremendous advantages of maintaining the vital pulp.
         (2) Time between the accident and treatment—in the 24 hours after a traumatic injury, the initial reaction of the pulp is proliferative with no more than 2 mm pulp inflammation. After 24 hours, chances of direct bacterial contamination increase.
         (3) Concomitant periodontal injury—a periodontal injury compromises the nutritional supply of the pulp.
         (4) Restorative treatment plan—if a more complex restoration is to be placed, root canal therapy is recommended.

C. Root fracture—limited to fracture involving roots only (cementum, dentin, and pulp). It could be horizontal, which may show bleeding from the sulcus.
   1. Horizontal root fracture.
      a. Biologic consequences.
         (1) When a root fractures horizontally, the coronal segment is displaced, but generally the apical segment is not displaced.
         (2) Pulp necrosis of the coronal segment (25%) may result from displacement.
         (3) Because the apical pulp circulation is not disrupted, pulpal necrosis in the apical segment is rare.
      b. Diagnosis.
         (1) Because root fractures are usually oblique (facial to palatal), one periapical radiograph may miss it.
         (2) Radiographic examination should include an occlusal film and three periapical films (one at 0 degrees, then one each at + and − 15 degrees from the vertical axis of the tooth).
         (3) Healing patterns—Andreasen and Hjorting-Hansen described four types of healing. The first three types are considered successful. The fourth is typical when the coronal segment loses its vitality.
            (a) Healing with calcified tissue.
               (i) Ideal healing is calcific healing. A calcific callus is formed at the fracture site on the root surface and inside the canal wall.
            (b) Healing with interproximal connective tissue.
            (c) Healing with bone and connective tissue.
            (d) Interproximal inflammatory tissue without healing.
      c. Treatment.
         (1) With root fractures that have maintained the vitality of the pulp, the main goal of treatment is to enhance the healing process. Prognosis improves with quick treatment, close reduction of the root segments, and splinting. Splint as soon as possible, depending on location of the fracture and mobility.
         (2) Coronal root fracture.
            (a) Poor prognosis—if the fracture occurs at the level of or coronal to the crest of the alveolar bone, the prognosis is extremely poor.
            (b) Stabilize coronal fragment with rigid splint for 6 to 12 weeks.
            (c) If reattachment of the fractured fragments is impossible, extraction of the coronal segment is indicated. The apical segment may be carried out by orthodontic forced eruption or by periodontal surgery.

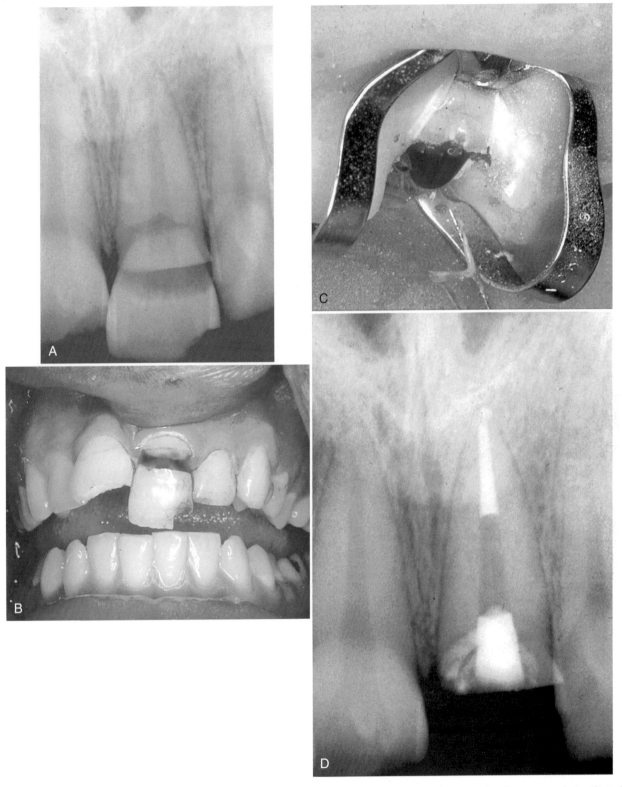

Figure 1-5 Complicated crown fracture. **A,** Complicated coronal fracture is deep into the dentin, and pulp is exposed. **B,** Clinical view. **C** and **D,** Tooth is treated with complete pulpectomy and root canal filling. *(From Gutmann JL, Lovdahl PE:* Problem Solving in Endodontics, *ed 5. St Louis, Mosby, 2011.)*

(3) Midroot fracture.
  (a) Stabilize for 3 weeks.
  (b) Pulp necrosis occurs in 25% of root fractures. For the most part, the necrosis is limited to the coronal segment. The pulp lumen is wide at the apical extent of the coronal segment, so apexification may be indicated.
  (c) In rare cases when both coronal and apical pulps are necrotic, endodontic treatment through the fracture is difficult. Necrotic apical segments can be removed surgically.
(4) Apical root fracture—horizontal fractures in the apical one third (portion of the root closest to the root tip) have the best prognosis. The pulp is mostly vital, and the tooth has little or no mobility.
  d. Prognosis.
    (1) Improves as fracture approaches apex.
    (2) Horizontal is better than vertical.
    (3) Nondisplaced is better than displaced.
    (4) Oblique is better than transverse.

Displacement Injuries

A. Luxation—dislocation of a tooth from its alveolus resulting from acute trauma (Ellis class V).
B. Concussion.
  1. Description and diagnosis—no displacement, normal mobility, sensitive to percussion; generally responds to pulp testing. Pulp blood supply is likely to recover.
  2. Treatment.
    a. Baseline vitality tests and radiographs.
    b. Occlusal adjustment.
    c. No immediate treatment is needed. Let the tooth "rest" (avoid bite), then follow-up.
C. Subluxation.
  1. Description and diagnosis—The tooth is loosened but not displaced.
  2. Treatment.
    a. Baseline vitality tests and radiographs.
    b. Occlusal adjustment.
    c. Splint for 1 to 2 weeks if mobile.
  3. Pulpal outcome.
    a. Pulpal necrosis rate of 6% with closed apices.
    b. Pulpal outcome more favorable with open apices.
D. Extrusive or lateral luxation.
  1. Description and diagnosis.
    a. Tooth is partially extruded from its socket.
    b. Occasionally this is accompanied by alveolar fracture.
    c. Lateral extrusion—usually the crown was displaced palatally, and the root apex was displaced labially.
  2. Treatment.
    a. Radiographs.
    b. Reposition teeth.

    c. Physiologic splint.
    d. Endodontic treatment if necessary (or observe for revascularization for open apices).
  3. Pulp outcome.
    a. Mature teeth with closed apices.
      (1) Extrusive luxation—65% rate of pulpal necrosis.
      (2) Lateral luxation—80% rate of pulpal necrosis.
E. Intrusive luxation.
  1. Description and diagnosis—apical displacement of the tooth.
  2. Treatment.
    a. Immature teeth with open apices—allow to reerupt.
    b. Mature teeth (close apices).
      (1) Orthodontic reposition.
      (2) Surgical reposition.
      (3) Endodontic treatment.
  3. Pulp outcome—96% rate of pulpal necrosis.

4.3 Avulsion

A. Avulsion (exarticulation)—complete separation of a tooth from its alveolus by traumatic injury (Ellis class VI) (Figure 1-6).

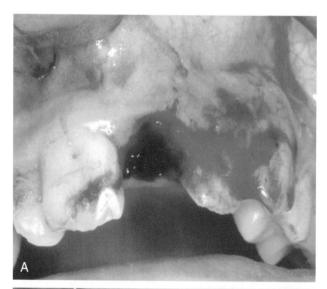
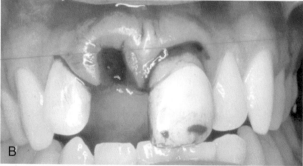

Figure 1-6 A and **B,** Two cases of tooth avulsion. Sometimes the damage to the surrounding tissues can be extensive. *(From Gutmann JL, Lovdahl PE: Problem Solving in Endodontics, ed 5. St Louis, Mosby, 2011.)*

B. Treatment—first priority is to protect the viability of the PDL.
  1. Reimplantation immediately if possible.
    a. Immediate reimplantation → improve PDL healing → prevent root resorption.
  2. If on-site reimplantation not possible, extraalveolar dry time must be considered.
    a. Critical extraalveolar dry time, success rate.
      (1) Less than 15 minutes, 90%.
      (2) 30 minutes, 50%.
      (3) More than 60 minutes, less than 10%.
    b. Storage media.
      (1) Optimal storage environment—maintain and reconstitute metabolites.
        (a) Viaspan.
        (b) Hank's Balanced Salt Solution.
      (2) Wet—just maintains viability.
        (a) Milk.
        (b) Saline.
        (c) Saliva (hypotonic—cell lysis).
        (d) Water—*least* desirable (hypotonic—cell lysis and inflammation).
  3. Management in the dental office.
    a. Closed apex with extraoral dry time less than 60 minutes and tooth stored in a special storage medium, milk, or saliva.
      (1) Do not handle the root surface and do not curette the socket.
      (2) Remove coagulum from socket with saline and examine alveolar socket.
      (3) Reimplant tooth slowly with slight digital pressure.
      (4) Stabilize with a semirigid (physiologic) splint for 7 to 10 days.
      (5) Administer systemic antibiotic (penicillin 4× per day for 7 days or doxycycline 2× per day for 7 days at appropriate dose for patient age and weight).
      (6) Refer to physician to evaluate need for tetanus booster.
    b. Closed apex with extraoral dry time more than 60 minutes.
      (1) Remove debris and necrotic PDL.
      (2) Remove coagulum from socket with saline and examine alveolar socket.
      (3) Immerse tooth in a 2.4% sodium fluoride solution with pH of 5.5 for 5 minutes.
      (4) Reimplant tooth slowly with slight digital pressure.
      (5) Stabilize with a semirigid (physiologic) splint for 7 to 10 days.
      (6) Administer systemic antibiotic (penicillin 4× per day for 7 days or doxycycline 2× per day for 7 days at appropriate dose for patient age and weight).
      (7) Refer to physician to evaluate need for tetanus booster.
    c. Open apex with extraoral dry time less than 60 minutes and tooth stored in a special storage medium, milk, or saliva.
      (1) If contaminated, clean the root surface and apical foramen with a stream of saline.
      (2) Place the tooth in doxycycline (1 mg/20 mL saline).
      (3) Remove coagulum from socket with saline and examine alveolar socket.
      (4) Reimplant tooth slowly with slight digital pressure.
      (5) Stabilize with a semirigid (physiologic) splint for 7 to 10 days.
      (6) Administer systemic antibiotic (penicillin 4× per day for 7 days or doxycycline 2× per day for 7 days at appropriate dose for patient age and weight).
      (7) Refer to physician to evaluate need for tetanus booster.
    d. Open apex with extraoral dry time more than 60 minutes.
      (1) Reimplantation usually is not indicated.
  4. Endodontic treatment—7 to 10 days after reimplantation.
    a. Extraoral time less than 60 minutes.
      (1) Closed apex.
        (a) Endodontic treatment is initiated at 7 to 10 days.
        (b) If endodontic treatment is delayed or signs of resorption are present, "long-term" calcium hydroxide treatment is given before root canal filling.
      (2) Open apex.
        (a) Endodontic treatment should be avoided, and signs of revascularization should be checked.
        (b) At the first sign of an infected pulp, the apexification procedure is begun.
    b. Extraoral time more than 60 minutes.
      (1) Close apex.
        (a) Same protocol as with dry time less than 60 minutes.
      (2) Open apex (if reimplanted).
        (a) If endodontic treatment was not performed out of the mouth, the apexification procedure is initiated.

4.4 Biologic Consequences of Traumatic Injuries

A. Attachment damage (Table 1-3)—external resorption.
  1. Surface resorption.
    a. Transient phenomenon that is extremely common, self-limiting, and reversible.
    b. As a result of mechanical damage to the cementum surface, the root surface undergoes spontaneous destruction and repair.

Table 1-3

External Root Resorption

	INFLAMMATORY ROOT RESORPTION	REPLACEMENT ROOT RESORPTION
Radiographs	Resorptive defect on root surface is separated from bone by radiolucency	PDL separating bone and tooth surface is absent
Cause	Root canal bacteria and their by-products move through the wide dentinal tubules to root surface	Trauma to PDL
Pulp	Necrosis	No known relationship between pulp vitality and replacement resorption
Progress	Rapid, but can be arrested	Can be delayed, but cannot be stopped
Treatment and prognosis	Immediate root canal treatment is required. Removing infected pulp halts resorption	In the absence of adverse signs and symptoms, no pulpal treatment is indicated, but radiographic follow-up is essential

PDL, Periodontal ligament.

c. Repair occurs within 14 days. This is not clinically significant.
2. Replacement resorption (ankylosis).
    a. Cause.
        (1) PDL damage (nonviable PDL).
        (2) Occurs in 61% of reimplanted teeth (Andreason, 1995).
    b. Radiographic evidence.
        (1) Continuous replacement of lost root with bone, no radiolucency (loss of cementum, dentin, and PDL with ingrowth and fusion of bone to the root defect).
    c. Clinical evidence.
        (1) Progressive submergence with growth (leading to infraocclusion).
        (2) Irreversible—dental treatment cannot stop progression of ankylosis.
        (3) Metallic sound on percussion.
3. Cervical resorption (extracanal invasive resorption, subepithelial external root resorption).
    a. Cause—sulcular infection from the following.
        (1) Physical injuries.
            (a) Trauma.
            (b) Orthodontics.
            (c) Periodontal treatment.
        (2) Chemical injuries—nonvital bleaching.
        (3) Idiopathic.
    b. Radiographic evidence.
        (1) Mesiodistal—it mimics the appearance of cervical caries adjacent to an infrabony defect.
        (2) Buccolingual—it shows a radiolucency over the well-defined outline of the canal.
        (3) Ragged, asymmetric, and irregular "moth-eaten" appearance.
        (4) Most misdiagnoses of resorptive defects are made between internal root resorptions, cervical caries, and cervical resorption.

c. Clinical evidence.
    (1) Crestal bony defect associated with the lesion.
    (2) Pink spot possible (owing to the granulation tissue in the cervical dentin undermining the crown enamel).
    (3) Pulp vitality testing is within normal limits.
d. Location.
    (1) At the attachment level of the tooth.
    (2) Usually begins at cementoenamel junction.
e. Treatment—surgical removal of granulation tissue and repair with restoration.
B. Apical neurovascular supply damage.
1. Pulp canal obliteration—calcific metamorphosis.
    a. 27% of complications after luxation.
    b. Occurs with increased likelihood with immature teeth (open apices), intrusions, and severe crown fractures.
2. Pulpal necrosis.
    a. Frequency of pulpal necrosis.
        (1) Type of injury—concussion (2%) < subluxation (6%) < extrusion (65%) < lateral luxation (80%) < intrusion (96%).
        (2) Stages of root development—incomplete (17%) < complete (68%).
3. Inflammatory resorption (Table 1-4; see Table 1-3).
    a. Cause—pulp necrosis.
        (1) Bacteria and toxins enter into the dentinal tubules.
        (2) pH is lowered, and inflammatory root resorption ensues.
    b. Radiographic evidence.
        (1) Bowl-shaped resorption involving cementum and dentin.
        (2) Occurs 3 weeks after trauma.
    c. Location—at apical one third of the root, sometimes progresses to entire root.

Table 1-4

Internal Root Resorption versus External Root Resorption

	INTERNAL ROOT RESORPTION	EXTERNAL ROOT RESORPTION
Definition	Destructive process initiated within **root canal** system	Destructive process initiated in **periodontium**

Etiology	"Inflammation" from:
	1. Caries
	2. Attrition, abrasion, erosion
	3. Cracked teeth
	4. Trauma
	5. $Ca(OH)_2$ pulpotomy
	6. Crown preparation
	7. Idiopathic
		1. IRR: necrotic pulp, bacteria and bacterial by-products initiate and follow ports of exit to affect periodontium
		2. RR: trauma to periodontium
		3. CR: sulcular infection from:
		   a. Physical injuries: trauma, orthodontic or periodontal treatment
		   b. Chemical injuries: nonvital bleaching
		   c. Idiopathic

Location	1. Occurs at any location along the root canal 2. Rare in permanent teeth	1. IRR: occurs at apical and lateral aspects of root 2. RR: occurs at any location along root 3. CR: at attachment level of the tooth (usually begins at cementoenamel junction)
Clinical manifestations	1. Generally asymptomatic (usually first recognized clinically through routine radiographs) 2. Pink spot possible (owing to granulation tissue in coronal dentin undermining crown enamel 3. Most misdiagnoses of resorptive defects are made between internal root resorptions and subepithelial external resorption (CR)	RR: 1. Characteristic high-pitched, "metallic" sound to percussion 2. Progressive submergence with growth CR: 1. Crestal bony defect associated with lesion 2. Pink spot possible
Radiographic appearance	1. Margins are sharp, smooth, and clearly defined 2. Oval, walls of root canal appear to balloon out 3. Usually symmetrical 4. Uniform in density 5. Unaltered canal or chamber cannot be followed through the lesion: loss of canal anatomy (defect appears as an expansion of pulp chamber or canal) 6. Does not move with angled radiographs	IRR and CR: 1. Margins are less well defined, ragged, and irregular 2. "Moth-eaten" appearance 3. Usually asymmetrical 4. Variations in density that may appear striated 5. Unaltered canal configuration can be followed through the area of lesion (root canal outline can be seen "running through" radiolucent defect) 6. Moves with angled radiographs RR: 1. More radiopaque than radiolucent 2. Disappearance of PDL space followed by bone replacement

Vitality testing	1. Usually a positive response (for internal resorption to be active, at least part of the pulp must be vital)
	2. Sometimes a negative response because:
	   a. Coronal pulp is necrotic and active resorbing cells are more apical in the canal
	   b. Pulp becomes nonvital after a period of active resorption
		1. IRR: negative (nonvital) response
		2. RR: not related
		3. CR: normal response

Treatment	Prompt endodontic therapy stops the process	1. IRR: nonsurgical endodontic treatment 2. RR: root canal therapy is of little value. No reliable techniques or medicaments 3. CR: surgical removal of granulation tissue and repair with restoration

CR, Cervical resorption; *IRR*, inflammatory root resorption; *PDL*, periodontal ligament; *RR*, replacement resorption.

4.5 Inflammatory Root Resorption versus Replacement Root Resorption

Inflammatory resorption and replacement resorption are most commonly associated with luxation injuries.

5.0 Adjunctive Endodontic Treatment

Outline of Review

5.1 Dental-Pulp Complex
5.2 Vital Pulp Therapy
5.3 Bleaching Discolored Teeth

5.1 Dentin-Pulp Complex

A. Pulp biology.
  1. Pulp consists of loose, fibrous connective tissue.
  2. There is a lack of collateral circulation.
  3. Pulp does not expand owing to rigidity of the dentin.
  4. Within the pulp are odontoblasts, fibroblasts, nerves, blood vessels, and lymphatics.
B. Reparative dentin.
  1. After injury or irritation, primary odontoblasts may die.
  2. Secondary odontoblasts can form and produce reparative dentin as a defense.
  3. Odontoblasts form reparative dentin at the site of an irritant.
  4. The pulp can defend itself against most nonmicrobial irritants.
  5. When the irritant is too great, deposition of reparative dentin may be insufficient, and pulp defenses become overwhelmed.
  6. When bacteria enter the pulp with sufficient quantity or virulence, complete pulpal necrosis is imminent and irreversible.
C. Caries and microleakage.
  1. Bacteria from dental caries are the main cause of more serious pulpal injury and the main cause of pulpitis.
  2. This can be initial caries or caries developing under defective restorations (recurrent decay).
  3. Bacteria can penetrate beyond the more obvious carious lesion through dentinal tubules.

5.2 Vital Pulp Therapy

A. Materials for vital pulp therapy dressing—can stimulate dentinal bridge formation.
  1. Calcium hydroxide.
    a. Used as a pulp capping material since the 1930s and has a solid history of clinical documentation.
    b. Its inherent high pH of 12.5 cauterizes tissue and causes superficial necrosis.
    c. This material develops a sterile necrotic zone that encourages the pulp to induce hard tissue repair with secondary odontoblasts.

2. MTA.
  a. Portland cement derivative made of primarily fine hydrophilic particles.
  b. Consists of calcium phosphate and calcium oxide.
  c. Sets in presence of moisture.
  d. Long setting time (approximately 2 hours, 45 minutes).
  e. Nonresorbable quality makes it a great sealing agent.
  f. MTA used as a filling material appears to be able to induce cementoblastic cells to produce hard tissue.
B. Vital pulp therapy—indirect pulp capping, direct pulp capping, partial pulpotomy, pulpotomy, and apexogenesis.
  1. Indirect pulp cap.
    a. Definition.
      (1) Procedure in which a material is placed on a thin partition of remaining carious dentin that, if removed, might expose the pulp in permanent immature teeth.
    b. Indications.
      (1) When teeth have deep carious lesions approximating the pulp but no signs or symptoms of pulpal degeneration or apical disease.
    c. Clinical objective.
      (1) To arrest the carious process and allow remineralization.
      (2) Wait for 6 to 8 weeks to allow deposition of reparative dentin (at the rate of 1.4 μm/day).
      (3) Remove the remaining caries leaving healthy, dentin and permanently restore the tooth.
  2. Direct pulp cap.
    a. Definition.
      (1) Dental material placed directly on a mechanical or traumatic vital pulp exposure.
    b. Indications.
      (1) Pulp has been exposed less than 24 hours.
      (2) Healthy pulp exposures during an operative procedure.
      (3) Asymptomatic.
      (4) Small exposure site.
    c. During follow-up visits.
      (1) Test for palpation, percussion, thermal pulp testing, and periapical radiograph.
      (2) A hard tissue barrier may be visualized 6 weeks postoperatively.
    d. Prognosis—survival of the pulp depends on the following.
      (1) Quality of the bacteria-tight seal provided by the restoration.
      (2) Degree of bleeding.
      (3) Disinfection of the superficial pulp and dentin or elimination of any inflamed zone of pulp.
  3. Partial pulpotomy (also known as *Cvek pulpotomy* and *shallow pulpotomy*).

a. Definition—surgical removal of a small portion of coronal pulp tissue to preserve the remaining coronal and radicular pulp tissues (described by Cvek in 1978).

b. Indications.

(1) Inflammation is greater than 2 mm into the pulp chamber but has not reached the root orifices.

(2) Traumatic exposures longer than 24 hours or mechanical exposures.

(3) Immature permanent tooth or mature tooth with simple restorative plan.

c. Follow-up.

(1) Same as pulp capping.

(2) Sensitivity test is unavailable because of loss of coronal pulp.

(3) Use radiograph to assess continuation of root formation or development of periapical lesion.

d. Prognosis—good prognosis depends on the following.

(1) Adequate removal of inflamed pulp.

(2) Good disinfection of dentin and pulp.

(3) Ability to avoid blood clot formation after amputation.

(4) Bacteria-tight seal of restoration.

4. Pulpotomy.

a. Definition.

(1) Surgical removal of the coronal portion of a vital pulp to preserve the vitality of the remaining radicular pulp.

(2) The level of pulp amputation is chosen arbitrarily but usually at the level of the root orifices.

b. Indications.

(1) Vital pulp in immature teeth with carious, mechanical exposure or traumatic exposures after 72 hours.

(2) No history of spontaneous pain.

(3) No abscess, radiographic bone loss, or mobility.

c. Potential problems—operators cannot determine whether all diseased tissue has been removed.

5. Apexogenesis.

a. Definition—maintenance of pulp vitality to allow continued development of the entire root. Apical closure occurs approximately 3 years after eruption.

b. Clinical objectives.

(1) The key is to allow the body to make a stronger root.

(2) This procedure relates to teeth with retained viable pulp tissue in which the pulp tissue is protected, treated, or encouraged to permit the process of normal root lengthening, root wall thickening, and apical closure.

(3) Nonsurgical endodontic therapy can be performed more safely and effectively to treat the pulpal disease.

c. Indications.

(1) Immature tooth with incomplete root formation and with damaged coronal pulp and healthy radicular pulp.

d. Contraindications.

(1) Avulsed teeth.

(2) Unrestorable teeth.

(3) Teeth with severe horizontal fracture.

(4) Necrotic teeth.

e. Prognosis—good when pulp capping or shallow pulpotomy is done correctly; conventional pulpotomy is not as successful.

f. Success rate depends on the following.

(1) Extent of pulpal damage.

(2) Restorability of the tooth.

C. Pulpectomy.

1. Pulpectomy is *not* vital pulp therapy because the tooth is pulpless.

2. Definition—to remove coronal and radicular pulp tissues.

3. Applications.

a. Temporary pain relief on teeth with irreversible pulpitis until nonsurgical endodontic treatment can be performed.

D. Apexification.

1. Apexification is *not* vital pulp therapy because the tooth is pulpless.

2. Definition—method to stimulate the formation of calcified tissue at the open apex of pulpless teeth.

3. Indication—infected teeth with open apices in which standard instrumentation techniques cannot create an apical stop to facilitate effective obturation of the canal.

4. Technique—disinfection of canal followed by induction or placement of an acceptable apical barrier.

a. Calcium hydroxide and MTA have been used to create an apical barrier.

(1) Calcium hydroxide may be used to induce apical hard tissue formation. A thick paste of calcium hydroxide must be placed in the canal and replaced every 3 months until a hard tissue barrier forms, against which gutta-percha may be placed to fill the canal. This traditional technique may require 1 year for hard tissue formation.

(2) MTA can be packed into the apical 3 mm of the canal, and the remainder of the canal can be filled with gutta-percha at the same appointment.

(3) MTA has established biologic outcomes in terms of healing and root-end closure at least comparable to teeth treated with calcium hydroxide.

b. Advantages of MTA compared with calcium hydroxide—treatment can be completed in less time, improved patient compliance, reduced cost of clinical time.

5.3 Bleaching Discolored Teeth

A. Causes of discoloration.
   1. Pulp necrosis (or remnants of pulp tissue)—tissue disintegration by-products are released and penetrate tubules.
   2. Intrapulpal hemorrhage.
   3. Calcific metamorphosis—extensive formation of tertiary dentin gives tooth a yellow color.
   4. Age.
   5. Fluorosis—gives teeth a mottled white-to-gray appearance.
   6. Systemic drugs.
   7. Defects in tooth formation.
   8. Blood dyscrasias.
   9. Obturation materials—from zinc oxide–eugenol, plastics, or metallic components of sealers.
B. Intracoronal (nonvital or internal) bleaching techniques.
   1. Thermocatalytic technique.
      a. Place oxidizing agent (30% hydrogen peroxide [Superoxol]) in the chamber and apply heat.
      b. Complications—external cervical resorption because irritation diffuses through the dentinal tubules to cementum and PDL. Heat combined with chemicals may cause necrosis of the cementum and inflammation of the PDL.
   2. Walking bleach.
      a. Place mix of sodium perborate and water in the chamber. Because Superoxol is not used, 2-mm protective cement barrier is unnecessary.
      b. Return in 2 to 6 weeks.

6.0 Posttreatment Evaluation

Outline of Review

6.1 Restoration of Endodontically Treated Teeth
6.2 Success and Failure

6.1 Restoration of Endodontically Treated Teeth

A. Coronal leakage.
   1. Major cause of endodontic failure.
      a. More endodontically treated teeth are lost because of restorative factors than because of failure of the root canal treatment itself.
      b. After root canal therapy, the internal chambers of the tooth may become reinfected if coronal leakage occurs. Saliva contamination with bacteria and endotoxins can cause endodontic failure, a risk that increases with the duration of saliva exposure.
   2. The temporary restoration does not provide complete protection against occlusal forces. When an immediate restoration is impossible, a bonded temporary restoration at the canal orifice can be used.
   3. Permanent restorations are best placed as soon as possible after obturation to seal the internal aspect of the tooth from contamination.
   4. When the root canal space has been grossly recontaminated, retreatment should be considered.
B. Structural considerations.
   1. Endodontically treated teeth do *not* become brittle. The moisture content of endodontically treated teeth is not reduced even after 10 years.
   2. Teeth are weakened by loss of tooth structure.
      a. Loss of marginal ridges is a major contributor to reduced cuspal strength.
      b. The loss of structural integrity with access preparation (rather than changes in dentin) leads to a higher occurrence of fractures in endodontically treated teeth compared with vital teeth.
      c. The most important part of the restored tooth is the tooth itself.
      d. No combination of restorative materials can substitute for tooth structure.
   3. Ferrule.
      a. When a crown is needed, the axial walls of the crown engage the axial walls of the prepared tooth, forming the ferrule. The ferrule is a band that encircles the external dimension of the residual tooth, similar to the metal bands around a barrel. It is formed by the walls and margins of the crown.
      b. A longer ferrule increases resistance to fracture.
         (1) Fracture resistance (to cervical tensile strength) increases significantly with an increasing amount of sound tooth structure.
         (2) A longer ferrule increases fracture resistance and resists lateral forces from posts and leverage from the crown in function.
         (3) Crown preparations with 1-mm coronal extension of dentin above the margin have double the fracture resistance compared with when the core terminates immediately above the margin.
      c. The ferrule must encircle a vertical wall of sound tooth structure above the margin and must not terminate on restorative core material.
      d. Insufficient remaining tooth structure to construct a ferrule should be evaluated for crown lengthening surgery or orthodontic extrusion to gain access to additional root surface.
   4. Post preparation.
      a. The primary purpose of the post is to retain a core in a tooth with extensive loss of coronal structure.
      b. The need for a post is dictated by the amount of remaining coronal tooth structure.

c. Posts do not reinforce the tooth but further weaken it by additional removal of dentin and by creating stress that predisposes to root fracture.

d. At least 5 to 7 mm of remaining gutta-percha is recommended.

6.2 Success and Failure

A. Causes of endodontic failures.
   1. Inadequate seal of the root canal system.
      a. Coronal seal is more important than apical seal in long-term.
      b. Historically, obturation has been accorded the role of the most critical step and the cause of most treatment failures. However, the two events are associated but not by cause and effect because poorly obturated canals are usually poorly débrided as well.
   2. Poor access cavity.
   3. Inadequate débridement.
   4. Missed canals.
   5. Vertical fractures.
   6. Procedure errors (perforation, ledging, loss of length).
   7. Leaking temporary or permanent restoration.
   8. Periodontal involvement.
   9. Resorption.
   10. Compromised host factors (systemic conditions).
   11. Misdiagnosis.
B. Factors influencing success rate.
   1. Apical pathosis.
      a. The presence of an apical lesion before treatment reduces the success rate of endodontic treatment by 10% to 20%.
   2. Bacterial status of the canal.
      a. The presence of bacteria in the canal before obturation results in a poorer prognosis.
   3. Quality of endodontic work.
   4. Quality of coronal seal.
C. Principles of successful endodontics (note: factors 1 through 3 represent the traditional endodontic triad).
   1. Microbial disinfection.
   2. Débridement—the key to success.
   3. Obturation.
   4. Diagnosis.
   5. Treatment plan.
   6. Knowledge of anatomy of morphology.
   7. Restoration.

Sample Questions

1. An 8-year-old girl presents to the office with an Ellis class II fracture. In an effort to determine a pulpal diagnosis, which of the following tests is the *least* accurate?
   A. Percussion
   B. Palpation
   C. Electrical pulp test
   D. Cold test

2. Symptomatic irreversible pulpitis pain in which of the following sites is *most* likely to radiate to the ear?
   A. Maxillary premolar
   B. Maxillary molar
   C. Mandibular premolar
   D. Mandibular molar

3. Which of the following statements regarding external root resorption is *not* true?
   A. It is a destructive process initiated in the periodontium.
   B. There are three main types: inflammatory root resorption, replacement resorption, and cervical resorption.
   C. It can be located anywhere along the root canal.
   D. The margins are sharp, smooth, and well defined.

4. Which of the following statements *most* likely applies to a cracked tooth?
   A. The direction of the crack usually extends mesiodistally.
   B. The direction of the crack usually extends faciolingually.
   C. Radiographic examination is the best way to detect a cracked tooth.
   D. Choices A and C only
   E. Choices B and C only

5. Which of the following statements regarding treatment of a tooth manifesting with a sinus tract is *true*?
   A. Treat with conventional (nonsurgical) endodontic therapy.
   B. Antibiotics are not needed.
   C. The sinus tract should heal in 2 to 4 weeks after conventional root canal therapy.
   D. If the sinus tract persists after root canal therapy, perform root end surgery with root end filling.
   E. All of the above

6. The major objectives of access preparation include all of the following *except* one. Which one is the *exception*?
   A. Attainment of direct straight-line access to canal orifices
   B. Confirmation of clinical diagnosis
   C. Conservation of tooth structure
   D. Attainment of direct straight-line access to the apical root

7. Which of the following is *not* a property of NaOCl?
   A. Chelation
   B. Tissue dissolution at higher concentrations
   C. Microbicidal activity
   D. Flotation of debris and lubrication

8. While performing nonsurgical endodontic therapy, you detect a ledge. What should you do?

A. Use a smaller instrument and get by the ledge
B. Fill as far as you have reamed
C. Use a small round bur and remove the ledge
D. Continue working gently to remove the ledge

9. Which perforation location has the *best* prognosis?
A. Coronal third of root
B. Apical third of root
C. Chamber floor
D. Middle third of root

10. A classic teardrop-shaped apical lesion on a radiograph can indicate a vertical root fracture. The prognosis of a vertical root fracture is hopeless, and the tooth should be extracted.
A. The first statement is *true*, and the second statement is *false*.
B. The first statement is *false*, and the second statement is *true*.
C. Both statements are *true*.
D. Both statements are *false*.

11. A patient presents with a chief complaint of swelling in the mandibular left quadrant that started 2 days ago and developed quickly. The patient has a mild fever with malaise, and clinical examination revealed localized fluctuant swelling in the buccal vestibule of teeth #18 and #19. Tooth #19 is nonresponsive to thermal testing and exhibits moderate pain to percussion. Radiographic findings reveal a slight widened PDL space. Based on these findings, the *most* likely apical diagnosis is _____.
A. Acute apical abscess
B. Irreversible necrotic apical periodontitis
C. Asymptomatic irreversible pulpitis
D. Symptomatic apical periodontitis

12. Prolonged, unprovoked night pain suggests which of the following conditions of the pulp?
A. Pulpal necrosis
B. Mild hyperemia
C. Reversible pulpitis
D. Periodontal abscess

13. The pathognomonic symptom of symptomatic apical periodontitis is _____.
A. Swelling
B. Intermittent pain
C. Tenderness to palpation
D. Tenderness to percussion

14. In differentiating between an endodontic abscess and periodontal abscess, first test _____.
A. Pulp vitality
B. Probing depths
C. Percussion sensitivity
D. Degree of mobility

15. Which of the following statements is *not* consistent with cracked tooth syndrome?
A. Symptoms are often variable because of direction, location, and extent of the crack.

B. Teeth with cracks may have erratic pain on mastication.
C. Pain is associated with release of pressure rather than increased biting force.
D. Pain, especially in response to cold, is a telltale sign.
E. Absence of pain rules out the presence of a crack.

16. In a tooth with a primary periodontal lesion with secondary endodontic involvement, proceed first with _____.
A. Periodontal treatment
B. Nonsurgical endodontic treatment
C. Antibiotic treatment
D. Incision and drainage

17. A patient calls late Saturday night because of severe, throbbing pain in a mandibular premolar aggravated by "heat, biting, and touching." What procedure is recommended?
A. Instruct the patient to apply ice intermittently, take aspirin, and call Monday for an appointment
B. See the patient at the office and initiate endodontic treatment
C. See the patient at the office, remove the carious dentin, and place a sedative zinc oxide–eugenol cement temporary restoration
D. Prescribe an analgesic and refer the patient to an endodontist
E. Refer the patient to the hospital oral surgery department for extraction

18. In an emergency patient, symptomatic irreversible pulpitis and symptomatic apical periodontitis of tooth #12 is diagnosed. Which of the following is the *best* treatment protocol for this patient?
A. Anesthesia followed by incision and drainage
B. Anesthesia followed by extraction
C. Anesthesia followed by pulpectomy
D. Prescribe antibiotic for 1 week and follow with nonsurgical endodontic treatment

19. In which of the following conditions is elective root canal therapy contraindicated?
A. AIDS
B. Recent MI
C. Leukemia
D. Radiotherapy
E. Second trimester of pregnancy

20. What is the best timing for performing incision and drainage at an area of infection?
A. When the swelling is hard and diffuse
B. When the area is the most painful
C. When the area is large
D. When the swelling is localized and fluctuant

21. Endodontic infection usually is polymicrobial. What is the predominate type of microorganism found in a tooth that requires endodontic therapy?
A. Aerobic bacteria
B. Facultative bacteria

C. Obligate anaerobic bacteria

D. Yeast microorganisms

22. The "danger zone" of mandibular molar for perforations during canal instrumentation is ____.
    A. The periphery at the level of the dentinocemental junction
    B. Within 2 mm of the apex
    C. The furcation area
    D. The periphery of the access at the level of the cementoenamel junction

23. What is the treatment of choice for an 8-year-old patient who has a 1-mm intrusion injury of tooth #8?
    A. Extract the tooth
    B. Perform pulpotomy immediately
    C. Splint the tooth for 10 to 14 days immediately
    D. Allow the tooth to reerupt

24. On routine radiographic survey of a new patient, you notice a circle-shaped radiolucency midroot and over the pulpal outline of tooth #6. You take a second mesially angulated radiograph and confirm the radiolucency is part of the pulp canal outline. After a vital response to cold testing, your diagnosis and subsequent treatment plan are ____.
    A. Internal resorption and completion of nonsurgical endodontic treatment
    B. Internal resorption and surgical repair of the defect
    C. External root resorption and forced orthodontic eruption to expose the defect
    D. External root resorption and extraction

25. During a nonvital bleaching procedure, if a barrier material is not placed between the root canal filling and bleaching material, the tooth can be subjected to ____.
    A. External cervical resorption
    B. Demineralization of tooth structure
    C. Gingival inflammation
    D. Poor color improvement

26. A healthy 32-year-old man presents with localized fluctuant swelling associated with a necrotic pulp and an apical diagnosis of acute apical abscess for tooth #5. The principal modality or modalities for treating a localized fluctuant swelling include which of the following?
    A. Administration of antibiotics
    B. Achievement of drainage
    C. Removal of the source of infection
    D. Both A and C
    E. Both B and C

27. Which of the following statements *most* accurately describes the manufacturing process for a K-type hand instrument?
    A. Grinding a stainless steel wire to a tapered square or rhomboid cross section
    B. Twisting a square or rhomboid (cross section) non-tapered silver metal blank

C. Grinding a silver metal blank to a nontapered square or rhomboid cross section

D. Both B and C

E. All of the above

28. Benefits of intracanal irrigation include all of the following *except* one. Which one is the *exception*?
    A. Dissolves organic debris
    B. Disinfects complex anatomy that is not accessible by instrumentation
    C. Removes the smear layer
    D. Facilitates obturation

29. The bacterial flora of an infected previously treated endodontic tooth is best characterized as:
    A. Gram negative strict anaerobes
    B. Gram positive facultative anaerobes
    C. Gram negative facultative aerobes
    D. Gram positive strict aerobes

30. Because of its mesial concavity the following tooth is vulnerable to iatrogenic perforation:
    A. The mandibular first premolar
    B. The mandibular second premolar
    C. The maxillary first premolar
    D. The maxillary second premolar

31. Which of the following is not an accepted treatment protocol for a NaOCl accident?
    A. Instructions to minimize swelling with the use of cold compresses within the first 24 hours
    B. Irrigation with hydrogen peroxide
    C. Analgesics for pain control
    D. Antibiotics for patients at increased risk of secondary infection

32. Ethylenediaminetetraacitic acid or EDTA is best characterized as a ____ with a primary mode of action best described as ____:
    A. Chelating agent; removing the inorganic portion of the smear layer
    B. Emulsifying agent; removing the organic portion of the smear layer
    C. Chelating agent; removing the organic portion of the smear layer
    D. Emulsifying agent; removing the inorganic portion of the smear layer

33. Of the following clinical diagnostic tests which is the most accurate in determining the state of pulpal health?
    A. Electric pulp test (EPT)
    B. Heat test
    C. Cold test
    D. Both b and c

34. What constitutes the largest portion of gutta-percha obturation material?
    A. Gutta-percha
    B. Zinc oxide
    C. Waxes and resins
    D. Heavy metal salts

35. Which is the most likely to cause pulp necrosis?
    A. Subluxation
    B. Extrusion
    C. Avulsion
    D. Concussion
36. Which of the following statement(s) is(are) true regarding treatment of a tooth presenting with a sinus tract?
    A. Treat with conventional root canal therapy.
    B. Antibiotics are not needed.
    C. The sinus tract should heal in 2 to 4 weeks after conventional root canal therapy.
    D. If the tract persists post-root canal therapy, do root-end surgery with root-end filling.
    E. All of the above choices are true.
37. Features of focal sclerosing osteomyelitis often include:
    A. A nonvital pulp test.
    B. A history of recent restoration of the tooth in question.
    C. A radiolucent lesion which, in time, becomes radiopaque.
    D. None of the choices is true.
38. Once the root canal is obturated, what usually happens to the organism that had previously entered periradicular tissues from the canal?
    A. They persist and stimulate formulation of a granuloma.
    B. They are eliminated by the natural defenses of the body.
    C. They reenter and reinfect the sterile canal unless root-end surgery is performed.
    D. They will have been eliminated by various medicaments that were used in the root canal.

Operative Dentistry

ANDRÉ V. RITTER*

Operative dentistry is the art and science of the diagnosis, treatment, and prognosis of defects of teeth that do not require full coverage restorations for correction. Such treatment should result in the restoration of proper tooth form, function, and esthetics, while maintaining the physiologic integrity of the teeth in harmonious relationship with the adjacent hard and soft tissues, all of which should enhance the general health and welfare of the patient.

1.0 Dental Caries

Outline of Review

1.1. Introduction and Etiology
1.2. Pathogenesis and Diagnosis
1.3. Prevention
1.4. Treatment Overview
1.5. Summary

1.1 Introduction and Etiology

A. Objective—to understand and manage dental caries not only at the tooth level but also at the total patient level, diagnosing and treating the underlying caries

*Adapted from Heymann HO, Swift EJ, Ritter AV: *Sturdevant's Art & Science of Operative Dentistry,* ed 6. St. Louis, Mosby, 2013. Original contents were created by authors of that edition. The author also acknowledges the contributions of Dr. Theodore "Ted" M. Roberson to the previous edition(s) of the present chapter and the aforementioned textbook.

process (caries management based on risk assessment) (Figures 2-1 and 2-2).
B. Definition—dental caries is a multifactorial, transmissible infectious oral disease caused primarily by the complex interaction of cariogenic oral flora (biofilm) with fermentable dietary carbohydrates on the tooth surface over time. However, dental caries onset and activity are much more complex than this three-way interaction because not all people with teeth and biofilm who consume carbohydrates have caries over time. Several modifying risk and protective factors influence the dental caries process (Figure 2-3).
C. The caries balance—at the tooth level, caries activity is characterized by localized demineralization and loss of tooth structure. Cariogenic bacteria in the biofilm metabolize refined carbohydrates for energy and produce organic acid by-products. These organic acids, if present in the biofilm ecosystem for extended periods of time, can lower the pH in the biofilm to below a critical level (5.5 for enamel, 6.2 for dentin). The low pH drives calcium and phosphate from the tooth to the biofilm in an attempt to reach equilibrium, resulting in a net loss of minerals by the tooth, or *demineralization.* When the pH in the biofilm is restored and the concentration of soluble calcium and phosphate is supersaturated relative to that in the tooth, mineral can be added back to partially demineralized enamel in a process called *remineralization.* At the tooth surface and subsurface level, dental caries results from a dynamic process of attack (demineralization) and restitution (remineralization) of the tooth matter. These events occur several times a day over the life of the tooth and are modulated by many factors, including number and type of microbial flora in the biofilm, diet, oral hygiene, genetics, dental anatomy, use of fluorides and other chemotherapeutic agents, salivary flow and buffering capacity, and inherent resistance of the tooth structure and composition, all of which differ from person to person, tooth to tooth, and tooth surface to tooth surface. The balance between demineralization and remineralization has been illustrated in terms of

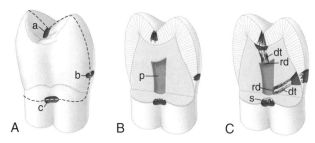

Figure 2-1 A, Caries may originate at many distinct sites: pits and fissures *(a)*, smooth surface of crown *(b)*, and root surface *(c)*. Proximal-surface lesion of crown is not illustrated here because it is a special case of smooth-surface lesion. Histopathology and progress of facial (or lingual) and proximal lesions are identical. *Dotted line* indicates cut used to reveal cross sections illustrated in **B** and **C**. **B,** In cross section, the three types of lesions show different rates of progression and different morphology. Lesions illustrated here are intended to be representative of each type. No particular association between the three lesions is implied. Pit-and-fissure lesions have small sites of origin visible on the occlusal surface but have a wide base. The overall shape of a pit-and-fissure lesion is an inverted "V." In contrast, a smooth-surface lesion is V-shaped with a wide area of origin and apex of the V directed toward pulp *(p)*. Root caries begins directly on dentin. Root-surface lesions can progress rapidly because dentin is less resistant to caries attack. **C,** Advanced caries lesions produce considerable histologic change in enamel, dentin, and pulp. Bacterial invasion of the lesion results in extensive demineralization and proteolysis of the dentin. Clinically, this necrotic dentin appears soft, wet, and mushy. Deeper pulpally, dentin is demineralized, but it is not invaded by bacteria, and it is structurally intact. This tissue appears to be dry and leathery in texture. Two types of pulp-dentin response are illustrated. Under pit-and-fissure lesions and smooth-surface lesions, odontoblasts have died, leaving empty tubules called dead tracts *(dt)*. New odontoblasts have been differentiated from pulp mesenchymal cells. These new odontoblasts have produced reparative dentin *(rd)*, which seals off dead tracts. Another type of pulp-dentin reaction is sclerosis *(s)*—occlusion of the tubules by peritubular dentin. This is illustrated under a root-caries lesion. *(From Heymann HO, Swift EJ, Ritter AV: Sturdevant's Art and Science of Operative Dentistry, ed 6. St. Louis, Mosby, 2013.)*

pathologic factors (i.e., factors favoring demineralization) and protective factors (i.e., factors favoring remineralization). Individuals in whom the balance tilts predominantly toward protective factors (remineralization) are much less likely to develop dental caries than individuals in whom the balance is tilted toward the pathologic factors (demineralization). Understanding the balance between demineralization and remineralization is key to caries management (Figure 2-4).

D. Specific plaque hypothesis—not all of the 300 species of bacteria in the oral cavity can cause caries. Bacteria that generate plaque biofilm resulting in caries are considered to be *cariogenic* organisms. All plaque biofilm is not cariogenic.

E. *Streptococcus mutans*—a nonmotile, gram-positive bacterium, *S. mutans* is a cariogenic bacterium.

1. *S. mutans* is believed to be the primary causative agent of initial caries.
   a. *S. mutans* adheres to enamel. Its glucosyltransferase enzyme causes the formation of an extracellular polysaccharide, which allows it to stick to smooth tooth surfaces. It converts sucrose into fructans and glucans, which extrude from the bacterium and stick to the tooth.
   b. *S. mutans* produces and tolerates acid. It metabolizes sucrose to an end product of lactic acid.
   c. *S. mutans* thrives in a sucrose-rich environment secondary to converting sucrose for adherence and acid production.
   d. *S. mutans* produces bacteriocins, which kill off competing organisms.

F. Enamel caries—ion transfer continuously occurs at the biofilm-enamel interface. The initial decalcification occurs at the subsurface. It may be 1 to 2 years before enough decalcification occurs to cause surface integrity loss—that is, a "cavity."

G. Dentinal caries—once enamel cavitation has occurred, the underlying dentin has already been affected by the progression of the destruction, and the *Lactobacillus* organism becomes a primary agent for further destruction of the dentin.

H. Saliva—if sugars are the key to success of cariogenic bacteria (a major pathologic factor), saliva is a major block barring those same bacteria (a major protective factor).

I. Protective mechanisms of saliva.
   1. Bacterial clearance.
      a. Glycoproteins (large carbohydrate-protein molecules) in saliva cause some bacteria to agglutinate (clump together) and then be removed by swallowing the 1.5 L of saliva formed each day.
   2. Buffering action.
      a. Saliva contains urea and other buffers that help to dilute any plaque acids.
   3. Antimicrobial actions.
      a. Various proteins, enzymes, and antibodies in saliva discourage or even kill bacterial growth.
      b. Lysozyme—destroys cell walls and causes membrane permeability of bacteria.
      c. Lactoferrin—actively binds iron, which is important for bacterial enzyme production and function. It may also destroy *S. mutans*.
      d. Lactoperoxidase—inactivates some bacterial enzymes.
      e. Type A secretory immunoglobulins—antibodies secreted by saliva, which fight against *S. mutans* attacks.
   4. Remineralization.
      a. Calcium, phosphate, potassium, and varying concentrations of fluoride ions in saliva are readily available to assist with remineralization. Some salivary proteins, such as statherin, cystatins,

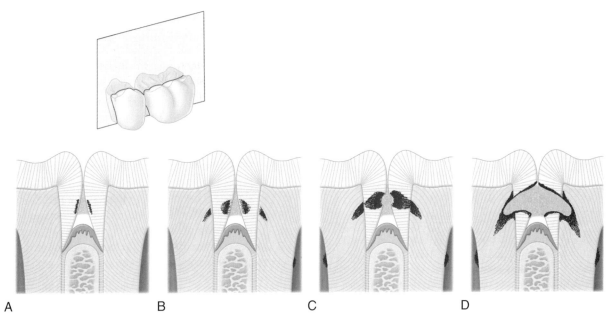

A   B   C   D

Figure 2-2 Longitudinal sections (see *inset* for **A**) showing initiation and progression of caries on interproximal surfaces. **A,** Initial demineralization (indicated by shading in the enamel) on the proximal surfaces is not detectable clinically or radiographically. All proximal surfaces are demineralized to some degree, but most are remineralized and become immune to further attack. The presence of small amounts of fluoride in the saliva virtually ensures that remineralization and immunity to further attack will occur. **B,** When proximal caries first becomes detectable radiographically, the enamel surface is likely still to be intact. An intact surface is essential for successful remineralization and arrest of the lesion. Demineralization of the dentin (indicated by shading in the dentin) occurs before cavitation of the surface of the enamel. Treatment designed to promote remineralization can be effective up to this stage. **C,** Cavitation of the enamel surface is a critical event in the caries process in proximal surfaces. Cavitation is an irreversible process and requires restorative treatment and correction of the damaged tooth surface. Cavitation can be diagnosed only by clinical observation. The use of a sharp explorer to detect cavitation is problematic because excessive force in application of the explorer tip during inspection of the proximal surfaces can damage weakened enamel and accelerate the caries process by creating cavitation. Separation of the teeth can be used to provide more direct visual inspection of suspect surfaces. Fiberoptic illumination and dye absorption also are promising new evaluation procedures, but neither fiberoptic illumination nor dye absorption is specific for cavitation. **D,** Advanced cavitated lesions require prompt restorative intervention to prevent pulpal disease, limit tooth structure loss, and remove the nidus of infection of odontopathic organisms. *(From Heymann HO, Swift EJ, Ritter AV: Sturdevant's Art and Science of Operative Dentistry, ed 6. St. Louis, Mosby, 2013.)*

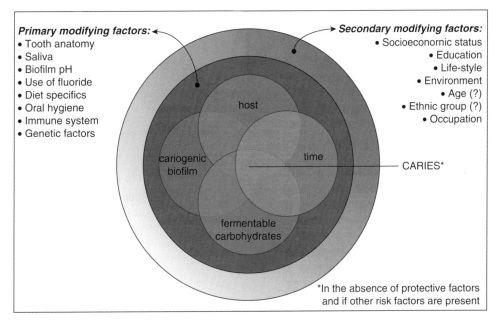

Primary modifying factors:
- Tooth anatomy
- Saliva
- Biofilm pH
- Use of fluoride
- Diet specifics
- Oral hygiene
- Immune system
- Genetic factors

Secondary modifying factors:
- Socioeconornic status
- Education
- Life-style
- Environment
- Age (?)
- Ethnic group (?)
- Occupation

host

cariogenic biofilm

time

fermentable carbohydrates

CARIES*

*In the absence of protective factors and if other risk factors are present

Figure 2-3 Modified Keyes-Jordan diagram. In simple terms, dental caries is a result of the interaction of cariogenic oral flora (biofilm) with fermentable dietary carbohydrates on the tooth surface (host) over time. However, dental caries onset and activity are much more complex because not all persons with teeth and biofilm who consume carbohydrates have caries over time. Modifying risk factors and protective factors influence the dental caries process. *(Modified from Keyes PH, Jordan HV: Factors influencing initiation, transmission and inhibition of dental caries. In Harris RJ, editor: Mechanisms of Hard Tissue Destruction. New York, Academic Press, 1963.)*

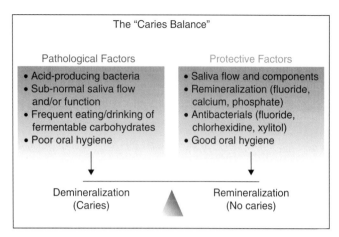

Figure 2-4 The caries balance. The balance between demineralization and remineralization is illustrated in terms of pathologic factors (i.e., factors favoring demineralization) and protective factors (i.e., factors favoring remineralization). *(Modified from Featherstone JDB: Prevention and reversal of dental caries: role of low level fluoride. Community Dent Oral Epidemiol 27:31-40, 1999.)*

histatins, and proline-rich proteins, promote remineralization.
J. Reduced salivary flow problems.
   1. Prolonged pH depression (decreased buffering).
   2. Decreased antibacterial effects.
   3. Decrease in ions available for remineralization.
   4. Decreased elimination of microorganisms.

1.2 Pathogenesis and Diagnosis

A. Objectives.
   1. Identify caries lesions that need surgical treatment.
   2. Identify caries lesions that need nonsurgical treatment.
   3. Identify patients who are at high risk for caries and need special preventive treatment.
   4. Emphasis must shift from detection only of cavitations to the detection of high caries risk and predictions of caries progression.
B. Identification of high-risk patients.
   1. Definition—identification of patients who have factors that place them at increased risk to develop dental caries. There is no exact mechanism to make this determination.
   2. Option for high-risk identification (Box 2-1).
      a. High *S. mutans* counts.
      b. Any two of the following.
         (1) Two or more active caries lesions.
         (2) Large numbers of restorations.
         (3) Poor dietary habits.
         (4) Low salivary flow.
         (5) Poor oral hygiene.
         (6) Suboptimal fluoride exposure.
         (7) Unusual tooth morphology.

1.3 Prevention

A. Objectives.
   1. Improve biofilm conditions to favor remineralization and hinder demineralization.
   2. Realize that the repair of a caries lesion does not cure the disease caries.
B. Antimicrobial.
   1. Intense application on a short-term basis.
C. Fluoride.
   1. Beneficial effects of fluoride.
      a. Bactericidal.
      b. Provides fluoride ion for remineralization forming fluorapatite (which is more resistant to acid attack than hydroxyapatite enamel).
   2. Types and sources.
      a. Community fluoridated water systems.
      b. Rinses.
      c. Gels.
      d. Varnishes.
      e. Toothpastes.
D. Saliva.
   1. Alter saliva-reducing medications if possible.
   2. Use saliva stimulants.
      a. Sugar-free gums and lozenges.
      b. Saliva substitutes.
      c. Encourage diet high in protein and vegetables.
      d. Use pilocarpine hydrochloride or cevimeline hydrochloride if needed.
E. Sucrose.
   1. Must decrease frequency—more important than decreasing quantity.

2. A single exposure to sucrose for a caries-active mouth can result in pH being reduced below the 5.5 level for a sustained period because of the rapid metabolism by *S. mutans*.

F. Xylitol (note: the evidence for xylitol as a caries preventive agent is controversial).

1. Natural sugar from birch trees (five-carbon sugar).
2. Keeps sucrose molecule from binding with *S. mutans*.
3. *S. mutans* cannot ferment xylitol.

G. Oral hygiene—disrupts plaque biofilm formation.

H. Sealants—remove habitats for *S. mutans*.

I. Restorations.

1.4 Treatment Overview

A. Objectives—first remove nidi of infection by restoring large caries lesions and placing sealants. Assess patient's caries risk, and institute individualized preventive measures (Table 2-1).

B. Restorations—when cavitated lesions are present, they should be restored first, usually before any antimicrobial agents are used. If antimicrobials are used first, they disrupt the normal flora and allow the virulent organisms in the protected (cavitated) areas to flourish on now-unprotected tooth surfaces.

1. Restorations remove large nidi of infectious organisms, but, more importantly, they remove habitats for more bacterial adherence.

2. If many cavitated lesions are present, caries-control restorations (with glass-ionomer) are required. These may eventually be replaced with permanent restorations (with composite, amalgam, or indirect materials).

3. Restorations alone do not cure the disease caries.

C. Sealants—sealants should be applied to at-risk molars and premolars.

D. Intense, short-term use of agents.

1. Chlorhexidine (note: the evidence for chlorhexidine as a caries preventive agent is controversial).
2. Fluoride varnishes.

E. Continuous, long-term use of agents.

1. Xylitol products (e.g., xylitol lozenge).
2. Calcium phosphate products (e.g., CPP-ACP paste or rinse).

F. Fluoride rinses (over-the-counter).

1. Begin after chlorhexidine is finished.
2. Use at different times than for brushing twice a day.
3. Increase remineralization.

G. Recall (3 months after chlorhexidine or fluoride varnish application).

1. Identify *S. mutans* counts.
2. Clinical examination.
   a. Check sealants (if they fail, they usually come off early) and caries control restorations, if used.
   b. 3-month recalls.

Table 2-1

*Suggested Risk-Based Interventions for Adults**

CARIES RISK CATEGORY	OFFICE-BASED INTERVENTIONS	HOME-BASED INTERVENTIONS
High	• 3-month recare examination and oral prophylaxis • Fluoride varnish at each recare visit • Individualized oral hygiene instructions and use of specialized cleaning aids (e.g., powered toothbrush, Waterpik) • Dietary counseling • Bite-wing radiographs every 6-12 months†	• Brush with prescription fluoride dentifrice (e.g., 1/1%/5000 ppm NaF) • Use sugar substitutes (e.g., xylitol, sorbitol) • Apply calcium-phosphate compounds (e.g., MI Paste) • Use antimicrobial agents (e.g., xylitol gum or lozenge, chlorhexidine rinse) • If xerostomic, increase salivary function (e.g., xylitol gum, rinses, oral moisturizers)
Moderate	• 4-6 month recare examination and oral prophylaxis • Fluoride varnish at each recall • Reinforce proper oral hygiene • Dietary counseling	• Brush with fluoride dentifrice (e.g., 1450 ppm fluoride) • OTC fluoride rinse (e.g., 0.05% NaF)
Low	• 9-12 month recare examination and oral prophylaxis • Reinforce good oral hygiene	• Brush with fluoride dentifrice

Modified from Shugars DA, Bader JD: *MetLife Quality Resource Guide,* ed 3. Bridgewater, NJ, Metropolitan Life Insurance, Co., 2009-2012, p 6.

NaF, Sodium fluoride; *OTC,* over-the-counter; *ppm,* parts per million.

*These are general guidelines and should be customized based on the specific needs of the patient and the weight of individual risk factors uncovered with a caries risk assessment instrument.

†Data from U.S. Department of Health and Human Services, Public Health Service, Food and Drug Administration; and American Dental Association, Council on Dental Benefit Programs, Council on Scientific Affairs: The selection of patients for dental radiographic examinations. Rev. ed. 2004. Available at: www.ada.org/prof/resources/topics/radiography.asp. Accessed January 20, 2012.

1.5 Summary

A. Caries is a bacterial infection.
B. Efforts must be made to identify the *cause* of the patient's caries problem.
C. Efforts must be made to identify patients at high risk for caries.
D. Early diagnosis of caries is important.
E. Nonsurgical treatment of incipient lesions should be used.
F. Understanding the balance between demineralization and remineralization is key to caries management.
G. Restoring a tooth does not cure the disease caries.

2.0 Patient Assessment, Examination, Diagnosis, and Treatment Planning

Pretreatment considerations consisting of patient assessment, examination and diagnosis, and treatment planning are the foundation of sound dental care. These considerations follow a systematic progression because the diagnosis and treatment plan depend on thorough assessment and examination of the patient.

Outline of Review

2.1 Patient Assessment Considerations
2.2 Examination and Diagnosis
2.3 Treatment Planning
2.4 Summary

2.1 Patient Assessment Considerations

A. Infection control.
B. Chief complaint.
C. Medical review.
  1. Communicable diseases.
  2. Allergies and medications.
  3. Systemic diseases and cardiac abnormalities.
  4. Physiologic changes associated with aging.
D. Sociologic and psychological review.
E. Dental history.
F. Risk assessment.

2.2 Examination and Diagnosis

A. General considerations.
  1. Charting and records, preferably electronic.
  2. Tooth denotation system.
  3. Preparation for clinical examination.
  4. Interpretation and use of diagnostic tests.
B. Examination of orofacial soft tissues.
  1. As with the other aspects of the clinical examination, soft tissue evaluation requires a systematic approach.
    a. Submandibular glands and cervical nodes.
    b. Masticatory muscles.

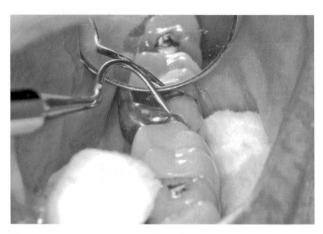

Figure 2-5 An accurate clinical examination requires a clean, dry, well-illuminated mouth. Cotton rolls are placed in the vestibular space and under the tongue to maintain dryness and enhance visibility. *(From Heymann HO, Swift EJ, Ritter AV: Sturdevant's Art and Science of Operative Dentistry, ed 6. St. Louis, Mosby, 2013.)*

    c. Cheeks, vestibules, mucosa, lips, lingual and facial alveolar mucosa, palate, tonsillar areas, tongue, and floor of the mouth.
C. Examination of teeth and restorations (Figures 2-5 to 2-8).
  1. Clinical examination for caries.
    a. Traditionally, dental caries has been diagnosed by one or all of the following.
      (1) Visual changes in tooth surface texture or color.
      (2) Tactile sensation when an explorer is used judiciously.
      (3) Radiographs.
      (4) Transillumination.
    b. Over the past decade, several technologies have emerged that show promising results for the clinical diagnosis of caries.
      (1) Laser fluorescence (DIAGNOdent).
      (2) Digital imaging fiberoptic transillumination (DIFOTI).
      (3) Quantitative light-induced fluorescence (QLF).
      (4) Electrical conductance or impedance measurement.
    c. Because no test currently available is completely accurate, the dentist cannot rely solely on one test to make a decision whether to treat surgically or chemically.
    d. Caries is most prevalent in the pits and fissures of the occlusal surfaces where the developmental lobes of the posterior teeth failed to coalesce, partially or completely. Use of an explorer to diagnose fissure caries is strongly discouraged because injudicious use of an explorer may cause fracture of the surface enamel that has been weakened by subsurface demineralization. An occlusal surface is examined visually and radiographically. The visual

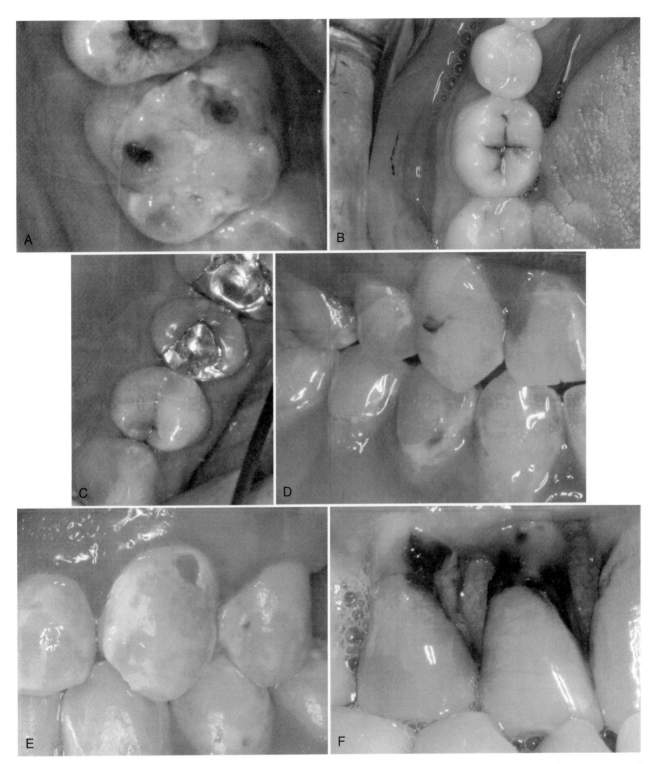

Figure 2-6 Caries can be diagnosed clinically by careful inspection. **A,** Carious pit on cusp tip. **B,** Loss of translucency and change in color of occlusal enamel resulting from a carious fissure. **C,** White chalky appearance or shadow under marginal ridge. **D,** Incipient smooth-surface caries lesion, or a white spot, has intact surface. **E,** Smooth-surface caries can appear white or dark, depending on the degree of extrinsic staining. **F,** Root-surface caries. *(From Heymann HO, Swift EJ, Ritter AV: Sturdevant's Art and Science of Operative Dentistry, ed 6. St. Louis, Mosby, 2013.)*

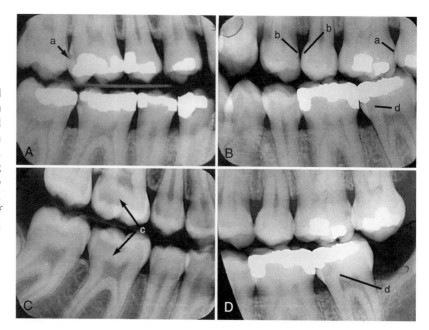

Figure 2-7 Caries can be diagnosed radiographically as translucencies in the enamel or dentin. **A** and **B,** Proximal caries tends to occur bilaterally *(a)* and on adjacent surfaces *(b)*. **C,** Occlusal caries *(c)*. **D,** Recurrent caries gingival to an existing restoration *(d)*. Same recurrent caries *(d)* also is shown in **B**. *(From Heymann HO, Swift EJ, Ritter AV: Sturdevant's Art and Science of Operative Dentistry, ed 6. St. Louis, Mosby, 2013.)*

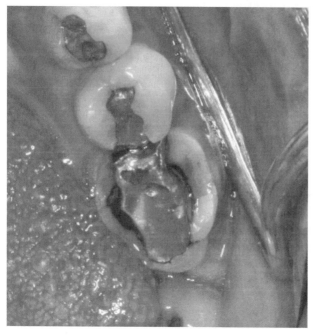

Figure 2-8 Extensively restored teeth with weakened and fractured cusps. Note the distal developmental fissure in the second molar, which further predisposes the distal cusps to fracture. *(From Heymann HO, Swift EJ, Ritter AV: Sturdevant's Art and Science of Operative Dentistry, ed 6. St. Louis, Mosby, 2013.)*

examination is conducted in a dry, well-illuminated field. Through direct vision and reflecting light through the occlusal surface of the tooth, the occlusal surface is diagnosed as carious if there is chalkiness or apparent softening or cavitation of tooth structure forming the fissure or pit or brown-gray discoloration radiating peripherally from the fissure or pit. Radiographic diagnosis should be made from a bite-wing radiograph when radiolucency is apparent beneath the occlusal enamel surface emanating from the dental enamel junction. In contrast, a noncarious occlusal surface has either grooves or fossae that have shallow, tight fissures that exhibit superficial staining with no radiographic evidence of caries.

e. Precarious or carious pits are occasionally present on cusp tips, on the occlusal two thirds of the facial or lingual surface of the posterior teeth, and on the lingual surface of maxillary incisors. Typically, these pits are the result of developmental enamel defects.

f. Proximal-surface caries, one form of smooth-surface caries, is usually diagnosed radiographically. However, it also may be detected by careful visual examination either after tooth separation or through fiberoptic transillumination.

g. Brown spots on intact, hard proximal-surface enamel adjacent and usually gingival to the contact area are often seen in older patients whose caries activity is low. These discolored areas are a result of extrinsic staining during earlier caries demineralization-remineralization cycles. Such a spot is no longer carious and is usually more resistant to caries as a result of fluorhydroxyapatite formation. Restorative treatment is not indicated. These arrested lesions sometimes challenge the diagnosis because of faint radiographic evidence of the remineralized lesion.

h. Proximal coefficient of thermal expansion surface caries in anterior teeth may be identified by radiographic examination, visual inspection (transillumination optional), or probing with an explorer.

i. Smooth-surface caries occur on the facial and lingual surfaces of the teeth, particularly in gingival areas that are less accessible for cleaning. The earliest clinical evidence of incipient caries on these surfaces is a white spot that is visually different from the adjacent translucent enamel and, in contrast to enamel hypocalcification white lesions, partially or totally disappears from vision by wetting. Both types of white spots are undetectable tactilely because the surface is intact, smooth, and hard. For the carious white spot, preventive treatment should be instituted to promote remineralization of the lesion.

(1) The presence of several facial (or lingual) smooth-surface caries lesions in the same patient suggests a high caries rate. In a caries-susceptible patient, the gingival third of the facial surfaces of maxillary posterior teeth and the gingival third of the facial and lingual surfaces of the mandibular posterior teeth should be evaluated carefully because these teeth are at a greater risk for caries. Advanced smooth-surface caries exhibits discoloration and demineralization and feels soft to penetration by the explorer. The discoloration ranges from white to dark brown, with rapidly progressing caries usually being light in color. With slowly progressing caries in a patient with low caries activity, darkening occurs over time because of extrinsic staining, and remineralization of decalcified tooth structure occasionally may harden the lesion. Such an arrested lesion may sometimes be rough, although cleanable, and a restoration may not be indicated except for esthetics. The dentin in an arrested remineralized lesion is termed *sclerotic*.

j. Root-surface caries—early in its development, root caries appears as a well-defined discolored area adjacent to the gingival margin, typically near the cementoenamel junction (CEJ). Root caries is found to be softer than the adjacent sound tissue, and lesions typically spread laterally around the CEJ. Active root caries is detected by the presence of softening and cavitation. Although root-surface caries may be detected on radiographic examination, a careful, thorough clinical examination is critical. A difficult diagnostic challenge is a patient who has attachment loss with no gingival recession, limiting accessibility for clinical inspection. These rapidly progressing lesions are best diagnosed using vertical bite-wing radiographs. However, differentiation of a caries lesion from cervical burnout radiolucency is essential.

k. Regardless of the location or type of caries lesions, a careful, thorough clinical examination is critical in the diagnosis of caries and for confirmation of radiographic evidence of the disease.

2. Clinical examination of amalgam restorations.

a. Evaluation of all restorations must be done systematically in a clean, dry, well-lighted field. Clinical evaluation of amalgam restorations requires visual observation, application of tactile sense with the explorer, use of dental floss, interpretation of radiographs, and knowledge of the probabilities that a given condition is sound or at risk for further breakdown. At least 11 distinct conditions may be encountered when amalgam restorations are evaluated, including amalgam "blues," proximal overhangs, marginal ditching, voids, fracture lines, lines indicating the interface between abutted restorations, improper anatomic contours, marginal ridge incompatibility, improper proximal contacts, recurrent caries, and improper occlusal contacts.

b. Amalgam blues or discolored areas are often seen through the enamel in teeth that have amalgam restorations. This bluish hue results either from the leaching of corrosion products of amalgam into the dentinal tubules or from the color of underlying amalgam as seen through translucent enamel. The latter occurs when the enamel has no dentin support, such as in undermined cusps, marginal ridges, and regions adjacent to proximal margins. When other aspects of the restoration are sound, amalgam blues are not indicative of caries, do not warrant classifying the restoration as defective, and require no further treatment. However, replacement of the restoration may be considered for esthetics or for areas under heavy functional stress that may require a cusp capping restoration to prevent possible tooth fracture.

c. Proximal overhangs are diagnosed visually, tactilely, and radiographically.

d. Marginal gap or ditching—shallow ditching less than 0.5 mm deep usually is not a reason for restoration replacement because such a restoration usually looks worse than it really is. The self-sealing property of amalgam allows the restoration to continue serving adequately if it can be satisfactorily cleaned and maintained. However, if the ditch is too deep to be cleaned or it jeopardizes the integrity of the remaining restoration or tooth structure, the restoration should be replaced.

e. Voids—accessible small voids in other marginal areas where the enamel is thicker may be corrected by recontouring or repairing with a small restoration.

f. Fracture lines are detected by clinical examination.

g. Lines indicating the interface between abutted restorations are detected by clinical examination and are acceptable.

h. Improper anatomic contours—amalgam restorations should duplicate the normal anatomic contours of the teeth. Restorations that have improper anatomic contours, are impinging on the soft tissue, present recurrent caries, have inadequate occlusal contacts, have inadequate embrasure form or proximal contact, or prevent the use of dental floss should be classified as defective.

3. Clinical examination of composite and other tooth-colored restorations—similar to amalgam except that more emphasis is given to esthetics when examining anterior restorations. Corrective procedures include recontouring, polishing, repairing, or replacing.

4. Clinical examination of cast restorations—similar to amalgam and composite.

5. Radiographic examination of teeth and restorations—as a general rule, patients at higher risk for caries or periodontal disease should receive more frequent and more extensive radiographic surveys.

a. For diagnosis of proximal-surface caries, restoration overhangs, or poorly contoured restorations, posterior bite-wing and anterior periapical radiographs are most helpful. When interpreting the radiographic presentation of proximal tooth surfaces, it is necessary to know what the normal anatomy looks like in a radiograph before any abnormalities can be diagnosed. In a radiograph, proximal caries appears as a dark area or a radiolucency in the proximal enamel at or gingival to the contact of the teeth. This radiolucency is typically triangular and has its apex toward the dentinoenamel junction (DEJ).

2.3 Treatment Planning

A. Introduction.
   1. General considerations.
      a. A treatment plan is a carefully sequenced series of services designed to eliminate or control etiologic factors; repair existing damage; and create a functional, maintainable environment. A sound treatment plan depends on thorough patient evaluation, dentist expertise, understanding of indications and contraindications, and a prediction of the patient's response to treatment.
      b. The development of a dental treatment plan for a patient consists of four steps.
         (1) Examination and problem identification.
         (2) Decision to recommend intervention.
         (3) Identification of treatment alternatives.
         (4) Selection of the treatment with the patient's involvement.
      c. Notes: treatment plans are influenced by patient preferences, motivation, systemic health, emotional status, and financial capabilities. A treatment plan also can be modified by the dentist's knowledge, experience, and training; laboratory support; dentist-patient compatibility; availability of specialists; and functional, esthetic, and technical demands. Even when modification is necessary, the practitioner is ethically and professionally responsible for providing the best level of care possible. A treatment plan is not a static list of services. Rather, it is a multiphase and dynamic series of events. Its success is determined by its suitableness to meet the patient's initial and long-term needs.

   2. Treatment plan sequencing—generally, the concept of greatest need guides the order in which treatment is sequenced. This concept dictates that what the patient needs most is performed first.
      a. Urgent phase.
      b. Control phase.
      c. Reevaluation phase.
      d. Definitive phase.
      e. Maintenance phase.
   3. Interdisciplinary considerations in operative treatment planning.
      a. Endodontics.
      b. Periodontics.
      c. Orthodontics.
      d. Oral surgery.
      e. Occlusion.
      f. Fixed and removable prosthodontics.

B. Indications for operative treatment (Tables 2-2 and 2-3).
   1. Operative preventive treatment—this preventive program should include altering the oral environment to encourage remineralization of incipient smooth-surface lesions and treating caries-prone pits and fissures with sealants. As bacterial habitats are disrupted daily, diet is improved, and fluoride is incorporated into the enamel, there is a decrease in the occurrence of new lesions, along with remineralization of incipient lesions. Also, extensive acute caries should be immediately eradicated by either a definitive restoration or a caries-control restoration to help suppress the infectious process.
   2. Treatment of incipient lesions—incipient caries lesions are contained entirely within enamel and have not spread to the underlying dentin. Assuming that an incipient lesion has been properly identified, there are two basic options available to the dentist.
      a. First and more preferred is targeted remineralization followed by regular monitoring. This approach is based on the facts that incipient caries lesions usually do not progress rapidly, and changing the oral environment combined with the application of fluoride varnish and self-administered fluoride can lead to remineralization of these lesions.
      b. The second strategy used to treat incipient lesions is restoration. This option is the last resort for managing incipient lesions. Many new caries detection

Table 2-2

Pit-and-Fissure Caries Treatment Decision Making*

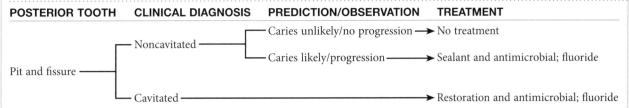

Cavitated means that extensive enamel demineralization has led to destruction of the walls of the pit or fissure and bacterial invasion has occurred. Demineralization of the underlying dentin is usually extensive by the time the cavitation has occurred.

Noncavitated (caries-free):
- No radiolucency below occlusal enamel
- Deep grooves may be present
- Superficial staining may be present in grooves
- Mechanical binding of explorer may occur

Cavitated (diseased):
- Chalkiness of enamel on walls and base of pit or fissure
- Softening at the base of a pit or fissure
- Brown-gray discoloration under enamel adjacent to pit or fissure
- Radiolucency below occlusal enamel

From Roberson TM, Heymann HO, Swift EJ: Sturdevant's Art & Science of Operative Dentistry, ed 5. St. Louis, Mosby, 2006.

*If a cavitated lesion exists in a pit or fissure, it must be restored. If the pit or fissure is not cavitated but at risk, it should be sealed. The pits and fissures of molar teeth in children should be sealed routinely as soon as possible after eruption. Pits and fissures in adults should be sealed if the adult is found to have multiple active lesions or found to be at high risk.

Table 2-3

Proximal Caries Treatment Decision Making*

POSTERIOR TOOTH	CLINICAL DIAGNOSIS	PREDICTION/OBSERVATION	TREATMENT
Proximal surface	Noncavitated	Caries unlikely/no progression	No treatment
		Caries likely/progression	Antimicrobial/fluoride
	Cavitated		Restoration and antimicrobial/fluoride

Noncavitated:
- Surface intact; use of an explorer to judge surface must be done with caution because excessive force can cause penetration of intact surface over demineralized enamel
- Opacity of proximal enamel may be present
- Radiolucency may be present
- Marginal ridge is not discolored
- Opaque area may be seen in enamel by translumination

Cavitated:
- Surface broken, detectable visually or tactilely; temporary mechanical separation of the teeth may aid diagnosis
- Marginal ridge may be discolored
- Opaque area in dentin on translumination
- Radiolucency is present

From Roberson TM, Heymann HO, Swift EJ: Sturdevant's Art & Science of Operative Dentistry, ed 5. St. Louis, Mosby, 2006.

*Proximal surfaces are difficult to judge clinically. The critical event in the caries process is surface cavitation. A cavitated surface must be restored, whereas a demineralized noncavitated surface can be treated only by antimicrobial and fluoride agents. Bite-wing radiographs can reveal a decrease in density, but radiolucencies alone are not diagnostic of cavitation. Restoration of all radiolucent surfaces results in excessive, unnecessary restorative treatment.

devices have high rates of false-positive findings, which can lead to the misdiagnosis of otherwise healthy teeth as diseased and planned for restoration. When a restoration is indicated, the preparation should be done as conservatively as possible. In other words, only enough tooth structure should be removed to ensure that the lesion is eliminated and that the resulting preparation retains the chosen restoration.

C. Criteria for restoring.
1. Elevated caries risk (see Box 2-1).
2. Low frequency of routine dental care because of lack of motivation.
3. Lesion extends to DEJ.
4. Esthetic treatment—these treatments include esthetic recontouring of the anterior teeth, vital and nonvital tooth bleaching, microabrasion, diastema closures, and other composite additions by means other than extensive full-coverage restorations. Also, porcelain veneers are available for esthetically prominent anterior teeth.
5. Treatment of abrasion, erosion, attrition, and abfraction.
   a. Abrasion—mechanical wear secondary to abnormal forces (toothbrushing).
   b. Erosion—wear secondary to chemical presence.
   c. Attrition—normal tooth wear.
   d. Abfraction—biomechanical loading causing loss of tooth structure in the cervical area. This is usually due to occlusal forces causing the tooth to bend, making microfractures in the cervical thin enamel, which is removed even more rapidly as a result of additional toothbrushing abrasion. A pattern of the lesion often is seen below an occlusal cusp tip wear pattern.
6. Areas of significant attrition that are worn into dentin and are sensitive or compromise esthetics or function should be considered for restoration. However, before cast restorations are used, a complete occlusal analysis and an in-depth interview with the patient regarding the etiology should be conducted to reduce contributing factors. Also, bite guard therapy should be considered. Abraded or eroded areas should be considered for restoration only if one or more of the following exists.
   a. The area has caries involvement.
   b. The defect is sufficiently deep to compromise the structural integrity of the tooth.
   c. Intolerable sensitivity exists and is unresponsive to conservative desensitizing measures.
   d. The defect contributes to a periodontal problem.
   e. The area is to be involved in the design of a removable partial denture.
   f. The depth of the defect is judged to be close to the pulp.
   g. The patient desires esthetic improvements.

7. Treatment of root-surface caries—care must be exercised to distinguish the active root-surface caries lesion from the root-surface lesion that previously was active but has become inactive (arrested). The latter lesion shows eburnated dentin (sclerotic dentin) that has darkened from extrinsic staining, is firm to the touch of an explorer, may be rough but is cleanable, and is seen in patients (usually older) whose oral hygiene and diet in recent years are good. If it is determined that the lesion needs restoration, it can be restored with amalgam or tooth-colored materials.

D. Treatment of root-surface hypersensitivity.
1. The most accepted theory of the cause of root-surface hypersensitivity is the hydrodynamic theory, which postulates that the pain results from indirect innervation caused by dentinal fluid movement in the tubules that stimulates mechanoreceptors near the predentin. Some of the causes of such fluid shifts are temperature change, air-drying, and osmotic pressure. *Any treatment that can reduce these fluid shifts by partially or totally occluding the tubules may help reduce the sensitivity.*
2. Numerous forms of treatment have been used to provide relief, such as topical fluoride, fluoride rinses, oxalate solutions, dentin bonding agents, sealants, iontophoresis, and desensitizing toothpastes. Although all of these methods have met with varying degrees of success, dentin-bonding agents provide the best rate of success. When these conservative methods fail to provide relief, restorative treatment is indicated.

E. Repairing and resurfacing existing restorations—resurfacing or repair of composites and amalgam and repair of cast restorations have been shown to be effective. If a restoration has an isolated defect, and it can be confirmed when explored operatively that all carious tooth structure has been removed, it is acceptable and often preferable to repair or recontour.

F. Replacement of existing restorations—indications for replacing restorations include the following.
1. The restoration has significant discrepancies.
2. The tooth is at risk for caries or fracture.
3. The restoration is a negative etiologic factor to adjacent teeth or tissue.
4. A marginal void, especially in the gingival one third, cannot be repaired.
5. Poor proximal contour or a gingival overhang that contributes to periodontal breakdown is present.
6. A marginal ridge discrepancy contributes to food impaction.
7. Overcontour of a facial or lingual surface results in plaque gingival to the height of contour and resultant inflammation of gingiva overprotected from the rubbing-cleansing action of a food bolus or toothbrush.

8. Poor proximal contact is either open (resulting in interproximal food impaction and inflammation of impacted gingival papilla) or improper in location or size.

9. Recurrent caries cannot be adequately treated by a repair restoration.

10. Ditching deeper than 0.5 mm of the occlusal amalgam margin is judged carious or caries-prone. The presence of shallow ditching around an amalgam restoration by itself is not an indication for replacement.

11. Esthetics is unacceptable for tooth-colored restorations. Restorations that have only light marginal staining and are judged noncarious can be corrected by a shallow, narrow, marginal repair restoration.

12. In many instances, recontouring or resurfacing the existing restoration can delay replacement.

G. Indications for direct composite and other tooth-colored restorations—the American Dental Association has both supported the use of composite for many class I and II restorations and indicated that such restorations should have a clinical longevity similar to amalgam restorations. Direct composite restorations are appropriately indicated for most clinical applications, anteriorly and posteriorly.

H. Indications for indirect tooth-colored restorations—tooth-colored restorations that are indirectly fabricated out of the mouth may be indicated for class I and II restorations because of esthetics, strength, and other bonding benefits. However, they are usually more costly than direct tooth-colored restorations. Indirect tooth-colored restorations include the following.

1. Processed composite—although processed composite restorations possess improved wear resistance over direct composites, they are indicated primarily for conservative class I and II preparations in areas with low to moderate stress.

2. Feldspathic porcelain—feldspathic porcelain inlays and onlays for class I and II restorations are highly esthetic but are associated with a relatively high incidence of fracture, especially if subjected to heavy occlusal forces. Porcelain restorations also have the potential to wear opposing tooth structure.

3. Cast ceramic—cast ceramic inlays and onlays for class I and II preparations offer excellent marginal fit, low abrasion to opposing tooth structure, and superior strength compared with processed composite or feldspathic porcelain. They offer an excellent esthetic alternative to cast metal restorations.

4. Computer-generated (computer-aided design [CAD]/computer-aided manufacturing [CAM]) inlays and onlays—onlays and inlays can be generated with CAD/CAM. Because these restorations are fabricated chairside, only one appointment is required for placement compared with two appointments required for the other types of indirectly fabricated tooth-colored restorations.

I. Indications for cast metal restorations—although indications for intracoronal castings are few, a gold onlay that caps all of the cusps and includes some of the axial tooth line angles is an excellent restoration. Cast metal restorations may be the treatment of choice for patients undergoing occlusal rehabilitation. Also, teeth with deep subgingival margins are well treated with cast restorations because they provide a better opportunity for control of proximal contours and for restoration of the difficult subgingival margin compared with amalgam and composite restorations.

2.4 Summary

A. Proper diagnosis and treatment planning play a critical role in the quality of dental care. Each patient must be evaluated individually in a thorough and systematic fashion. After the patient's condition is understood and recorded, a treatment plan can be developed and rendered.

B. A successful treatment plan carefully integrates and sequences all necessary procedures indicated for the patient. There are few absolutes in treatment planning; the available information must be considered carefully and incorporated into a plan to fit the needs of the individual. Patients should have an active role in the process; they should be made aware of the findings, be advised of the risks and benefits of the proposed treatment, and be given the opportunity to help decide the course of treatment.

C. Examination, diagnosis, and treatment planning are extremely challenging and rewarding for both the patient and the dentist if done thoroughly and properly with the patient's best interest in mind.

3.0 Instrumentation for Operative Dentistry Procedures

Outline of Review

3.1 Hand Instruments for Cutting
3.2 Overview of Powered Cutting Instruments
3.3 Rotary Cutting Instruments
3.4 Cutting Mechanisms
3.5 Hazards with Cutting Instruments

3.1 Hand Instruments for Cutting

Modern hand instruments, when properly used, produce beneficial results for both the operator and the patient. Some of these results can be satisfactorily achieved only with hand instruments and not with rotary instruments. Preparation form dictates some circumstances in which hand instruments are to be used, whereas accessibility dictates others.

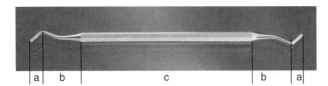

Figure 2-9 Double-ended instrument illustrating three component parts of hand instruments: blade *(a)*, shank *(b)*, and handle *(c)*. *(Modified from Boyd LRB: Dental Instruments: A Pocket Guide, ed 4. St. Louis, Saunders, 2012.)*

A. Terminology and classification.
   1. Instrument categories.
      a. Cutting (excavators, chisels, and others).
      b. Noncutting (amalgam condensers, mirrors, explorers, probes, and others).
   2. Instrument design—most hand instruments, regardless of use, are composed of three parts: handle, shank, and blade (Figure 2-9). For many noncutting instruments, the part corresponding to the blade is termed the *nib*. The end of the nib, or working surface, is known as the *face*. The blade or nib is the working end of the instrument and is connected to the handle by the shank. Some instruments have a blade on both ends of the handle and are known as *double-ended instruments*. The blades are of many designs and sizes, depending on the function they are to perform.
   3. Operative cutting instrument formulas—cutting instruments have formulas describing the dimensions and angles of the working end. These are placed on the handle using a code of three or four numbers separated by dashes or spaces (e.g., 10-8.5-8-14). The first number indicates the width of the blade or primary cutting edge in tenths of a millimeter (0.1 mm). The second number of a four-number code indicates the primary cutting edge angle, measured from a line parallel to the long axis of the instrument handle in clockwise centigrades. The angle is expressed as a percent of 360 degrees. The instrument is positioned so that this number always exceeds 50. If the edge is locally perpendicular to the blade, this number is normally omitted, resulting in a three-number code. The third number (second number of a three-number code) indicates the blade length in millimeters. The fourth number (third number of a three-number code) indicates the blade angle, relative to the long axis of the handle in clockwise centigrade. For these measurements, the instrument is positioned so that this number is always 50 or less.

B. Cutting instrument applications—cutting instruments are used to cut hard or soft tissues of the mouth. Excavators are used for removal of caries and refinement of the internal parts of the preparation. Chisels are used primarily for cutting enamel.

   1. Excavators—four subdivisions.
      a. Ordinary hatchets—the ordinary hatchet has the cutting edge of the blade directed in the same plane as that of the long axis of the handle and is bibeveled; it is used primarily on anterior teeth for preparing retentive areas.
      b. Hoes—the hoe has the primary cutting edge of the blade perpendicular to the axis of the handle and is used for planing tooth preparation walls and forming line angles.
      c. Angle-formers—the angle-former is used primarily for sharpening line angles and creating retentive features in dentin. It also may be used in placing a bevel on enamel margins. It is a monangle instrument and has the primary cutting edge at an angle (other than 90 degrees) to the blade. It may be described as a combination of a chisel and gingival margin trimmer. It is available in pairs (right and left).
      d. Spoons—spoon excavators are used for removing caries. The blades are slightly curved, and the cutting edges are either circular or clawlike. The circular edge is known as a *discoid*, whereas the clawlike blade is termed a *cleoid*. The shanks may be binangled or triple-angled to facilitate accessibility.
   2. Chisels—chisels are intended primarily for cutting enamel.
      a. Straight, slightly curved, or binangle—the straight chisel has a straight shank and blade, with the bevel on only one side. Its primary edge is perpendicular to the axis of the handle. It is similar in design to a carpenter's chisel. The shank and blade of the chisel also may be slightly curved (Wedelstaedt design) or may be binangled. The force used with all of these chisels is essentially a straight thrust.
      b. Enamel hatchets—enamel hatchets are used for cutting and planning enamel surfaces.
      c. Gingival margin trimmers—the gingival margin trimmer is designed to produce a proper bevel on gingival enamel margins of proximo-occlusal preparations. It is similar in design to the enamel hatchet except the blade is curved (similar to a spoon excavator), and the primary cutting edge is at an angle (other than perpendicular) to the axis of the blade. It is made as right and left types.
   3. Other cutting instruments—other hand cutting instruments, such as the knife, file, and discoid-cleoid instrument, are used for trimming and carving restorative material rather than for cutting tooth structure.

C. Hand instrument techniques.
   1. Modified pen grasp.
   2. Inverted pen grasp.
   3. Palm-and-thumb grasp.
   4. Modified palm-and-thumb grasp.

5. Rests.

6. Guards.

3.2 Overview of Powered Cutting Instruments

A. Rotary speed ranges (Figure 2-10)—the rotational speed of an instrument is measured in revolutions per minute (rpm). Three speed ranges are generally recognized: low or slow speeds (<12,000 rpm), medium or intermediate speeds (12,000 to 200,000 rpm), and high or ultrahigh speeds (>200,000 rpm). Most useful instruments are rotated at either low or high speed. The crucial factor for some purposes is the surface speed of the instrument, which is the velocity at which the edges of the cutting instrument pass across the surface being cut. This is proportional to both the rotational speed and the diameter of the instrument, with large instruments having higher surface speeds at any given rate of rotation.

B. Laser equipment—lasers are increasingly used in dentistry. Current units are expensive and must be used frequently in a dental practice to justify the expense. At the present time, lasers are used primarily for either soft tissue applications or hard tissue surface modification. They generally are not used for tooth preparations because it is difficult to generate a defined margin or tooth preparation surface.

C. Air-driven particle abrasion equipment—Contemporary air-driven particle abrasion equipment (commonly known simply as air abrasion) is helpful for stain removal, débriding pits and fissures before sealing, and micromechanical roughening of surfaces to be bonded (enamel, cast metal alloys, or porcelain). This approach works well when organic material is being removed and when only a limited amount of enamel or dentin is involved. Although promoted for caries excavation, air abrasion cannot produce well-defined preparation wall and margin details that are possible with conventional rotary cutting techniques.

3.3 Rotary Cutting Instruments

A. Common design characteristics—despite the great variation among rotary cutting instruments, they share certain design features. Each instrument consists of

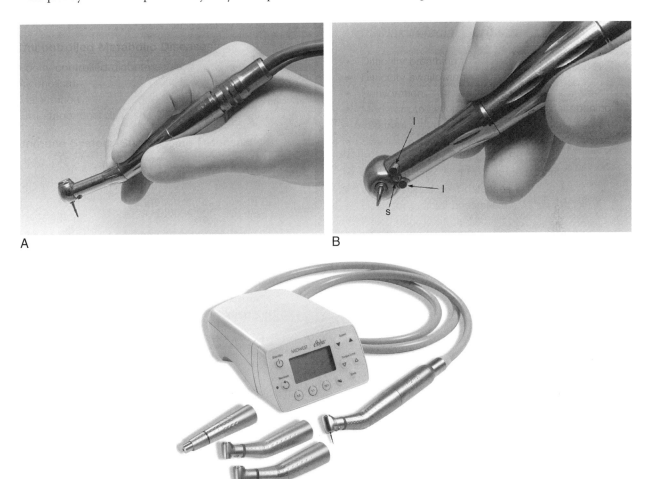

A

B

C

Figure 2-10 A, Contrangle air-turbine handpiece connected to the air-water supply line. **B,** Ventral view of the handpiece showing four port for air-water spray *(S)* onto bur at cutting site and epoxied end of fiberoptic bundle *(l)* to shine light at cutting site. **C,** Electrical handpieces and unit. *(**C,** courtesy of DENTSPLY International, York, PA.)*

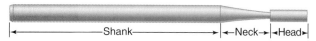

|←————————Shank————————→|←Neck→|←Head→|

Figure 2-11 Normal designation of three parts of rotary cutting instruments. *(From Heymann HO, Swift EJ, Ritter AV: Sturdevant's Art and Science of Operative Dentistry, ed 6. St. Louis, Mosby, 2013.)*

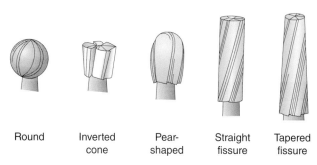

| Round | Inverted cone | Pear-shaped | Straight fissure | Tapered fissure |

Figure 2-12 Basic bur head shapes. *(From Finkbeiner BL, Johnson CS: Mosby's Comprehensive Dental Assisting. St. Louis, Mosby, 1995.)*

three parts: shank, neck, and head. Each has its own function, influencing its design and the materials used for its construction. There is a difference in the meaning of the term *shank* as applied to rotary instruments and to hand instruments (Figure 2-11).

B. Dental burs—the term *bur* is applied to all rotary cutting instruments that have bladed cutting heads.
   1. Bur classification systems—to facilitate the description, selection, and manufacture of burs, it is highly desirable to have some agreed-on shorthand designation that represents all variables of a particular head design by some simple code (Figure 2-12).
   2. Shapes—the term *bur shape* refers to the contour or silhouette of the head. Although there are a variety of different bur shapes and blade configurations, the basic head shapes are round, inverted cone, pear, straight fissure, and tapered fissure.
      a. A round bur is spherical and is customarily used for initial entry into the tooth, extension of the preparation, preparation of retention features, and caries removal.
      b. An inverted cone bur is a portion of a short tapered cone with the apex of the cone directed toward the bur shank. Head length is approximately the same as the diameter. This shape is particularly suitable for providing undercuts in tooth preparations.
      c. A pear-shaped bur is a portion of a tapered cone with the small end of the cone directed toward the bur shank. The end of the head either is continuously curved or is flat with rounded corners where the sides and flat end intersect. A long-length pear bur (length three times the width) is advocated for tooth preparations.

   d. A straight fissure bur is an elongated cylinder. Some clinicians advocate this shape for amalgam tooth preparation. Modified burs of this design with slightly curved tip angles are available.
   e. A tapered fissure bur is a portion of a tapered cone with the small end of the cone directed away from the bur shank. This shape is used for tooth preparations for indirect restorations for which freedom from undercuts is essential for successful withdrawal of patterns and final seating of the restorations. Tapered fissure burs can have a flat end with the tip corners slightly rounded.

C. Diamond abrasive instruments—abrasive rotary dental cutting instruments are based on small, angular particles of a hard substance held in a matrix of softer material.
   1. Terminology—diamond instruments consist of three parts: metal blank, powdered diamond abrasive, and metallic bonding material that holds the diamond powder onto the blank. The blank in many ways resembles a bur without blades. It has the same essential parts: head, neck, and shank. Various shapes and designs of diamond cutting instruments are available (Figure 2-13).
   2. Diamond particle factors—the clinical performance of diamond abrasive instruments depends on the size, spacing, uniformity, exposure, and bonding of the diamond particles. Increased pressure causes the particles to dig into the surface more deeply, leaving deeper scratches and removing more tooth structure.
      a. Diamond particle size is commonly categorized as coarse, medium, fine, and very fine for diamond preparation instruments. The clinical performance of diamond instruments is strongly affected by the technique used to take advantage of the design factors for each instrument.
      b. Diamond finishing instruments use even finer diamonds to produce smooth surfaces for final finishing. Clinically smooth surfaces can be routinely attained by using a series of finer and finer polishing steps.

3.4 Cutting Mechanisms

Effective and efficient cutting requires a powered handpiece, air-water spray for cooling, high operating speed (>200,000 rpm), light pressure, and a new carbide bur or diamond instrument. Carbide burs are better for end-cutting, produce lower heat, and have more blade edges per diameter for cutting. They are effectively used for punch cuts to enter tooth structure, intracoronal tooth preparation, amalgam removal, small preparations, and secondary retention features. Diamond instruments have greater hardness, and coarse diamonds have very high cutting effectiveness. Diamonds are more effective than burs for both intracoronal and extracoronal tooth preparations,

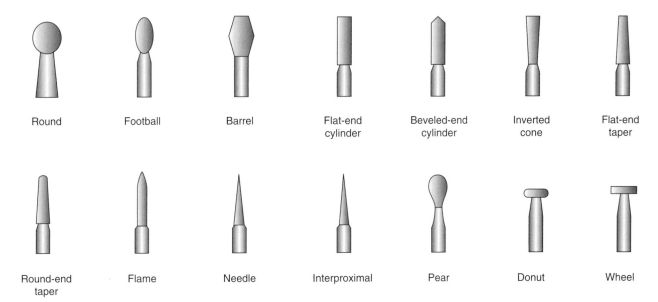

Round Football Barrel Flat-end cylinder Beveled-end cylinder Inverted cone Flat-end taper

Round-end taper Flame Needle Interproximal Pear Donut Wheel

Figure 2-13 Characteristic shapes and designs for a range of diamond cutting instruments. *(From Heymann HO, Swift EJ, Ritter AV: Sturdevant's Art and Science of Operative Dentistry, ed 6. St. Louis, Mosby, 2013.)*

beveling enamel margins on tooth preparations, and enameloplasty.

3.5 Hazards with Cutting Instruments

Almost everything done in a dental office involves some risk to the patient, dentist, or auxiliary personnel. For the patient, there are pulpal dangers from the tooth preparation and restoration procedures. There are also soft tissue dangers. Everyone is potentially susceptible to eye, ear, and inhalation dangers. However, careful adherence to standard precautions can eliminate or minimize most risks associated with cutting instrument use.

A. Pulpal precautions—the use of cutting instruments can harm the pulp by exposure to mechanical vibration, heat generation, desiccation and loss of dentinal tubule fluid, and transection of odontoblastic processes. As the thickness of remaining dentin decreases, the pulpal insult (and response) from heat or desiccation increases.

B. Soft tissue precautions—the lips, tongue, and cheeks of the patient are the most frequent areas of soft tissue injury. The handpiece should never be operated unless there is good access and vision to the cutting site. A rubber dam is very helpful in isolating the operating site. When the dam is not used, the dentist and dental assistant can retract the soft tissue with a mouth mirror, cotton roll, or saliva ejector.

C. Eye precautions—the operator, assistant, and patient should wear glasses with side shields to prevent eye damage from airborne particles during operative procedures using rotary instrumentation. When using high speeds, particles of old restorations, tooth structure, bacteria, and other debris are discharged at high speeds from the patient's mouth.

D. Ear precautions—an objectionable high-pitched whine is produced by some air-turbine handpieces at high speeds. Aside from the annoying aspect of this noise, there is some possibility that hearing loss can result from continued exposure.
  1. Potential damage to hearing from noise depends on the intensity or loudness (decibels), frequency (Hz), duration (time) of the noise, and susceptibility of the individual.
  2. Increased age, existing ear damage, disease, and medications are other factors that can accelerate hearing loss.

E. Inhalation precaution—aerosols and vapors are a health hazard to all present and are created by cutting tooth structure and restorative materials. The aerosols are fine dispersions in air of water, tooth debris, microorganisms, and restorative materials. Aerosols and vapors should be eliminated as much as possible by careful evacuation near the tooth being operated on.
  1. A rubber dam protects the patient against oral inhalation of aerosols or vapors, but nasal inhalation of vapor and finer aerosol may still occur.
  2. Disposable masks worn by dental office personnel filter out bacteria and all but the finest particulate matter.

4.0 Preparation of Teeth

Outline of Review

4.1 Introduction
4.2 Stages and Steps in Tooth Preparation
4.3 Moisture Control

4.4 Tooth Preparation for Amalgam Restorations

4.5 Tooth Preparation for Composite Restorations

4.1 Introduction

A. Why teeth need to be restored.
  1. Remove caries.
  2. Correct fracture.
  3. Correct erosive tooth wear.
  4. Reduce risk of pulp damage.
  5. Improve or correct esthetics.
  6. Improve or correct contour or function.
B. Definition of tooth preparation.
  1. Mechanically altering a tooth to remove diseased or weakened tooth structure.
  2. Mechanically altering a tooth to receive the appropriate restorative material (Figure 2-14).
    a. For maximum strength.
    b. For maximum form, function, and esthetics.
C. Objectives of tooth preparation.
  1. Remove all defects.
  2. Protect the pulp.
  3. Be as conservative as possible.
  4. Make tooth and restoration strong.
  5. Make restoration functional and esthetic.
D. Factors affecting tooth preparation.
  1. General factors.
    a. Diagnosis.
    b. Patient desires.
    c. Multitreatment needs.
  2. Emphasis on conservation of tooth structure.
    a. Examples.
      (1) Supragingival margins.
      (2) Minimal pulpal depth.
      (3) Minimal faciolingual width.
      (4) Rounded internal line angles.
    b. Benefits of smaller preparations.
      (1) Less removal of tooth structure.
      (2) Better esthetics.
      (3) Less trauma to pulp.
      (4) Stronger remaining tooth structure.
      (5) More easily retained material.
  3. Type of restorative material to be used.
    a. Gold, porcelain, amalgam, or composite—each require different preparation forms (Table 2-4).
  4. Biologic considerations.
    a. Pulpal effects of preparation.
    b. Fracture potential of undermined enamel.
    c. Tooth strength considerations.
E. Considerations in tooth preparations (Box 2-2).

4.2 Stages and Steps in Tooth Preparation

A. Initial (primary) tooth preparation—extension of the preparation walls to sound tooth structure in all directions except pulpally.
  1. Outline form and initial depth (Figure 2-15).
    a. Definition—extension to sound tooth structure at an initial depth of 0.2 to 0.75 mm into dentin.
    b. Principles.
      (1) Place margins where finishable.
      (2) Remove unsupported, weakened tooth structure.
      (3) Include all faults.
    c. Dictated by the following.
      (1) Caries.
      (2) Old material.
      (3) Size of defect.
      (4) Occlusion.
      (5) Marginal configuration.
      (6) Adjacent tooth or contour.
    d. Features.
      (1) Preserve cuspal strength.
      (2) Preserve marginal ridge strength.
      (3) Keep faciolingual width narrow.
      (4) Connect two close (0.5 mm) preparations.
      (5) Restrict depth to 0.2 to 0.75 mm into dentin.
      (6) Use enameloplasty.

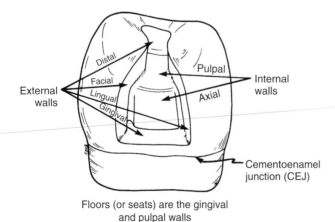

Floors (or seats) are the gingival and pulpal walls

Figure 2-14 External and internal walls for an amalgam tooth preparation.

Box 2-2
Considerations in Tooth Preparations

Extent of caries	Pulp protection
Extent of old material	Patient cooperation
Occlusion	Fracture lines
Extent of defect	Bone support
Pulpal involvement	Caries activity
Esthetic needs	Economics
Tooth contours	Patient desires
Patient age	Material limitations
Bur design	Radiographic findings
Patient's homecare	Overall diagnosis
Gingival status	Anesthesia

Table 2-4

Tooth Preparation: Amalgam versus Composite

	AMALGAM	COMPOSITE
Outline form	Include fault May extend to break proximal Include adjacent suspicious area	Same Same No Seal these areas
Pulpal depth	Uniform 1.5 mm	Remove fault; not usually uniform
Axial depth	Uniform 0.2-0.5 mm inside DEJ	Remove fault; not usually uniform
Cavosurface margin	Create 90-degree amalgam margin	≥90 degrees
Bevels	None (except possibly gingival)	Large preparation, esthetics, and seal
Texture of prepared walls	Smoother	Rough
Cutting instrument	Burs	Diamonds
Primary retention form	Convergence occlusally	None (roughness/bonding)
Secondary retention form	Grooves, slots, locks, pins, bonding	Bonding; grooves for very large or root-surface preparation
Resistance form	Flat floors, rounded angles, box-shaped floors, perpendicular or occlusal forces (?)	Same for large preparations; no special form for small-to-moderate size preparations
Base indications	Provide ~2 mm between pulp and amalgam	Not needed
Liner indications	Ca(OH)$_2$ over direct or indirect pulp caps	Same
Sealer	Gluma desensitizer when not bonding	Sealed by bonding system used

From Roberson TM, Heymann HO, Swift EJ: Sturdevant's Art & Science of Operative Dentistry, ed 5. St. Louis, Mosby, 2006.

Ca(OH)$_2$, Calcium hydroxide.

e. Occlusal preparations.
  (1) Extend margin to sound tooth structure.
  (2) Extend to include all of the fissure that is not eliminated by enameloplasty.
  (3) Restrict depth to 0.2 mm into dentin.
  (4) Join two preparations if less than 0.5 mm remaining.
  (5) Extend to provide access for preparing, inserting material, and finishing the restoration.
f. Smooth-surface preparations.
  (1) Proximal surfaces.
    (a) Extend until no friable enamel remains.
    (b) Do not stop margins on cusp heights or ridge crests.
    (c) Get enough access.
    (d) Axial wall depth restricted to 0.2 mm inside DEJ to 0.75 mm depth from external surface.
    (e) Extend gingival margin to get 0.5 mm clearance.
    (f) Extend facial and lingual proximal walls to clearance. If it is necessary to extend the facial and lingual walls 1 mm or more to break the contact arbitrarily, the proximal margin is left in the contact.
  (2) Gingival walls of class V. Outline is governed only by extent of lesion except pulpally.
g. Enameloplasty—removal of a defect by recontouring or reshaping the enamel when the defect is no deeper than one quarter the thickness of enamel. When the defect is greater than one third the thickness of enamel, the wall must be extended.
2. Primary resistance form.
  a. Definition—prevention of tooth or restoration fracture from occlusal forces along the long axis of the tooth.
  b. Factors affecting primary resistance form.
    (1) Occlusal contacts.
    (2) Amount of remaining tooth structure.
    (3) Type of restorative material.
  c. Features.
    (1) Flat floors, pulpal, and gingival.
    (2) Box shape.
    (3) Preserve marginal ridges.
    (4) Preserve cuspal strength.
    (5) Remove weakened tooth structure.
    (6) Cap cusps as indicated (Figure 2-16).
    (7) Rounded internal line angles.
    (8) Adequate thickness of material.

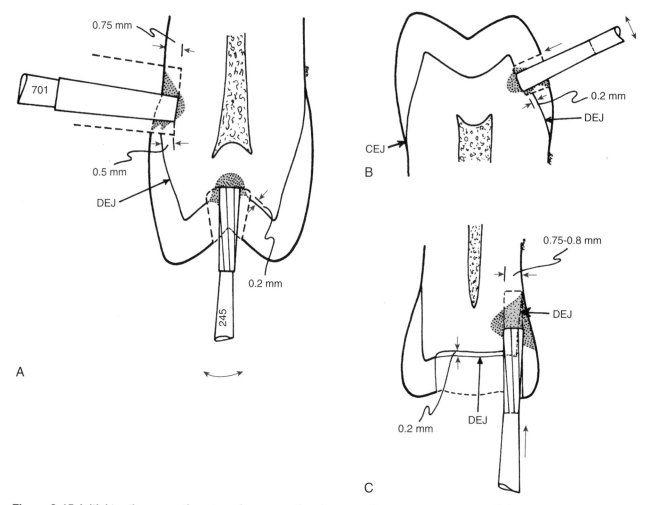

Figure 2-15 **Initial tooth preparation stage for conventional preparations. A-C,** Extensions in all directions are to sound tooth structure, while maintaining a specific limited pulpal or axial depth regardless whether the end (or side) of bur is in dentin, caries, old restorative material, or air. Dentinoenamel junction *(DEJ)* and cementoenamel junction *(CEJ)* are indicated in **B**. In **A**, initial depth is approximately two thirds of 3-mm bur head length, or 2 mm, as related to prepared facial and lingual walls, but is half the No. 245 bur head length, or 1.5 mm, as related to central fissure location.

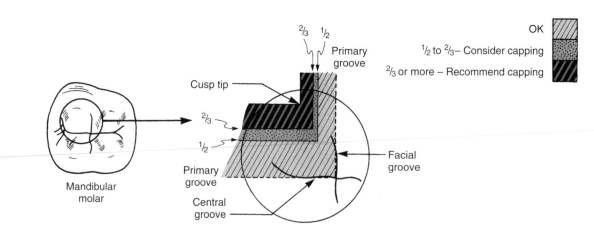

Figure 2-16 **Rule for cusp capping.** If extension from a primary groove toward the cusp tip is no more than half the distance, no cusp capping should be done. If this extension is one half to two thirds of the distance, consider cusp capping. If the extension is more than two thirds of the distance, usually cusp capping is done.

3. Primary retention form.
   a. Definition—prevention of dislodgment of the material.
   b. Features.
      (1) Preparation wall configuration—shape, height, form.
4. Convenience form.
   a. Alterations to improve access and visibility for preparing and restoring the cavity.
B. Final tooth preparation—completing the tooth preparation.
   1. Removing remaining caries.
      a. Objective—remove all microorganisms (infected dentin).
         (1) Initial preparation may remove all caries.
         (2) Deep excavation, questionable dentin near pulp (indication for indirect pulp cap).
            (a) Leave last bit of leathery carious dentin, place reinforced glass-ionomer as caries-control restoration.
            (b) May or may not use calcium hydroxide liner.
            (c) May or may not reenter to reexcavate after 6 to 8 weeks (note: evidence is controversial).
            (d) After follow-up period (approximately 6 to 8 weeks), restore with definitive restoration.
         (3) Pulpal communication (exposure)—indications for direct pulp cap.
            (a) Small mechanical (noncarious) exposure (<1 mm).
            (b) Asymptomatic tooth.
            (c) Isolated area.
            (d) Hemorrhage controlled.
            (e) Use calcium hydroxide for reparative dentin.
            (f) Place resin-modified glass ionomer (RMGI) base over liner.
            (g) Remove coronal portion of exposed pulpal tissue in pulp chamber, and place calcium hydroxide liner and RMGI base.
         (4) Endodontic treatment (root canal)—indications.
            (a) Large and carious exposure (>1 mm).
            (b) Symptomatic tooth.
            (c) Area contaminated (saliva, debris).
            (d) Purulent exudate.
   2. Secondary resistance and retention forms—secondary resistance and retention forms may be performed *after* placement of liners and bases (see Section 5.1, Sealers, Liners, and Bases).
      a. Mechanical or preparation features.
         (1) Retentive locks, grooves, coves (primarily for metallic restorations).
         (2) Groove extensions (may be for any restoration).
         (3) Skirts (primarily for cast restorations).
         (4) Beveled enamel margins (primarily for cast and composite restorations).
         (5) Pins, slot, steps, amalgam pins (primarily for amalgam restorations).
      b. Bonding.
      c. Cement (for cast restorations).
   3. Finishing the external walls.
      a. Definition—establishing the design and smoothness of the cavosurface margin.
      b. Objectives.
         (1) Best seal between tooth and material.
         (2) Smooth junction between tooth and material.
         (3) Maximum strength for tooth and material.
      c. Features.
         (1) Bevels.
         (2) Butt joints.
      d. Considerations.
         (1) Direction of enamel rods.
         (2) Support of enamel rods.
         (3) Type of material.
         (4) Location of margin.
         (5) Degree of smoothness desired.
   4. Final procedures—cleaning, inspecting, sealing, and applying surface treatments.
      a. Readying the preparation for the material.
      b. Removing any debris.
      c. Sealing or bonding.

4.3 Moisture Control

A. Isolation of the operating field—the goals of operating field isolation are the following.
   1. Moisture control—moisture control refers to excluding sulcular fluid, saliva, and gingival bleeding from the operating field. It also refers to preventing the handpiece spray and restorative debris from being swallowed or aspirated by the patient. The rubber dam, suction devices, and absorbents have variable effectiveness in moisture control.
   2. Retraction and access—the rubber dam, high-volume evacuator, absorbents, retraction cord, and mouth prop are used for retraction and access.
   3. Harm prevention—prevention from harm is provided as much by the manner in which these devices are used as by the devices themselves.
   4. Local anesthesia—local anesthetics play a role in eliminating the discomfort of dental treatment and controlling moisture.
B. Rubber dam—the rubber dam is used to define the operating field by isolating one or more teeth from the oral environment. The dam eliminates saliva from the operating site and retracts the soft tissue. Also, there are fewer interruptions to replace cotton rolls to

maintain isolation. When excavating a deep carious lesion and risking pulpal exposure, use of the rubber dam is strongly recommended to prevent pulpal contamination from oral fluids.

1. Advantages.
   a. Increased access and visibility.
   b. Isolates area.
   c. Keeps area dry.
   d. Protects patient and operator.
   e. Retracts soft tissue.
   f. Preserves and protects materials.
2. Disadvantages.
   a. Some patients object.
   b. Some situations do not work.
   c. Partially erupted teeth.
   d. Extremely malpositioned teeth.
C. Cotton roll isolation and cellulose wafers.
   1. Absorbents, such as cotton rolls and cellulose wafers, can also provide isolation. Absorbents are isolation alternatives when rubber dam application is not used and when absorbents can be as effective as rubber dam isolation. In conjunction with profound anesthesia, absorbents provide acceptable moisture control for most clinical procedures. Using a saliva ejector in conjunction with absorbents may abate salivary flow further.
D. Other isolation devices.
   1. Numerous new and innovative isolation devices have been introduced more recently, some of them incorporating illumination and suction capabilities to the usual cheek or tongue retraction.

4.4 Tooth Preparation for Amalgam Restorations

A. Clinical technique.
   1. Initial clinical procedures—a complete examination, diagnosis, and treatment plan must be finalized before the patient is scheduled for operative appointments (emergencies are an exception). A brief review of the chart (including medical factors), treatment plan, and radiographs should precede each restorative procedure. At the beginning of each appointment, the dentist should also examine the operating site carefully and assess the occlusion, particularly of the tooth or teeth scheduled for treatment.
   a. Local anesthesia (when needed).
   b. Isolation of the operating site—isolation for amalgam restorations can be accomplished with a rubber dam or cotton rolls.
   c. Other preoperative considerations.
      (1) A wedge placed preoperatively in the gingival embrasure is useful when restoring a posterior proximal surface. This step causes separation of the operated tooth from the adjacent tooth and may help protect the rubber dam and the interdental papilla.
      (2) A preoperative assessment of the occlusion also should be made. This step should occur before rubber dam placement and should identify not only the occlusal contacts of the tooth to be restored but also the contacts on opposing and adjacent teeth. For smaller amalgam restorations, the projected facial and lingual extensions of a proximal box should be visualized before preparing the occlusal portion of the tooth, reducing the chance of overpreparing the cuspal area, while maintaining a butt joint form of the facial or lingual proximal margins.
   d. Requirements—as noted previously, appropriate tooth preparation (Figure 2-17) for an amalgam restoration depends on both tooth and material factors.
      (1) 90-degree or greater amalgam margin (butt joint form).
      (2) Adequate depth (thickness of amalgam).
      (3) Adequate mechanical retention form (undercut form).
   e. Principles of tooth preparation.
      (1) Initial stage.
         (a) Place the tooth preparation extension into sound tooth structure at the marginal areas (not pulpally or axially).

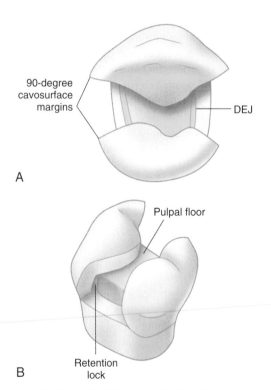

Figure 2-17 A and **B,** Diagrams of class II amalgam tooth preparations illustrating uniform pulpal and axial wall depths, 90-degree cavosurface margins, and convergence of walls or prepared retention form or both. *DEJ,* Dentinoenamel junction. *(From Heymann HO, Swift EJ, Ritter AV: Sturdevant's Art and Science of Operative Dentistry, ed 6. St. Louis, Mosby, 2013.)*

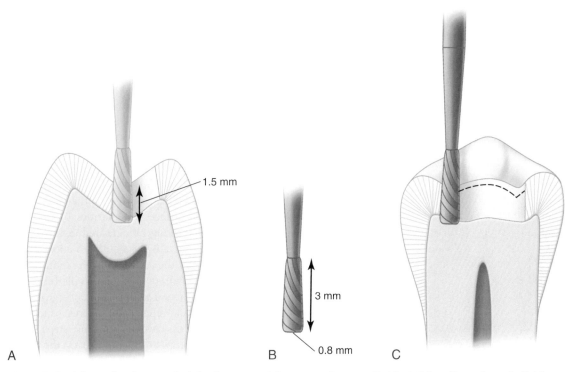

Figure 2-18 Pulpal floor depth. A, Pulpal depth measured from central groove. **B,** No. 245 bur dimensions. **C,** Guides to proper pulpal floor depth: (1) one half the length of the No. 245 bur, (2) 1.5 mm, or (3) 0.2 mm inside (internal to) dentinoenamel junction. *(From Heymann HO, Swift EJ, Ritter AV: Sturdevant's Art and Science of Operative Dentistry, ed 6. St. Louis, Mosby, 2013.)*

(b) Extend the depth (pulpally or axially or both) to a prescribed, uniform dimension.

(c) Provide an initial form that retains the amalgam in the tooth.

(d) Establish the tooth preparation margins in a form that results in a 90-degree amalgam margin when the amalgam is inserted.

(2) The final stage of tooth preparation removes any remaining defect (caries or old restorative material) and incorporates any additional preparation features (slots, pins, steps, or amalgam pins) to achieve appropriate retention and resistance form.

f. Initial tooth preparation depth—all initial depths of a tooth preparation for amalgam relate to the DEJ except when the occlusal enamel has been significantly worn thinner and when the preparation extends onto the root surface. The initial depth pulpally is 0.2 mm inside (internal to) the DEJ or 1.5 mm as measured from the depth of the central groove—whichever results in the greatest thickness of amalgam. The initial depth of the axial wall form is 0.2 mm inside the DEJ when retention locks are not used and 0.5 mm inside the DEJ when retention locks are used. The deeper extension allows placement of the retention locks without undermining marginal enamel. However,

axial depths on the root surface should be 0.75 to 1 mm deep, providing room for a retention groove or cove, while providing for adequate thickness of the amalgam (Figure 2-18).

g. Outline form—the initial extension of the tooth preparation should be visualized preoperatively by estimating the extent of the defect, the preparation form requirements of the amalgam, and the need for adequate access to place the amalgam into the tooth. Otherwise, the enamel is subject to fracture. For enamel strength, the marginal enamel rods should be supported by sound dentin.

(1) When making the preparation extensions, every effort should be made to preserve the strength of cusps and marginal ridges. When possible, the outline form should be extended around cusps and avoid undermining the dentinal support of the marginal ridge enamel.

(2) When viewed from the occlusal, the facial and lingual proximal cavosurface margins of a class II preparation should be 90 degrees (i.e., perpendicular to a tangent drawn through the point of extension facially and lingually). In most instances, the facial and lingual proximal walls should be extended just into the facial or lingual embrasure. This extension provides adequate access for performing the preparation

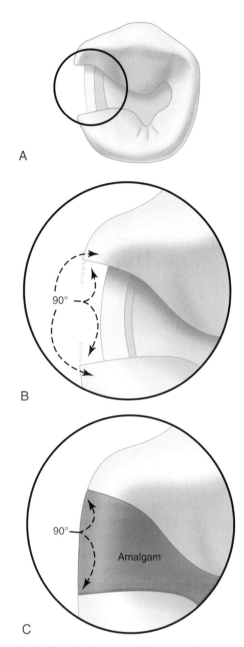

Figure 2-19 Proximal cavosurface margins. A, Facial and lingual proximal cavosurface margins prepared at 90-degree angles to a tangent drawn through the point on the external tooth surface. **B,** A 90-degree proximal cavosurface margin produces a 90-degree amalgam margin. **C,** 90-degree amalgam margins. *(From Heymann HO, Swift EJ, Ritter AV: Sturdevant's Art and Science of Operative Dentistry, ed 6. St. Louis, Mosby, 2013.)*

(with decreased potential to mar the adjacent tooth), easier placement of the matrix band, and easier condensation and carving of the amalgam. Such extension provides clearance between the cavosurface margin and the adjacent tooth. For the more experienced operator, extending the proximal margins beyond the proximal contact into the respective embrasure is not always necessary (Figure 2-19).

(3) Factors dictating outline form include caries, old restorative material, inclusion of the entire defect, proximal or occlusal contact relationship, and need for convenience form.
h. Cavosurface margin—if either enamel or amalgam has marginal angles less than 90 degrees, they are subject to fracture because both are brittle structures.
i. Primary retention form—retention form preparation features lock or retain the restorative material in the tooth. Amalgam retention form is provided by the following.
   (1) Mechanical locking of the inserted amalgam into surface irregularities of the preparation (even though the desired texture of the preparation walls is smooth) to allow good adaptation of the amalgam to the tooth.
   (2) Preparation of vertical walls (especially facial and lingual walls) that converge occlusally.
   (3) Special retention features, such as locks, grooves, coves, slots, pins, steps, or amalgam pins, that are placed during the final stage of tooth preparation—the first two of these are considered primary retention form features and are provided by the orientation and type of the preparation instrument. The third is a secondary retention form feature and is discussed in a subsequent section. An inverted cone carbide bur (No. 245) provides the desired wall shape and texture.
j. Primary resistance form—resistance form preparation features help the restoration and tooth resist fracturing as a result of occlusal forces.
   (1) Resistance features that assist in preventing the tooth from fracturing.
      (a) Maintaining as much unprepared tooth structure as possible (preserving cusps and marginal ridges).
      (b) Having pulpal and gingival walls prepared perpendicular to occlusal forces, when possible.
      (c) Having rounded internal preparation angles.
      (d) Removing unsupported or weakened tooth structure.
      (e) Placing pins into the tooth as part of the final stage of tooth preparation (note: this strategy is considered a secondary resistance form feature).
   (2) Resistance form features that assist in preventing the amalgam from fracturing.
      (a) Adequate thickness of amalgam (1.5 to 2 mm in areas of occlusal contact and 0.75 mm in axial areas).
      (b) Marginal amalgam of 90 degrees or greater.

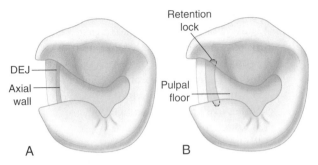

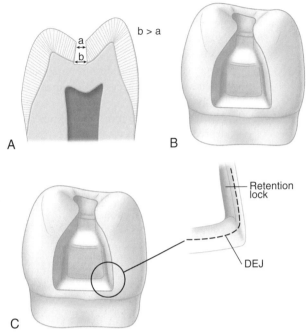

Figure 2-20 Axial wall depth. A, If no retention grooves needed, axial depth 0.2 mm inside (internal to) dentinoenamel junction *(DEJ).* **B,** If retention grooves needed, axial depth 0.5 mm inside (internal to) DEJ. *(From Heymann HO, Swift EJ, Ritter AV: Sturdevant's Art and Science of Operative Dentistry, ed 6. St. Louis, Mosby, 2013.)*

Figure 2-21 Typical amalgam tooth preparation retention form features. **A** and **B,** Occlusal convergence of prepared walls (primary retention form). **C,** Retention grooves in proximal box (secondary retention form). *DEJ,* Dentinoenamel junction. *(From Heymann HO, Swift EJ, Ritter AV: Sturdevant's Art and Science of Operative Dentistry, ed 6. St. Louis, Mosby, 2013.)*

(c) Boxlike preparation form, which provides uniform amalgam thickness.

(d) Rounded axiopulpal line angles in class II tooth preparations.

(3) Many of these resistance form features can be achieved using the No. 245 bur, which is an inverted cone design with rounded corners.

k. Convenience form—convenience form preparation features are features that make the procedure easier or the area more accessible. Convenience form may include arbitrary extension of the outline form so that marginal form can be established; caries can be accessed for removal; matrix can be placed; or amalgam can be inserted, carved, and finished. Convenience form features also may include extending the proximal margins to provide clearance from the adjacent tooth and extension of other walls to provide greater access for caries excavation.

l. Removal of remaining fault and pulp protection—if caries or old restorative material remains after the initial preparation, it should be located only in the axial or pulpal walls (the extension of the peripheral preparation margins should have already been to sound tooth structure).

m. Secondary resistance and retention form—if it is determined (based on clinical judgment) that insufficient retention or resistance forms are present in the tooth preparation, additional preparation is indicated. Many features that enhance retention form also enhance resistance form. Such features include the placement of grooves, locks, coves, pins, slots, or amalgam pins. Usually, the larger the tooth preparation, the greater the need for secondary resistance and retention forms (Figures 2-20 and 2-21).

n. Final procedures—after the previous steps are performed, the tooth preparation should be viewed from all angles. Careful assessment should be performed to ensure that all caries has been removed, depths are proper, margins provide for the correct amalgam and tooth preparation angles, and the tooth is cleaned of any residual debris.

4.5 Tooth Preparation for Composite Restorations

A. Clinical technique.

1. Preliminary considerations.

a. Occlusion assessment of both operated and adjacent teeth.

b. Clean tooth with flour of pumice (only if no tooth preparation is done).

c. Select shade (before teeth are dried).

(1) Shade tab.

(2) Place composite on tooth surface, cure, and then remove.

d. Area isolation (rubber dam or cotton roll-retraction cord).

2. Tooth preparation.

a. General considerations.

(1) Include all faults.

(2) Remove most weakened tooth structure (friable enamel).

(3) Pulp protection (if needed).

(4) Minimal mechanical retention needed except in the following cases.
    (a) No enamel (root surface, need more retention).
    (b) Large restoration (need more retention).
(5) Roughen enamel (or place bevel, only on facial, visible margins).
    (a) Bevel, usually 0.5 mm wide and at 45 degrees.
    (b) Coarse diamond.
    (c) Increased surface area = increased retention.
(6) Floors prepared perpendicular to long axis of tooth when concerned about resistance form or have large preparation.

b. Conventional—root surface preparations.
  (1) Remove fault.
  (2) Roughen or bevel enamel (if available).
  (3) Nonenamel areas.
    (a) 90-degree margins.
    (b) Mechanical retention.

c. Beveled conventional—replacement preparations (Figure 2-22).

(1) Maintain preparation form of restoration.
(2) Bevel or roughen enamel (coarse diamond).
(3) May need to place retention if on root (¼ round bur used to make cove).

d. Modified—initial preparations (Figure 2-23).
  (1) Fault dictates outline form.
  (2) Remove only fault, scooped out.
  (3) Roughen or bevel enamel.
  (4) Etch enamel.
  (5) Etch and prime dentin.

e. Controversial or new approaches.
  (1) Box-only preparations.
  (2) Tunnel preparations (not recommended).
  (3) Sandwich technique.
  (4) Bonding a weakened tooth.
    (a) Arbitrary extension of grooves or walls.
    (b) Arbitrarily leaving weakened tooth structure.
    (c) These features may help in increasing the strength of the remaining weakened tooth structure because of the micromechanical bond of the material reinforcing the tooth.

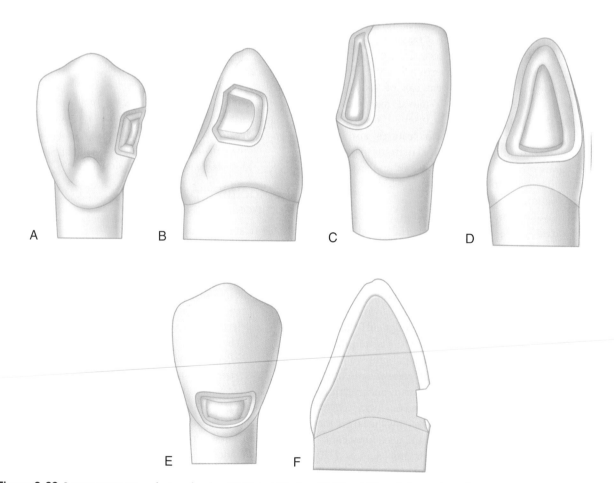

Figure 2-22 Larger preparation designs for class III (**A** and **B**), class IV (**C** and **D**), and class V (**E** and **F**) restorations. *(From Heymann HO, Swift EJ, Ritter AV: Sturdevant's Art and Science of Operative Dentistry, ed 6. St. Louis, Mosby, 2013.)*

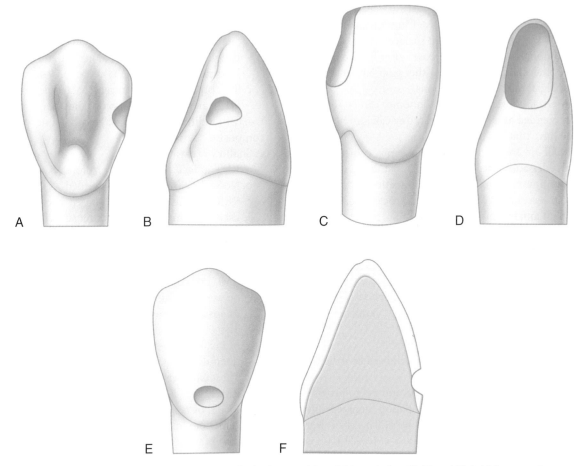

Figure 2-23 Preparation designs for class III (**A** and **B**), class IV (**C** and **D**), and class V (**E** and **F**) initial composite restorations (primary caries). *(From Heymann HO, Swift EJ, Ritter AV: Sturdevant's Art and Science of Operative Dentistry, ed 6. St. Louis, Mosby, 2013.)*

5.0 Restoration of Teeth

Outline of Review

5.1 Sealers, Liners, and Bases

A. Sealers.
1. Occlusion of the dentinal tubules limits the potential for tubular fluid movement and resultant sensitivity.
2. Sealers (also referred to as desensitizers) are effective disinfectants, provide cross-linking of any exposed dentin matrix and occlude ("plug") dentinal tubules by cross-linking tubular proteins.
3. Sealers are typically aqueous solutions.
4. Some sealers may contain glutaraldehyde, hydroxy-ethylmethacrylate (HEMA), benzalkonium chloride, chlorhexidine, or other desensitizers. Historically, copal varnish was used as a liner under amalgam restorations.

B. Liners.
1. Liners are thin layers of material used primarily to provide a barrier to protect the dentin from residual reactants diffusing out of a restoration, from oral fluids, or from both, which may penetrate leaky tooth-restoration interfaces.
2. Liners also contribute initial electrical insulation; generate some thermal protection; and, in some formulations, provide pulpal treatment.
3. Liners are used to cover a direct or near pulpal exposure and to line very deep areas of a tooth preparation in vital teeth.
4. Calcium hydroxide and RMGI are examples of typical liners used with direct restorations.

C. Bases.
1. Bases (cement bases, typically 1 to 2 mm) are used to provide thermal protection for the pulp and to

supplement mechanical support for the restoration by distributing local stresses from the restoration across the underlying dentin surface.

2. Additional bulk (from the base) affords mechanical and thermal protection to the pulp under metal (amalgam or gold) restorations.

3. RMGI or conventional glass-ionomer cement is recommended as a base to overlay any calcium hydroxide liner that has been placed.

4. RMGI or conventional glass-ionomer cement base provides additional strength to resist amalgam condensation pressure as well as protection of the liner from dissolution during bonded procedures.

D. Use with amalgam restorations.
   1. Shallow excavations.
      a. Remaining dentin thickness (RDT) is 2 mm or more.
      b. Use a dentin sealer/desensitizing agent such as Gluma Desensitizer or G5. Sealers/desensitizers replace the traditional use of copal varnish.
   2. Moderately deep excavations.
      a. RDT is judged to be 0.5 to 2 mm.
      b. Use a light-cured RMGI base, followed by a dentin sealer/desensitizing agent.
      c. The objective of the base application is to provide approximately 2 mm of insulation between the restorative material and the pulp. The shallower the excavation, the less thickness of RMGI base is required. This replaces the traditional approach of using a zinc oxide–eugenol base material followed by a copal varnish.
   3. Deep excavations.
      a. Noncarious (mechanical) pulpal exposure less than 1.0 mm in diameter or excavations where the RDT is judged to be less than 0.5 mm such that a microexposure of the pulp is suspected.
      b. Use a thin (0.5 to 0.75 mm) layer of calcium hydroxide liner on the suspected exposure site followed by RMGI base to seal the immediate site of the exposure.
      c. The objectives are to prohibit bacterial infiltration and protect the liner from dissolution.
      d. A dentin sealer/desensitizing agent or, if the operator chooses, an appropriate amalgam bonding agent is placed on the remaining dentin.

E. Use with composite restorations.
   1. Shallow to moderately deep excavations.
      a. RDT is judged to be 0.5 mm or more.
      b. No liner or base material is indicated.
      c. Only a dentin bonding system along with the composite restorative material is needed.
   2. Deep excavations.
      a. Noncarious (mechanical) pulpal exposure less than 1.0 mm in diameter or excavations where the RDT is judged to be less than 0.5 mm such that a microexposure of the pulp is suspected.
      b. Use a thin (0.5 to 0.75 mm) layer of calcium hydroxide liner placed on the suspected exposure site followed by RMGI base and the proper application of a bonding agent along with the composite restorative material.
      c. The objective is to prevent bacterial infiltration, while avoiding dissolution of the liner.

F. Use with indirect restorations (gold, ceramic, processed composite).
   1. Shallow excavations.
      a. RDT judged to be 2 mm or more.
      b. No sealer, liner, or base is needed.
      c. RMGI cement or a resin-based cement may be used for cementation, providing excellent dentinal sealing.
   2. Moderately deep excavations.
      a. RDT judged to be 0.5 to 2 mm.
      b. RMGI or conventional glass-ionomer cement may be used to restore axial or pulpal wall contour and to ensure an adequate thermal barrier.
      c. The objective is to provide approximately 2 mm of insulation between the restorative material and the pulp.
      d. The shallower the excavation, the less thickness of RMGI base is required.
      e. RMGI or resin-based material is recommended for cementation.
   3. Deep excavations.
      a. Noncarious (mechanical) pulpal exposure less than 1.0 mm in diameter or excavations where RDT is judged to be less than 0.5 mm such that a microexposure of the pulp is suspected.
      b. Use thin (0.5 to 0.75 mm) layer of calcium hydroxide liner on the suspected exposure site followed by RMGI base to restore axial or pulpal wall contour, ensure an adequate thermal barrier, and seal the exposure site.
      c. The objective is to prevent bacterial infiltration, while avoiding the base from dissolution.
      d. In these cases, given the much higher cost of the indirect restoration compared with a direct amalgam or composite restoration and the risk of endodontic complications secondary to the pulp exposure, strong consideration should be given to performing endodontic therapy before completion of the indirect restoration.
      e. Occasionally, it may be deemed more efficient simply to block out the excavated area on the die during laboratory procedures, allowing the cement to fill in the area of excavation during cementation.

5.2 Amalgam Restorations

A. Introduction.
   1. Types.
      a. Low copper—generally inferior, seldom used.
      b. High copper.

(1) Spherical.
   (a) Greater leakage.
   (b) Greater postoperative sensitivity.
(2) Admix.
2. Properties.
  a. The linear coefficient of thermal expansion of amalgam is greater than that of tooth structure.
  b. The compressive strength of high-copper amalgam is similar to tooth structure.
  c. The tensile strength of high-copper amalgam is lower than tooth structure.
  d. Amalgams are brittle and have low edge strength.
  e. High-copper amalgams exhibit no clinically relevant creep or flow.
  f. Amalgam is a high thermal conductor.
3. Clinical performance.
  a. Marginal fracture.
  b. Bulk fracture.
  c. Secondary caries.
4. Handling.
  a. Operator preference regarding using admix or spherical alloys.
  b. Mercury hygiene—very important as described subsequently.
5. Uses.
  a. Nonesthetic cervical lesions.
  b. Large class I and II preparations where heavy occlusion would be on the material.
  c. Class I and II preparations where isolation problems exist for bonding.
  d. Temporary or caries-control restorations.
  e. Foundations.
  f. Patient sensitivity to other materials.
  g. Where cost is a factor.
  h. Inability to do a good composite.
6. Advantages.
  a. Strength.
  b. Wear resistance.
  c. Easy to use.
  d. Less technique-sensitive.
  e. Self-sealing margins over time.
  f. History of use.
  g. Lower fee.
  h. Long-term clinical longevity.
7. Disadvantages.
  a. Not esthetic.
  b. Conductivity.
  c. Tooth preparation more demanding, less conservative.
8. Mercury controversy.
  a. There is a lack of scientific evidence that amalgam poses health risks to humans except for rare allergic reactions.
  b. Efforts are under way to reduce the environmental mercury to which people are exposed to lessen their total mercury exposure.
  c. There is no evidence ensuring that alternative materials pose a lesser health hazard.
  d. True allergies to amalgam rarely have been reported (50 cases since 1900).
  e. Estimate of human uptake of mercury vapor from amalgams is 5 $\mu g/m^3$.
9. Requirements for a successful amalgam restoration.
  a. Appropriately indicated clinical situation.
  b. High-copper material.
  c. Adequate tooth preparation.
  d. 90-degree cavosurface margins.
  e. Thickness of amalgam (1 to 2 mm).
  f. Mechanical retention form.
  g. Seal dentinal tubules.
  h. Good condensation (including lateral condensation).
  i. Appropriate development of contours and contacts.
B. Restorative technique—after the tooth preparation for most amalgam restorations, a sealer is placed on the prepared dentin before amalgam insertion to occlude the dentinal tubules. This step may occur before or after the matrix application.
1. Matrix placement—a matrix primarily is used when a proximal surface is to be restored.
  a. The objectives of a matrix are the following.
   (1) Provide proper contact.
   (2) Provide proper contour.
   (3) Confine the restorative material.
   (4) Reduce the amount of excess material.
  b. For a matrix to be effective, it should have the following characteristics.
   (1) Be easy to apply and remove.
   (2) Extend below the gingival margin.
   (3) Extend above the marginal ridge height.
   (4) Resist deformation during material insertion.
  c. The matrix should be stabilized with a wooden wedge to close any gaps that may develop between the matrix band and the gingival margin of the preparation and to provide stability to the matrix during the condensation and initial carving of the restoration. Care should be exercised to place the wedge securely apical to the gingival margin of the preparation, not to push the matrix band into the tooth preparation area resulting in undercontour of the restoration (Figure 2-24).
2. Mixing (triturating) the amalgam material—the manufacturer's directions should be followed when mixing the amalgam material. Both the speed and the time of mix are factors in the setting reaction of the material; alterations in either may cause changes in the properties of the inserted amalgam.
3. Inserting the amalgam.
  a. Proper condensation is very important to ensure confluence of the amalgam with the margins.

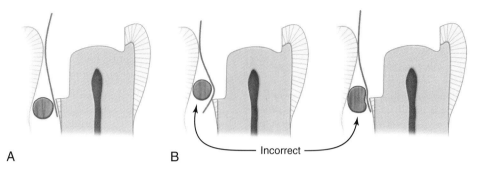

A   **B**   — Incorrect —

Figure 2-24 **A,** Correct wedge position. **B,** Incorrect wedge positions. *(From Heymann HO, Swift EJ, Ritter AV: Sturdevant's Art and Science of Operative Dentistry, ed 6. St. Louis, Mosby, 2013.)*

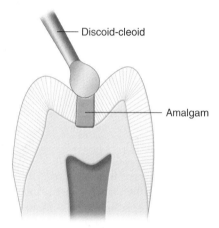

Discoid-cleoid

Amalgam

Figure 2-25 Carving occlusal margins. *(From Heymann HO, Swift EJ, Ritter AV: Sturdevant's Art and Science of Operative Dentistry, ed 6. St. Louis, Mosby, 2013.)*

    b. Spherical amalgam is more easily condensed than admixed (lathe-cut) amalgam.

    c. As a general rule, use smaller amalgam condensers first. This allows the amalgam to be properly condensed into the internal line angles and secondary retention features. Subsequently, larger condensers are used.

    d. Place amalgam to slight excess with condensers.

    e. Precarve burnish with a large, egg-shaped burnisher to finalize the condensation, remove excess mercury, and initiate the carving process.

4. Carving the amalgam—when precarve burnishing has been done, the remainder of the accessible restoration must be contoured to achieve proper form and function.

    a. Occlusal areas.

      (1) A discoid-cleoid instrument is used to carve the occlusal surface of an amalgam restoration. The rounded end (discoid) is positioned on the unprepared enamel adjacent to the amalgam margin and pulled parallel to the margin (Figure 2-25). When the pit and groove anatomy is initiated with the cleoid end of the instrument, the instrument is switched, and the discoid end is used to smooth out the anatomic form. A small Hollenbeck carver also can be used to carve amalgam restorations. The amalgam is not deeply carved; some semblance of pits and grooves is necessary to provide appropriate sluiceways for the escape of food from the occlusal table.

      (2) It may be beneficial to ensure that the mesial and distal pits are carved to be inferior to the marginal ridge height, helping prevent food from being wedged into the occlusal embrasure. Having definite but rounded occlusal anatomy also helps provide sluiceways for the escape of food from the occlusal table. For large class II or foundation restorations, the initial carving of the occlusal surface should be rapid, concentrating primarily on the marginal ridge height and occlusal embrasure areas. These areas are developed with an explorer tip or carving instrument by mimicking the adjacent tooth. The explorer tip is pulled along the inside of the matrix band, creating the occlusal embrasure form. When viewed from the facial or lingual, the created embrasure form should be identical to that of the adjacent tooth, assuming the adjacent tooth has appropriate contour. Likewise, the height of the amalgam marginal ridge should be the same as that of the adjacent tooth. If both of these areas are developed properly, the potential for fracture of the marginal ridge area of the restoration is significantly reduced.

      (3) When the initial occlusal carving has occurred, the matrix is removed to provide access to the other areas of the restoration that require carving.

    b. Facial and lingual areas—most facial and lingual areas are accessible and can be carved directly after the matrix band and wedge have been removed. A Hollenbeck carver is useful in carving these areas. The base of the amalgam knife (scaler 34/35) is also

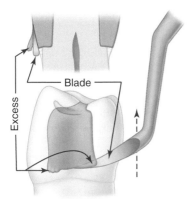

Figure 2-26 Gingival excess may be removed with amalgam knives. *(From Heymann HO, Swift EJ, Ritter AV: Sturdevant's Art and Science of Operative Dentistry, ed 6. St. Louis, Mosby, 2013.)*

appropriate. For cervical areas, it is important to remove any excess and develop the proper contour of the restoration. Usually, the contour is convex; care in carving this area is necessary. The convexity is developed by using both the occlusal and the gingival unprepared tooth structure adjacent to the preparation as guides for initiating the carving. The marginal areas are blended, resulting in the desired convexity and providing the physiologic contour that promotes good gingival health.

c. Proximal embrasure areas.

(1) The development of the occlusal embrasure already has been described. The amalgam knife (or scaler) is an excellent instrument for removing proximal excess and developing proximal contours and embrasures (Figure 2-26). The knife is positioned below the gingival margin, and excess is carefully shaved away. The knife is drawn occlusally to refine the proximal contour (below the contact) and the gingival embrasure form. The sharp tip of the knife also is beneficial in developing the facial and lingual embrasure forms. Care must be used to prevent carving away any of the desired proximal contact. If the amalgam is hardening, the amalgam knife must be used to shave, rather than cut, the excess away. If a cutting motion is used, the possibility of breaking or chipping the amalgam is increased.

(2) The proximal portion of the carved amalgam can be evaluated by visual assessment (reflecting light into the contact area to confirm a proximal contact) and placement of dental floss into the area. If dental floss is used, it must be used judiciously, ensuring that the contact area is not inadvertently removed. A piece of floss can be inserted through the contact and into the gingival embrasure area by initially wrapping the floss around the adjacent tooth

and exerting pressure on that tooth rather than the restored tooth, while moving the floss through the contact area. Once the floss is into the gingival embrasure area, it is wrapped around the restored tooth and moved occlusally and gingivally both to determine whether excess exists and to smooth the proximal amalgam material. If excess material is felt along the gingival margin, the amalgam knife should be used again until a smooth margin is obtained.

5. Finishing the amalgam restoration—when the carving is completed, the restoration is visualized from all angles, and an assessment of the thoroughness of the carving is made. If spacing is seen between the adjacent teeth and their opposing teeth, the area of premature occlusal contact on the amalgam should be identified and relieved. Articulating paper is used to adjust the contacts more precisely until the proper occlusal relationship is generated. After the occlusion is adjusted, the discoid-cleoid can be used to smooth the accessible areas of the amalgam. A lightly moistened cotton pellet held in the operative pliers can be used to smooth the accessible parts of the restoration. If the carving and smoothing are done properly, no subsequent polishing of the restoration is needed, and good long-term clinical performance results.

6. Repairing an amalgam restoration—if an amalgam restoration fractures during insertion, the defective area must be prepared again as if it were a small restoration. Appropriate depth and retention form must be generated, sometimes entirely within the existing amalgam restoration. If necessary, another matrix must be placed. A new mix of amalgam can be condensed directly into the defect and adheres to the amalgam already present if no intermediary material has been placed between the two amalgams. The sealer material can be placed on any exposed dentin, but it should not be placed on the amalgam preparation walls.

C. Common problems—causes and potential solutions.

1. Following is a list of common problems associated with amalgam restorations. Subsequent technique chapters may refer back to these problems.

a. Postoperative sensitivity—causes.

(1) Lack of adequate condensation, especially lateral condensation in the proximal boxes.

(2) Lack of proper dentinal sealing with sealer or pulp protection.

b. Marginal voids—causes.

(1) Inadequate condensation.

(2) Material pulling away or breaking from the marginal area when carving bonded amalgam.

c. Marginal ridge fractures—causes.

(1) Axiopulpal line angle not rounded in class II tooth preparations.

(2) Marginal ridge left too high.

(3) Occlusal embrasure form incorrect.

(4) Improper removal of matrix.

(5) Overzealous carving.

d. Amalgam scrap and mercury collection and disposal problems—causes.

(1) Careless handling.

(2) Inappropriate collection technique.

2. Potential solutions.

a. Careful attention to proper collection and disposal.

b. Following the Best Management Practices for Amalgam Waste as presented by the American Dental Association (available at www.ada.org).

D. Controversial issues—because the practice of operative dentistry is dynamic, constant changes are occurring. As new products and techniques are developed, their effectiveness cannot be assessed until appropriately designed research protocols have tested their worth. Many such developments are occurring at any time, many of which do not have the necessary documentation to prove their effectiveness, even though they receive very positive publicity. Several examples of such controversies follow.

1. Amalgam restoration safety—amalgam restorations are safe. The U.S. Public Health Service has reported the safety of amalgam restorations. Even recognizing these assessments, the mercury contained in current amalgam restorations still causes concerns, both legitimate and otherwise. Proper handling of mercury during mixing of the amalgam material, condensing and carving of the amalgam restoration, removal of old amalgam restorations, and amalgam scrap disposal is very important.

2. Spherical or admixed amalgam—spherical materials have advantages in providing higher earlier strength and permitting the use of less pressure. Admixed materials permit easier proximal contact development because of higher condensation forces.

3. Bonded amalgam restorations—bonded amalgam restorations are no longer recommended, even though some operators may select them for large restorations. If bonding an amalgam, the use of typical secondary retention form preparation features (e.g., grooves, locks, pins, slots) is still required. Small to moderate amalgam restorations should not be bonded.

4. Proximal retention locks—proximal retention locks for large amalgam restorations may be beneficial, although their use for smaller restorations is not deemed necessary. Correct placement of proximal retention locks is difficult.

5.3 Enamel and Dentin Bonding

A. Introduction.

1. Advantages of bonding to the tooth structure.

a. Less microleakage.

b. Less marginal staining.

c. Less recurrent caries.

d. Less pulpal sensitivity.

e. More conservative tooth preparation.

f. Improved retention.

g. Reinforcement of remaining tooth structure.

h. Reduced sensitivity in noncarious cervical lesions.

i. More conservative treatment of root-surface carious lesions.

2. Uses of adhesive techniques.

a. Change shape and color of anterior teeth.

b. Restore class I, II, III, IV, V, and VI lesions.

c. Improve retention for metallic or porcelain fused to metal crowns.

d. Bond ceramic restorations.

e. Bond indirect composite restorations.

f. Seal pits and fissures.

g. Bond orthodontic brackets.

h. Bond periodontal splints.

i. Bond conservative tooth-replacement restorations.

j. Repair existing restorations (composite, amalgam, ceramic, metal).

k. Provide foundations for crowns or onlays.

l. Desensitize exposed root surfaces.

m. Impregnate dentin and enamel to make them less susceptible to caries.

n. Bond fragments of anterior teeth.

o. Bond prefabricated and cast posts.

p. Reinforce remaining enamel and dentin after tooth preparation. Reinforcement of remaining tooth structure by bonding is believed to be temporary.

3. Status of bonding to tooth structure.

a. Enamel bonding.

(1) 10- to 15-second acid etch (with 30% to 40% phosphoric acid) is sufficient to etch enamel.

(2) Is fast, reliable, predictable, and strong.

(3) Microleakage is virtually nonexistent at etched enamel margins.

(4) Resists polymerization shrinkage forces of composite.

b. Dentin bonding.

(1) Is accomplished with either etch-and-rinse (simultaneous with enamel etch) or self-etch (with a self-etching primer or all-in-one adhesive) techniques.

(2) Is less reliable, less durable, and not as predictable as enamel bonding.

(3) May have some microleakage, especially after aging of the restoration.

(4) May have similar or higher bond strengths than enamel.

(5) May not resist polymerization shrinkage forces.

4. Factors that affect the ability to bond to dentin versus enamel.

a. Microstructural features of enamel and dentin.
  (1) Composition.
      (a) Enamel—90% mineral (hydroxyapatite).
      (b) Dentin—much less mineral, more organic (type I collagen), and more water.
  (2) Structural variations.
      (a) Enamel prisms and interprismatic areas—all etched and bondable.
  (3) Dentin-tubules—peritubular, intratubular, and intertubular channels.
      (a) Tubules from pulp to DEJ.
      (b) Contain the odontoblastic extensions and fluid.
      (c) Much larger (2.4 µm) and numerous (45,000/mm^2) near pulp than near DEJ (0.6 µm, 20,000/mm^2).
      (d) Fluid movement inside that is dictated by pulpal pressure.
      (e) Sclerosis—dentin that is aging, below a caries lesion, or exposed to oral fluids exhibits increased mineral content and is much more resistant to acid-etching, and the penetration of dentin adhesive is limited.
      (f) Smear layer—the debris left on the surface after cutting and consists of hydroxyapatite and altered denatured collagen and fills the orifices of the tubules (forming smear plugs), decreasing dentin permeability by 86%. Etching that removes the smear layer results in greater fluid flow onto the dentinal surface, which may interfere with adhesion.
      (g) Linear coefficient of thermal expansion—for dentin, is altered four times less than the composite material when subjected to thermal changes.
b. Material factors—composites shrink as they polymerize, creating stresses up to 7 megapascals (1 MPa = 150 lb/in^2).
c. Preparation factors—preparations with multiple walls or boxlike shapes (configuration) have limited stress relief opportunity for the composite material (polymerization shrinkage), and the high configuration factor (C-factor) may result in internal bond disruption and marginal gaps.
  (1) C-factor is determined by the ratio of prepared (bonded) versus unprepared (unbonded) walls within a tooth preparation.
  (2) High C-factor may indicate increased chance for postoperative sensitivity.
B. Current adhesive systems used for bonding.
  1. Etch-and-rinse, previously called total-etch (etch enamel and dentin)—this concept advocated the etching of dentin with acids along with the etching of enamel.

a. Etch-and-rinse three-step systems, also known as multibottle or fourth-generation systems (etchant, primer, adhesive)—1990s.
  (1) General considerations—these remain the gold standard.
      (a) How the systems work.
          (i) The tooth structure is etched with an acid to demineralize enamel and dentin selectively, increase the surface area, and clean the surface of debris. Etched enamel appears chalky; dentin does not. Etched dentin exposes a layer of collagen. The primer serves to increase the collagen, and the adhesive flows between the collagen and interlocks with it to form a sandwich or hybrid or resin-reinforced layer.
      (b) Most bond strength is from the formation of the hybrid layer. The surface layer is only a few microns thick, creating a demineralized layer of dentin intermingled with resin.
      (c) Seals the dentin—decreases postoperative sensitivity.
      (d) Good dentin bonding strengths—same or better than enamel bond (note: must have bond strength of 17 to 21 MPa to resist polymerization contraction force of composite).
  (2) Steps.
      (a) Etch enamel and dentin for 10 to 15 seconds.
          (i) Etches enamel.
          (ii) Removes smear layer.
          (iii) Opens and widens dentin tubules.
          (iv) Demineralizes dentin surface.
          (v) Etches out mineral (hydroxyapatite) but leaves collagen fibrils (these have low surface energy).
      (b) Rinse well and leave moist or rewet (Aqua Prep or Gluma Desensitizer).
      (c) Apply two to three layers of primer HEMA/biphenyl dimethacrylate.
          (i) Resin monomer wetting agent.
          (ii) Dissolved in acetone, ethanol, and water.
          (iii) Bifunctional—wets dentin (increases the surface tension) and bonds to overlying resin.
          (iv) Acts as a solvent.
      (d) Apply adhesive (bonding agent)—bisphenol A-glycidyl methacrylate or other methacrylate.
          (i) May also contain HEMA or other primer constituents to enhance bonding.
          (ii) Penetrates primed intertubular dentin and tubules.

(iii) Provides a polymerized surface layer.

(iv) Bonds primer and composite.

(e) Place composite.

b. Etch-and-rinse two-step systems, also known as one-bottle or fifth-generation systems (primer and adhesive are combined but still need etchant).

(1) General considerations.

(a) Primer and adhesive combined.

(b) Still require etchants—remove the smear layer.

(c) Most require wet bonding.

(d) Bond mechanism is the hybrid layer formation.

(e) Generally, bond strengths not as high as multibottle systems, but this is likely not clinically significant.

(f) Very technique-sensitive—must follow manufacturer's directions exactly.

(g) Must have dentin wettability just right.

(h) Use primarily for direct procedures.

(i) Not faster than multibottle materials.

(2) Steps.

(a) Etch for 10 seconds.

(b) Rinse well and leave moist or rewet.

(c) Apply two to three layers of primer/adhesive, thin gently with air, and light-cure (surface should appear shiny).

(d) Reapply adhesive, thin, and light-cure.

(e) Place composite.

2. Self-etching systems—etchant and primer or etchant, primer, and adhesive combined, the objective being to remove the operator variables (rinsing and drying).

a. General considerations.

(1) They do not completely remove the smear layer, which is probably why they have less postoperative sensitivity.

(2) They need to be refrigerated owing to reactive components.

(3) Use carbide burs, not diamonds, because diamonds leave a much thicker smear layer, which makes bonding more difficult.

(4) These do not etch enamel as well as phosphoric acid.

(5) Enamel etching with phosphoric acid may be beneficial, but do not etch dentin because it decreases dentin bond.

(6) Agitate the application, and place multiple coats.

(7) Air dry at least 10 seconds because material must have some water and needs to have a longer drying time to remove the water.

b. Types.

(1) Self-etch one-step systems, also known as all-in-one—most risky category.

(a) General considerations.

(i) Most research and development are in this area.

(ii) Does not remove smear layer.

(iii) Very simple to use.

(iv) Initial poor clinical research but getting better.

(v) Not as good a bond to dentin (25 MPa).

(2) Self-etch two-step (self-etch primer and then a bonding adhesive).

(a) General considerations.

(i) Requires approximately five coats.

(ii) Does not remove smear layer.

(iii) Fast and easy to use.

(iv) No rinsing; no worry about moisture.

(v) Very low postoperative sensitivity.

(vi) Beginning to get good clinical results.

(vii) Does not bond well to uncut enamel—12 MPa; must roughen enamel, and consider etching.

c. Advantages of self-etch systems.

(1) Easy to use.

(2) Eliminates variables with wet bonding.

(3) Depth of etch is self-limiting.

(4) Sensitivity is reduced.

d. Disadvantages of self-etch systems.

(1) Bond strengths to enamel and dentin generally lower.

(2) Some do not adequately etch uncut enamel.

(3) Bond strengths to autocuring composites are poor.

(4) Clinical performance not proven.

(5) Bond durability questionable.

C. Conclusions.

1. Technique suggestions.

a. Use microbrushes to apply primer/adhesive.

b. Place bonding agent in a small well to minimize evaporation.

c. Replace caps quickly and tightly.

d. Dispense only 1 to 2 drops for each tooth.

2. Technique factors for optimum bond.

a. Must have proper isolation of the field.

b. Roughen sclerotic dentin—increases surface area and removes some of the sclerotic dentin.

c. May still need mechanical retention.

d. Bevel or roughen and etch enamel.

e. Must have dentin moist (or rewet) for etch-and-rinse systems.

f. Dispense adhesives just before use; otherwise, the solvent evaporates.

g. Apply and dry primer adequately; otherwise, may have gross leakage and postoperative sensitivity (gently dry with air syringe). Too much primer is better than too little.

(1) Do not overthin the bonding agent (adhesive) too much; otherwise, may get an air-inhibited layer only, and it does not bond as well.

(2) Fill incrementally and cure in appropriate thicknesses (1 to 2 mm); may no longer be as critical a factor with offsetting polymerizaton shrinkage.

(3) Follow directions.

3. Longevity of resin-dentin bonds.

a. Laboratory results show a loss of bond strength over time.

(1) Perhaps from hydrolysis of the adhesive resin or the collagen fibers or both.

(2) The all-in-one types show the worst results.

(3) Bond durability is much greater when the peripheral margin is all in enamel.

D. Summary.

1. Dentin and enamel bonding strengths are similar for most etch-and-rinse systems.

2. Most etch-and-rinse adhesive systems bond better to moist dentin (i.e., leave dentin moist or remoisten with water or a sealer/desensitizer).

3. Self-etch systems are promising but not proven.

4. One-bottle systems may be simpler but are not better; three-step systems may still be best.

5. Dentin variability remains a problem—sclerosis, tubule size, tubule location.

6. Proper clinical technique is critical to success.

7. Enamel bonding is fast, strong, and long-lasting.

8. Dentin bonding may be strong but may not be long-lasting.

5.4 Composite Restorations

A. Introduction.

1. Types.

a. Macrofilled composites.

(1) Average particle size (APS) = 10 μm.

(2) "First-generation" restorative composites.

(3) Paste-paste, chemical cure.

(4) Limited shade-matching capabilities.

(5) Poor physical and mechanical properties.

(6) Poor esthetics.

b. Microfilled composites.

(1) APS = 0.04 μm (40 nm).

(2) Light-cured.

(3) Suboptimal fracture toughness—not strong for occlusal bearing areas.

(4) Excellent esthetics and polishability.

(5) Lower elastic modulus—better in class V situations.

(6) Use primarily in anterior restorations.

c. Hybrid (midifill, minifill) composites.

(1) APS = 1 μm (0.001 mm).

(2) Light-cured.

(3) Good properties.

(4) Good esthetics but not as polishable as microfills.

(5) Universal use—anterior and posterior restorations.

d. Microhybrid composites.

(1) APS = 0.4 to 0.8 μm (500 to 800 nm).

(2) Light-cured.

(3) Retain good properties of hybrids (strength), with improved handling.

(4) Polishability almost equal to microfills.

(5) Universal use—anterior and posterior restorations.

e. Nanofilled/nanohybrid composites.

(1) Filler characteristics—vary with brand but typically 20 nm nanomers and 0.6 to 1.5 μm nanoclusters.

(2) Light-cured.

(3) Excellent handling.

(4) Highly polishable.

(5) Low shrinkage.

(6) Universal use—anterior and posterior restorations.

f. Flowable composites.

(1) High matrix/filler ratio content.

(2) Higher polymerization shrinkage.

g. Packable composites.

(1) Increased viscosity.

(2) No documented benefits.

2. Properties.

a. High coefficient of thermal expansion = percolation, recurrent caries, stain.

b. High water absorption = deterioration of material.

c. All composites undergo polymerization shrinkage.

d. Wear resistance has improved substantially with research and development.

e. Surface texture is a function of filler size (smaller = smoother) and type.

3. Clinical performance.

a. Marginal fracture—microfilled composites.

b. Bulk fracture—rare.

c. Secondary caries.

d. Wear—when used in heavy occlusal load areas.

e. Marginal leakage heavily dependent on bonding.

4. Handling—method of polymerization.

a. Auto (chemical) cured—no longer used.

b. Light-cured.

(1) Requires light source.

(2) Controlled insertion time.

(3) Less finishing time required.

(4) Less porosity.

c. Types of curing lights.

(1) Quartz/tungsten/halogen.

(2) Light-emitting diode lights are more promising light systems available today.

5. Uses.

a. Class I, II, III, IV, V, and VI preparations.

b. Sealants.

c. Esthetic enhancements.

d. Hypocalcified areas.

e. Partial veneers.

f. Full veneers.

g. Anatomic additions.

h. Resin-bonded bridges.

i. Luting agent.

j. Diastema closure.

k. Foundation.

6. Advantages.

a. Esthetics.

b. Insulation.

c. Bonding to tooth structure.

d. Conservation of tooth structure.

e. Less mechanical retention form needed.

f. Strengthening of remaining tooth structure—reinforcement of remaining tooth structure by bonding is believed to be temporary.

g. Minimal to no microleakage—decreased interfacial staining, recurrent caries, or postoperative sensitivity.

7. Disadvantages.

a. Wear potential—only when all of occlusal contact on composite.

b. Very technique-sensitive; must have dry field; difficult to do; takes more time.

c. Polymerization shrinkage—may cause contraction gaps on root surfaces between composite and root.

d. C-factor may cause sensitivity, especially in class I lesions.

8. Requirements for a successful composite restoration.

a. Etched or primed enamel and dentin and adhesive placement.

b. All occlusion should not be on composite.

c. Must not contaminate operating area.

d. Adequate technical skill of operator.

B. Restorative technique—all composite restorations are bonded in with a dental adhesive. A liner or base or both may be needed depending on the RDT, as discussed previously. When a matrix is used (class II, III, and IV), typically the liner or base is placed before matrix placement, whereas the dental adhesive is placed after matrix placement.

1. Matrix placement—a matrix primarily is used when a proximal surface is to be restored. For composites, a thin Mylar strip matrix is used for most class III and IV restorations, whereas a precontoured metal matrix (sectional or not) is used for most class II restorations.

a. Objectives of a matrix.

(1) Provide proper contact.

(2) Provide proper contour.

(3) Confine the restorative material.

(4) Reduce the amount of excess material.

b. For a matrix to be effective, it should have the following characteristics.

(1) Be easy to apply and remove.

(2) Extend below the gingival margin.

(3) Extend above the marginal ridge height in posterior restorations and the incisal edge in anterior restorations.

c. The matrix should be stabilized with a wooden wedge to close any gaps that may develop between the matrix and the gingival margin of the preparation and to provide stability to the matrix during insertion of the composite. Care should be exercised to place the wedge securely apical to the gingival margin of the preparation, not to push the matrix band into the tooth preparation area resulting in undercontour of the restoration.

2. Placing adhesive system on enamel and dentin.

a. Follow manufacturer's directions.

b. See previous section relative to adhesive systems.

3. Inserting the composite (Figure 2-27).

a. Apply matrix if not already applied.

b. Proper incremental placement is important to ensure adaptation to tooth preparation and margins and to avoid voids or gaps in between increments.

c. Insertion instruments.

(1) Composite hand instruments (plastic or metal).

(2) Syringe.

d. Use incremental portions.

(1) Light cures only to 2- to 3-mm depth in most composites and curing units.

(2) Large restorations require multiple increments.

e. Cure each increment for the time prescribed by the manufacturer (varies with composite type, shade, and opacity).

f. Use dentin and enamel shades in esthetic cases.

g. Try to develop contour on last increment as close as possible to final anatomy of the tooth. Keep excess to a minimum.

h. Remove matrix (if used).

(1) Check for voids and undercontour, and repair (add composite) if needed.

(2) Cure again from other angles.

4. Contouring and finishing the restoration—good insertion technique significantly reduces the amount of finishing required. Usually only a slight excess of material is present that must be removed to provide the final contour and smooth finish.

a. Use medium-coarse diamond instruments to remove gross excess.

b. Use fine diamond finishing instruments, 12-bladed carbide finishing burs, and abrasive finishing discs to obtain proper contour.

c. Select instrument that fits surface being contoured and finished, amount of contour needed, and desired finish level.

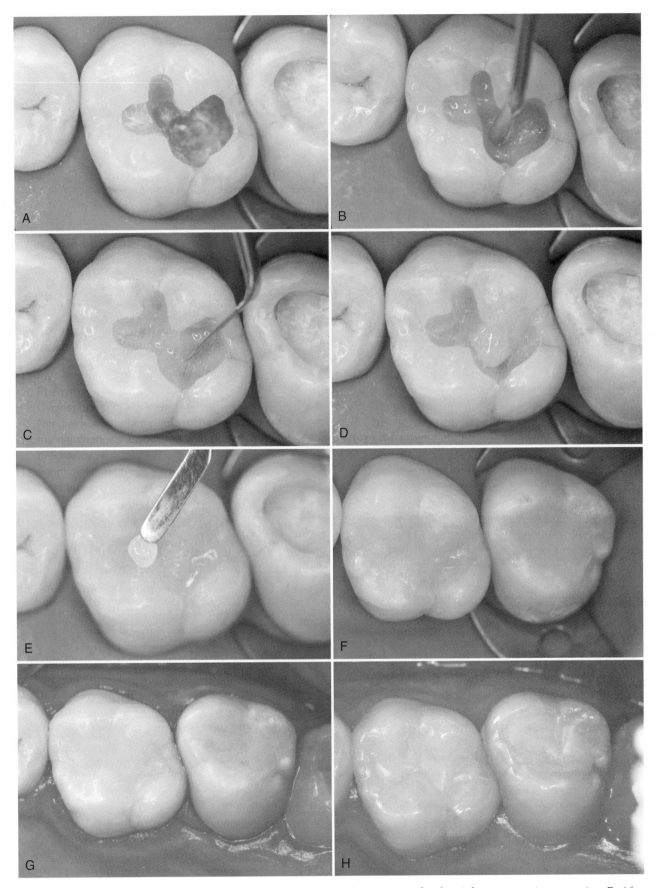

Figure 2-27 Class I composite incremental insertion. **A,** Tooth preparation for class I direct composite restoration. **B,** After resin-modified glass-ionomer base is placed, the first composite increment is inserted and light-activated. **C-F,** Composite is inserted and light-activated incrementally, using cusp inclines as anatomic references to sculpt the composite before light activation. **G,** Completed restorations. **H,** At 5-year follow-up. *(From Heymann HO, Swift EJ, Ritter AV: Sturdevant's Art and Science of Operative Dentistry, ed 6. St. Louis, Mosby, 2013.)*

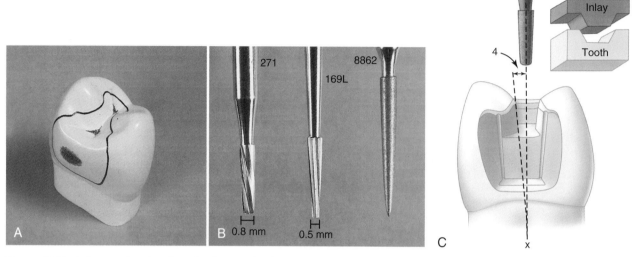

Figure 2-28 A, Proposed outline form for disto-occlusal preparation. **B,** Dimensions and configuration of No. 271, No. 169L, and No. 8862 instruments. **C,** Conventional 4-degree divergence from line of draw *(line xy). (From Heymann HO, Swift EJ, Ritter AV: Sturdevant's Art and Science of Operative Dentistry, ed 6. St. Louis, Mosby, 2013.)*

d. Flexible abrasive discs and finishing strips are suitable for convex and flat surfaces.

e. Finishing points and oval-shaped finishing burs are more suitable for concave surfaces.

f. Finishing cups can be used in both convex and concave surfaces.

g. Use medium speed with light intermittent brush strokes and air coolant for contouring and finishing.

h. Check occlusion after the rubber dam is removed, if one was used.

5.5 Gold Inlay and Onlay Restorations

A. Introduction (Figure 2-28).

1. Definition—intracoronal cast metal restorations (inlay) that cap (cover) all cusps (onlay).

2. Advantages.

a. Excellent track record.

b. Good fit.

c. Excellent method to restore occlusal relationship.

d. Structurally sound material.

3. Disadvantages.

a. Nonesthetic.

b. Complicated tooth preparation.

c. Complicated marginal finishing.

d. Need adequate laboratory support.

e. Cost.

4. Indications.

a. Large occlusal surface needs.

b. Tooth contour needs.

c. Fractures.

d. Splinting.

e. Bracing for teeth with root canal treatment.

f. Bridge retainers.

g. Partial retainers.

5. Requirements for a successful gold onlay.

a. Tooth preparation.

(1) Draw/draft (divergence to the external surface of 2 to 5 degrees per prepared wall).

(2) Removal of weakened tooth structure.

(3) Beveled finish lines.

(4) Pulpal protection.

(5) Soft tissue management.

(a) Causes of inadequate tissue management.

(i) Careless, traumatic preparation.

(ii) Poor-fitting temporary restoration.

(iii) Temporary cement irritation.

(iv) Careless use of retraction cord.

(b) Problems resulting from bleeding or unhealthy tissues.

(i) Access, vision impairment.

(ii) Impression difficulty.

(iii) Temporary fabrication difficulty.

(iv) Cementation difficulty.

b. Laboratory fabrication.

(1) Accurate impression.

(2) Appropriate waxing.

(3) Adherence to laboratory protocol.

c. Cementation.

(1) Adequate marginal finishing.

(2) Proper manipulation of luting agent.

B. Clinical procedure—tooth preparation.

1. Introduction.

a. Draw/draft.

(1) 0.2 to 5 degrees per wall.

(2) The longer the wall, the greater the amount of draw/draft.

(3) Must draw for casting to seat on tooth.

(4) More parallel = more retention.

b. Retention.

(1) Primary retention.
    (a) Draw/draft.
    (b) Length of longitudinal (vertical) walls.
(2) Secondary retention.
    (a) Retention grooves (proximally).
    (b) Skirts.
    (c) Groove extensions.
c. Objectives for beveled margins.
  (1) Good fit of gold to tooth.
  (2) Strong tooth margin.
    (a) Usually strongest enamel margin.
  (3) Burnishable gold margin.
    (a) Can bend a 30- to 50-degree gold margin.
    (b) Less than 30 degrees may be too thin and may break.
    (c) Greater than 50 degrees may be too thick and will not bend.
d. Pulp protection.
  (1) Caries removal.
  (2) Liners, bases, and build-ups.
    (a) Must be retained in preparation for impression, temporary, try-in, cementation.
2. Tooth preparation.
  a. Initial tooth preparation.
    (1) Occlusal extensions.
      (a) Cap cusps as soon as possible.
        (i) Use depth cuts.
        (ii) Removes weakened tooth structure.
        (iii) Increases access.
        (iv) Increases visibility.
      (b) Preserve noncapped cusps.
      (c) Preserve noninvolved marginal ridges.
      (d) Smooth outline form.
    (2) Wall design.
      (a) No. 271 bur.
      (b) 2- to 5-degree taper per wall.
      (c) Increased wall height increases retention.
      (d) Increased draw decreases retention.
    (3) Proximal box.
      (a) Gingival extension (to include all faults and obtain clearance with adjacent tooth).
      (b) Draw (same 2 to 5 degrees).
      (c) Facial and lingual extension (to include all faults and obtain clearance with adjacent tooth).
      (d) Cavosurface margin (30 to 40 degrees).
      (e) Blend with other bevels.
  b. Final tooth preparation.
    (1) Removing remaining caries.
    (2) Pulp protection, base, and build-up.
    (3) Secondary retention form—retention grooves, skirts, and groove extensions.
    (4) Margination and bevels.
      (a) General rules.
        (i) Use diamond (fine).
        (ii) Cut dry for final marginating for better vision.

      (b) Occlusal bevel.
        (i) 0.5-mm width.
        (ii) Want 40-degree gold margin.
        (iii) On occlusal surface.
        (iv) May not need because angulation of the facial and lingual cusps may provide for the fabrication of a 40-degree gold margin without preparation.
      (c) Groove extension bevel.
        (i) Lingual/facial groove extension.
        (ii) 0.5-mm width.
        (iii) Want 40-degree gold margin.
      (d) Cusp counterbevel.
        (i) 0.5- to 1.0-mm width.
        (ii) Want 30-degree gold margin.
        (iii) For nonesthetic capped cusps.
      (e) Stubbed margin.
        (i) 0.25- to 0.5-mm width.
        (ii) Perpendicular to long axis of crown.
        (iii) For esthetic capped cusps.
      (f) Secondary flare.
        (i) Extends facial and lingual proximal margin into facial and lingual embrasure.
        (ii) Want 40-degree gold margin.
        (iii) Diamond held perpendicular to long axis of preparation.
        (iv) Occlusogingival width is not uniform.
      (g) Collar.
        (i) Beveled shoulder design around a capped cusp.
        (ii) Provides bracing.
        (iii) Shoulder prepared with No. 271 bur.
        (iv) 0.5-mm bevel prepared with diamond.
      (h) Skirt.
        (i) Extends casting around line angle.
        (ii) Increases retention form.
        (iii) Increases resistance form.
        (iv) "Minicrown prep."
        (v) Use diamond.
        (vi) Facial and lingual finish lines result in 40-degree gold margin.
        (vii) Gingival finish line is a chamfer with a minimum depth (not uniform) of 0.5 mm and extended into the gingival one third of the crown.
      (i) Gingival bevel.
        (i) 0.5- to 1-mm width.
        (ii) Want 30-degree gold margin.
        (iii) All bevels must blend with each other.
c. View preparation from all angles (Figures 2-29 and 2-30).
  (1) Check draw.
  (2) Check reduction.
  (3) Check margin continuity.
  (4) Ensure all of fault removed.

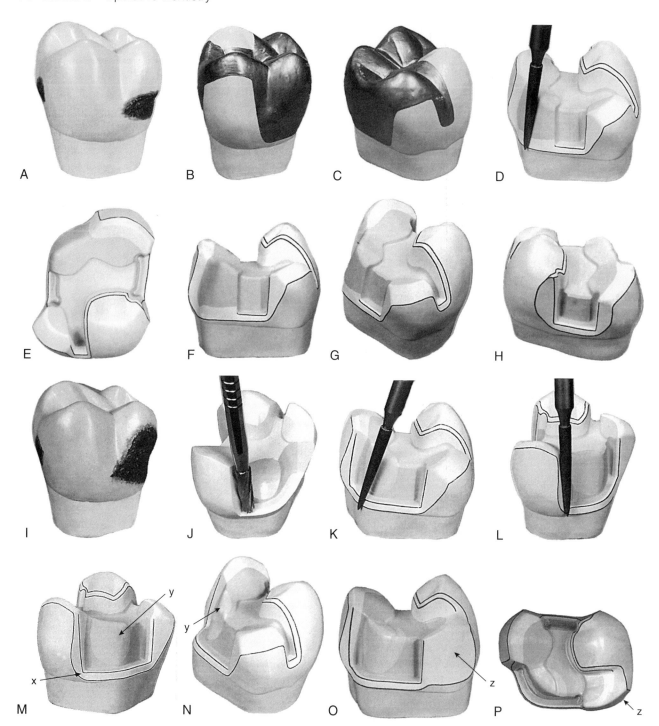

Figure 2-29 A, Maxillary molar with caries on distofacial corner and mesial surface. **B** and **C,** Completed mesio-occlusal, distofacial, and distolingual inlay for treating caries shown in **A**: facio-occlusal view (**B**) and distolinguo-occlusal view (**C**). **D-H,** Preparation for treating caries illustrated in **A**: disto-occlusal view with diamond instrument being applied (**D**), occlusal view (**E**), distal view (**F**), distolinguo-occlusal view (**G**), and mesio-occlusal view (**H**). **I,** Maxillary molar with deeper caries on distofacial corner and with mesial caries. **J,** Preparation (minus bevels and flares) for mesio-occlusal, distofacial, and distolingual inlay to restore the carious molar shown in **I**. No. 271 carbide bur is used to prepare the gingival shoulder and the vertical wall. **K** and **L,** Beveling margins. **M** and **N,** Completed preparation for treating caries shown in **I**. Gingival and facial bevels blend at *x*, and *y* is the cement base. **O** and **P,** When the lingual surface groove has not been prepared and when the facial wall of the proximal box is mostly or totally missing, forces directed to displace the inlay facially can be opposed by lingual skirt extension *(z)*. *(From Heymann HO, Swift EJ, Ritter AV: Sturdevant's Art and Science of Operative Dentistry, ed 6. St. Louis, Mosby, 2013.)*

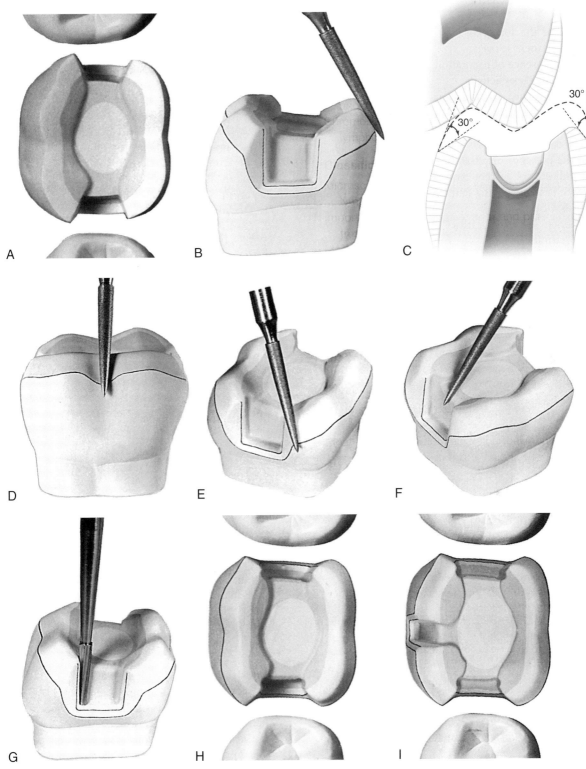

Figure 2-30 A, Caries has been removed, and the cement base has been inserted. **B,** Counterbeveling facial and lingual margins of reduced cusps. **C,** Section of **B. D,** The fissure that extends slightly gingival to the normal position of the counterbevel may be included by slightly deepening the counterbevel in the fissured area. **E,** Junctions between the counterbevels and the secondary flares are slightly rounded. **F,** Axiopulpal line angle is lightly beveled. **G,** Improving the retention form by cutting proximal grooves. **H,** Completed mesio-occlusodistal onlay preparation. **I,** Completed mesio-occlusodistofacial onlay preparation showing extension to include the facial surface groove or fissure. *(From Heymann HO, Swift EJ, Ritter AV: Sturdevant's Art and Science of Operative Dentistry, ed 6. St. Louis, Mosby, 2013.)*

Sample Questions

1. Which of the following statements regarding caries risk assessment is *true*?
   A. The presence of restorations is a good indicator of current caries activity.
   B. The presence of restorations is a good indicator of past caries activity.
   C. The presence of plaque biofilm is a good indicator of current caries activity.
   D. The presence of pit-and-fissure sealants is a good indicator of current caries activity.

2. Which of the following statements about indirect pulp caps is *false*?
   A. Some leathery caries may be left in the preparation.
   B. A liner is generally recommended in the excavation.
   C. The operator should wait at least 6 to 8 weeks before reentry (if then).
   D. The prognosis of indirect pulp cap treatment is poorer than that of direct pulp caps.

3. Smooth-surface caries refers to _____.
   A. Facial and lingual surfaces
   B. Occlusal pits and grooves
   C. Mesial and distal surfaces
   D. A and C

4. The use of the rubber dam is best indicated for _____.
   A. Adhesive procedures
   B. Quadrant dentistry
   C. Teeth with challenging preparations
   D. Difficult patients
   E. All of the above

5. For a dental hand instrument with a formula of 10-8.5-8-14, the number 10 refers to the _____.
   A. Width of the blade in tenths of a millimeter
   B. Primary cutting edge angle in centigrades
   C. Blade length in millimeters
   D. Blade angle in centigrades

6. When placement of proximal retention locks in class II amalgam preparations is necessary, which of the following statements is *not* correct?
   A. One should not undermine the proximal enamel.
   B. One should not prepare locks entirely in the axial wall.
   C. Even if deeper than ideal, one should use the axial wall as a guide for proximal lock placement.
   D. One should place locks 0.2 mm inside the DEJ to ensure that the proximal enamel is not undermined.

7. Which of the following statements about class V amalgam restorations is *not* correct?
   A. The outline form is usually kidney-shaped or crescent-shaped.
   B. Because the mesial, distal, gingival, and incisal walls of the tooth preparation are perpendicular to the external tooth surface, they usually diverge facially.
   C. Using four corner coves instead of two full-length grooves conserves dentin near the pulp and may reduce the possibility of a mechanical pulp exposure.
   D. If the outline form approaches an existing proximal restoration, it is better to leave a thin section of tooth structure between the two restorations (<1 mm) than to join the restorations.

8. In the conventional class I composite preparation, retention is achieved by which of the following features?
   1. Occlusal convergence
   2. Occlusal bevel
   3. Bonding
   4. Retention grooves
   A. 2 and 4
   B. 1 and 3
   C. 1 and 4
   D. 2 and 3

9. Many factors affect tooth/cavity preparation. Which of the following would be the *least* important factor?
   A. Extent of the defect
   B. Size of the tooth
   C. Fracture lines
   D. Extent of the old material

10. Which of the following statements about an amalgam tooth/cavity preparation is *true*?
    A. The enamel cavosurface margin angle must be 90 degrees.
    B. The cavosurface margin should provide for a 90-degree amalgam margin.
    C. All prepared walls should converge externally.
    D. Retention form for class V preparations can be placed at the DEJ.

11. Causes of postoperative sensitivity with amalgam restorations include all of the following *except* one. Which one is the *exception*?
    A. Lack of adequate condensation, especially lateral condensation in the proximal boxes
    B. Voids
    C. Extension onto the root surface
    D. Lack of dentinal sealing

12. When carving a class I amalgam restoration, which of the following statements is *false*?
    A. Carving may be made easier by waiting 1 or 2 minutes after condensation before it is started.
    B. The blade of the discoid carver should move parallel to the margins resting totally on the partially set amalgam.
    C. Deep occlusal anatomy should not be carved.
    D. The carved amalgam outline should coincide with the cavosurface margins.

13. The setting reaction of dental amalgam proceeds primarily by _____.

A. Dissolution of the entire alloy particle into mercury
B. Dissolution of the copper from the particles into mercury
C. Precipitation of tin-mercury crystals
D. Mercury reaction with silver on or in the alloy particle

14. Restoration of an appropriate proximal contact results in all of the following *except* one. Which one is the *exception*?
    A. Reduction or elimination of food impaction at the interdental papilla
    B. Provides appropriate space for the interdental papilla
    C. Provides increased retention form for the restoration
    D. Maintenance of the proper occlusal relationship

15. Major differences between etch-and-rinse (previously known as total-etch) and self-etching primer adhesive systems include all of the following *except* one. Which one is the *exception*?
    A. Time necessary to apply the materials
    B. Amount of smear layer removed
    C. Bond strengths to enamel
    D. Need for wet bonding

16. A casting may fail to seat on the prepared tooth owing to all of the following factors *except* one. Which one is the *exception*?
    A. Temporary cement still on the prepared tooth after the temporary restoration has been removed
    B. Proximal contacts of casting too heavy or too tight
    C. Undercuts present in prepared tooth
    D. The occlusal of the prepared tooth was underreduced

17. All of the following reasons are likely to indicate the need for restoration of a cervical notch *except* one. Which one is the *exception*?
    A. Patient age
    B. Esthetic concern
    C. Tooth is symptomatic
    D. Deeply notched axially

18. All of the following statements about slot-retained complex amalgams are true *except* one. Which one is the *exception*?
    A. Slots should be at least 1.5 mm in depth.
    B. Slots should be 1 mm or more in length.
    C. Slots may be segmented or continuous.
    D. Slots should be placed at least 0.5 mm inside the DEJ.

19. Which one of the following acids is generally recommended for etching tooth structure?
    A. Maleic acid
    B. Polyacrylic acid
    C. Phosphoric acid
    D. Tartaric acid
    E. Ethylenediaminetetraacetic acid

20. Triturating a dental amalgam _____.
    A. Reduces the size of the alloy particles
    B. Coats the alloy particles with mercury
    C. Reduces the crystal sizes as they form
    D. Dissolves the alloy particles in mercury

21. Which of the following materials has the highest linear coefficient of thermal expansion?
    A. Amalgam
    B. Direct gold
    C. Tooth structure
    D. Composite resin

22. A cervical lesion should be restored if it is _____.
    A. Carious
    B. Very sensitive
    C. Causing gingival inflammation
    D. All of the above

23. Compared with amalgam restoration, composite restorations are _____.
    A. Stronger
    B. More technique-sensitive
    C. More resistant to occlusal forces
    D. Not indicated for class II restorations

24. The one constant contraindication for a composite restoration is _____.
    A. Occlusal factors
    B. Inability to isolate the operating area
    C. Extension onto the root surface
    D. Class I restoration with a high C-factor

25. Which of the following statements regarding the choice between doing a composite or amalgam restoration is *true*?
    A. Establishing restored proximal contacts is easier with composite.
    B. The amalgam is more difficult and technique-sensitive.
    C. The composite generally uses a more conservative tooth/cavity preparation.
    D. Amalgam should be used for class II restorations.

26. Match each condition of tooth loss with the most closely linked type of tooth loss.

A. Mechanical wear secondary to abnormal forces (s.a. toothbrushing) ___	1. Abfraction
B. Normal tooth wear ___	2. Attrition
C. Wear secondary to chemical presence ___	3. Erosion
D. Tooth loss in the cervical area secondary to biomechanical loading ___	4. Abrasion

27. From the following list, select the reasons to consider the restoration of abraded or eroded (noncarious) cervical lesions. (Choose four.)
    A. Caries develops in the lesion.
    B. The defect is shallow and does not compromise the structural integrity of the tooth.

C. Intolerable sensitivity exists and is unresponsive to conservative desensitizing measures.

D. The defect contributes to a phonetic problem.

E. The area is to be involved in the design of a removable partial denture.

F. Teeth are endodontically treated.

G. The patient desires an esthetic improvement.

28. From the following list, select the reasons associated with replacement of existing restorations. (Choose four.)

A. Marginal ridge discrepancy that contributes to food impaction

B. Existing restoration has significant discrepancies and is a negative etiologic factor to adjacent teeth or tissue

C. Light marginal staining not compromising esthetics and judged noncarious

D. Poor proximal contour or a gingival overhang that contributes to periodontal breakdown

E. Recurrent caries that can be adequately treated by a repair restoration

F. Presence of shallow ditching around an amalgam restoration

G. For tooth-colored restorations, unacceptable esthetics

29. Match each pulpal condition with the most closely linked recommended pulp therapy.

A. Mechanical pulp exposure, noncarious (<1.0 mm) ___   1. Endodontic therapy

B. Remaining dentin thickness greater than 2.0 mm over vital pulp ___   2. No pulp therapy required

C. Carious pulp exposure (>1.0 mm) with purulent exudate ___   3. Direct pulp cap

D. Residual questionable dentin near pulp, asymptomatic tooth ___   4. Indirect pulp cap

30. Place the following steps for the application of an etch-and-rinse (total-etch) three-step dental adhesive in correct sequence.

A. Apply adhesive ___

B. Rinse etchant and leave surface wet ___

C. Complete tooth preparation ___

D. Apply two to three layers of primer ___

E. Etch enamel and dentin with phosphoric acid for 10 to 15 seconds ___

F. Light-cure ___

31. Place the following steps for a class II amalgam restoration in correct sequence.

A. Check occlusion of restoration and adjust if necessary ___

B. Place matrix and wedge ___

C. Carve amalgam material ___

D. Mix amalgam material ___

E. Complete tooth preparation ___

F. Condense amalgam material ___

32. From the following list, select the functions of skirts in gold onlay tooth preparations. (Choose two.)

A. Increase retention form

B. Provide bracing

C. Increase resistance form

D. Enhance esthetics

E. Provide pulp protection

F. Improve draw

Oral and Maxillofacial Surgery and Pain Control

LARRY L. CUNNINGHAM, JR.

PHILIP LIN

KENNETH L. REED

OUTLINE

1.0 Oral and Maxillofacial Surgery

Larry L. Cunningham, Jr., Philip Lin

This chapter reviews the basic aspects of oral and maxillofacial surgery to help prepare dental students for the National Board Dental Examination. As with the other chapters in this text, this chapter is not meant to be all-inclusive. This review is based on topics found in *Contemporary Oral and Maxillofacial Surgery* (see References). Questions that arise from the use of this review should be researched in that text and other, more in-depth references.

Outline of Review

1.1 Principles of Surgery

Many surgical techniques exist, as you have learned from your training, and these are reviewed here. All of these techniques should be used with specific principles in mind.
A. Visualization—requirements for adequate visualization.
   1. Assistance.
   2. Access.
B. Aseptic technique.
C. Incisions.
D. Flap design.
E. Tissue handling.
F. Hemostasis.

1.2 Dentoalveolar Surgery

There are many indications for the removal of teeth. Although performing a dental extraction is most often a minor surgery, it is still a surgery. Any invasive procedure requires that the practitioner have complete knowledge of the patient's history and perform a head and neck physical examination. Thorough documentation of the history and physical examination, indications for the procedure, and the patient's informed consent is the standard of care.
A. Indications for dental extractions.
   1. Severe caries—teeth that cannot be restored.
   2. Pulpal necrosis and irreversible pulpitis when endodontics is not an option.
   3. Severe periodontal disease—with irreversible bone loss and tooth mobility.
   4. Orthodontic prescriptions—commonly extracted teeth are the maxillary and mandibular first premolars and third molars.
   5. Malposed teeth—teeth that cause mucosal trauma and cannot be repositioned with orthodontics; teeth in hyperocclusion that are unopposed and interfering with other restorative care.
   6. Cracked teeth.
   7. Preprosthetic extractions—when a patient's treatment plan includes complete dentures or when certain teeth interfere with planned prosthetic treatment.
   8. Impacted teeth—teeth that will not erupt into proper occlusion.
   9. Supernumerary teeth.
   10. Teeth associated with pathology.
   11. Radiation therapy—patients needing radiation therapy for head and neck cancer should be evaluated for the health of the dentition. Questionable teeth should be extracted before radiation therapy.

B. Contraindications.
   1. Overview—there are few true contraindications to the extraction of teeth. Elective dentoalveolar surgery in extremely ill patients should be carefully considered by the practitioner. In some instances, a patient's health may be so compromised that the patient cannot withstand a surgical procedure.
   2. Examples.
      a. Severe uncontrolled metabolic diseases (brittle diabetes).
      b. End-stage renal disease.
      c. Advanced cardiac conditions (unstable angina).
      d. Leukemia and lymphoma—patients with these conditions should be treated before dental extractions.
      e. Hemophilia or platelet disorders—patients with these conditions should be treated before dental extractions.
      f. Head and neck radiation—extractions in patients with a history of head and neck radiation can lead to osteoradionecrosis. These patients commonly are treated with hyperbaric oxygen therapy before dentoalveolar surgery.
      g. Intravenous bisphosphonate treatment—patients treated with intravenous bisphosphonates (e.g., for treatment of bone malignancies or severe osteoporosis) are at increased risk of osteonecrosis of the jaw.
      h. Pericoronitis—pericoronitis is an infection of the soft tissues (cellulitis) around a partially erupted mandibular third molar. Generally, this infection should be cleared before extracting the involved tooth; antibiotics, irrigation, and removal of the maxillary third molar should be considered as part of the treatment of pericoronitis.
   3. Other relative contraindications to oral surgery are acute infectious stomatitis and malignant disease.
C. Radiographic examination.
   1. Relationship of associated vital structures.
   2. Configuration of roots.
   3. Condition of surrounding bone.
   4. Mechanical principles involved in tooth extraction.
D. Indications for surgical extractions—more difficult extractions can often be predicted from the examination or from preoperative radiographs. Surgeons should consider performing an elective surgical extraction when they perceive a possible need for excessive force to extract a tooth.
   1. Examples.
      a. After initial attempts at forceps extraction have failed.
      b. When the patient has especially dense bone.
      c. In older patients, owing to less elastic bone.
      d. Short clinical crowns with severe attrition (bruxism).
      e. Hypercementosis or widely divergent roots.
      f. Extensive decay or crown loss.
E. Surgical extractions and impactions—an impacted tooth is one that fails to erupt into the dental arch within the expected time. The tooth becomes impacted because adjacent teeth, dense overlying bone, or excessive soft tissue prevents eruption. Because impacted teeth do not erupt, they are retained for the patient's lifetime unless surgically removed. The most commonly impacted teeth are the mandibular third molars, maxillary third molars, and maxillary canines. The term *unerupted* includes both impacted teeth and teeth that are in the process of erupting. The term *embedded* is occasionally used interchangeably with the term *impacted*. Inadequate arch length is the primary reason that teeth fail to erupt. The most common teeth to become impacted are the third molars because they are the last to erupt.
   1. All impacted teeth should be considered for removal at the time of diagnosis for the following reasons.
      a. Prevention of periodontal disease in teeth adjacent to impacted teeth.
      b. Prevention of dental caries.
      c. Prevention of pericoronitis.
      d. Prevention of root resorption of adjacent teeth.
      e. Prevention of odontogenic cysts and tumors.
      f. Treatment of pain of unexplained origin.
      g. Prevention of jaw fractures.
      h. Facilitation of orthodontic treatment.
   2. Contraindications to extraction of impacted teeth.
      a. Extremes of age (preteen or asymptomatic full bony impaction in patients >35 years old).
      b. Compromised medical status.
      c. Likely damage to adjacent structures.
F. Classifications of impacted teeth.
   1. Angulation—mesioangular (least difficult), horizontal, vertical, distoangular (most difficult).
   2. Pell and Gregory classification.
      a. Relationship to anterior border of ramus.
         (1) Class 1—normal position anterior to the ramus.
         (2) Class 2—one half of the crown is within the ramus.
         (3) Class 3—entire crown is embedded within the ramus.
      b. Relationship to occlusal plane.
         (1) Class A—tooth at the same plane as other molars.
         (2) Class B—occlusal plane of third molar is between the occlusal plane and the cervical line of the second molar.
         (3) Class C—third molar is below the cervical line of the second molar.
   3. Factors relating to difficulty of extraction (Boxes 3-1 and 3-2).
G. Surgical principles.

BOX 3-1

Factors That Make Impaction Surgery Less Difficult

1. Mesioangular position
2. Pell and Gregory class 1 ramus
3. Pell and Gregory class A depth
4. Roots one third to two thirds formed*
5. Fused conical roots
6. Wide periodontal ligament*
7. Large follicle*
8. Elastic bone*
9. Separated from second molar
10. Separated from inferior alveolar nerve*
11. Soft tissue impaction

From Hupp JR, Tucker MR, Ellis E: *Contemporary Oral and Maxillofacial Surgery,* ed 6. St. Louis, Mosby, 2013.

*Present in young patients.

BOX 3-2

Factors That Make Impaction Surgery More Difficult

1. Distoangular
2. Pell and Gregory class 2 or 3 ramus
3. Pell and Gregory class B or C depth
4. Long, thin roots*
5. Divergent curved roots
6. Narrow periodontal ligament*
7. Thin follicle*
8. Dense, inelastic bone*
9. Contact with second molar
10. Close to inferior alveolar canal
11. Complete bony impaction

From Hupp JR, Tucker MR, Ellis E: *Contemporary Oral and Maxillofacial Surgery,* ed 6. St. Louis, Mosby, 2013.

*Present in older patients.

---

1. Exposure—whether removing third molars or other difficult extractions, there are several important principles for surgical extractions. The first is that the surgeon must have adequate visibility of the surgical site. There must be exposure with an adequate-sized flap. An envelope flap is most often used, but releasing incisions are common. The base (vestibular) portion of the flap should always be wider than the apex (crestal) portion of the flap to maintain adequate blood supply to the released soft tissues. Care should be taken in developing this flap for mandibular third molars. The mandible posterior to the third molar thins and diverges laterally. An incision made too far medially could damage the lingual nerve, causing numbness on that half of the tongue.

BOX 3-3

Prevention of Soft Tissue Injuries

1. Pay strict attention to the soft tissues to prevent injuries.
2. Develop adequate-sized flaps.
3. Use minimal force for retraction of soft tissue.

Modified from Hupp JR, Tucker MR, Ellis E: *Contemporary Oral and Maxillofacial Surgery,* ed 4. St. Louis, Mosby, 2003.

---

2. Bone removal—removal of bone is often needed for atraumatic extractions. It is better to remove some bone with a surgical bur than to fracture off an entire buccal cortex because of the use of too much force. The amount of bone removed is usually much greater for an impacted third molar than for a normal surgical extraction. A trough of bone on the buccal aspect of the tooth down to the cervical line should be removed initially. Additional bone removal may be required depending on the tooth position and root morphology. Care should be taken not to injure the lingual cortex of the mandible.

3. Tooth sectioning—sectioning of tooth may also be needed to avoid radical removal of mandibular bone or injury to other vital structures. The mandibular third molars frequently require sectioning of the tooth, but other teeth may also need to be sectioned to avoid fracture of the buccal alveolus. The tooth is delivered in pieces after it is sectioned.

4. Irrigation of the wound—copious irrigation is important to avoid the presence of fractured tooth or bone spicules below the soft tissue flap, which may lead to a subperiosteal abscess. Replacement of the soft tissue flaps completes the procedure (Box 3-3).

5. Complications.
   a. Tearing of the mucosal flap can be avoided by initially creating an appropriately sized incision. Any significant mucosal tears should be repaired at the end of the procedure.
   b. Puncture wounds in the palate, tongue, or other soft tissue areas are caused by the application of excessive and uncontrolled force to the instruments. These wounds are treated with pressure to stop any bleeding and are left open to heal by secondary intent. Consideration should be given to antibiotic coverage, depending on the injury.
   c. Oral-antral communications should be managed with a figure-of-eight suture over the socket, sinus precautions, antibiotics, and a nasal spray to prevent infection and keep the ostium open.
   d. Root fracture.
   e. Tooth displacement.
      (1) Maxillary molar root into the maxillary sinus.
      (2) Maxillary third molars into the infratemporal fossa.

(3) Mandibular molar roots forced into the sub-mandibular space through the buccal cortical bone.

(4) Tooth lost into the oropharynx.

(a) May result in airway obstruction.

(b) Patient should be transported to an emergency department for chest and abdominal radiographs.

f. Injury to adjacent teeth.

(1) Fracture of teeth or restorations.

(2) Luxation of adjacent teeth.

g. Alveolar process fractures and fractures of maxillary tuberosity can occur when excessive force is used to remove teeth.

h. Trauma to the inferior alveolar nerve may occur in the area of the roots of the mandibular third molars, causing numbness to the lower lip and chin. The lingual nerve travels very near the lingual cortex of the mandible adjacent to the mandibular third molars and can be affected by cortical fracture during third molar removal. This injury would cause loss of sensation and taste on that side of the tongue. Patients with numbness lasting more than 4 weeks should be referred for microneurosurgical evaluation.

i. Bleeding is an uncommon complication of dental extractions. Causes of excessive bleeding are injury to the inferior alveolar artery during extraction of a mandibular tooth (usually the third molar); a muscular arteriolar bleed from the elevation of a mucoperiosteal flap for third molar removal; or bleeding related to the patient's hemostasis. Examples of patients with altered hemostasis are patients who are taking warfarin or drugs for platelet inhibition, patients who have hemophilia or von Willebrand's disease, and patients who have chronic liver insufficiency.

j. Infections are uncommon in healthy patients. Whenever a mucoperiosteal flap is elevated for a surgical extraction, there is the possibility for a subperiosteal abscess. All surgical flaps should be irrigated liberally before suturing. Treatment for a subperiosteal abscess is drainage of the abscess and antibiotic treatment.

k. Localized osteitis (dry socket) can occur in 3% of mandibular third molar extractions but does not require antibiotics; it heals with irrigation of the socket and local treatment for pain control.

H. Alveoplasty—alveoplasty is indicated for the removal of any area that may cause difficulty in denture construction or in the patient's satisfaction with the prosthesis. An intraoral and extraoral examination of the patient should include an assessment of the existing tooth relationships, if any remain; the amount and contour of remaining bone; the quality of soft tissue overlying the primary denture-bearing area; the vestibular depth; the location of muscle attachments; the jaw relationships; and the presence of soft tissue or bony pathologic conditions. This examination should include the use of palpation, radiographs, and models of the patient. Alveoplasty can be minor and may include only the thin and sharp edges of the alveolus after tooth extraction, or it may be more aggressive and include removing undercuts and sharp edges from areas such as the mylohyoid ridge.

I. Tori removal—exostoses and palatal tori are overgrowths of bone on the lateral surfaces of the alveolar ridges or in the palate. Exostoses can grow to great sizes but are considered a variation of normal and need to be removed only when there is a need for denture or partial denture construction or because of repeated trauma to the area.

J. Soft tissue surgery—sometimes the bone is well contoured for denture or partial denture construction, but the soft tissues limit the ability to achieve appropriate thickness of denture material or interfere with appropriate fit of the prosthesis. Areas for soft tissue surgery may include the following.

1. Mandibular retromolar pad.

2. Maxillary tuberosity.

3. Excessive alveolar ridge tissue.

4. Inflammatory fibrous hyperplasia.

5. Labial and lingual frenum.

K. Reconstructive dentoalveolar surgery.

1. Implant dentistry is currently the state of the art for replacement of lost dentition. Implants are used for the replacement of one or multiple teeth and to retain complete prostheses in an overdenture fashion. Dental implants are made of titanium that osteointegrates with bone. Whether used as single tooth replacements or as an anchor for a denture, several principles are important for success of the dental implant.

a. Primary stability.

b. Quantity and quality of bone.

(1) Denser cortical bone (e.g., at the anterior mandible) has a higher implant success rate than loose cancellous bone and thin cortical bone (e.g., at the posterior maxilla).

(2) There are four types of bone quality (Figure 3-1). Regardless of implant height, types I through III bones are associated with higher implant success rates compared with type IV bone, which is mostly marrow with thin cortical bone.

c. Anatomic structures (Table 3-1).

(1) Sinus.

(2) Adjacent teeth.

(3) Inferior alveolar nerve and mental nerve.

2. When teeth have been missing for an extended time, alveolar bone resorbs, leaving a flattened and, in

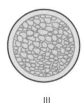

I II III IV

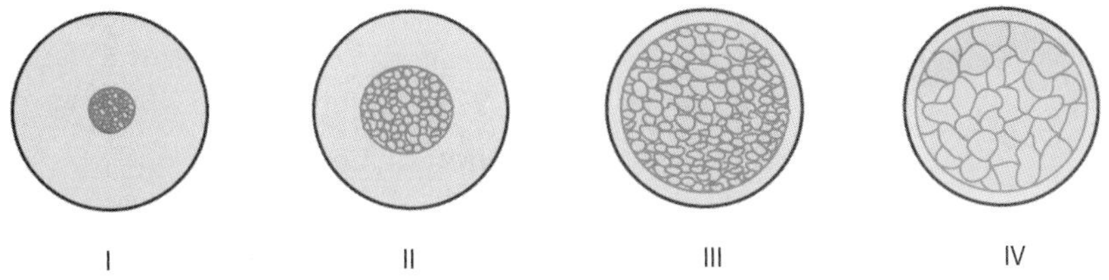

Figure 3-1 Bone types based on quantity of cortical bone and density of cancellous marrow. *(From Hupp JR, Tucker MR, Ellis E: Contemporary Oral and Maxillofacial Surgery, ed 6. St. Louis, Mosby, 2013.)*

Table 3-1	
Anatomic Limitations to Implant Placement	
STRUCTURE	**MINIMUM REQUIRED DISTANCE BETWEEN IMPLANT AND INDICATED STRUCTURE**
Buccal plate	1 mm
Lingual plate	1 mm
Maxillary sinus	1 mm
Nasal cavity	1 mm
Incisive canal	Avoid midline maxilla
Interimplant distance	3 mm between outer edge of implants
Inferior alveolar canal	2 mm from superior aspect of bony canal
Mental nerve	5 mm from anterior or bony foramen
Inferior border	1 mm
Adjacent natural tooth	1.5 mm

Modified from Peterson LJ, et al: *Contemporary Oral and Maxillofacial Surgery*, ed 4. St. Louis, Mosby, 2003.

some cases, depressed alveolar ridge that is inadequate for denture retention. This bone resorption occurs commonly in the mandibular arch, where the surface area for prosthesis retention is comparatively smaller. Alveolar ridges can be augmented for prosthesis retention in different ways.

a. Grafting of the alveolus—this can be accomplished with various grafting materials.

(1) Autogenous bone.

(a) Cortical bone can be obtained from numerous areas for reconstruction of alveolar ridges, depending on the amount of bone needed. The most common graft sites for this purpose include the following.

(i) Anterior cortex of the symphysis (when the volume of bone needed is smaller).

(ii) Lateral cortex of the ramus and external oblique ridge.

(iii) Iliac crest.

(iv) Rib.

(b) Biocompatibility is the greatest advantage of autograft. The disadvantage of autograft is the requirement of a second surgical site (i.e., the donor site).

(2) Allograft—this graft material is obtained from cadaver bone that is processed to ensure sterility and to decrease substances in the bone that can trigger host immune response. However, this process destroys the osteoinductive capability of the bone, whereas the osteoconductive property of the graft remains. Although allograft avoids the need for a second surgical site, a greater amount of the grafted material is resorbed compared with autografts.

(3) Xenograft—xenograft is acquired from a genetically different species than the recipient. Bovine bone is an example of xenograft. Xenografts and allografts have similar advantages and disadvantages, including elimination of a donor site and significant resorption after grafting.

(4) Bone morphogenetic protein (BMP)—BMP belongs to a family of proteins that can induce bone formation and enhance graft healing. Recombinant human BMP (rhBMP-2) has been used in maxillofacial skeleton reconstruction. To reconstruct a larger bony defect, BMP is sometimes combined with allograft, using the osteoinductive and osteoconductive properties from both graft materials.

b. Distraction osteogenesis (DO)—DO is a biologic process of new bone deposition and formation between osteotomized bone surfaces that are separated by gradual traction. Because DO uses the body's innate ability to generate new bone, no grafting materials are needed. This process is useful to provide height or length to bone but is less satisfactory for providing width of bone.

3. Alveolar ridge preservation (i.e., socket preservation) maintains height and width of alveolar ridge after teeth removal. The success of alveolar ridge preservation depends on atraumatic extraction without compromising buccal and lingual bone. The extraction site is thoroughly cleaned to remove debris and granulation tissues. Grafting materials such as allograft or xenograft are placed in the socket covered by resorbable collagen membrane. Resorbable sutures are used to secure grafting material and membrane, and primary closure at the surgical site is usually unnecessary.

Classification of Dentoalveolar Injuries

Crown Craze or Crack (i.e., Infraction)

Crack or incomplete fracture of the enamel without a loss of tooth structure

Horizontal or Vertical Crown Fracture

Confined to enamel
Enamel and dentin involved
Enamel, dentin, and exposed pulp involved
Horizontal or vertical
Oblique (involving the mesioincisal or distoincisal angle)

Crown-Root Fracture

No pulp involvement
Pulp involvement

Horizontal Root Fracture

Involving apical third
Involving middle third
Involving cervical third
Horizontal or vertical

Sensitivity (i.e., Concussion)

Injury to the tooth-supporting structure, resulting in sensitivity to touch or percussion but without mobility or displacement of the tooth

Mobility (i.e., Subluxation or Looseness)

Injury to the tooth-supporting structure, resulting in tooth mobility but without tooth displacement

Tooth Displacement

Intrusion (displacement of tooth into its socket—usually associated with compression fracture of socket)
Extrusion (partial displacement of tooth out of its socket—possibly no concomitant fracture of alveolar bone)
Labial displacement (alveolar wall fractures probable)
Lingual displacement (alveolar wall fractures probable)
Lateral displacement (displacement of tooth in mesial or distal direction, usually into a missing tooth space—alveolar wall fractures probable)

Avulsion

Complete displacement of tooth from its socket (may be associated with alveolar wall fractures)

Alveolar Process Fracture

Fracture of alveolar bone in the presence or absence of a tooth or teeth

From Hupp JR, Tucker MR, Ellis E: *Contemporary Oral and Maxillofacial Surgery,* ed 6. St. Louis, Mosby, 2013.

1.3 Trauma Surgery

A. Tooth fractures—classifications of tooth fractures have been well described (Box 3-4). When tooth fractures involve the pulp chamber, treatment usually includes root canal therapy. Nonrestorable teeth should be extracted. See Section 1 on Endodontics for more information.

B. Facial fractures—facial fractures require a very thorough physical examination. Signs of a bone fracture are pain, contour deformity, ecchymosis, laceration, abnormal mobility of the bone, numbness, crepitation, and hematoma. Fractures should always be considered and ruled out with a history of a motor vehicle collision, an altercation, a fall, or a sports accident.

C. Mandible fractures—mandible fractures can almost always be identified on a panoramic radiograph. Suspected fractures should always be visualized in at least two radiographs, including panoramic view, Towne's view, posterior-anterior skull view, or lateral oblique view.

1. The most common sites for the mandible to fracture are the condyle, the angle, and the symphysis. Frac-

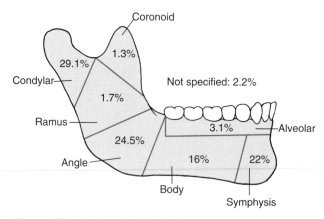

Figure 3-2 Anatomic distribution of mandibular fractures. *(From Hupp JR, Tucker MR, Ellis E: Contemporary Oral and Maxillofacial Surgery, ed 6. St. Louis, Mosby, 2013.)*

tures can be classified as greenstick, simple, comminuted, and compound (open) (Figures 3-2 and 3-3).

2. Contemporary treatment for mandible fractures that are displaced and mobile is with open reduction and internal fixation using titanium bone plates and screws. If the patient has teeth, the occlusion is used

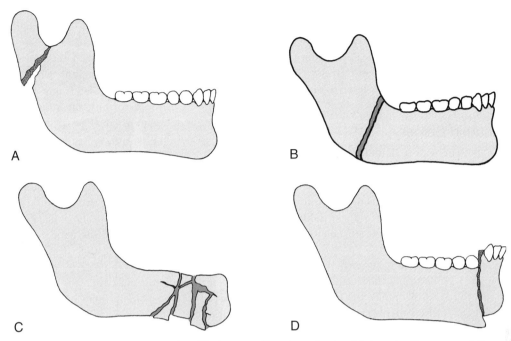

Figure 3-3 Types of mandible fractures classified according to extent of injury in the area of the fracture site. **A,** Greenstick. **B,** Simple. **C,** Comminuted. **D,** Compound. Bone would be exposed through the mucosa near teeth. *(From Hupp JR, Tucker MR, Ellis E: Contemporary Oral and Maxillofacial Surgery, ed 6. St. Louis, Mosby, 2013.)*

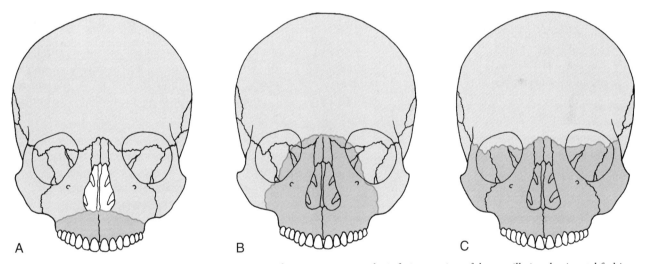

Figure 3-4 Le Fort midfacial fractures. **A,** Le Fort I fracture separating the inferior portion of the maxilla in a horizontal fashion, extending from the piriform aperture of the nose to the pterygoid maxillary suture area. **B,** Le Fort II fracture involving separation of the maxilla and nasal complex from the cranial base, zygomatic orbital rim area, and pterygoid maxillary suture area. **C,** Le Fort III fracture (i.e., craniofacial separation), which is complete separation of the midface at the level of the naso-orbital-ethmoid complex and zygomaticofrontal suture area. Fracture also extends through the orbits bilaterally. *(From Hupp JR, Tucker MR, Ellis E: Contemporary Oral and Maxillofacial Surgery, ed 6. St. Louis, Mosby, 2013.)*

to guide the surgeon during the repair of the fracture. Other methods of repair include lingual splinting (pediatric patients) and intermaxillary fixation (wiring the jaws closed).

D. Midface fractures—midface fractures are best evaluated with computed tomography (CT) scans of the face. Two orientations (axial and coronal) are needed for full evaluation of fractures of the midface, which can involve the maxilla, zygoma, nose, and orbits.

1. Maxillary fractures have been described as Le Fort levels I, II, and III (Figure 3-4). As with mandible fractures, midface fractures are described by the bone involved as simple (closed), compound (open), or comminuted.

2. Maxillary Le Fort fractures, orbital fractures, and zygomatic fractures usually require internal rigid fixation. Isolated zygomatic arch fractures can often be reduced with a minor surgical procedure and without the use of bone plates and screws. Simple nasal fractures are repaired with internal and external splints.

1.4 Orthognathic Surgery

Evaluation of a patient with a dentofacial deformity is guided by the principle of balance and symmetry. Orthognathic surgery is performed to correct severe skeletal discrepancies that prevent appropriate dental occlusion and most often is done in conjunction with orthodontics. Dental health and oral hygiene are important considerations in these patients.

A. Patients are evaluated according to normal facial proportions (Figure 3-5). Vertically, the face is divided into relatively equal thirds. Horizontally, the face is divided into relatively equal fifths. Patients can be described as having concave or convex profiles.

B. Angle classifications of occlusion are used to describe the dental arch relationships as well as the facial profile.
   1. Angle class I—normal dental occlusion with a straight (orthognathic) profile.
   2. Angle class II—mandibular first molars and canines are in a posterior position relative to the maxillary counterparts, and the face appears posteriorly convergent (retrognathic).
   3. Angle class III—mandibular first molars and canines are in an anterior position relative to the maxillary counterparts, and the face appears to be anteriorly convergent (prognathic).

C. Imaging—lateral cephalograms are the main images used in treatment planning for orthognathic surgery, although panoramic radiographs, anterior-posterior cephalograms, and periapical radiographs are taken as needed. Cephalometric analysis, when combined with facial evaluation, helps determine the jaw primarily involved in the deformity, direction of growth of the jaws, and the most ideal procedure for the patient's diagnosis (Figure 3-6).

D. Diagnosis—the primary diagnoses in patients with dentofacial deformity are maxillary hyperplasia or hypoplasia and mandibular hyperplasia or hypoplasia. Other common descriptive terms are apertognathic (anterior open bite), vertical maxillary excess (when the maxilla is too long, and the patient has an excessively gummy smile), horizontal transverse discrepancy (when the patient is in posterior crossbite), and macrogenia or microgenia (when the chin is too big or too small). Some patients may have a *cant* or a vertical asymmetry in addition to the other diagnoses.

E. Surgery—surgical treatment depends on the specific diagnosis and the facial evaluation. Generally, when a diagnosis of a deficient or excessive jaw is made, surgery is performed to correct the problem. Surgical work-up typically includes radiographs and cephalometric analysis and a prediction tracing, model surgery, and construction of an acrylic splint to be used intraoperatively.
   1. Maxillary surgery—maxillary surgeries are referred to as Le Fort I osteotomies. The maxilla can be moved forward and down more easily than it can be moved up or back. It can also be segmented into two or three pieces to position the occlusion better.

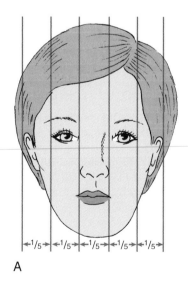

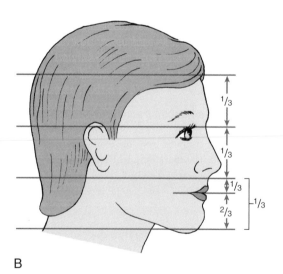

A   B

Figure 3-5 Normal facial proportions. A, Full-face view of proportional relationships. Relationships of medial intercanthal distance, alar base width, and lip proportions to remainder of facial structures are demonstrated. **B,** Normal profile proportions demonstrate relationships of upper, middle, and lower thirds of face and proportional relationships of lip and chin morphology within lower third of face. *(From Hupp JR, Tucker MR, Ellis E: Contemporary Oral and Maxillofacial Surgery, ed 6. St. Louis, Mosby, 2013.)*

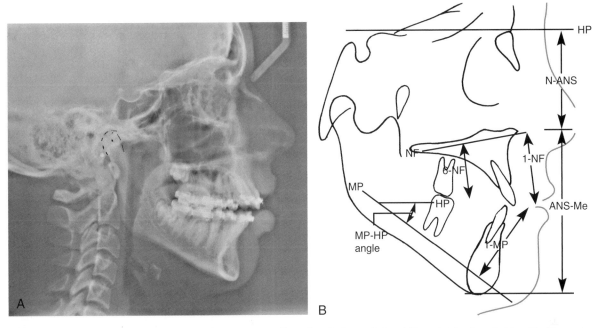

Figure 3-6 A, Lateral cephalometric radiograph. **B,** Tracing of lateral cephalometric head film, with landmarks identified for evaluating facial, skeletal, and dental abnormalities by using a system of cephalometrics for orthognathic surgery. *(A, From Hupp JR, Tucker MR, Ellis E: Contemporary Oral and Maxillofacial Surgery, ed 6. St. Louis, Mosby, 2013. B, From Burstone CJ, et al: Cephalometrics for orthognathic surgery. J Oral Surg 36:269, 1978.)*

2. Mandibular surgery—mandibular surgery is most often done using one of two osteotomies: bilateral sagittal split osteotomy (Figure 3-7) or vertical ramus osteotomy (Figure 3-8). The mandible can be moved anteriorly to correct retrognathia or posteriorly to correct prognathism. In addition, the chin can be moved using a genial osteotomy (genioplasty) to correct macrogenia or microgenia.

3. DO—with DO, oral and maxillofacial surgeons have much greater flexibility in treating difficult deformities of the facial skeleton. Patients with deformities such as cleft lip and palate and hemifacial microsomia previously required difficult surgeries. DO involves cutting an osteotomy to separate segments of bone and the application of an appliance that facilitates the gradual and incremental separation of bone segments (Figure 3-9).

1.5 Facial Pain and Neuropathology and Osteonecrosis of the Jaw

A. Overview.
1. The differential diagnosis of facial pain includes pathology of dental structures, muscles, joints, blood vessels, salivary glands, sinuses, eyes, ears, and central and peripheral nervous systems.
2. The perception of pain has physiologic and psychological aspects. For pain to be experienced from a physiologic perspective, transduction (activation of A-delta and C fibers to the spinal cord or brainstem),

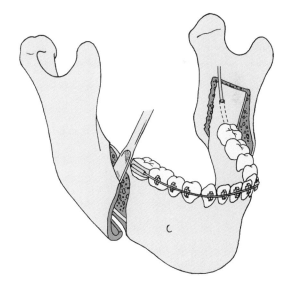

Figure 3-7 Sagittal split osteotomy. Ramus of mandible is divided by the creation of a horizontal osteotomy on the medial aspect and a vertical osteotomy on the lateral aspect of the mandible. These are connected by an anterior ramus osteotomy. The lateral cortex of the mandible is separated from the medial aspect, and the mandible is advanced or set back for correction of mandibular deficiency or excess, respectively. *(From Hupp JR, Tucker MR, Ellis E: Contemporary Oral and Maxillofacial Surgery, ed 6. St. Louis, Mosby, 2013.)*

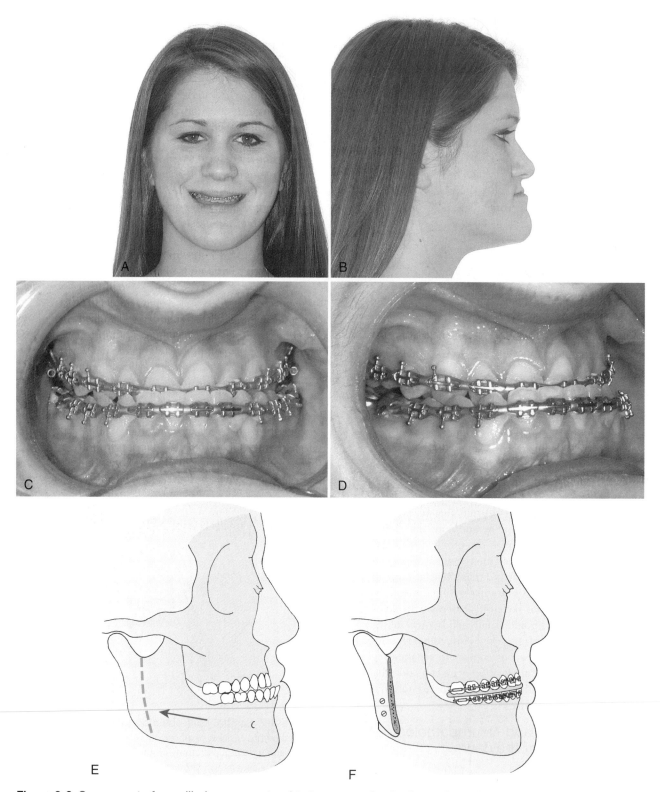

Figure 3-8 Case report of mandibular excess. **A** and **B,** Preoperative facial esthetics photos demonstrate typical features of class III malocclusion resulting from mandibular excess. **C** and **D,** Presurgical occlusal photos. **E** and **F,** Diagrams of intraoral vertical ramus osteotomy with posterior positioning of mandible and rigid fixation.

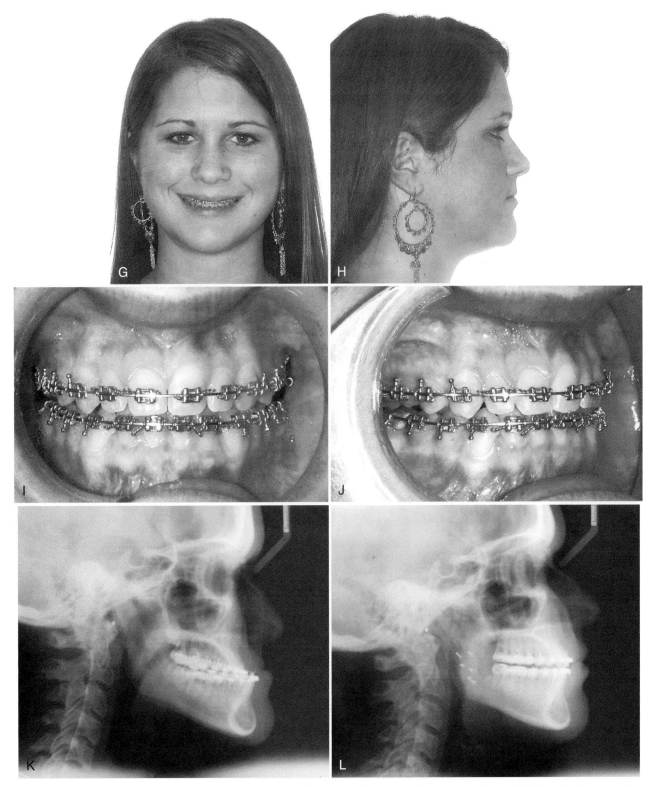

Figure 3-8, cont'd G and H, Postoperative frontal and profile views of the patient (compare with **A** and **B**). I and J, Postoperative occlusion (compare with **C** and **D**). **K** and **L**, Preoperative and postoperative radiographs. *(From Hupp JR, Tucker MR, Ellis E: Contemporary Oral and Maxillofacial Surgery, ed 6. St. Louis, Mosby, 2013.)*

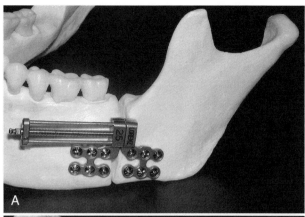

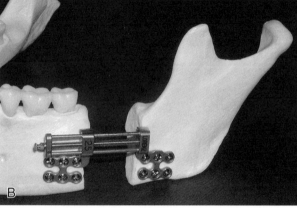

Figure 3-9 Distractor appliance used for mandibular advancement. A, Osteotomy of posterior mandibular body and ramus area with distractor in place. **B,** Distraction appliance fully expanded. Regenerated bone fills the intrabone gap during slow incremental activation of distractor that slowly separates the segments. *(From Hupp JR, Tucker MR, Ellis E: Contemporary Oral and Maxillofacial Surgery, ed 6. St. Louis, Mosby, 2013.)*

Table 3-2	
Classifications of Orofacial Pain	
PAIN TYPE	**SOURCE**
Somatic (increased stimulus yields increase in pain)	Musculoskeletal (TMJ, periodontal, muscles)
	Visceral (salivary gland, dental pulp)
Neuropathic (pain independent of stimulus intensity)	Damage to pain pathways (TN, trauma, stroke)
Psychogenic	Intrapsychic disturbance (conversion reaction, psychotic delusion, malingering)
Atypical	Facial pain of unknown cause/diagnosis pending

Data from Peterson LJ, et al: *Contemporary Oral and Maxillofacial Surgery,* ed 4. St. Louis, Mosby, 2003.

TMJ, Temporomandibular joint; *TN,* trigeminal neuralgia.

transmission (pain information in the central nervous system sent to the thalamus and cortical centers for processing of sensory and emotional aspects), and modulation (limitation of rostral flow of pain information from the spinal cord and trigeminal nucleus to higher cortical centers) must occur. The human experience of pain is the sum total of these physiologic processes and the psychological factors of higher thought and emotions (Figure 3-10).

3. When pain lasts longer than 4 to 6 months, it is defined as chronic, and the psychological aspects are especially important in patient treatment and management.

B. Classifications of orofacial pain (Table 3-2).

1. Neuropathic pain.

a. The prototypic neuropathic facial pain is trigeminal neuralgia (tic douloureux). There is classically a trigger point, and the pain typically manifests as electrical, sharp, shooting, and episodic (seconds to minutes in duration) followed by refractory periods. It is most commonly seen in patients older than 50 years. Trigeminal neuralgia is treated medically with anticonvulsant drugs (e.g., carbamazepine, oxcarbazepine, gabapentin) and surgically (microvascular decompression [Jannetta procedure], stereotactic radiosurgery, percutaneous needle rhizotomy, entry zone balloon root compression).

b. Odontalgia secondary to deafferentation (atypical odontalgia) occurs as a result of trauma or surgery (endodontic therapy or extraction). These procedures result in damage to the afferent pain transmission system. Proposed mechanisms include peripheral hyperactivity at the surgical site and central nervous system hyperactivity secondary to changes in the second-order nerve in the trigeminal nucleus.

c. Postherpetic neuralgia is a potential sequela of a herpes zoster infection. The pain is classically described as burning, aching, or electric shock–like. It is treated medically with anticonvulsants, antidepressants, or sympathetic blocks. Ramsay Hunt syndrome is a herpes zoster infection of the sensory and motor branches of cranial nerves VII and VIII resulting in facial paralysis, vertigo, deafness, and cutaneous eruption of the external auditory canal.

d. Neuromas may occur after nerve injury. The proximal section of the transected nerve (if no connection to the distal nerve fragment is present) forms sprouts filled with Schwann's cells and other neural elements. This area (neuroma) can become very sensitive to stimuli and can cause chronic neuropathic pain.

e. Burning mouth syndrome is most commonly seen in postmenopausal women. Patients complain of

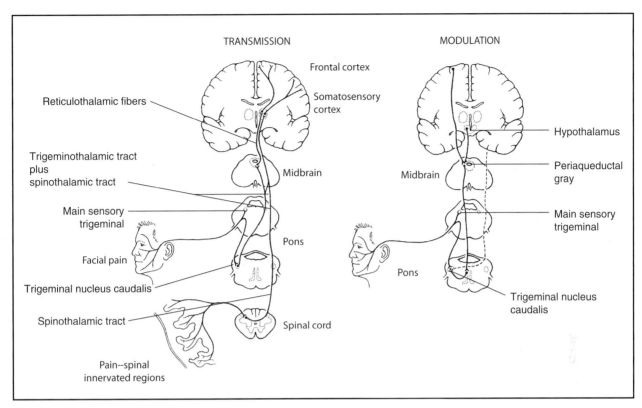

Figure 3-10 Trigeminal and spinal pain transmission pathways *(left)* and trigeminal pain modulation system *(right)*. *Dotted line* indicates decreased pain transmission. *(From Hupp JR, Tucker MR, Ellis E: Contemporary Oral and Maxillofacial Surgery, ed 6. St. Louis, Mosby, 2013.)*

pain, dryness, and burning of the mouth and tongue. They may also complain of altered taste sensation. This syndrome is believed to be secondary to a defect in pain modulation. In 50% of patients, the symptoms resolve without treatment over a 2-year period. Hormonal therapy has not been proven to be efficacious, and anticonvulsants and antidepressants have not yielded consistent results.

   f. Chronic headache is categorized as being migraine, tension type, or cluster.

   g. The presenting symptoms of temporal arteritis (giant cell arteritis) are often difficult to differentiate from other causes of jaw and head pain, and a delay in diagnosis often leads to blindness in the affected side (Table 3-3).

1.6 Temporomandibular Disorders

A. Overview—classifications of temporomandibular disorders include myofascial pain, disc displacement disorders, degenerative joint disease (DJD), systemic arthritic conditions, chronic recurrent dislocation, ankylosis, neoplasia, and infections.

B. Types.

   1. Myofascial pain disorder (MPD) is the most common cause of masticatory pain and compromised function. MPD is characterized by diffuse, poorly localized pain in the preauricular region, often involving other muscles of mastication. Pain and tenderness develop as a result of abnormal muscle function and hyperactivity. A parafunctional habit (clenching, posturing, and bruxing) may be etiologically related to this clinical entity. It can also be the result of disc displacement disorders and degenerative arthritis. Wear facets may be seen in these patients; in patients with a nocturnal parafunctional habit, symptoms are often worse in the morning.

   2. Disc displacement disorders are seen with and without reduction (the return of the normal disc-to-condyle relationship). When reduction is present, normal interincisal opening without deviation can be seen despite joint and muscle tenderness. The opening click corresponds to the condyle moving over the posterior area of the anteriorly displaced disc, resulting in reduction. The reciprocal click (closing click) occurs when the jaw is closed and the disc fails to maintain its normal reduced relationship to the condyle. Nonreduction disc displacement disorders result in limited range of motion and resultant ipsilateral deviation on opening (Figure 3-11).

   3. Systemic arthritic conditions include rheumatoid arthritis, systemic lupus erythematosus, and crystalline arthropathies including calcium pyrophosphate dihydrate deposition (pseudogout). There are usually

Table 3-3

Differential Diagnoses of Common Headaches

	TEMPORAL ARTERITIS	MIGRAINE	CLUSTER	TENSION
Onset	Acute or chronic	Acute	Acute	Chronic
Location	Localized	Unilateral (40%)	Unilateral	Global, unilateral
Associated symptoms	Weight loss, polymyalgia, rheumatic, fever, decreased vision, jaw claudication	Nausea, vomiting, photophobia, phonophobia	Rhinorrhea, lacrimation of ipsilateral side	Multisomatic complaints
Pain character	Severe throbbing over affected area	Throbbing	Sharp stabbing	Aching
Duration	Prolonged	Prolonged	30 min–2 hr	Daily
Prior history	–	+	+	+
Diagnostic test	ESR (+)	None—history	None—history	None—history
PE	Tender temporal arteries, myalgias, fever	Nausea, vomiting, photophobia, phonophobia	Unilateral, rhinorrhea, lacrimation, partial Horner's syndrome	–

From Hupp JR, Tucker MR, Ellis E: *Contemporary Oral and Maxillofacial Surgery,* ed 6. St. Louis, Mosby, 2013.

ESR, Erythrocyte sedimentation rate; *PE,* physical examination.

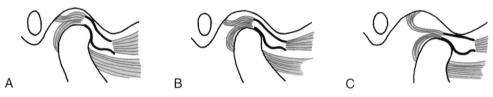

Figure 3-11 Anterior disc displacement without reduction. A, Disc that has been chronically anteriorly displaced now has an amorphous shape rather than a distinct biconcave structure. **B,** When the condyle begins to translate forward, the disc remains anterior to the condyle. **C,** In maximum open position, disc tissue continues to remain anterior to the condyle, with posterior attachment tissue interposed between the condyle and the fossa. *(From Hupp JR, Tucker MR, Ellis E: Contemporary Oral and Maxillofacial Surgery, ed 6. St. Louis, Mosby, 2013.)*

other clinical systemic signs and symptoms with these conditions.

4. Chronic recurrent dislocation occurs when the mandibular condyle translates anterior to the articular eminence and requires mechanical manipulation to achieve reduction. It is associated with pain and muscle spasm. When the problem becomes chronic (multiple recurrences), interventions include botulinum toxin A (Botox) injection of lateral pterygoids or surgery.

5. Ankylosis can occur intracapsularly or extracapsularly and can be fibrous or bony. Bony ankylosis results in more limitation of motion. Trauma is the most common cause of ankylosis; however, surgery, radiation therapy, and infection can also result in temporomandibular joint (TMJ) ankylosis. A patient with ankylosis presents with severely restricted range of motion that may be accompanied by pain. Patients are often able to demonstrate limited translation on the affected side but nonetheless have severe limitation in interincisal opening.

C. Nonsurgical therapy for TMJ dysfunction.

1. Overview—nonsurgical therapy classically includes patient education, physical therapy, pharmacotherapy, and occlusal considerations. Treatment objectives are to decrease pain symptoms and improve function. In cases of ankylosis and severe symptomatic DJD, surgery may be the preferred initial treatment of choice. For most cases of DJD, MPD, and internal derangement (reducing and nonreducing), the nonsurgical approach is preferred for initial management (Figure 3-12).

2. Counseling—parafunctional habits (e.g., nail biting) can be associated with MPD, and the patient should be counseled concerning any such habits. Stress may also be related to MPD and pain from internal derangement, and the patient should be counseled by an appropriately trained professional if indicated.

3. Medical therapy—medications used for treatment of TMJ disorders include nonsteroidal antiinflammatory drugs, steroids, narcotic and nonnarcotic analgesics, antidepressants, and muscle relaxants. The

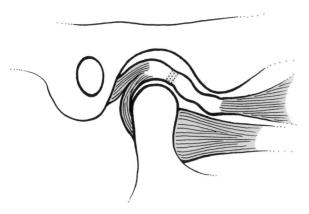

Figure 3-12 Anteriorly displaced disc results in stress on retrodiscal tissue. Subsequent fibrosis provides adaptation, producing a functional, although anatomically different, interpositional disc. *(From Hupp JR, Tucker MR, Ellis E: Contemporary Oral and Maxillofacial Surgery, ed 6. St. Louis, Mosby, 2013.)*

choice of medication should be based on the diagnosis, cause of the symptoms, and medical comorbidities associated with the individual patient.

4. Physical therapy—physical therapy modalities can be very helpful in the nonsurgical management of patients with TMJ disorders. Biofeedback, ultrasound, transcutaneous electrical nerve stimulation (TENS), massage, thermal treatment, exercise, and iontophoresis may be considered. Many of these modalities result in increased circulation to the affected region, facilitating the removal of painful metabolic by-products and delivering therapeutic medications. It is believed that TENS may override pain input or that it results in the release of endogenous endorphins.

5. Occlusion—splints usually can be classified as either autorepositioning or anterior repositioning. The autorepositioning splint is used for muscle and joint pain when no specific anatomically based pathologic entity can be identified. It is hypothesized to work by reducing intraarticular pressure. It is designed to have no working or balancing interferences with full arch contact. The anterior repositioning splint protrudes the mandible into a forward position, hypothetically recapturing the normal disc-to-condyle relationship (this has not been shown to be a valid or reliably efficacious modality). Occlusal modification may be accomplished via equilibration, prosthetic restoration, orthodontics, and orthognathic surgery. The role of occlusion in temporomandibular disorders is unclear.

6. Arthrocentesis has been shown to be beneficial in patients with internal derangement. One or two needles are placed into the superior joint space. A few milliliters of saline or lactated Ringer's solution is injected. Some surgeons advocate lavage at this time as well. It is hypothesized that the efficacy of the modality is based on distention of the joint capsule, release of adhesions, and potential for removal of chemical mediators associated with joint pathology.

D. Surgical treatments.

1. Overview—surgical treatments of the TMJ include arthrocentesis, arthroscopy, disc repositioning, disc repair or removal, condylotomy, and total joint replacement.

2. Arthroscopy involves the placement of two cannulas to allow access for intracapsular instrumentation of the superior joint space. Disc manipulation, disc release, posterior band cautery, and disc repositioning and stabilization techniques all have been described. Arthroscopy appears to be an effective modality in a select group of surgical patients and offers a potentially less morbid access to the joint.

3. Disc repositioning surgery (open arthroplasty) is used in patients with painful, persistent clicking-popping and closed lock. The disc is mobilized, and a posterior wedge may be removed, with suturing used to reposition the disc into a more anatomically desirable position. Generally, good results are seen initially, but 10% to 15% of patients report no benefit or worsening symptoms postoperatively.

4. Disc repair or removal (discectomy) is indicated when the disc is severely damaged. There is wide variation in the reported results with this procedure, ranging from excellent resolution to severe degeneration and associated pain and dysfunction. When the disc is removed, recommendations for replacement have been made. Some prosthetic materials have proven to be problematic, so there is a tendency to favor autogenous materials. Preferred tissues include temporalis muscle and fascia, fat, and auricular cartilage.

5. Condylotomy is accomplished by performing an intraoral vertical ramus osteotomy. The proximal segment is not fixated; this theoretically allows the soft tissues to reposition the condyle and disc passively into a more functionally neutral position. This technique has been described for treatment of internal derangement with and without reduction, DJD, and chronic dislocation.

6. Total joint replacement is indicated for severely pathologic joints, as is seen in rheumatoid arthritis, severe DJD, ankylosis, neoplasia, and posttraumatic destruction. Costochondral bone graft reconstruction is the most common autogenous material used. However, this material does not address fossa pathology, which may be significant and must be addressed in pathologic joints associated with the use of some prosthetic materials. Total prosthetic joint reconstructions usually involve a prosthetic condyle and fossa. Results with this technique have been variable and may reflect the complexity and diversity of the cases studied.

1.7 Odontogenic Infections

A. Pathophysiology—the microbiology of odontogenic infections represents the flora of the head and neck, mouth, teeth, and gingiva. These infections are polymicrobial. The most common organisms are aerobic gram-positive cocci, anaerobic gram-positive cocci, and anaerobic gram-negative rods (Tables 3-4 and 3-5).

B. Organisms—the pathologic mechanism by which these complex infections develop has been well described. The highly virulent aerobic *Streptococcus* species initiate the infectious process after inoculation into deep tissues. Cellulitis occurs, followed by proliferation of anaerobic organisms. The aerobic organisms consume oxygen, making the microenvironment favorable for the anaerobes.

C. Progression—the natural history of the progression of odontogenic infections relates to their origin as either pulp necrosis and periapical abscess or periodontal infections. Once the infection is into deep tissues, it follows the path of least resistance. It may travel through the intramedullary space or perforate through a thin area of bone cortex and directly enter an anatomic space. The most common space involved is the vestibular space. These often drain spontaneously and result in an asymptomatic, chronic draining fistula.

D. Fascial spaces—fascial spaces (Table 3-6) involved in odontogenic infections commonly include the vestibular, buccal, canine, sublingual, submandibular, submental, masticator (pterygomandibular, masseteric, superficial temporal, deep temporal), and lateral pharyngeal spaces. They are referred to as *potential spaces* because under healthy conditions there is no space; abscess formation causes cavities along these anatomic planes. These spaces are contiguous; as the abscess matures and spreads, more of these spaces become involved, resulting in increased pain, trismus, dysphagia, and dysphonia. Canine space infections and deep temporal space infections can result in cavernous sinus thrombosis via the ophthalmic veins. Lateral pharyngeal infections can traverse the retropharyngeal and prevertebral spaces and spread into the mediastinum. All of these infections should be considered life-threatening medical emergencies (Figures 3-13 to 3-17).

E. Treatment principles—treatment of odontogenic infections requires adherence to six principles.
 1. Determine the severity of infection through history and physical examination. The history should specify

Table 3-4

Role of Anaerobic Bacteria in Odontogenic Infection

	%
Anaerobic only	50
Mixed anaerobic and aerobic	44
Aerobic only	6

Data from Brook I, Frazier EH, Gher ME: *Aerobic and anaerobic microbiology of periapical abscess.* Oral Microbiol Immunol 6:123-125, 1991. IN Hupp JR, Tucker MR, Ellis E: *Contemporary Oral and Maxillofacial Surgery,* ed 6. St. Louis, Mosby, 2013.

Table 3-5

Major Pathogens in Odontogenic Infections

	PERCENT OF CASES	
MICROORGANISM	**SAKAMOTO ET AL (1998)**	**HEIMDAHL ET AL (1985)**
Streptococcus milleri group	65	31
Peptostreptococcus species	65	31
Other anaerobic streptococci	9	38
Prevotella species (e.g., *P. oralis* and *P. buccae*)	74	35
Porphyromonas species (e.g., *P. gingivalis*)	17	—
Fusobacterium species	52	45

From Hupp JR, Tucker MR, Ellis E: *Contemporary Oral and Maxillofacial Surgery,* ed 6. St. Louis, Mosby, 2013.

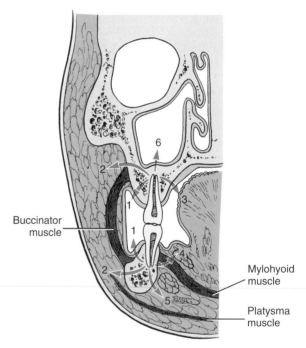

Figure 3-13 As infection erodes through bone, it can express itself in various places, depending on the thickness of overlying bone and the relationship of muscle attachments to the site of perforation. Six possible locations are illustrated: vestibular abscess *(1)*, buccal space *(2)*, palatal abscess *(3)*, sublingual space *(4)*, submandibular space *(5)*, and maxillary sinus *(6)*. *(From Cummings CW, et al: Otolaryngology: Head and Neck Surgery, ed 3, vol 4. St. Louis, Mosby, 2006.)*

Table 3-6

Borders of the Deep Fascial Spaces of the Head and Neck

SPACE	ANTERIOR	POSTERIOR	SUPERIOR	INFERIOR	SUPERFICIAL OR MEDIAL*	DEEP OR LATERAL†
Buccal	Corner of mouth	Masseter muscle Pterygomandibular space	Maxilla Infraorbital space	Mandible	Subcutaneous tissue and skin	Buccinator muscle
Infraorbital	Nasal cartilages	Buccal space	Quadratus labii superioris muscle	Oral mucosa	Quadratus labii superioris muscle	Levator anguli oris muscle Maxilla
Submandibular	Anterior belly digastric muscle	Posterior belly digastric muscle Stylohyoid muscle Stylopharyngeus muscle	Inferior and medial surfaces of mandible	Digastric tendon	Platysma muscle Investing fascia	Mylohyoid muscle Hyoglossal muscle Superior constrictor muscles
Submental	Inferior border of mandible	Hyoid bone	Mylohyoid muscle	Investing fascia	Investing fascia	Anterior bellies of digastric muscles†
Sublingual	Lingual surface of mandible	Submandibular space	Oral mucosa	Mylohyoid muscle	Muscles of tongue*	Lingual surface of mandible†
Pterygomandibular	Buccal space	Parotid gland	Lateral pterygoid muscle	Inferior border of mandible	Medial pterygoid muscle*	Ascending ramus of mandible†
Submasseteric	Buccal space	Parotid gland	Zygomatic arch	Inferior border of mandible	Ascending ramus of mandible*	Masseter muscle†
Lateral pharyngeal	Superior and middle pharyngeal constrictors	Carotid sheath and scalene fascia	Skull base	Hyoid bone	Pharyngeal constrictors and retropharyngeal space*	Medial pterygoid muscle†
Retropharyngeal	Superior and middle pharyngeal constrictor muscles	Alar fascia	Skull base	Fusion of alar and prevertebral fasciae at C6–T4		Carotid sheath and lateral pharyngeal space†
Pretracheal	Sternothyroid-thyrohyoid fascia	Retropharyngeal space	Hyoid cartilage	Superior mediastinum	Sternothyroid-thyrohyoid fascia	Visceral fascia over trachea and thyroid gland

From Flynn TR: *Anatomy of oral and maxillofacial infections.* IN Topazian RG, Goldberg MH, Hupp JR, editors: Oral and Maxillofacial Infections, ed. 4, Philadelphia, 2002, WB Saunders.

*Medial border.

†Lateral border.

a chief complaint and determine time and circumstances of onset, duration of symptoms, speed of progression, and critical systemic symptoms (e.g., dysphagia, dysphonia, trismus, fever, chills, malaise, numbness of face, headache, meningeal signs, altered vision). The physical examination should include vital signs to determine evidence of sepsis, airway compromise, probable cause, and specific anatomic space involvement.

2. Evaluate the state of the patient's host defense mechanisms with a thorough history and physical examination. Certain metabolic diseases (e.g., diabetes),

Figure 3-14 A, Buccal space lies between the buccinator muscle and the overlying skin and superficial fascia. This potential space may become involved via maxillary or mandibular molars *(arrows).* **B,** Typical buccal space infection, extending from the level of the zygomatic arch to the inferior border of the mandible and from the oral commissure to the anterior border of the masseter muscle. *(From Flynn TR: The swollen face. Emerg Med Clin North Am 15:481-519, 2000.)*

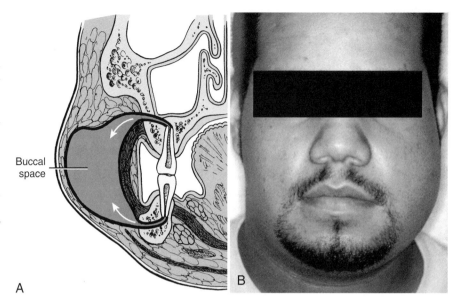

Buccal space

A

B

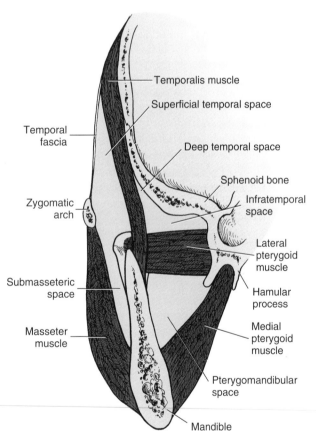

Temporalis muscle

Superficial temporal space

Temporal fascia

Deep temporal space

Sphenoid bone

Infratemporal space

Zygomatic arch

Lateral pterygoid muscle

Hamular process

Submasseteric space

Medial pterygoid muscle

Masseter muscle

Pterygomandibular space

Mandible

Figure 3-15 The masticator space is bounded by the fascia overlying the masseter muscle, the medial pterygoid muscle, the temporalis muscle, and the skull. The superficial and deep temporal spaces are separated from each other by the temporalis muscle. The lateral pterygoid muscle divides the pterygomandibular space from the infratemporal portion of the deep temporal space, and the zygomatic arch divides the submasseteric space from the superficial temporal space. *(Redrawn from Cummings CW, et al: Otolaryngology: Head and Neck Surgery, ed 3, vol 4. St. Louis, Mosby, 2006.)*

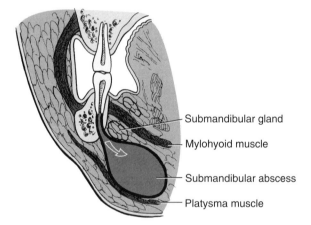

Submandibular gland

Mylohyoid muscle

Submandibular abscess

Platysma muscle

Figure 3-16 The submandibular space lies between the mylohyoid muscle and anterior layer of the deep cervical fascia, just deep to the platysma muscle, and includes the lingual and inferior surfaces of the mandible below the mylohyoid muscle attachment. *(From Cummings CW, et al: Otolaryngology: Head and Neck Surgery, ed 3, vol 4. St. Louis, Mosby, 2006.)*

malnutrition, obesity, and drug use may increase or disguise the severity of these infections (Box 3-5).

3. Determine whether the patient should be treated by a general dentist or a specialist. Some odontogenic infections are life-threatening and require aggressive medical and surgical intervention. However, most can be treated with minor surgical procedures and commonly used antibiotics (Box 3-6).

4. Treating the infection surgically is fundamental in the management of odontogenic infections. Removal of the source of infection and decompression and drainage of purulence are the goals of surgery.

   a. Surgical interventions may vary in spectrum from pulpotomy to transfacial incision and drainage of multiple fascial spaces.

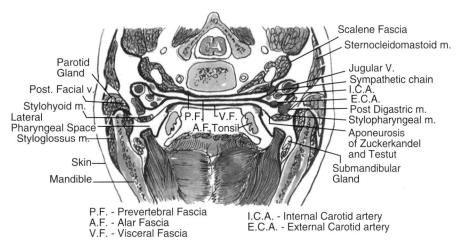

P.F. - Prevertebral Fascia
A.F. - Alar Fascia
V.F. - Visceral Fascia

I.C.A. - Internal Carotid artery
E.C.A. - External Carotid artery

Figure 3-17 The lateral pharyngeal space is located between the medial pterygoid muscle laterally and the superior pharyngeal constrictor medially. The retropharyngeal and danger spaces lie between the pharyngeal constrictor muscles and the prevertebral fascia. The retropharyngeal space lies between the superior constrictor muscle and the alar fascia. The danger space lies between the alar layer and the prevertebral fascia. *(From Flynn TR: Anatomy and surgery of deep fascial space infections. In Kelly JJ, editor: Oral and Maxillofacial Surgery Knowledge Update 1994. Rosemont, IL: American Association of Oral and Maxillofacial Surgeons, 1994.)*

Compromised Host Defenses

Uncontrolled Metabolic Diseases

Poorly controlled diabetes
Alcoholism
Malnutrition
End-stage renal disease

Immune System–Suppressing Diseases

HIV/AIDS
Lymphomas and leukemias
Other malignancies
Congenital and acquired immunologic diseases

Immunosuppressive Therapies

Cancer chemotherapy
Corticosteroids
Organ transplantation

From Hupp JR, Tucker MR, Ellis E: *Contemporary Oral and Maxillofacial Surgery,* ed 6. St. Louis, Mosby, 2013.

Criteria for Referral to an Oral-Maxillofacial Surgeon

- Difficulty breathing
- Difficulty swallowing
- Dehydration
- Moderate to severe trismus (interincisal opening <20 mm)
- Swelling extending beyond the alveolar process
- Elevated temperature (>101°F)
- Severe malaise and toxic appearance
- Compromised host defenses
- Need for general anesthesia
- Failed prior treatment

From Hupp JR, Tucker MR, Ellis E: *Contemporary Oral and Maxillofacial Surgery,* ed 6. St. Louis, Mosby, 2013.

---

b. The goal is to obtain adequate drainage so that the spread of infection can be brought under control and the offending agent can be treated with either extraction or endodontic or periodontal management.

c. Before incision and drainage, a specimen for culture and sensitivity should be obtained. Ideally, the specimen is obtained before the initiation of antibiotics. It can be done under local or general anesthesia, depending on the severity of the infection.

d. Usually at least 2 mL of purulent aspirate is adequate and can be obtained with the use of a 5- to 10-mL syringe and an 18-gauge needle. The site of aspiration should be surgically prepared before obtaining the sample.

e. Depending on the microbiology laboratory policy, the specimen either should be capped with a rubber stopper after the removal of any evidence of air in the specimen or should be immediately placed into an anaerobic specimen tube and sent without delay to the laboratory for processing.

f. Gram stains also should be obtained to guide antibiotic management.

5. Support the patient medically with adequate airway management, hydration and electrolytes, antibiotic

Box 3-7

Indications for Culture and Antibiotic Sensitivity Testing

- Infection spreading beyond the alveolar process
- Rapidly progressive infection
- Previous therapy with multiple antibiotics
- Nonresponsive infection (after >48 hours)
- Recurrent infection
- Compromised host defenses

From Hupp JR, Tucker MR, Ellis E: *Contemporary Oral and Maxillofacial Surgery,* ed 6. St. Louis, Mosby, 2013.

Box 3-8

Bone Vascularity Factors

- Radiation therapy
- Osteoporosis
- Osteopetrosis
- Paget's disease of bone
- Fibrous dysplasia
- Bone malignancy
- Bone necrosis (heavy metals, bisphosphonates)

From Hupp JR, Tucker MR, Ellis E: *Contemporary Oral and Maxillofacial Surgery,* ed 4. St. Louis, Mosby, 2003.

management, nutritional considerations, analgesics, and identification of medical comorbidities and their possible role in the infection.

6. Choose and prescribe appropriate antibiotics. The use of antibiotics has benefits and risks. Consequently, the *determination that there is a need* must first be established. Generally, if there is evidence of bacterial invasion into underlying tissues that is greater than host defenses can resist, antibiotics should be used. The clinical presentation of bacterial invasion can vary substantially based on previously mentioned host defense capacities. The following criteria have been recommended as indications for antibiotic use (Box 3-7).

7. Odontogenic infection.
   a. Bacterial targets—because the causative bacteria seen in odontogenic infections are highly predictable, *routine empiric therapy is acceptable.* The choice should be effective against streptococci and oral anaerobes.
   b. Antibiotics—penicillin V is often the preferred drug. If the patient is penicillin-allergic, clindamycin and clarithromycin are good choices. *Narrow-spectrum antibiotics are preferable over broad-spectrum antibiotics* because they are less likely to alter the normal flora with associated symptoms and impact on development of resistant strains. The selected antibiotic should have the *lowest incidence of toxicity and side effects; bactericidal agents are preferred to bacteriostatic* (particularly in immunocompromised hosts), and responsible use must take into consideration the *cost of the selected agent.*

8. Osteomyelitis.
   a. Definition—osteomyelitis means inflammation of the medullary portion of bone.
   b. Progression—infection, inflammation, and ischemia are the mechanisms by which osteomyelitis spreads until surgical and medical interventions can bring the process under control. The most common initiating causes are odontogenic infections and trauma, and they follow a contiguous path. The infection usually begins in the medullary space involving the cancellous bone. The cortical bone, periosteum, and soft adjacent tissues eventually become involved.
   c. Occurrence—osteomyelitis is relatively rare and is more commonly seen in the mandible than in the maxilla secondary to the difference in blood supply. Hematogenous spread of infection to bone can also result in osteomyelitis; however, this mechanism is rarely seen in the jaw. Patients with host defense suppression are more likely to get osteomyelitis (see Box 3-5).

F. Microbiology—the causative bacteria in osteomyelitis are similar to the bacteria that cause odontogenic infections (streptococci, anaerobic cocci, and gram-negative rods). Treatment of osteomyelitis is medical and surgical. Adequate débridement, use of appropriate antibiotics, and medical assessment to rule out and treat any host factors that may predispose the patient to developing osteomyelitis all play a part in the proper management of this complex infection.

1.8 Bisphosphonate-Related Osteonecrosis of the Jaws

A. Overview—bisphosphonate medications inhibit osteoclast activities, resulting in decreased bone resorption. They also affect osteoblast activities, which indirectly influences osteoclasts. Because of their effectiveness, bisphosphonates have been used in treating bony diseases such as multiple myeloma, Paget's disease of bone, and metastatic diseases. However, increasing evidence has demonstrated postoperative complications associated with bisphosphonate use, including chronic bony exposure that does not heal and spontaneous exposure of alveolar bones. This process is known as bisphosphonate-related osteonecrosis of the jaws (BRONJ).

Box 3-9

Stage-Specific BRONJ Treatment Recommendations

At risk category	• No surgical or medical treatment indicated
	• Patient education and routine dental care
Stage 1	• Antibacterial mouth rinse
	• Clinical Follow-up on a quarterly basis
	• Patient education and review of indications for continues bisphosphonate therapy
Stage 2	• Oral antibacterial mouth rinse
	• Symptomatic treatment with oral antibiotics and pain medication
	• Only superficial débridements to relieve soft tissue irritation
Stage 3	• Antibacterial mouth rinse
	• Antibiotic therapy and pain control
	• Surgical debridement or resection for longer term palliation of infection and pain

From Fonseca RJ: Oral and maxillofacial surgery, 2e, Saunders, St. Louis, 2009.

B. Diagnosis—the criteria for diagnosis of BRONJ include nonhealing bony exposure in jaws for at least 8 weeks and current or previous bisphosphonate use without history of radiation therapy to the jaws.

C. Oral versus intravenous bisphosphonates—oral bisphosphonates have been used to manage milder bony diseases such as osteoporosis, whereas intravenous bisphosphonates have been effective in treating bone metastases and hypercalcemia resulting from malignancy. BRONJ has a greater association with intravenous bisphosphonate use than with oral therapy.

D. Patient management—owing to insufficient scientific data, current recommendations for BRONJ management are based on expert opinions. Before initiating bisphosphonate therapy, patients should have a thorough dental evaluation and plan to extract teeth that are nonrestorable or with guarded prognosis, to remove tori, and to perform alveoloplasty. The goal is to reduce factors that can initiate BRONJ. When possible, bisphosphonate therapy should be delayed to allow adequate healing time after oral surgery, usually about 2 to 3 weeks.

1. Duration of bisphosphonate therapy—the risk of BRONJ is increased as duration of bisphosphonate therapy exceeds 3 years. No treatment adjustments are needed for patients who take oral bisphosphonates less than 3 years and who have no comorbid risk factors. A 3-month drug holiday is recommended for patients taking oral bisphosphonates for longer than 3 years. To prevent dental problems that eventually require oral surgery, it is important to emphasize good oral hygiene with patients who have a recent history of bisphosphonate use or who are currently receiving bisphosphonate therapy. If possible, surgeries and dental implant placement should be avoided, and endodontic treatments should be considered before extractions.

2. Stage-dependent treatment recommendations for patients with BRONJ—BRONJ is separated into stages, and treatments are modified based on the severity of each stage (Box 3-9).

1.9 Biopsies

A. Overview—four types of biopsies are cytology, aspiration, incisional, and excisional. The indications vary based on history, anatomy, differential diagnosis, and morbidities in the specific clinical setting.

B. Biopsy techniques.

1. Overview—soft tissue biopsy techniques and principles conform to standard surgical principles. Block anesthesia is preferable because injection into the lesion from which the biopsy specimen will be taken can distort the architecture and sometimes make diagnosis difficult. Tissue stabilization is necessary so that accurate surgical incisions can be made. Hemostasis is important so that high-volume suction is not needed.

a. Suction—a gauze-wrapped suction tip on a low-volume suction device has been recommended to avoid the possibility of aspirating the biopsy specimen into the evacuation device.

b. Incision—the incision is preferably done with a sharp scalpel because it is less damaging to the specimen and adjacent soft tissue. With this technique, margins are most clearly defined, and the anatomic architecture of the lesion has the least chance of being altered.

c. Laser—a carbon dioxide laser in the super-pulsed mode with a small, focused beam is acceptable when concerns for homeostasis are significant; however, a fine peripheral zone of necrosis does occur.

d. Handling and tagging—the tissue specimen must be handled with care to avoid mechanical trauma that can render the specimen nondiagnostic. A traction suture can help with this issue. If a malignancy is suspected, a tissue tag (identification of surgical margin) should be used to help identify the orientation of the specimen. If a margin is found to be positive, further resection can be appropriately directed. Proper specimen care requires that the tissue be placed in 10% formalin in a volume 20 times that of the specimen.

e. Wound management—wound management requires either a primary closure (if possible) or placement of periodontal dressings in cases of gingival or palatal biopsies in which secondary healing would be necessary.

f. Records—a biopsy data sheet should be accurately filled out, including pertinent history and clinical findings. Margin markers should be noted, illustrations used when needed, and radiographs or clinical photos included when warranted. It is the dentist's responsibility to understand the nature and implications of the diagnosis. If the histopathologic diagnosis is inconsistent with the clinical diagnosis, this must be reconciled before further surgical intervention. Further discussion with the pathologists, additional biopsy specimens, or second opinions from an expert in oral and maxillofacial pathology may be required.

2. Oral brush cytology.

a. Uses—detecting cancerous and precancerous lesions. It may be useful for monitoring or screening lesions in an adjunctive role to observation.

b. Method—the cytology brush is placed over the suspicious lesion and rotated 5 to 10 times to obtain cells from all three epithelial layers. The collected cells are transferred to a glass slide where a fixative is placed. When the specimen is dried, it is sent to a laboratory for computer and human analysis. One of three categories is assigned to the cellular specimen: negative, positive (definitive evidence of cellular atypia or carcinoma), or atypical (abnormal epithelium). All positive and atypical findings should undergo definitive scalpel biopsy.

3. Aspiration biopsy or fine-needle aspiration.

a. Method—a technique that uses a special syringe and needle to collect cells from a clinically or radiographically identified mass.

b. Uses—relatively low morbidity and high diagnostic accuracy for most lesions. Other uses of aspiration techniques include simple aspiration of a hard or soft tissue lesion to determine if the lesion is solid, cystic, or vascular. This use of aspiration is indicated in any intraosseous lesion before surgical exploration.

4. Incisional biopsy is a technique used when a lesion is large (>1 cm), polymorphic, suspicious for malignancy, or in an anatomic area with high morbidity. The specimen must be obtained in a representative area of the lesion, avoiding areas of necrosis, with adequate depth to make a definitive histologic diagnosis.

5. Excisional biopsy is used on smaller lesions (<1 cm) that appear benign and on small vascular and pigmented lesions. It entails the removal of the entire lesion and a perimeter of surrounding uninvolved tissue (margin).

6. Hard tissue or intraosseous biopsy techniques and principles.

a. Origin—most intraosseous lesions are of odontogenic origin, usually inflammatory. When this is not the case, biopsy is usually indicated unless the history suggests otherwise.

b. Method—a good history and physical examination are imperative before treatment. Hard tissue biopsies follow the same surgical principles as soft tissue lesions; however, there are some special considerations secondary to anatomic issues. All radiolucent lesions that require biopsy should be aspirated first. Aspiration provides the dentist with valuable information regarding the nature of the lesion (i.e., solid, cystic, fluid-filled, air-filled, vascular). It helps determine whether further studies are needed (e.g., arteriogram) or whether surgery should proceed (e.g., for a fluid-filled cyst).

c. Flaps—mucoperiosteal flaps are always used for intraosseous lesions and should be full thickness, over sound bone allowing 4- to 5-mm margins, and avoid major neurovascular structures.

d. Osseous windows.

(1) Osseous windows may be necessary for central lesions of the jaw and are determined by size of the lesion, cortical perforations, and proximity to teeth and neurovascular structures.

(2) The bony structure should be identified for the pathologist and submitted for histopathologic examination with the underlying specimen.

(3) Specimen removal depends on whether the biopsy is excisional or incisional. In the case of excisional biopsy, care should be taken to remove the specimen thoroughly while paying attention to the anatomy of adjacent teeth and neurovascular structures.

(4) After the lesion is removed, 1 mm of adjacent osseous tissue should be removed by curettage in all directions. In an incisional biopsy, the desired section of specimen is removed, and the wound is closed after irrigation. Specimen care is similar to care of soft tissue biopsy specimens.

1.10 Surgical Management of Cysts and Tumors

A. Overview—goals of surgical management are eradication of the pathologic entity and esthetic functional rehabilitation. For this to occur, issues that affect final reconstruction and return to function must be taken into consideration at the initiation of treatment. Things to consider are patient expectations and physical and emotional tolerances, methods and indications for grafting, soft tissue management, dental rehabilitation, and strength and range-of-motion rehabilitation. Considerations for nerve preservation are predicated on the anatomy and cell type and biologic characteristics of the lesion.

B. Cysts and cystlike lesions can be classified as fissural or odontogenic. Odontogenic keratocysts tend to act more aggressively and have higher rates of recurrence than fissural cysts and cysts of odontogenic inflammatory origin. Cysts of the jaw are treated by enucleation, marsupialization, a staged combination of enucleation and marsupialization, or enucleation and curettage (Table 3-7).

C. Tumors of the jaws.
1. Overview—jaw tumors vary in their natural history, origin, duration, and clinical behavior. Depending on these factors, taking into consideration the anatomic location and size, enucleation and curettage or resection may be an option. Categories of resection are marginal, partial thickness, total, and composite. Table 3-8 summarizes in general terms the primary treatment modalities for tumors of the jaw based on histologic criteria.
2. Malignant tumors.
   a. Most common are epidermoid carcinomas (squamous cell).
   b. The salivary glands, blood vessels, lymphatics, muscle, bone, and other connective tissue can also give rise to primary malignancies of the head and neck.
   c. Cancer of the breast, prostate, lung, kidney, thyroid, hematopoietic system, and colon can metastasize to the head and neck region.
   d. When a primary cancer of the head and neck is diagnosed, clinical staging should be performed before definitive treatment. Staging may include (in addition to a thorough history and physical examination) CT scans, positron emission tomography scans, chest radiographs, and panendoscopies.
   e. Combinations of surgery, radiation therapy, and chemotherapy are used for treating this class of disease.
   f. Decisions for treatment of head and neck malignancies are driven by histologic type, stage, location, and whether it is a primary or metastatic lesion. In addition, before any definitive treatment, the patient's wishes and medical comorbidities must be taken into consideration.
3. Reconstruction.
   a. The decision to reconstruct after jaw resection is ideally made before definitive surgery as part of a comprehensive treatment plan that takes into account patient expectations, medical comorbidities, prognosis, and the functional and esthetic considerations based on the anatomic deformity.
   b. Treatment options range from no reconstruction with wound management and secondary healing (possible removable prosthetic use) to complex microvascular osteocutaneous reconstruction with placement of endosseous implants.
   c. The timing of the reconstruction varies among medical centers.

Table 3-7

Treatment of Cysts of the Jaws

TECHNIQUE	DESCRIPTION	INDICATIONS	PROS/CONS
Enucleations	Shelling out without rupture	Treatment of choice should be used when it can safely be done without sacrificing adjacent structures	Often definitive treatment, easier postoperative wound care/may weaken jaw, damage structure
Marsupialization	Surgical window decompression evacuation	When enucleation would damage adjacent structures. Morphology of lesion makes enucleation unlikely to be successful	Simple and may spare vital structure/difficult wound care, pathologic tissue is left
Staged enucleation and marsupialization	1st-degree marsupialization/ 2nd-degree enucleation	See above if cyst is not totally obliterated after marsupialization heals	See above
Enucleation and curettage	Shelling out without rupture, followed by 1- to 2-mm curettage of adjacent bone	Odontogenic keratocysts. Any cyst that recurs after enucleation	May recur, more destructive to adjacent structures

Data from Peterson LJ, et al: *Contemporary Oral and Maxillofacial Surgery,* ed 4. St. Louis, Mosby, 2003.

Table 3-8

Types of Jaw Tumors and Primary Treatment Modalities

ENUCLEATION OR CURETTAGE OR BOTH	MARGINAL OR PARTIAL RESECTION	COMPOSITE RESECTION*
Odontogenic Tumors		
Odontoma	Ameloblastoma	Malignant ameloblastoma
Ameloblastic fibroma ameloblastic fibro-odontoma	Calcifying epithelial odontogenic tumor	Ameloblastic fibrosarcoma
		Ameloblastic odontosarcoma
Adenomatoid odontogenic tumor	Myxoma	Primary intraosseous carcinoma
Calcifying odontogenic cyst	Ameloblastic odontoma	
Cementoblastoma	Squamous odontogenic tumor	
Central cementifying fibroma		
Fibro-osseous Lesions		
Central ossifying fibroma	Benign chondroblastoma	Fibrosarcoma
Fibrous dysplasia (if necessary)		Osteosarcoma
Cherubism (if necessary)		Chondrosarcoma
Central giant cell granuloma		Ewing's sarcoma
Aneurysmal bone cyst		
Osteoma		
Osteoid osteoma		
Osteoblastoma		
Other Lesions		
Hemangioma	Hemangioma	Lymphomas
Eosinophilic granuloma		Intraosseous salivary gland malignancies
Neurilemoma		
Neurofibroma		Neurofibrosarcoma
Pigmented neuroectodermal tumor		Carcinoma that has invaded jaw

From Hupp JR, Tucker MR, Ellis E: *Contemporary Oral and Maxillofacial Surgery,* ed 6. St. Louis, Mosby, 2013.

Note: These are generalities. Treatment is individualized for each patient and each lesion.

*These lesions are malignancies and may be treated variably. For lesions totally within the jaw, partial resection may be performed without adjacent soft tissue and lymph node dissections. Radiotherapy and chemotherapy may also play a role in overall therapy.

d. Cases involving reconstruction are complex and benefit from a multidisciplinary team approach from the time of definitive treatment through reconstruction.

2.0 Local Anesthesia

Kenneth L. Reed

Outline of Review

2.1 Local Anesthetic Drug Overview
2.2 Local Anesthesia Techniques

2.1 Local Anesthetic Drug Overview

A. Selected pharmacology of local anesthetics (see Section 8 on Pharmacology for further details).
  1. Definition—a local anesthetic is a drug that reversibly blocks the conduction of nerve impulses when applied locally in a concentration without toxic effects. We are concerned with sensory nerves dentally; however, local anesthetics also block motor nerves if the concentration is sufficient.

B. Pharmacodynamics of local anesthetics (block sodium channels).
  1. Differential nerve blockade (concept of critical length).
    a. In 1942, Takeuchi and Tasaki reported that complete anesthesia occurs when three consecutive nodes of Ranvier are blocked (assuming myelinated nerves), and this finding continues to be reported in dental textbooks today. This principle of "critical length" also applies to unmyelinated nerves.
    b. Studies have demonstrated that anesthetic blockade can be cumulative along the axon length, resulting in a gradual reduction in conduction velocity that eventually leads to a complete

blockade. Increasing the length of the nerve exposed to the local anesthetic may increase the success of clinical anesthesia. This finding might suggest that if an inferior alveolar nerve block fails, the clinician may wish to perform a second injection via the Gow-Gates technique because this would lead to an increase in the length of inferior alveolar nerve bathed in local anesthetic.

  c. All nerves are susceptible to blockade, regardless of their function.

   (1) Motor and sensory.

  d. Sensations disappear and reappear in a definite order.

   (1) Pain.

   (2) Temperature.

   (3) Touch.

   (4) Pressure.

C. Pharmacokinetics of local anesthetics (see Section 8 on Pharmacology).

 1. Redistribution is affected by the following.

  a. Diffusion away from the site of action.

  b. Vascularity of the injection site.

   (1) Increased blood flow—shorter duration of action.

  c. Protein binding characteristics of the local anesthetic that are directly related to lipid solubility.

   (1) Increased protein binding—increased lipid solubility (increased duration of action).

 2. Principles.

  a. Duration of action of local anesthetics is directly proportional to protein binding and lipid solubility.

  b. The lower the pK_a of the drug (closer to physiologic pH), the faster the onset of action.

D. Systemic toxicities.

 1. Initial clinical signs and symptoms.

  a. Mild to moderate toxicity.

   (1) Talkativeness, apprehension, excitability, slurred speech, dizziness, and disorientation.

  b. Severe toxicity.

   (1) Seizures, respiratory depression, coma, death.

 2. Allergic responses.

  a. Esters have a high incidence (approximately 5% of the population).

  b. Amides have a low incidence (<1% of the population).

  c. Note: an allergy to a local anesthetic packaged in a dental cartridge before 1985 may have been due to an allergy to methylparaben, not the local anesthetic agent itself. For patients allergic to esters and amides, diphenhydramine (Benadryl) may be an alternative choice; however, the package insert for diphenhydramine specifically warns against this.

  d. Metabisulfite.

   (1) An antioxidant, not a preservative, with a low incidence of allergenicity.

   (2) Protects the vasoconstrictor from oxidation.

   (3) Present only in local anesthetic cartridges with a vasopressor (epinephrine or levonordefrin).

 3. Methemoglobinemia.

  a. Essentially unique to prilocaine when exceeding 600 mg (for a 70-kg adult), but a lower dose applies in a patient with hereditary methemoglobinemia. The second most common local anesthetic to cause this is articaine.

E. Potency.

 1. Potency and clinical efficacy are separate issues.

  a. When used for inferior alveolar nerve blocks, all local anesthetics have been demonstrated to have equal efficacy; there is no one local anesthetic that has been shown to be superior.

  b. All local anesthetic manufacturers have adjusted the concentration of their drugs such that 1 mL of drug "A" is equivalent to 1 mL of drug "B" with respect to potency (and toxicity).

  c. For two drugs that reach the same therapeutic effect per volume, a drug in 1 mg/mL is more potent than a drug in 2 mg/mL.

  d. Bupivacaine is the most potent local anesthetic packaged for dentistry, and prilocaine and articaine are the least potent.

F. Addition of vasoconstrictors (see Section 8 on Pharmacology).

 1. Primary rationale.

  a. Increase the duration of effect.

 2. Secondary rationales.

  a. Reduce systemic toxicity by decreasing the rate of systemic absorption of a given dose of local anesthetic.

  b. Reduce bleeding by decreasing blood flow into the operative area.

   (1) This applies to infiltration into the local area— *not* epinephrine used in a nerve block (given distant from the site).

 3. Drug interactions.

  a. Antidepressants—tricyclic (e.g., amitriptyline [Elavil]) and newer atypical drugs (e.g., duloxetine [Cymbalta]).

   (1) Increased sensitivity to epinephrine.

  b. Nonspecific β blockers—propranolol (Inderal).

   (1) Enhance peripheral α_1-adrenergic effects with β_2 blockade (unopposed α).

    (a) β blockade decreases heart rate.

    (b) Epinephrine increases blood pressure.

    (c) The net result is likely to be an increase in blood pressure without tachycardia.

  c. Normal, healthy (American Society of Anesthesiologists [ASA] 1) patient.

   (1) Maximum of 200 μg of epinephrine.

  d. Patients with cardiovascular compromise or patients taking tricyclic or atypical antidepressants or nonselective β blockers.

(1) Limit epinephrine to no more than 40 μg per appointment.

G. Pregnancy and lactation.
  1. Pregnancy class C drugs—articaine, bupivacaine, mepivacaine, epinephrine.
  2. Pregnancy class B—lidocaine, prilocaine.

H. Pediatrics.
  1. If safety of a local anesthetic is based on the number of milliliters that may be administered to a pediatric patient of a given size, 2% lidocaine with 1:100,000 epinephrine is the safest local anesthetic for use in children.
  2. Bupivacaine is not approved by the U.S. Food and Drug Administration for use in children younger than 12 years.
  3. The maximum recommended doses of local anesthetics for adults are as follows.

Drug	pK_a	Maximum Recommended Dose (mg/kg)*	Maximum Total Dose (mg)*
Articaine (4%)	7.7	7	—
Bupivacaine (0.5%)	8.1	—	90
Lidocaine (2%)	7.7	7†	500†
Mepivacaine (2%, 3%)	7.6	6.6	400
Prilocaine (4%)	7.8	8	600

*Lower of the two values.

†Based on combination with 1:100,000 epinephrine.

2.2 Local Anesthesia Techniques

A. Needle dimensions.
  1. Length—short needles average 20 mm and long needles average 32 mm.
  2. Outside diameter.
    a. 30-gauge averages 0.3 mm.
    b. 27-gauge averages 0.4 mm.
    c. 25-gauge averages 0.5 mm.
  3. Needle gauge.
    a. Positive aspiration is directly correlated to needle gauge.
    b. Larger gauge needles do not deflect as often.
    c. Larger gauge needles do not break as often. (There have been hundreds of lawsuits that have gone to court concerning needle breakage. About 97% of needle breaks have involved breakage of a 30-gauge needle.)
    d. Patients cannot tell the difference between 25-gauge, 27-gauge, and 30-gauge needles.

B. Posterior superior alveolar nerve block.
  1. Area of anesthesia—from the maxillary third molar anteriorly to the maxillary first molar with the possible exception of the mesiobuccal aspect of the maxillary first molar. This injection does not anesthetize palatal tissue.

2. Technique—position of the needle.
    a. Distal to the malar process.
    b. At 45 degrees to the mesiodistal plane.
    c. At 45 degrees to the buccolingual plane.
    d. With a 15- to 16-mm depth of penetration.
    e. Deposit 1.0 mL of local anesthetic (cartridge volume = 1.8 mL) slowly after aspiration.

C. True anterior superior alveolar nerve block.
  1. Area of anesthesia—from the midline of the maxilla to the mesiobuccal aspect of the maxillary first molar.
    a. Anesthetizes the anterior superior alveolar, middle superior alveolar, inferior palpebral, lateral nasal, and superior labial nerves.
    b. Does not anesthetize palatal tissue.
  2. The entrance to the infraorbital foramen is located just inferior to the infraorbital rim at the infraorbital notch along an imaginary line from the pupil of the eye to the ipsilateral commissure of the lip.
    a. Needle penetration is over the maxillary first premolar.
    b. Needle penetration is in the long axis of the tooth, 15 mm deep and lateral to or at the height of the buccal vestibule.
    c. The needle touches bone as an endpoint.
    d. After aspiration, 0.9 mL (½ cartridge) of anesthetic is injected slowly.
      (1) Note: 2a-d describes the infraorbital nerve block, which guarantees only anesthesia of the soft tissue. To convert the infraorbital nerve block to the true anterior superior alveolar nerve block that guarantees anesthesia of the pulps of teeth, add the next step.
    e. Pressure applied for 2 minutes (by the clock).

D. Greater palatine.
  1. Area of anesthesia—on the palate from the canine distally to the posterior aspect of the hard palate and from the gingival margin to the midline.
  2. The greater palatine foramen is generally located roughly halfway between the gingival margin and midline of the palate and approximately 5 mm anterior to the junction of hard and soft palate.
  3. Technique.
    a. Topical anesthesia.
    b. Pressure anesthesia—20 seconds minimum.
    c. Angulation of needle insertion is immaterial.
    d. Depth of penetration: to bone (generally about 5 mm).
    e. Inject 0.5 mL (approximately ⅓ cartridge) after aspiration.

E. Nasopalatine.
  1. Area of anesthesia—palatal soft tissue from canine to canine, bilaterally (the premaxilla).
  2. Technique.
    a. Topical anesthesia.
    b. Pressure anesthesia—20 seconds minimum.

c. Needle tip at a 45-degree angle to the palatal soft tissue; penetration is at the junction of the palate and incisive papilla.

d. Endpoint—bone.

e. Inject 0.5 mL after aspiration.

F. Local anesthesia—mandibular techniques.

1. Mental or incisive.

a. Area of anesthesia (mental nerve block)—soft tissue on the buccal of the premolars anteriorly to the midline lip, chin, periosteum, and bone in the affected area.

b. Topical anesthesia.

c. Insert needle in the depth of the buccal vestibule opposite the mandibular premolars.

d. 5-mm depth of insertion.

e. Deposit 0.9 mL (½ cartridge) local anesthetic.

(1) Note: 1a-e describes the mental nerve block, which guarantees only anesthesia of the soft tissue. To convert the mental nerve block to the incisive nerve block that guarantees anesthesia of the pulps of teeth, add the next stay.

f. Pressure for 2 minutes.

2. Inferior alveolar nerve block.

a. Area of anesthesia—pulps and buccal soft tissues of the mandibular teeth (except the area innervated by the buccal nerve), lip, chin, periosteum, and bone in the affected area.

b. Traditional (Halstead) block.

c. Approach from the contralateral premolars.

(1) 1.0 cm above the mandibular occlusal plane and parallel to it.

(2) With a needle endpoint 50% of the mesiodistal length of the ramus, distally.

d. *Alternatively*, higher mandibular block.

(1) Approach from the contralateral premolars.

(a) 1.5 cm above the mandibular occlusal plane and parallel to it.

(b) With a needle endpoint 60% of the mesiodistal length of the ramus, distally.

e. With either block.

(1) Advance a 25-gauge long needle until you hit bone (required).

(a) Withdraw 1 mm.

(b) Aspirate.

(c) Inject 1.5 mL (approximately ¾ of a cartridge) of local anesthetic over 2 minutes.

(d) Withdraw the needle halfway (approximately 10 to 15 mm).

(e) Aspirate.

(f) Slowly inject the lingual nerve.

(g) Save a few drops of anesthetic for the buccinator (long buccal) nerve if needed.

3. Vazirani-Akinosi technique.

a. First described in the literature in 1960 by Vazirani and again by Akinosi in 1977.

b. Anesthesia.

(1) Inferior alveolar.

(2) Lingual.

(3) Long buccal.

c. Useful for treating for the following.

(1) Uncooperative children.

(2) Patients with trismus.

d. Technique.

(1) A long needle is inserted parallel to the maxillary occlusal plane at the level of the maxillary buccal vestibule.

(a) Note: the original technique recommended at the level of the maxillary mucogingival junction.

(2) The depth of penetration is approximately one half the mesiodistal length of the ramus.

(a) About 25 mm in adults.

(b) Proportionately less in children.

(3) This endpoint is just superior to the lingula.

(4) The injection is performed blindly because no bony endpoint exists.

(5) In adult patients, a rule of thumb is that at the depth of needle penetration, the hub of the needle should be between the maxillary first and second molars.

4. Gow-Gates technique.

a. First described in the literature in 1973.

b. Originally the technique involved only extraoral landmarks.

c. Anesthesia.

(1) Inferior alveolar.

(2) Lingual.

(3) Auriculotemporal.

(4) Mylohyoid nerve.

(5) Long buccal (75% of the time).

d. Technique.

(1) Have the patient open the mouth as widely as possible to rotate and translate the condyle forward.

(2) The condyle is palpated with the fingers of the nondominant hand while the cheek is retracted with the thumb.

(3) Beginning from the contralateral canine, the needle is positioned so that a puncture point is made approximately at the location of the distobuccal cusp of the maxillary second molar.

(a) The needle is inserted slowly to a depth of 25 to 30 mm until bone is contacted.

(b) The injection must not be performed unless bone is contacted.

(c) The needle is withdrawn slightly, and the entire cartridge of local anesthetic solution is injected after aspiration.

(d) This injection is unique among intraoral injections because the operator does not attempt to get as close as possible to the nerve to be anesthetized.

    (e) The needle tip should be approximately 1.0 cm directly superior to the nerve, in the superior aspect of the pterygomandibular space.

References

Hupp JR, Tucker MR, Ellis E: *Contemporary Oral and Maxillofacial Surgery*, ed 6. St. Louis, Mosby, 2013.

Larsen P, Ghali GE, Waite P: *Peterson's Principles of Oral and Maxillofacial Surgery*, ed 3. Shelton, CT: People's Medical Publishing House, 2012.

Peterson LJ, et al: *Contemporary Oral and Maxillofacial Surgery*, ed 4. St. Louis, Mosby, 2003.

Sample Questions

1. Which of the following does *not* represent a fascial space for the spread of infection?
   A. Superficial temporal space
   B. Pterygomandibular space
   C. Masseteric space
   D. Rhinosoteric space
   E. Submental space

2. Which of the following classifications of impacted teeth must always involve both bone removal and sectioning during the surgical procedure?
   A. Mesioangular impaction
   B. Horizontal impaction
   C. Vertical impaction
   D. A and B only
   E. A, B, and C

3. Which of the following does *not* represent a possible finding of severe infection?
   A. Trismus
   B. Drooling
   C. Difficult or painful swallowing
   D. Swelling and induration with elevation of the tongue
   E. Temperature of 99° F

4. You are performing a 5-year follow-up on a 43-year-old patient with an implant. When comparing radiographs, you estimate that there has been almost 0.1 mm loss of bone height around the implant since it was placed. Which of the following is indicated?
   A. Removal of the implant and replacement with a larger size implant
   B. Removal of the implant to allow healing before another one can be placed 4 months later
   C. Remaking the prosthetic crown because of tangential forces on the implant
   D. The implant is doing well; this amount of bone loss is considered acceptable

5. On evaluation of an immediate postoperative panoramic film of a dental implant replacing tooth #30, you measure a distance of 1.5 mm from the apex of the implant to the inferior alveolar nerve canal. This is a titanium implant in an otherwise healthy patient. Which of the following actions is indicated?
   A. Proceed with immediate loading of the implant
   B. Continue but perform a two-stage procedure only
   C. Back the implant out approximately 0.5 mm to ensure a safe distance from the nerve
   D. Remove the implant and plan a repeat surgery after 4 months of healing

6. Myofascial pain dysfunction may be described as _____.
   A. Masticatory pain and limited function
   B. Clicking and popping of the joint
   C. An infectious process
   D. Dislocation of the disc

7. A 21-year-old man is referred for an orthognathic surgery consultation. After routine examination and review of radiographs, you note the following problem list: class III skeletal facial deformity with a negative overjet of 6 mm and significant maxillary crowding, missing left mandibular first molar owing to dental decay with multiple other early carious lesions, and calculus on the lingual surfaces of teeth #22 through #27 with gingival inflammation. Which of the following is the *most* appropriate order in which this patient's oral health needs should be sequenced?
   A. Definitive crown and bridge therapy, orthodontics to relieve crowding and to coordinate arches, caries management, surgery to correct the skeletal discrepancy, and periodontal therapy to control gingival inflammation
   B. Caries management, orthodontics to relieve crowding and to coordinate arches, definitive crown and bridge therapy, periodontal therapy to control gingival inflammation, and surgery to correct the skeletal discrepancy
   C. Periodontal therapy to control gingival inflammation, definitive crown and bridge therapy, orthodontics to relieve crowding and to coordinate arches, surgery to correct the skeletal discrepancy, and caries management
   D. Periodontal therapy to control gingival inflammation, caries management, orthodontics to relieve crowding and to coordinate arches, surgery to correct the skeletal discrepancy, and definitive crown and bridge therapy

8. Systemic effects of obstructive sleep apnea syndrome include all of the following *except* one. Which one is the *exception*?
   A. Hypertension
   B. Cor pulmonale
   C. Aortic aneurysm
   D. Cardiac arrhythmia

9. Which of the following is *not* a vital part of the physical examination for patients with TMJ complaints?
   A. Soft tissue symmetry
   B. Joint tenderness and sounds
   C. Soft palate length
   D. Range of motion of the mandible
   E. Teeth

10. Which of the following is considered the highest and most severe classification of maxillary fracture?
    A. Le Fort I
    B. Le Fort II
    C. Le Fort III
    D. Le Fort IV

11. Which of the following is *not* a relative contraindication for routine elective oral surgery?
    A. Unstable cardiac angina
    B. History of head and neck radiation
    C. Chronic sinusitis
    D. Hemophilia

12. Which of the following statements regarding temporomandibular disorders is true?
    A. The primary treatment for most patients with facial pain is TMJ surgery.
    B. Disc displacement without reduction can cause a decrease in interincisal opening.
    C. Myofascial pain is commonly related to parafunctional habits but not commonly related to stress.
    D. Systemic arthritic conditions do not affect the TMJ because it is not a weight-bearing joint.

13. Select from the following list correct applications and indications of antibiotic use in odontogenic infections. (Choose three.)
    A. Antibiotic should cover *Staphylococcus aureus* and aerobes
    B. β-Lactam antibiotics (e.g., penicillin V) are preferred
    C. No antibiotic coverage is indicated for patients with high-grade fever
    D. Clindamycin can be used if a patient is allergic to penicillin
    E. Broad-spectrum instead of narrow-spectrum antibiotic coverage is preferred
    F. Bactericidal agents are preferred to bacteriostatic agents in immunocompromised patients

14. Select from the following list factors that make surgical removal of impacted third molars more difficult. (Choose three.)
    A. Distoangular positioned third molar
    B. Mesioangular positioned third molar
    C. Narrow periodontal ligament
    D. Tooth roots are one half to one third formed
    E. Close proximity to inferior alveolar nerve
    F. Fused conical roots

15. For each clinical condition listed, select the most appropriate biopsy methods from the list provided.

   A. Soft tissue lesion is 0.5 cm in size __
   B. Osteomyelitis of the jaw __
   C. Soft tissue lesion is 4 cm in size __
   D. Cystic or vascular soft tissue lesions deep to mucosa __

   1. Excisional biopsy
   2. Incisional biopsy
   3. Aspiration or fine-needle biopsy
   4. Hard or tissue or intraosseous biopsy

16. Of the following anesthetics, which one is the least appropriate and which one is the most appropriate local anesthetic for use in children? (Choose two.)
    A. Articaine
    B. Bupivacaine
    C. Lidocaine
    D. Mepivacaine
    E. Prilocaine

17. Most injectable local anesthetics used in dentistry today are _____.
    A. Esters
    B. Amides
    C. Hybrids of both esters and amides
    D. None of the above

18. Which of the following local anesthetics is marketed for dentistry in the United States in more than one concentration?
    A. Articaine
    B. Bupivacaine
    C. Lidocaine
    D. Mepivacaine

19. The major factor determining whether aspiration can be reliably performed is the _____.
    A. Needle gauge
    B. Needle length
    C. Injection performed
    D. Patient

20. The _____ injection is recommended for palatal soft tissue anesthesia from canine to canine bilaterally in the maxilla.
    A. Posterior superior alveolar
    B. Inferior alveolar
    C. Long buccal
    D. Nasopalatine

21. Which of the following local anesthetics has the lowest pK_a?
    A. Lidocaine
    B. Prilocaine
    C. Mepivacaine
    D. Bupivacaine

22. Assuming a 1.8 mL-cartridge, three cartridges of 2% lidocaine with 1:100,000 epinephrine contain _____ lidocaine.
    A. 36 mg
    B. 54 mg
    C. 54 μg
    D. 108 mg

23. Which nerve block anesthetizes the distobuccal aspect of the mandibular first molar?
    A. Posterior superior alveolar
    B. Middle superior alveolar
    C. Anterior superior alveolar
    D. Inferior alveolar

24. Which of the following is the longest acting local anesthetic?
    A. Mepivacaine
    B. Lidocaine
    C. Prilocaine
    D. Bupivacaine

25. For a patient with a history of very significant liver disease, which of the following would be the safest local anesthetic?
    A. Articaine
    B. Prilocaine
    C. Lidocaine
    D. Bupivacaine

26. Which of the following injections has the highest degree of failure?
    A. Posterior superior alveolar
    B. Lingual

C. Nasopalatine
D. Inferior alveolar

27. Which of the following are possible reasons why some local anesthetic preparations have a longer duration of action than others? (Choose all that apply.)
    A. Presence of a vasoconstrictor
    B. Percent protein binding
    C. Degree of lipid solubility
    D. pK_a of the drug
    E. pH of the preparation
    F. Concentration of the local anesthetic solution as marketed

28. Which of the following apply to articaine? (Choose all that apply.)
    A. Has amide properties
    B. Has ester properties
    C. Is packaged in the lowest concentration of all local anesthetics in dentistry
    D. Is packaged in the highest concentration of all local anesthetics in dentistry
    E. Has hepatic biotransformation
    F. Has extrahepatic biotransformation

Oral Diagnosis

JEFFREY C.B. STEWART

SANJAY M. MALLYA

OUTLINE

1.0 Oral Pathology and Diagnosis

Jeffery Stewart

A working knowledge of oral pathology is fundamental to the recognition and diagnosis of oral and maxillofacial diseases in patients. This outline and the test questions that follow are intended to refresh and test the student's memory of clinical oral pathology. Some entities are simply listed, and some entities are not included because of their rarity. If students detect any areas of weakness, they are encouraged to consult a current textbook for detailed discussions of the entities and conditions that require additional study.

Outline of Review

The section editors acknowledge Drs. Joseph Regezi and Stuart C. White for their contributions as authors and editors of the Oral Diagnosis section of the first edition. Their outstanding efforts provided the foundation for this revision.

1.1 Developmental Conditions

Developmental conditions are soft tissue or hard tissue defects that occur during the development of the individual, either before or after birth. Most are easily recognizable.

A. Oral-facial clefts.
  1. Cleft lip.
    a. Unilateral (80%) or bilateral (20%).
    b. Defect between medial nasal process and maxillary process.
    c. Approximately 1 in 1000 births, but varies with race.
  2. Cleft palate.
    a. Lack of fusion between palatal shelves; approximately 1 in 2000 births.
    b. Cleft lip (25%), cleft palate (25%), cleft lip and palate (50%).
B. Lip pits.
  1. Invaginations at the commissures or near the midline.
C. Fordyce granules.
  1. Ectopic sebaceous glands.
  2. Commonly seen in buccal mucosa or lip.
D. Leukoedema.
  1. Bilateral opacification of the buccal mucosa.
  2. Common; no significance.
E. Macroglossia (Box 4-1).
F. Thyroid congenital abnormalities.
  1. Lingual thyroid.
    a. Thyroid tissue mass, midline tongue base.
    b. Caused by incomplete descent of thyroid anlage.
    c. May be patient's only thyroid.
  2. Thyroglossal tract cyst.
    a. Midline neck swelling secondary to cystic change of remnants of thyroid tissue.
    b. Located along embryonic path of thyroid descent.

Box 4-1

Causes of Macroglossia

Congenital hyperplasia/hypertrophy
Tumors—lymphangioma, vascular malformation,
    neurofibroma, multiple granular cell tumors, salivary
    gland tumors
Endocrine abnormality
Acromegaly, cretinism
Infections obstructing lymphatics
Beckwith-Wiedemann syndrome
Macroglossia, exophthalmos, gigantism
Amyloidosis

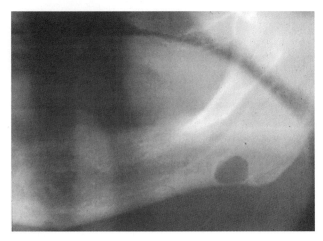

Figure 4-2 Stafne bone cyst. *(From Regezi JA, Scuibba JJ, Jordan RCK: Oral Pathology: Clinical Pathologic Correlations, ed 6. St. Louis, Saunders, 2012.)*

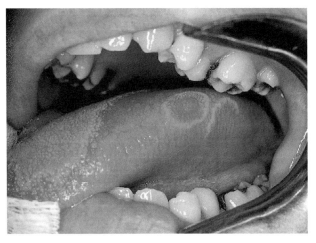

Figure 4-1 Geographic tongue. *(From Regezi JA, Scuibba JJ, Jordan RCK: Oral Pathology: Clinical Pathologic Correlations, ed 6. St. Louis, Saunders, 2012.)*

G. Geographic tongue (benign migratory glossitis, erythema migrans) (Figure 4-1).
  1. Common (2% of population) benign condition of the tongue of unknown cause.
  2. Appears as white annular lesions surrounding atrophic red central zones that migrate with time.
  3. Occasionally symptomatic (mild pain or burning).
  4. No treatment necessary.
H. Fissured tongue.
  1. Fissuring of tongue dorsum.
  2. Common (3% of population) and usually asymptomatic.
  3. Component of Melkersson-Rosenthal syndrome.
    a. Fissured tongue, granulomatous cheilitis, and facial paralysis.
I. Hemangioma.
  1. Congenital hemangioma.
    a. Focal proliferation of capillaries.
    b. Most lesions undergo involution; persistent lesions are excised.

  2. Vascular malformation.
    a. Persistent malformation of capillaries, veins, and arteries.
    b. Exhibits a thrill (palpate a pulse) and bruit (hear a pulse).
    c. Type of vascular malformation known as Sturge-Weber syndrome (encephalotrigeminal angiomatosis).
      (1) Lesions involve skin along one of the branches of the trigeminal nerve.
      (2) The leptomeninges of the cerebral cortex may be involved by the malformations, leading to mental retardation and seizures.
J. Lymphangioma.
  1. Congenital focal proliferation of lymphatic channels.
  2. When occurring in the neck, it is called *hygroma colli*.
K. Exostoses.
  1. Excessive cortical bone growth of unknown cause.
  2. Buccal exostoses, torus palatinus, torus mandibularis.
L. Developmental soft tissue cysts (including thyroglossal tract cyst).
  1. Dermoid cyst.
    a. Mass in midline floor of mouth if above mylohyoid muscle.
    b. Mass in upper neck if below mylohyoid muscle.
  2. Branchial cyst.
    a. Epithelial cyst within lymph node of the neck.
  3. Oral lymphoepithelial cyst.
    a. Cyst within lymphoid tissue that is the counterpart of branchial cyst of the neck.
    b. Nodule commonly in soft palate, oral floor, or lateral tongue.
M. Developmental jaw cysts and cystlike lesions (pseudocysts).
  1. Stafne (static) bone defect (Figure 4-2).
    a. Diagnostic radiolucency of the mandible secondary to invagination of the lingual surface of the jaw.

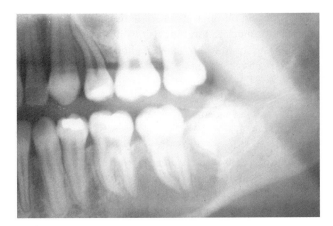

Figure 4-3 Traumatic bone cyst. *(From Regezi JA, Scuibba JJ, Jordan RCK: Oral Pathology: Clinical Pathologic Correlations, ed 6. St. Louis, Saunders, 2012.)*

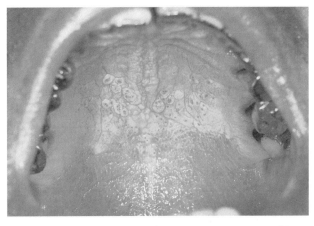

Figure 4-4 Nicotine stomatitis. *(From Regezi JA, Scuibba JJ, Jordan RCK: Oral Pathology: Clinical Pathologic Correlations, ed 6. St. Louis, Saunders, 2012.)*

  b. Located in the posterior mandible below the mandibular canal.
 2. Nasopalatine duct (canal) cyst.
  a. Lucency, often heart-shaped, in the nasopalatine canal.
  b. Caused by cystification of nasopalatine duct remnants.
 3. Globulomaxillary lesion.
  a. Clinical term denoting any pathologic radiolucency between the maxillary cuspid and the lateral incisor.
  b. Histopathologic analysis is required for definitive diagnosis because lesions in this location may represent a wide array of inflammatory lesions, odontogenic cysts and tumors, and nonodontogenic bone diseases.
 4. Traumatic (simple) bone cyst (Figure 4-3).
  a. Radiolucent dead space (no epithelial lining) in the mandible of teenagers.
  b. Some (not all) associated with jaw trauma.
 5. Focal osteoporotic bone marrow defect.
  a. Lucency in the jaw that contains hematopoietic bone marrow; often in an extraction site.

1.2 Mucosal Lesions— Physical-Chemical

Trauma and chemicals are frequent causes of oral lesions. Some of these lesions have an iatrogenic cause (i.e., caused by the dental practitioner).
A. Focal (frictional) hyperkeratosis.
 1. Common white lesion caused by chronic friction on mucosa.
 2. Differentiated from idiopathic leukoplakia because cause is known.
B. Linea alba.
 1. Type of frictional hyperkeratosis that appears as a linear white line in buccal mucosa.
C. Traumatic ulcer.

 1. Very common.
 2. Chronic ulcers mimic oral cancer and chronic infectious ulcers.
D. Chemical burn.
 1. Usually manifest as ulcers.
 2. May be caused by aspirin, hydrogen peroxide, silver nitrate, phenol, or other agents.
E. Nicotine stomatitis (Figure 4-4).
 1. White change in palate caused by smoking.
 2. Red dots in the lesion are inflamed salivary duct orifices.
 3. Not considered premalignant, unless related to "reverse smoking" (lighted end in mouth).
F. Amalgam tattoo.
 1. Traumatic implantation of amalgam particles into mucosa.
 2. Most common oral pigmented lesion.
G. Smoking-associated melanosis.
 1. Caused by a chemical in tobacco smoke that stimulates melanin production.
 2. Typically seen in the anterior gingival.
 3. Reversible if smoking is discontinued.
H. Melanotic macule.
 1. Most common melanocytic lesion.
 2. May be postinflammatory, syndrome-associated (primarily Peutz-Jeghers syndrome [freckles and benign intestinal polyps]), or idiopathic.
I. Drug-induced pigmentation.
 1. Most common culprits: minocycline, chloroquine, cyclophosphamide, azidothymidine (zidovudine).
J. Hairy tongue.
 1. Elongation of filiform papillae—of cosmetic significance only.
 2. Several causes, including extended use of antibiotics, corticosteroids, and hydrogen peroxide.
K. Dentifrice-associated slough.
 1. Superficial chemical burn of buccal mucosa caused by some dentifrices.

1.3 Mucosal Lesions—Infections

Oral infections are viral, bacterial, or fungal in nature. The most commonly encountered infections are viral, usually herpes simplex virus (HSV) infections. Clinical presentation of viral infections depends on viral type: herpes causes mucosal ulceration (preceded by vesicles), human papillomavirus (HPV) typically induces a verruciform (warty) lesion, and Epstein-Barr virus (EBV) causes a white lesion (hairy leukoplakia). Most bacterial and fungal infections manifest as chronic ulcers. The fungus *Candida albicans* can cause either white or red lesions.

A. Viral infections.
  1. HSV infections (Figure 4-5 and Table 4-1).
    a. High frequency of occurrence of infections.
    b. Primary disease predominantly in children.
    c. Severe in immunocompromised patients.
    d. Secondary disease is reactivation of latent virus in the trigeminal ganglion.
    e. Reactivation is triggered by sunlight, stress, or immunosuppression.

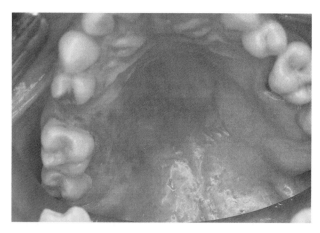

Figure 4-5 Secondary herpes simplex infection. *(From Regezi JA, Scuibba JJ, Jordan RCK: Oral Pathology: Clinical Pathologic Correlations, ed 6. St. Louis, Saunders, 2012.)*

    f. Lesion on finger is called *herpetic whitlow*.
    g. Intranuclear viral inclusions in epithelial cells are diagnostic when taken in clinical context.
  2. Varicella (chickenpox).
    a. Self-limiting childhood disease caused by varicella-zoster virus (VZV).
    b. Oral lesions are uncommon.
  3. Herpes zoster.
    a. This disease represents reactivation of latent VZV.
    b. The latent virus is believed to reside in the dorsal root and trigeminal ganglia.
  4. Coxsackievirus infections (hand-foot-and-mouth disease, herpangina).
    a. Both diseases are self-limiting childhood systemic infections, usually endemic.
    b. Sites of lesions in hand-foot-mouth disease: hands, feet, and mouth.
    c. Sites of lesions in herpangina: posterior oral cavity.
  5. Measles (rubeola).
    a. Self-limiting childhood systemic infection caused by measles virus.
    b. Fever, malaise, skin rash.
    c. Punctate buccal mucosa ulcers (Koplik's spots) precede skin rash.
  6. HPV infections.
    a. Papillomas.
      (1) Benign epithelial proliferations (pedunculated or sessile) of little significance.
      (2) Include verruca vulgaris (wart).
        (a) Warts much more prevalent in HIV-positive patients.
      (3) Most, if not all, caused by HPV.
    b. Condyloma acuminatum (genital warts).
      (1) Caused by HPV 6 and 11.
      (2) Oral lesions acquired by oral-genital contact.
      (3) Broad-based verruciform lesion.
    c. Focal epithelial hyperplasia (Heck's disease).
      (1) Most common in certain ethnic groups—Native Americans, Inuits, and Central Americans.

Table 4-1					
Common Herpes Infections					
	VIRUS	**LOCATION**	**SIGNS**	**SYMPTOMS**	**TREATMENT**
Primary herpes simplex	HSV 1	Perioral, oral, especially gingiva	Vesicles, ulcers	Fever, malaise, painful ulcers	Acyclovir, symptomatic
Secondary herpes simplex	HSV 1	Lips, hard palate, and gingiva	Vesicles, ulcers	Painful ulcers	Acyclovir, others
Varicella	Varicella-zoster virus	Trunk, head, and neck	Vesicles, ulcers	Fever, malaise, painful ulcers	Symptomatic, acyclovir
Herpes zoster	Varicella-zoster virus	Unilateral trunk, unilateral oral	Vesicles, ulcers	Painful ulcers	Acyclovir, Zoster vaccine

HSV, Herpes simplex virus.

(2) Multiple, small, dome-shaped warts on oral mucosa.

(3) Caused by HPV 13 and 32.

7. EBV infections (Box 4-2 and Figure 4-6).

a. Hairy leukoplakia.

(1) Opportunistic infection resulting in white patch or patches of the lateral tongue.

(2) Almost all associated with HIV (may be a pre-AIDS sign).

(3) Infrequently seen in patients with other immunosuppressed states; very rare in normal patients.

(4) Diagnosis is made from biopsy specimen showing intranuclear viral inclusions.

(5) Occurrence decreasing with use of new AIDS drugs.

Box 4-2

Oral Complications of AIDS

Infections
   Herpes simplex and herpes zoster
   EBV-associated hairy leukoplakia
   Cytomegalovirus
   HPV-associated warts
   Tuberculosis
   Histoplasmosis
   Candidiasis
Neoplasms
   Kaposi's sarcoma (human herpesvirus 8)
   High-grade lymphomas
Severe aphthous ulcers
Xerostomia
Gingivitis and periodontal disease

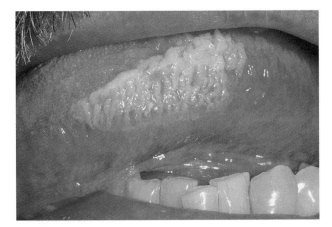

Figure 4-6 Hairy leukoplakia. *(From Regezi JA, Scuibba JJ, Jordan RCK: Oral Pathology: Clinical Pathologic Correlations, ed 6. St. Louis, Saunders, 2012.)*

b. Associated malignancies—Burkitt's lymphoma, nasopharyngeal carcinoma.

(1) There is good evidence that EBV has an etiologic role in these two malignancies.

B. Bacterial infections.

Acute bacterial infections are uncommon in oral mucosa, presumably owing to the protective effects (immunologic and physical) that saliva provides the stratified squamous epithelium lining the mouth. Acute pustular staphylococcal infections occasionally may appear after deep trauma or surgery. These infections are treated with appropriate antibiotics and surgical techniques (see Section 8 on Pharmacology and Section 3 on Oral and Maxillofacial Surgery and Pain Control). Chronic bacterial infections are also uncommon in oral mucosa, probably for the same reasons that acute infections are not often seen. The chronic infections outlined subsequently are uncommon to rare but are well known and distinctive.

1. Syphilis.

a. Caused by contact with patients infected with *Treponema pallidum.*

b. Primary lesion (chancre), secondary lesions (oral mucous patches, condyloma latum, maculopapular rash), and tertiary lesions (gummas, central nervous system involvement, cardiovascular involvement).

c. Congenital syphilis is an in utero infection with multiple stigmata, including Hutchinson's triad (notched incisors, deafness, ocular keratitis).

2. Tuberculosis.

a. Caused by inhalation of *Mycobacterium tuberculosis.*

b. Oral nonhealing chronic ulcers follow lung infection.

c. Incidence increasing secondary to overcrowding, debilitation, and AIDS.

d. Caseating granulomas with multinucleated giant cells (Langerhans' giant cells).

e. Multidrug therapy (e.g., isoniazid, rifampin, ethambutol).

3. Gonorrhea.

a. Sexually transmitted disease caused by *Neisseria gonorrhoeae.*

b. Oral manifestation is oral pharyngitis but is rarely seen.

4. Actinomycosis.

a. Opportunistic bacterium (*Actinomyces israelii*) found in oral flora of many patients.

b. Chronic jaw infection may follow dental surgery.

c. Head and neck infections are called *cervicofacial actinomycosis.*

d. Treated with long-term, high-dose penicillin.

5. Scarlet fever.

a. Systemic infection caused by some strains of group A streptococci.

b. In addition to the usual manifestation of "strep throat" (pharyngitis, fever, and malaise), children develop a skin rash caused by erythrogenic toxin.

c. Strawberry tongue (white-coated tongue with red, inflamed fungiform papillae).

d. Treated with penicillin to prevent complications of rheumatic fever.

C. Fungal infections.

  1. Deep fungi (histoplasmosis, coccidioidomycosis, blastomycosis, cryptococcosis).

    a. Histoplasmosis is endemic to the U.S. Midwest, and coccidioidomycosis (San Joaquin Valley fever) is endemic to the U.S. West.

    b. Deep fungal infections of the lung may lead to oral chronic granulomatous ulcers secondary to oral implantation of microorganisms.

    c. Oral lesions must be differentiated from oral cancer and chronic traumatic ulcers.

  2. Opportunistic fungi.

    a. Candidiasis (thrush, moniliasis) (Figure 4-7).

      (1) Caused by *C. albicans*, part of the normal flora in most patients.

      (2) Predisposing factors exist for fungal overgrowth (Box 4-3).

      (3) Acute lesions are white, which represent the fungal colonies growing in mucosa; removal leaves raw, bleeding surface.

      (4) Chronic lesions are erythematous.

      (5) Specific types of chronic candidiasis—denture sore mouth, angular cheilitis, and median rhomboid glossitis.

      (6) Topical treatment: nystatin, clotrimazole.

      (7) Systemic treatment: fluconazole, itraconazole, caspofungin.

    b. Aspergillosis, mucormycosis, *Rhizopus*.

      (1) These infections are caused by organisms that are found throughout the environment.

      (2) Patients who are medically debilitated or immunocompromised are at risk.

      (3) In the head and neck, most lesions appear as destructive ulcerations in the paranasal sinuses or nasal cavity.

      (4) Intense antifungal therapy is indicated, along with controlling the contributing condition.

1.4 Mucosal Lesions—Immunologic Diseases

These conditions are related to autoimmune or hyperimmune reactions to known or undetermined antigenic stimuli. Clinical manifestations include vesicles or bullae, ulcers, erythema, and white patches.

A. Aphthous ulcers (Figure 4-8, Box 4-4, and Table 4-2).

  1. Recurrent painful ulcers (not preceded by vesicles).

  2. Unknown cause, but probably related to a focal immune defect.

Box 4-3

Predisposing Factors for Candidiasis

Immune deficiency
Endocrine abnormality
  Diabetes mellitus
  Pregnancy
  Hypoparathyroidism
  Hypoadrenalism
Stress
Prolonged antibiotic therapy
Prolonged corticosteroid therapy
Chemotherapy for malignancies
Xerostomia
Poor oral hygiene

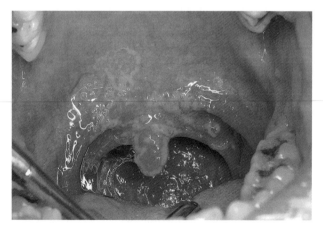

Figure 4-7 Acute candidiasis. *(From Regezi JA, Scuibba JJ, Jordan RCK: Oral Pathology: Clinical Pathologic Correlations, ed 6. St. Louis, Saunders, 2012.)*

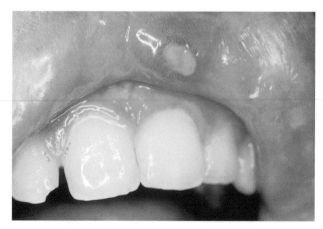

Figure 4-8 Minor aphthous ulcer. *(From Regezi JA, Scuibba JJ, Jordan RCK: Oral Pathology: Clinical Pathologic Correlations, ed 6. St. Louis, Saunders, 2012.)*

Clinical Types of Aphthous Ulcers

Minor Aphthous Ulcers

One to several painful oval ulcers <0.5 cm
Most common type
Duration of 7-10 days

Major Aphthous Ulcers

Up to 10 deep crateriform ulcers >0.5 cm
Very painful and may be debilitating
May take several weeks to heal

Herpetiform Aphthous Ulcers

Recurrent crops of minor aphthae
Painful, take 1-2 weeks to heal
May be found on any mucosal surface
Same cause as other aphthae (not viral)

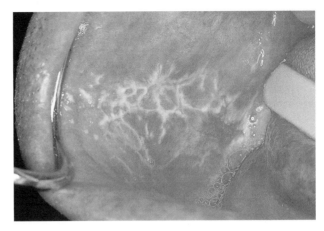

Figure 4-9 Lichen planus. *(From Regezi JA, Scuibba JJ, Jordan RCK: Oral Pathology: Clinical Pathologic Correlations, ed 6. St. Louis, Saunders, 2012.)*

Table 4-2

Systemic Diseases in Which Aphthous Ulcers Are Seen

	SYSTEMIC CONDITION	ORAL LESIONS
Crohn's disease	Granulomatous inflammation of GI tract	Minor aphthae
Behçet's syndrome	Immune dysfunction featuring vasculitis	Minor aphthae
Celiac sprue	Gluten-sensitive enteropathy	Minor aphthae
AIDS	Immunodeficiency	Major aphthae

GI, Gastrointestinal.

3. Appear on wet (not vermilion) nonkeratinized oral mucosa (i.e., not hard palate or hard gingiva).
4. Three clinical types—minor, major, herpetiform.
5. May be seen in association with some systemic diseases.
B. Behçet's syndrome.
   1. Multisystem disease believed to represent immune dysfunction in which vasculitis is a prominent feature.
   2. Oral and genital aphthous-type ulcers, conjunctivitis, uveitis (inflammation of the layers of the eye), arthritis, headache, and other central nervous system manifestations.
   3. Treated with corticosteroids and other immunosuppressive drugs.
C. Erythema multiforme.
   1. Self-limiting hypersensitivity reaction that affects skin or mucosa or both.

2. Minor form associated with secondary herpes simplex hypersensitivity; major form (Stevens-Johnson syndrome) often triggered by drugs.
D. Drug reactions and contact allergies.
   1. Potentially caused by any drug or foreign protein.
   2. May be a hyperimmune response or nonimmunologic (overdose, toxicity, irritant).
   3. Oral lesions include vesicular, ulcerative, erythematous, and lichenoid.
   4. Acquired angioedema is a specific type of allergic reaction.
      a. Precipitated by drugs or food (shellfish, nuts).
      b. Mediated by mast cell release of IgE.
      c. Results in characteristic soft, diffuse swelling of lips, neck, or face.
      d. Hereditary angioedema is a rare form that is an autosomal dominant trait.
E. Wegener's granulomatosis.
   1. Destructive granulomatous lesions with necrotizing vasculitis of unknown cause.
   2. Affects upper respiratory tract, lungs, and kidneys.
   3. Diagnosis based on biopsy and demonstration of antineutrophil cytoplasmic antibodies.
   4. Treatment is with cyclophosphamide and corticosteroids or rituximab; prognosis is good.
F. Midline granuloma.
   1. Destructive necrotizing midfacial phenomenon that clinically mimics lesions of Wegener's granulomatosis.
   2. Most cases represent peripheral T-cell lymphomas of the upper respiratory tract or mouth (perforation of the hard palate may be seen).
   3. Good prognosis when treated early with radiation.
G. Lichen planus (Figure 4-9 and Box 4-5).
   1. Common mucocutaneous disease (1% to 2% of adults affected).

Clinical Features of Lichen Planus

Oral Lesions

Oral lesions typically bilateral in the buccal mucosa, although tongue and gingival frequently affected

Lesions exhibit white (hyperkeratotic) lines

Clinical types

    Reticular: lesions consist of interlacing lines (Wickham's striae)

    Erosive: ulceration also present

    Erythematous or atrophic: lesions predominantly red

    Plaque: lesions predominantly plaquelike

Cutaneous Lesions

Cutaneous lesions characteristically purple pruritic papules on lower legs and arms

Lesions respond to corticosteroids

Erosive form may have slightly increased risk for malignant change

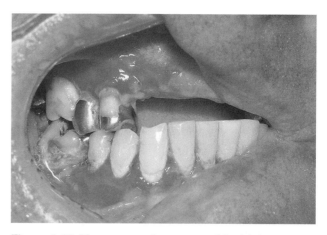

Figure 4-10 Mucous membrane pemphigoid. *(From Regezi JA, Scuibba JJ, Jordan RCK: Oral Pathology: Clinical Pathologic Correlations, ed 6. St. Louis, Saunders, 2012.)*

    2. T lymphocytes target (destroy) basal keratinocytes; the reason for this immunologically mediated phenomenon is unknown.

    3. Microscopy.

        a. Hyperkeratosis.

        b. Lymphocyte infiltrate at epithelial-connective tissue interface.

        c. Basal zone vacuolation secondary to basal keratinocyte destruction.

        d. Epithelium may exhibit a "saw tooth" pattern as it remodels after basal cell damage.

H. Lupus erythematosus.

    1. Autoimmune disease that occurs in either discoid or systemic form.

    2. Discoid (chronic) type.

        a. Affects skin (especially face and scalp) or oral mucosa (buccal mucosa, gingival, vermilion).

        b. Usually affects middle-aged adults, especially women.

        c. Lesions are erythematous; oral lesions mimic erosive lichen planus.

        d. No systemic signs or symptoms; rarely progresses to systemic form.

        e. Treated with corticosteroids and other drugs.

    3. Systemic (acute) type.

        a. Multiple organ involvement (heart, kidney, joints, skin, oral).

        b. Classic sign—butterfly rash over bridge of the nose.

        c. Autoantibodies directed against nuclear and cytoplasmic antigens.

        d. Serologic tests include antinuclear antibodies and lupus erythematosus cell test.

        e. Treated with corticosteroids and other immunosuppressive drugs.

I. Scleroderma.

    1. Autoimmune, multiorgan disease of adults, especially women.

    2. Fibrosis of tissues eventually leads to organ dysfunction.

    3. May occur concomitantly with other autoimmune diseases, such as lupus erythematosus, rheumatoid arthritis, dermatomyositis, and Sjögren's syndrome.

    4. Cutaneous changes include induration and rigidity, atrophy, and telangiectasias.

    5. Oral changes include restriction of orifice, uniform widening of periodontal membrane, and bony resorption of posterior margin of the mandibular ramus (best seen on a panogram).

J. Pemphigus vulgaris.

    1. Autoimmune, mucocutaneous disease in which antibodies are directed against desmosomal protein (desmoglein 3).

    2. Clinical features.

        a. Manifests as multiple, painful ulcers preceded by bullae that form within the epithelium.

        b. Positive Nikolsky's sign may be present (formation of blister with rubbing or pressure).

        c. Oral lesions precede skin lesions in about half of cases.

        d. Progressive clinical course; may be fatal if untreated.

    3. Treated with systemic corticosteroids or other immunosuppressive drugs.

K. Mucous membrane pemphigoid (Figure 4-10).

    1. Autoimmune disease of mucous membranes; antibodies directed against basement membrane antigens (e.g., laminin 5, BP180).

2. Clinical features.
   a. Affects older adults (typically >50 years old).
   b. Manifests as multiple, painful ulcers preceded by bullae that form below the epithelium at the basement membrane.
   c. Oral lesions may be found in any region, especially and sometimes exclusively in the attached gingival; ocular lesions can lead to blindness if untreated.
   d. Positive Nikolsky's sign may be present.
   e. Persistent disease.
3. Patients are managed with corticosteroids.

1.5 Mucosal Lesions— Premalignant Conditions

Patients with any of the following lesions are at risk for the development of squamous cell carcinoma. Some are caused by a known stimulus (especially tobacco), and some are idiopathic.

A. Idiopathic leukoplakia (Figure 4-11 and Box 4-6).
   1. White or opaque oral mucosa lesions that do not rub off and are not clinically diagnostic for any other white lesion.
   2. Cause is unknown, although tobacco and alcohol may be contributing factors.

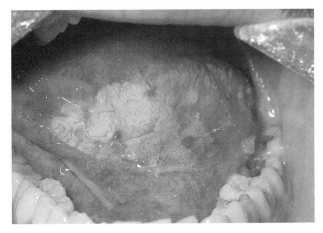

Figure 4-11 Idiopathic leukoplakia. *(From Regezi JA, Scuibba JJ, Jordan RCK: Oral Pathology: Clinical Pathologic Correlations, ed 6. St. Louis, Saunders, 2012.)*

3. Biopsy is mandatory because diagnosis cannot be made clinically.
   4. Transformation of benign lesions to squamous cell carcinoma is 5% to 15%.
   5. Treatment—excision; recurrence common.
B. Proliferative verrucous leukoplakia.
   1. High-risk form of leukoplakia.
   2. Cause is unknown, although some are associated with HPV 16 and 18.
   3. Lesions are recurrent or persistent and usually multiple.
   4. Lesions may start with a flat profile but progress to broad-based, wartlike (verruciform) lesions.
   5. High risk of malignant transformation to verrucous carcinoma or squamous cell carcinoma.
C. Erythroplakia (erythroplasia) (Box 4-7).
   1. High-risk, idiopathic red patch of mucosa.
   2. Most represent dysplasia or malignancy.
   3. Biopsy mandatory.
D. Actinic (solar) cheilitis.
   1. Cause—ultraviolet (UV) light, especially UVB, 2900 to 3200 nm.
   2. The lower lip shows epithelial atrophy and focal keratosis. The upper lip is minimally affected because it is more protected from UV light.
   3. The junction of vermilion and skin becomes indistinct.
   4. May progress to squamous cell carcinoma.
E. Oral submucous fibrosis.
   1. Irreversible mucosal change thought to be due to hypersensitivity to dietary substances, especially betel nut.
   2. Mucosa becomes opaque secondary to submucosal scarring.
   3. May progress to squamous cell carcinoma.
F. Smokeless tobacco–associated white lesion.
   1. White mucosal change resulting from direct effects of smokeless tobacco and additives.
   2. By definition, not idiopathic leukoplakia because cause is known and lesion is clinically diagnostic (however, it could be classified under a more generic designation of *leukoplakia* or *white patch*).

Box 4-6

Idiopathic Leukoplakia

Cause unknown, tobacco and alcohol add risk
Usually occurs >40 years old
High-risk sites (for malignant transformation): floor of mouth and tongue
Microscopy at time of first biopsy
  Hyperkeratosis (80%)
  Dysplasia (12%)
  In situ carcinoma (3%)
  Squamous cell carcinoma (5%)

Box 4-7

Erythroplakia (Erythroplasia)

Much less common than idiopathic leukoplakia
Cause unknown (idiopathic), some are tobacco related
Usually occurs between 50 and 70 years old
High-risk sites: floor of mouth, tongue, retromolar area
Microscopy
  Mild to moderate dysplasia (10%)
  Severe dysplasia/carcinoma in situ (40%)
  Squamous cell carcinoma (50%)

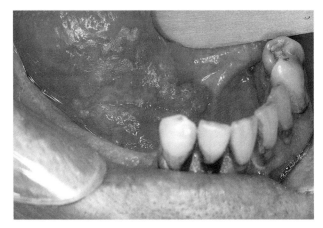

Figure 4-12 Squamous cell carcinoma. *(From Regezi JA, Scuibba JJ, Jordan RCK: Oral Pathology: Clinical Pathologic Correlations, ed 6. St. Louis, Saunders, 2012.)*

3. Seen in labial and buccal vestibules where tobacco is held.
4. May cause focal periodontal destruction, tooth abrasion, or hypertension. Malignant transformation is rare.

1.6 Mucosal Lesions—Malignancies

The various types of carcinomas can manifest as nonhealing ulcers, red patches, or irregular surface masses. Melanomas manifest as abnormally pigmented surface lesions that start at the junction of the epithelium and submucosa.

A. Verrucous carcinoma.
   1. Well-differentiated, slow-growing form of carcinoma that infrequently metastasizes.
   2. Tobacco and HPV 16 and 18 may have etiologic roles.
   3. Exhibits a broad-based verruciform architecture.
   4. Treated by surgical excision; good prognosis.
B. Squamous cell carcinoma (Figure 4-12 and Box 4-8).
   1. Etiology.
      a. Caused by mutation, amplification, or inactivation of oncogenes and tumor suppressor genes.
      b. Accumulation of genetic alterations results in loss of cell cycle control, abnormal signaling, increased cell survival, and cell motility.
      c. Causes of genetic alterations include tobacco and heredity.
      d. Increased incidence of oropharyngeal (including tonsillar) squamous cell carcinoma, many of which are associated with detection of oncogenic HPV infection (HPV 16 and 18).
      e. Increased risk of oral cancer in patients with Plummer-Vinson syndrome (mucosal atrophy, dysphagia, iron-deficiency anemia).
   2. Clinical features.
      a. May manifest as chronic, nonhealing ulcer, red or white patch, or mass.

Box 4-8

Clinical Features of Oral Squamous Cell Carcinoma

Most manifest as indurated nonpainful, nonhealing ulcer
Others manifest as white or red patch or mass
Males more frequently affected than females, 2:1
High-risk sites: posterior lateral tongue and floor of mouth

Treatment

Surgical excision of primary
Neck dissection with positive nodes or large primary lesion
Radiotherapy
Combination surgery and radiotherapy
Radiotherapy combined with chemotherapy
Overall 5-year survival 45%-50%

Prognosis

Good if lesion <2 cm in greatest dimension (stage I)
Fair if lesion 2-4 cm and no neck disease (stage II)
Poor if metastasis is found in neck (stages III and IV)

---

      b. Most commonly seen in posterior-lateral tongue and floor of mouth.
      c. In regard to patient prognosis, clinical stage is more important than microscopic classification.
   3. Treatment—excision or radiation; prognosis dependent mostly on stage.
      a. Overall 5-year survival is 45% to 50%; with neck metastasis, 25%.
C. Basal cell carcinoma.
   1. Common low-grade skin cancer that rarely metastasizes.
   2. Usually in sun-damaged skin; very rare in mucosa.
   3. Usually manifests as nonhealing, indurated chronic ulcer.
   4. Treated with surgery; very good to excellent prognosis.
D. Oral melanoma (Figure 4-13).
   1. Malignancy of melanocytes.
   2. High-risk sites are palate and gingiva.
   3. Some lesions have prolonged in situ phase preceding vertical (invasive) growth.
   4. Occurs almost always in adults; rarely seen in children.
   5. For oral mucosal lesions, 5-year survival is less than 20%; for skin lesions, greater than 65%.

1.7 Connective Tissue Tumors—Benign

Connective tissue tumors manifest as masses (lumps or bumps) within the submucosa. Overlying epithelium is

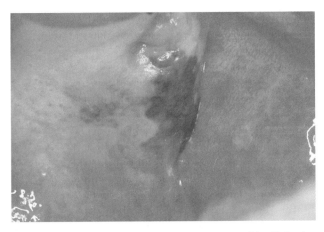

Figure 4-13 Melanoma. *(From Regezi JA, Scuibba JJ, Jordan RCK: Oral Pathology: Clinical Pathologic Correlations, ed 6. St. Louis, Saunders, 2012.)*

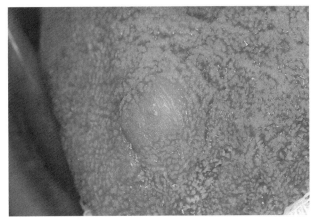

Figure 4-14 Granular cell tumor. *(From Regezi JA, Scuibba JJ, Jordan RCK: Oral Pathology: Clinical Pathologic Correlations, ed 6. St. Louis, Saunders, 2012.)*

BOX 4-9

Systemic Modifying Factors of Generalized Gingival Hyperplasia

Drugs
    Phenytoin (Dilantin)
    Cyclosporine
    Nifedipine and other calcium channel blockers
Hormonal changes associated with puberty and pregnancy
Leukemic infiltrates
Genetic factors

---

generally intact, unless ulceration occurs because of trauma to the lesion. These tumors generally fall into one of two groups: reactive or neoplastic.

A. Reactive.
  1. Fibrous lesions.
    a. Peripheral fibroma.
      (1) Fibrous hyperplasia of the gingiva.
      (2) Caused by trauma or chronic irritation.
    b. Generalized gingival hyperplasia.
      (1) Fibrous hyperplasia caused by local factors and modified by systemic conditions.
      (2) Phenytoin (Dilantin) for seizures and calcium channel blockers may contribute to gingival hyperplasia (Box 4-9).
    c. Focal fibrous hyperplasia.
      (1) Fibrous hyperplasia of oral mucosa.
      (2) Caused by chronic trauma or chronic irritation.
      (3) Also known as *traumatic fibroma*, *irritation fibroma*, and *hyperplastic scar*.
    d. Denture-induced fibrous hyperplasia.
      (1) Fibrous hyperplasia associated with ill-fitting dentures.
      (2) Usually seen in anterior labial vestibules.
      (3) Papillary hyperplasia (palatal papillomatosis) of the palate is another type of fibrous hyperplasia associated with ill-fitting dentures.
      (4) No malignant potential.
  2. Neural—traumatic neuroma.
    a. Entangled submucosal mass of neural tissue and scar.
    b. Caused by injury to nerve.
    c. Most commonly seen at mental foramen in oral cavity.
  3. Vascular—pyogenic granuloma.
    a. Hyperplasia of capillaries and fibroblasts.
    b. Caused by trauma or chronic irritation.
    c. Common in gingiva but can be seen anywhere there is mucosal (or skin) trauma.
B. Neoplastic.
  1. Fibrous.
    a. Nodular fasciitis.
      (1) Rare submucosal proliferation of fibroblasts.
      (2) Reactive lesion that exhibits rapid growth.
      (3) Treated with surgical excision, rare recurrence.
    b. Fibromatosis.
      (1) Although benign, this troublesome fibroblastic neoplasm is locally aggressive and infiltrative.
      (2) Difficult to eradicate and often recurs.
      (3) Behavior similar to low-grade fibrosarcoma.
  2. Neural.
    a. Granular cell tumor (Figure 4-14).
      (1) Benign, nonrecurring submucosal neoplasm of Schwann's cells.
      (2) Tumor cells have granular or grainy cytoplasm.
      (3) Overlying epithelium may exhibit pseudoepitheliomatous hyperplasia (microscopically mimics carcinoma).
      (4) Most commonly seen in tongue.
      (5) Infant counterpart—congenital granular cell tumor (congenital epulis).

(a) Occurs on gingiva only as pedunculated mass.

(b) No pseudoepitheliomatous hyperplasia.

(c) Surgical excision, no recurrence.

b. Schwannoma (neurilemoma).

(1) Benign neoplasm of Schwann's cells.

(2) Any site; tongue favored.

(3) Solitary; not syndrome-related.

c. Neurofibroma.

(1) Benign neoplasm of Schwann's cells and perineural fibroblasts.

(2) Any site, especially tongue and buccal mucosa.

(3) Solitary to multiple.

(4) Syndrome of neurofibromatosis 1.

(a) Multiple neurofibromas.

(b) Six or more café au lait macules (each >1.5 cm diameter).

(c) Axillary freckling (Crowe's sign) and iris freckling (Lisch spots).

(d) Malignant transformation of neurofibromas occurs in 5% to 15% of patients.

d. Mucosal neuromas of multiple endocrine neoplasia 2B.

(1) Autosomal dominant inheritance.

(2) Syndrome components.

(a) Oral mucosal neuromas (hamartomas).

(b) Medullary carcinoma of the thyroid.

(c) Pheochromocytoma of the adrenal gland.

3. Muscle.

a. Leiomyoma.

(1) Rare, benign neoplasm of smooth muscle origin.

b. Rhabdomyoma.

(1) Very rare, benign neoplasm of skeletal muscle origin.

4. Fat—lipoma.

a. Uncommon benign neoplasm of fat cell origin.

b. Buccal mucosa is characteristic site.

1.8 Connective Tissue Tumors—Malignant

Connective tissue tumors are rare tumors that arise from malignant conversion of connective tissue cells within the submucosa. They manifest as masses or ulcerated masses.

A. Fibrous—fibrosarcoma.

1. Rare sarcoma showing microscopic evidence of fibroblast differentiation.

B. Neural—malignant peripheral nerve sheath tumor (neurosarcoma).

1. Rare sarcoma showing microscopic evidence of neural differentiation.

2. May arise from preexisting neurofibroma or de novo (no preexisting lesion).

C. Vascular.

1. Kaposi's sarcoma.

a. Malignant proliferation of endothelial cells.

b. Human herpesvirus 8 has etiologic role.

c. Most commonly seen as a complication of AIDS; incidence markedly reduced by new antiretroviral therapies.

d. May also be seen as endemic African type or classic Mediterranean type.

D. Muscle.

1. Leiomyosarcoma.

a. Rare sarcoma showing microscopic evidence of smooth muscle differentiation.

2. Rhabdomyosarcoma.

a. Rare sarcoma showing microscopic evidence of skeletal muscle differentiation.

E. Fat—liposarcoma.

1. Rare sarcoma showing microscopic evidence of fat cell differentiation.

1.9 Salivary Gland Diseases— Reactive Lesions

Both major and minor salivary glands can be subject to numerous reactive influences. Causes of these changes include trauma, infection, metabolic changes, and immunologic dysfunction.

A. Mucous extravasation phenomenon.

1. Recurring submucosal nodule of saliva (often bluish in color) resulting from escape from duct of salivary gland.

2. Caused by traumatic severance of salivary excretory duct.

3. Common in lower lip (rare in upper lip) and buccal mucosa.

4. Recurrence if contributing gland is not removed.

B. Mucous retention cyst.

1. Submucosal nodule (often bluish in color) resulting from blockage of salivary duct by a salivary stone (sialolith).

2. Common in floor of mouth, palate, buccal mucosa, and upper lip (rare in lower lip).

3. Known as ranula when occurring in floor of mouth (Figure 4-15).

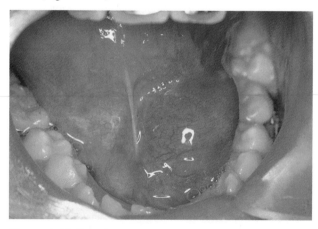

Figure 4-15 Ranula. *(From Regezi JA, Scuibba JJ, Jordan RCK: Oral Pathology: Clinical Pathologic Correlations, ed 6. St. Louis, Saunders, 2012.)*

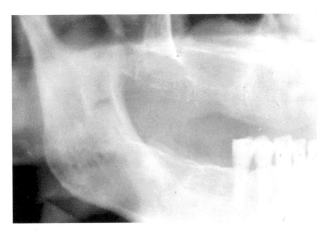

Figure 4-16 Maxillary sinus retention cyst. *(From Regezi JA, Scuibba JJ, Jordan RCK: Oral Pathology: Clinical Pathologic Correlations, ed 6. St. Louis, Saunders, 2012.)*

Box 4-10

Metabolic Conditions Associated with Bilateral Parotid Enlargement

Chronic alcoholism
Dietary deficiencies
Obesity
Diabetes mellitus
Hypertension
Hyperlipidemia
Sjögren's syndrome

C. Necrotizing sialometaplasia.
 1. Chronic ulcer of the palate secondary to ischemic necrosis of palatal salivary glands.
 2. Believed to be triggered by trauma, surgery, or local anesthesia.
 3. Heals in 6 to 10 weeks without treatment.
 4. Mimics carcinoma clinically and microscopically (squamous metaplasia of ducts).
D. Maxillary sinus retention cyst or pseudocyst (Figure 4-16).
 1. Common insignificant incidental finding in panoramic image.
 2. May represent blockage of sinus salivary gland or focal fluid accumulation of sinus mucosa.
 3. Lesions are asymptomatic and require no treatment.
E. Infectious sialadenitis.
 1. Infections of salivary glands may be acute or chronic, viral or bacterial.
 2. Viral infections.
  a. Mumps is an acute viral infection usually of the parotid glands.
  b. Cytomegalovirus infections are chronic and may be seen in immunosuppressed patients or (rarely) in infants via transplacental infection.
 3. Bacterial infections.
  a. Bacterial infections usually occur when salivary flow is reduced or impeded, especially in major glands, allowing bacterial overgrowth.
  b. Staphylococci and streptococci are the usual infecting agents.
F. Sarcoidosis.
 1. Chronic granulomatous disease of unknown cause, although bacteria (possibly mycobacteria) are suspected.
 2. This is predominantly a pulmonary disease, although many other organs may be affected, including salivary glands and mucosa.

 3. Granulomas (macrophage infiltrates) cause organ nodularity and loss of parenchyma.
 4. Diagnosis is made by biopsy, radiographic studies, and laboratory tests.
  a. Serum chemistry for hypercalcemia and elevated angiotensin-converting enzyme.
  b. Chest films for pulmonary involvement.
  c. Radiographs for bone involvement.
 5. Treated with corticosteroids and other immunomodulating drugs.
G. Metabolic enlargement of major salivary glands (Box 4-10).
 1. Bilateral parotid enlargement is associated with several systemic and metabolic conditions. The parotids generally feel soft to palpation.
H. Sjögren's syndrome.
 1. Chronic lymphocyte-mediated autoimmune disease affecting exocrine glands and other organ systems.
 2. Primary Sjögren's syndrome consists of keratoconjunctivitis sicca (dry eyes) and xerostomia (dry mouth).
 3. Secondary Sjögren's syndrome consists of dry eyes and mouth plus another autoimmune disease, usually rheumatoid arthritis.
 4. Diagnosis.
  a. Assessment of salivary function (usually labial salivary gland biopsy).
  b. Assessment of decrease in lacrimal function (Schirmer test).
  c. Laboratory tests for autoantibodies (rheumatoid factor, antinuclear antibodies, Sjögren's syndrome A, Sjögren's syndrome B).
 5. Cause is unknown, and treatment is symptomatic.
 6. Patients are at risk for development of lymphoma.
 7. Complication of cervical caries associated with dry mouth.

1.10 Salivary Gland Diseases— Benign Neoplasms

Benign salivary gland neoplasms manifest as asymptomatic connective tissue masses. Overlying mucosa or skin is typically intact (Table 4-3).

Table 4-3

Most Common Minor Salivary Gland Tumors

	USUAL SITE	PRESENTATION	MICROSCOPY	PROGNOSIS
Mixed tumor	Palate	Submucosal mass	Epithelial and mesenchymal cells	Excellent
Monomorphic adenomas	Palate, upper lip	Submucosal mass	Epithelial cells only	Excellent
Mucoepidermoid carcinoma	Palate	Mass and/or ulcer	Mucous cells and epithelial cells	Low-grade, excellent; high-grade, fair
Polymorphous low-grade adenocarcinoma	Palate	Mass and/or ulcer	Polymorphous epithelial cell patterns	Good
Adenoid cystic carcinoma	Palate	Mass and/or ulcer	Cribriform ("Swiss cheese") epithelial cell patterns	Poor

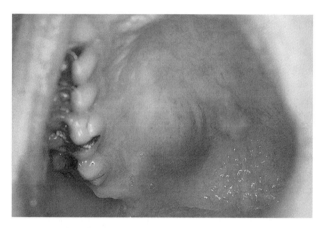

Figure 4-17 Mixed tumor. *(From Regezi JA, Scuibba JJ, Jordan RCK: Oral Pathology: Clinical Pathologic Correlations, ed 6. St. Louis, Saunders, 2012.)*

A. Mixed tumor (pleomorphic adenoma) (Figure 4-17).
   1. Most common benign salivary gland tumor (major and minor glands).
   2. Mixture of more than one cell type (epithelial and connective tissue elements) in many patterns (pleomorphic).
   3. Palate is most common site for minor gland lesions.
   4. Occasional recurrences associated with incomplete or poorly formed tumor capsule.
B. Monomorphic adenomas.
   1. Benign salivary tumors composed of a single cell type.
   2. Includes basal cell adenomas, canalicular adenomas, myoepitheliomas, and oncocytic tumors (oncocytes stain bright pink because of abundant mitochondrial proteins).
   3. Treated with surgical excision with infrequent recurrences.
C. Warthin's tumor.
   1. Warthin's tumor is an oncocytic tumor that also contains lymphoid tissue.
   2. Usually found in the parotid of older men.
   3. Occasionally bilateral.

1.11 Salivary Gland Diseases—Malignant Tumors

Malignancies of salivary gland origin have been classified into numerous types based on microscopic appearance, and not all are listed here. The behavior and prognosis associated with these tumors range from low-grade behavior with excellent prognosis to high-grade behavior with poor prognosis (see Table 4-3).

A. Mucoepidermoid carcinoma.
   1. Most common salivary malignancy in both minor and major glands.
   2. Palate is the most common intraoral site.
   3. Composed of mucous and epithelial cells.
   4. Microscopic low-grade lesions rarely metastasize and have an excellent prognosis.
   5. Microscopic high-grade lesions frequently metastasize and have a fair prognosis.
B. Polymorphous low-grade adenocarcinoma.
   1. Second most common minor salivary gland malignancy (rare in major glands).
   2. Palate most common site.
   3. Polymorphous microscopic patterns.
   4. Low-grade malignancy—good prognosis after surgical excision.
C. Adenoid cystic carcinoma.
   1. High-grade salivary malignancy.
   2. Palate most common site.
   3. Cribriform or "Swiss cheese" microscopic pattern.
   4. Spreads through perineural spaces.
   5. 5-year survival rate is 70%; 15-year survival rate is 10%.

1.12 Lymphoid Neoplasms

All lymphoid neoplasms are malignant. Hodgkin's lymphoma, characterized by Reed-Sternberg cells, is part of this group but is very rare in the oral cavity. Most lymphoid neoplasms occur in lymph nodes, although they occasionally arise in extranodal tissues, such as mucosa-associated lymphoid tissue (MALT). Oral manifestations include mass, ulcerated mass, and radiolucency.

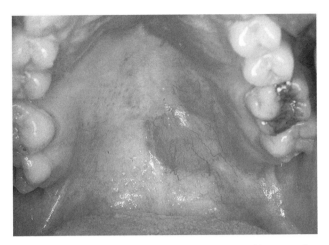

Figure 4-18 Lymphoma. *(From Regezi JA, Scuibba JJ, Jordan RCK: Oral Pathology: Clinical Pathologic Correlations, ed 6. St. Louis, Saunders, 2012.)*

A. Non-Hodgkin's lymphoma (Figure 4-18; Box 4-11).
  1. Malignancy of one of the cells making up lymphoid tissue.
  2. Microscopic classification of the various types of lymphomas currently follows the Revised European-American Lymphoma classification.
B. Multiple myeloma or plasma cell myeloma.
  1. Represents a monoclonal neoplastic expansion of immunoglobulin-secreting B cells (plasma cells) in what could be termed a *monoclonal gammopathy*.
  2. Clinical features.
    a. Multiple "punched-out" bone lucencies (solitary plasmacytoma invariably becomes multiple myeloma) in patients older than 50 years.
    b. Abnormal immunoglobulin protein peak (M protein) on serum electrophoresis.
    c. Urinary monoclonal light chains (Bence-Jones protein).
    d. Pain, swelling, and numbness.
    e. Anemia, bleeding, infection, and fracture associated with extensive marrow involvement.
    f. Treated with chemotherapy; poor prognosis.
  3. A form of amyloidosis occurs in 10% of patients with multiple myeloma.
    a. Amyloidosis in this context is due to formation of complex proteins in which immunoglobulin light chains are precursors.
    b. Amyloid protein is deposited in various organs and can lead to organ dysfunction (especially kidney, heart, gastrointestinal tract, liver, and spleen).
    c. Microscopically, amyloid proteins react with Congo red stain producing a green birefringence in polarized light.
    d. Other forms of amyloidosis (different precursor proteins).
      (1) Secondary amyloidosis developing in patients with chronic diseases such as rheumatoid

arthritis, chronic osteomyelitis, and chronic renal failure.
      (2) Single organ or localized amyloidosis (may be seen in the tongue).
C. Leukemias.
  1. Group of neoplasms of bone marrow (lymphocyte or myeloid precursors).

Box 4-11

Lymphomas

Cause

Undetermined for most lymphomas

EBV is important causative factor in immunodeficiency and in some Burkitt's lymphomas

Chromosome translocations are factors in some lymphomas, including Burkitt's lymphoma

Classification

Microscopic criteria used to separate various types of lymphoma

Important for predicting behavior and prescribing treatment

Most are B-cell type; T-cell lymphomas are very rare in the mouth

Staging

Determination of clinical extent of disease

Important factor for deciding type and intensity of therapy

Helps determine prognosis

Clinical Features

Lymphoma behavior patterns range from indolent to highly aggressive

Most head and neck tumors start in lymph nodes or in mucosa-associated lymphoid tissues (MALT lymphomas)

Tonsils and palate are most common intraoral sites

Bone involvement, especially in Burkitt's lymphoma, often results in swelling, pain, tooth mobility, and lip paresthesia

AIDS-associated lymphomas are typically high-grade B-cell tumors

Treatment

Dependent on lymphoma classification and stage

Typically, radiation is used for localized disease, and chemotherapy is used for extensive disease; chemoradiotherapy is also used

Some indolent low-grade lymphomas, known to respond poorly to therapeutic regimens, are not treated

2. Malignant cells occupy and replace normal marrow cells, including megakaryocytes (platelet-forming cells); malignant cells are also released into the peripheral blood.
3. Causes.
   a. Genetic factors, such as chromosome translocations.
   b. Environmental agents (e.g., benzene, radiation).
   c. Viruses (e.g., human T-lymphotropic virus 1).
4. Classification is based on cell lineage (myeloid or lymphoid) and whether the disease is acute or chronic.
5. Clinical features.
   a. Bleeding (owing to reduced platelets), fatigue (owing to anemia), and infection (owing to agranulocytosis) are important clinical signs of leukemias.
   b. Infiltration of gingival tissues by leukemic cells is common in chronic monocytic leukemia. Gingiva is red, boggy, and hemorrhagic.
   c. Treatment with chemotherapy is quite successful for acute leukemias but is less so for chronic leukemias.

1.13 Odontogenic Lesions— Odontogenic Cysts

Odontogenic cysts are derived from cells that are associated with tooth formation. Residual odontogenic epithelium may undergo cystification any time after tooth formation. Except for periapical cysts and some odontogenic keratocysts (keratocystic odontogenic tumors), the stimulus for cystic change is unknown (Table 4-4).
A. Periapical cyst (radicular cyst).
   1. Most common odontogenic cyst; always associated with nonvital tooth.
   2. Necrotic pulp causes periapical inflammation.
      a. If acute, a periapical abscess forms.
      b. If chronic, a dental granuloma (granulation tissue and chronic inflammatory cells) forms.

3. Rests of Malassez within a dental granuloma epithelialize the lesion, resulting in formation of a cyst.
4. Treated by root canal filling, apicoectomy, or tooth extraction with apical curettage.
B. Dentigerous cyst (Figure 4-19).
   1. Manifests as a lucency around the crown of an impacted tooth.
   2. Third molar and canines most often affected.
   3. Called *eruption cyst* if lesion occurs over tooth that has erupted into submucosa.
   4. Epithelial lining from reduced enamel epithelium has potential to transform into ameloblastoma.
C. Lateral periodontal cyst.
   1. Unilocular or multilocular lucency in the lateral periodontal membrane of adults.
   2. Most are found in the mandibular premolar region.
   3. Associated tooth is vital.
   4. Gingival cyst in an adult is soft tissue counterpart of this lesion.

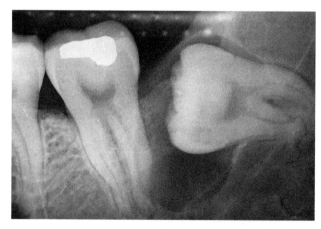

Figure 4-19 Dentigerous cyst. *(From Regezi JA, Scuibba JJ, Jordan RCK: Oral Pathology: Clinical Pathologic Correlations, ed 6. St. Louis, Saunders, 2012.)*

Table 4-4

Comparison of Odontogenic Cysts

	TOOTH VITAL?	EPITHELIAL SOURCE	INCIDENCE	RECURRENCE POTENTIAL?	SYNDROME-ASSOCIATED?
Periapical cyst	No	Rests of Malassez	Common	No	No
Dentigerous cyst	Yes	Reduced enamel epithelium	Common	No	No
Lateral periodontal cyst	Yes	Rests of dental lamina (Seres)	Uncommon	No	No
Gingival cyst	Yes	Rests of dental lamina (Seres)	Adults, rare; newborns, common	No	No
Odontogenic keratocyst	Yes	Rests of dental lamina (Seres)	Uncommon	Yes	Yes
Calcifying odontogenic cyst	Yes	Rests of dental lamina (Seres)	Rare	Yes	No
Glandular odontogenic cyst	Yes	Rests of dental lamina (Seres)	Rare	Yes	No

D. Gingival cysts of newborn.
   1. Multiple small gingival nodules resulting from cystification of rests of dental lamina.
   2. Also known as *Bohn's nodules*; inclusion cysts in the palates of infants are known as *Epstein's pearls*.
   3. No treatment necessary.
E. Odontogenic keratocyst (keratocystic odontogenic tumor) (Figure 4-20 and Box 4-12).
   1. Lesions may be clinically aggressive, recurrent, or associated with nevoid basal cell carcinoma (Gorlin) syndrome (multiple odontogenic keratocysts, numerous cutaneous basal cell carcinomas, skeletal abnormalities, calcified falx, and other stigmata).

Box 4-12

Odontogenic Keratocysts (Keratocystic Odontogenic Tumors)

Aggressive, recurrence risk, association with nevoid basal cell carcinoma syndrome

Solitary Cysts

5%-15% of all odontogenic cysts
10%-30% recurrence rate

Multiple Cysts (No Syndrome)

5% of all keratocysts
Recurrence rate greater than for solitary cysts

Syndrome-Associated Multiple Cysts

5% of all keratocysts
Recurrence rate greater than for multiple cysts (no syndrome)

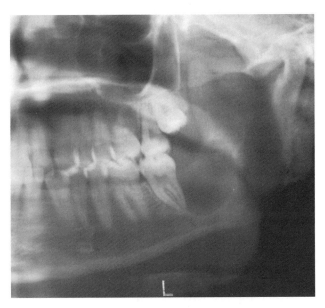

Figure 4-20 Odontogenic keratocyst. *(From Regezi JA, Scuibba JJ, Jordan RCK: Oral Pathology: Clinical Pathologic Correlations, ed 6. St. Louis, Saunders, 2012.)*

2. Mutation of the patched (*PTCH*) tumor suppressor gene is evident in syndrome-related cysts and probably in many solitary cysts. A proposed change of diagnostic terminology to keratocystic odontogenic tumor reflects the concept that the lesion is a neoplasm with cystic architecture rather than a developmental cyst.
   3. Lining epithelium is thin and parakeratinized.
   4. Less common orthokeratinized odontogenic cyst has much lower recurrence rate and is not syndrome-associated.
F. Calcifying odontogenic cyst.
   1. Rare odontogenic cyst of unpredictable behavior.
   2. Recurrence potential, especially for the solid variant.
   3. "Ghost cell" keratinization characterizes this cyst microscopically.
      a. Ghost cells may undergo calcification that may be detected radiographically (lucency with opaque foci).
   4. Cutaneous counterpart known as *Malherbe calcifying epithelioma* or *pilomatricoma*.
G. Glandular odontogenic cyst (sialo-odontogenic cyst).
   1. Rare odontogenic cyst that may be locally aggressive and exhibit recurrence potential.
   2. Name derived from glandlike spaces and mucous cells in epithelial lining.

1.14 Odontogenic Lesions— Odontogenic Tumors

Odontogenic tumors are bone tumors that are unique to the jaws. These lesions are derived from epithelial or mesenchymal cells involved in the formation of teeth. These lesions are almost always benign, although some may exhibit aggressive behavior and may have significant recurrence potential (Table 4-5). Some rare odontogenic tumors have not been included in this outline.
A. Ameloblastoma (Figure 4-21).
   1. Benign but aggressive odontogenic tumor with significant recurrence potential, especially if treated conservatively.

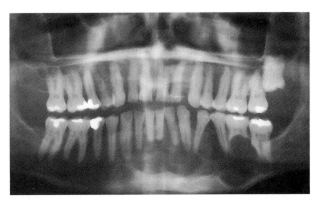

Figure 4-21 Ameloblastoma. *(From Regezi JA, Scuibba JJ, Jordan RCK: Oral Pathology: Clinical Pathologic Correlations, ed 6. St. Louis, Saunders, 2012.)*

Table 4-5

Characteristic Features of Odontogenic Tumors

	AGE (MEAN)	COMMON LOCATION	RADIOGRAPHIC CHANGES	BEHAVIOR
Ameloblastoma (solid type)	Adults (40 yr)	Molar—ramus	Unilocular or multilocular lucency	Benign, aggressive, recurrences
Calcifying epithelial odontogenic tumor	Adults (40 yr)	Molar—ramus	Unilocular or multilocular lucency; may have opaque foci	Benign, aggressive, may recur
Adenomatoid odontogenic tumor	Teens	Anterior jaws	Lucency, may have opaque foci	Benign, never recurs
Odontogenic myxoma	Adults (30 yr)	Either jaw	Unilocular or multilocular lucency	Benign, aggressive, recurrences
Ameloblastic fibroma and fibro-odontoma	Children and teens (12 yr)	Molar—ramus	Unilocular or multilocular lucency	Benign, rarely recurs
Odontoma	Children and teens	Compound type, anterior; complex type, posterior	Opaque	Benign, no recurrence

2. Cystic variant (cystic ameloblastoma) is less aggressive and is less likely to recur.

3. Peripheral or gingival ameloblastoma exhibits banal behavior.

4. Very rare malignant lesions are known as *malignant ameloblastoma* and *ameloblastic carcinoma*.

5. Several microscopic subtypes, all of which mimic to some degree the enamel organ, described for solid ameloblastomas; no difference in behavior.

6. Treatment ranges from wide excision to resection.

B. Calcifying epithelial odontogenic tumor (Pindborg tumor).

1. Rare odontogenic tumor with unusual microscopy (sheets of large epithelioid cells with areas of amyloid, some of which may become calcified).

2. Similar age distribution and location to ameloblastoma but less aggressive.

C. Adenomatoid odontogenic tumor.

1. Uncommon to rare odontogenic hamartoma that contains epithelial duct–like spaces and calcified enameloid material.

2. Two thirds in the maxilla, two thirds in females, two thirds in the anterior jaws, and two thirds over crown of impacted tooth.

3. Does not recur after conservative treatment.

D. Odontogenic myxoma (fibromyxoma).

1. Uncommon to rare tumor of myxomatous connective tissue (primitive-appearing connective tissue containing little collagen similar to dental pulp).

2. Either jaw affected.

3. Radiolucency, often with small loculations (honeycomb pattern).

4. Treated with surgical excision; moderate recurrence potential owing to lack of encapsulation and tumor consistency.

E. Central odontogenic fibroma.

1. Rare tumor of dense collagen with strands of epithelium.

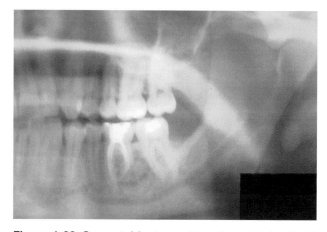

Figure 4-22 Cementoblastoma. *(From Regezi JA, Scuibba JJ, Jordan RCK: Oral Pathology: Clinical Pathologic Correlations, ed 6. St. Louis, Saunders, 2012.)*

2. Well-defined radiolucency in either jaw; often multilocular.

3. Treated with surgical excision; few recurrences.

F. Cementifying fibroma.

1. Can be considered similar or identical to ossifying fibroma.

2. Well-circumscribed lucency.

3. Some lesions are lucent with opaque foci.

4. Seen in adults and young adults, typically in the body of mandible.

5. Treated with curettage or excision; recurrences rare.

G. Cementoblastoma (Figure 4-22).

1. Well-circumscribed radiopaque mass of cementum and cementoblasts replacing root of a tooth.

2. Lesion is excised. The associated tooth is removed with lesion because of intimate association.

3. No recurrence after excision.

H. Periapical cemento-osseous dysplasia (Figure 4-23).

1. Reactive process of unknown cause that requires no treatment.

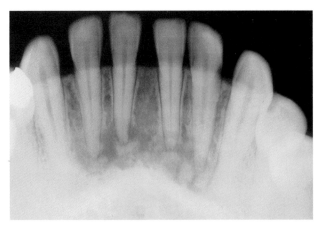

Figure 4-23 Periapical cemento-osseous dysplasia. *(From Regezi JA, Scuibba JJ, Jordan RCK: Oral Pathology: Clinical Pathologic Correlations, ed 6. St. Louis, Saunders, 2012.)*

2. Clinical features.
   a. Commonly seen at the apices of one or more mandibular anterior teeth.
   b. No symptoms; teeth vital.
   c. Most frequently seen in middle-aged women.
   d. Starts as circumscribed lucency, which gradually becomes opaque.
   e. An exuberant form that may involve the entire jaw is known as *florid osseous dysplasia*.
I. Ameloblastic fibroma and ameloblastic fibro-odontoma.
   1. The only difference between these lesions is the addition of an odontoma to the latter; they are otherwise the same lesion.
   2. Children and teens affected.
   3. Typically seen in mandibular molar region.
   4. Appears as a radiolucency (unilocular or multilocular) or as a radiolucency with an opacity (representing an odontoma).
   5. Microscopically, an encapsulated myxomatous connective tissue lesion containing strands of epithelium.
   6. Treated with enucleation or excision; rarely recurs.
J. Odontoma.
   1. Opaque lesion composed of dental hard tissues.
   2. Compound type contains miniature teeth; complex type composed of a conglomerate mass.
   3. Treated with curettage; no recurrence.

1.15 Bone (Nonodontogenic) Lesions— Fibro-osseous Lesions

Nonodontogenic lesions can occur in any bone of the skeleton. Fibro-osseous lesions are benign tumors composed of fibrous tissue in which new bony islands develop. These lesions have similar microscopic features, making diagnosis dependent on clinicopathologic correlation.
A. Ossifying fibroma.
   1. Common fibro-osseous lesion.

Microscopic Differential Diagnosis for Giant Cell Lesions of Bone

Central giant cell granuloma
Hyperparathyroidism
Aneurysmal bone cyst
Cherubism

2. Can be considered similar or identical to cementifying fibroma, although some may reach considerable size.
3. Clinical features.
   a. Radiographically appears as either a well-circumscribed lucency or a lucency with opaque foci.
   b. Seen in adults and young adults, typically in the body of the mandible.
   c. A variant known as *juvenile ossifying fibroma* occurs in younger patients and may exhibit an aggressive course.
4. Microscopically composed of fibroblastic stroma in which new bony islands or trabeculae are formed.
5. Treatment—curettage or excision; recurrences rare.
B. Fibrous dysplasia.
   1. Uncommon to rare unencapsulated fibro-osseous lesion associated with mutations of the *GNAS1* gene, affecting proliferation and function of osteoblasts and fibroblasts.
   2. Clinical features.
      a. Involves the entire half jaw; more common in the maxilla.
      b. Affects children and typically stops growing after puberty.
      c. Radiographic pattern is diffuse opacity (ground-glass appearance).
      d. McCune-Albright syndrome consists of polyostotic (more than one bone) fibrous dysplasia; cutaneous café au lait macules; and endocrine abnormalities, especially precocious puberty.
   3. Treated with surgical recontouring for cosmetic appearance.
C. Osteoblastoma.
   1. Circumscribed opaque mass of bone and osteoblasts.
   2. Young adults most commonly affected; 50% of patients have associated pain.
   3. Treated with surgical excision; few recurrences.

1.16 Bone (Nonodontogenic) Lesions— Giant Cell Lesions

Microscopically, bone (nonodontogenic) lesions have multinucleated giant cells in common; this makes clinicopathologic correlation important for diagnosis (Box 4-13).

A. Peripheral giant cell granuloma.
   1. Reactive red-to-purple gingival mass believed to be caused by local factors.
   2. Found in gingiva, typically anterior to permanent molar teeth.
   3. Composed of fibroblasts and multinucleated giant cells, similar to central counterpart.
   4. Treated with excision that extends to periosteum or periodontal ligament (PDL).
   5. Occasional recurrences are seen.
B. Central giant cell granuloma.
   1. Tumor that exhibits unpredictable clinical behavior; some are aggressive and have recurrence potential, whereas others have a bland course.
   2. Radiolucency, sometimes loculated, in teenagers; anterior mandible favored.
   3. Composed of fibroblasts and multinucleated giant cells.
   4. Treatment is excision, but occasional recurrences are encountered. Medical management (calcitonin or interferon) for large lesions is a possible option.
C. Aneurysmal bone cyst.
   1. Pseudocyst (cystlike spaces but no epithelial lining) that is composed of blood-filled spaces lined by fibroblasts and multinucleated giant cells.
   2. Multilocular lucency occurring typically in teenagers.
   3. Cause unknown; excision and occasional recurrences.
D. Hyperparathyroidism (von Recklinghausen's disease of bone).
   1. Multiple bone lesions resulting from effects of excessive levels of parathormone.
   2. May be caused by functioning parathyroid tumor or compensatory parathyroid hyperplasia secondary to renal failure, malabsorption, or vitamin D deficiency.
   3. Clinical features.
      a. Multiple radiolucent foci of fibroblasts and multinucleated giant cells as well as loss of lamina dura around tooth roots.
      b. Systemic signs include kidney stones, metastatic calcification, osteoporosis, neurologic problems, and arrhythmias (in addition to elevated parathormone and alkaline phosphatase).
E. Cherubism (Figure 4-24).
   1. Autosomal dominant condition of the jaws in children.
   2. Clinical features.
      a. Symmetrical (bilateral) swelling of one or both jaws.
      b. Stabilizes after puberty and requires no treatment.
      c. Loculated radiolucencies described as having "soap bubble" appearance.

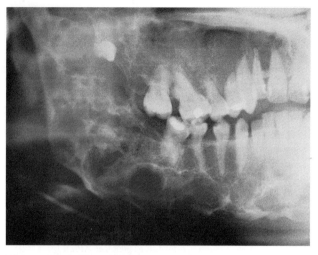

Figure 4-24 Cherubism. *(From Regezi JA, Scuibba JJ, Jordan RCK: Oral Pathology: Clinical Pathologic Correlations, ed 6. St. Louis, Saunders, 2012.)*

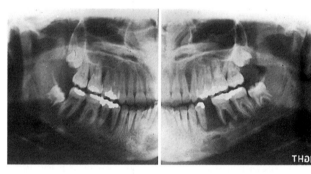

Figure 4-25 Langerhans' cell disease. *(From Regezi JA, Scuibba JJ, Jordan RCK: Oral Pathology: Clinical Pathologic Correlations, ed 6. St. Louis, Saunders, 2012.)*

Box 4-14

Classification of Langerhans' Cell Disease

Eosinophilic granuloma (chronic localized form)—
solitary or multiple bone lesions
Hand-Schüller-Christian disease (chronic disseminated form)—bone lesions, exophthalmos, and diabetes insipidus
Letterer-Siwe disease (acute disseminated form)—
bone, skin, and internal organ lesions

---

   3. Microscopically, this is another giant cell lesion. A distinctive perivascular collagen condensation may also be seen.
F. Langerhans' cell disease (idiopathic histiocytosis, Langerhans' granulomatosis) (Box 4-14 and Figure 4-25).
   1. All forms represent abnormal proliferation of Langerhans' cells.
   2. Clinical features.
      a. Radiographs show discrete "punched-out" lesions or lucencies around tooth roots ("floating teeth").

b. Treatment—variable, including excision, low-dose radiation, and chemotherapy.

3. Microscopically, eosinophils are mixed with the tumor Langerhans' cells. Some Langerhans' cells are multinucleated.

4. Prognosis very good when disease is localized; acute disseminated form is usually fatal.

G. Paget's disease.

1. Progressive metabolic disturbance of many bones (usually spine, femur, cranium, pelvis, and sternum).

2. Cause is unknown, and treatment is generally symptomatic.

3. Clinical features.

a. Adults older than 50 years affected.

b. Jaw involvement.

(1) Symmetrical enlargement.

(2) Dentures become too tight.

(3) Diastemas and hypercementosis may appear.

c. Bone pain, headache, altered vision and hearing (canal sclerosis).

d. Bleeding may complicate surgery because bone is highly vascular in early stages.

e. Jaw fracture and osteomyelitis are late complications secondary to bone sclerosis.

4. Microscopically, osteoblasts and multinucleated osteoclasts are found in abundance. As lesion advances, dense bone with numerous reversal or growth lines is seen, giving the tissue a mosaic pattern.

5. Treatment strategy is directed at suppression of bone resorption and deposition. Bisphosphonates—and to a lesser extent, calcitonin—have shown efficacy.

1.17 Bone (Nonodontogenic) Lesions—Inflammatory Diseases

Inflammation of bone (and bone marrow) or osteomyelitis is common in the jaws. Most lesions are associated with extension of periodontal or periapical inflammation. Others are associated with trauma to the jaws.

A. Acute osteomyelitis.

1. Acute inflammation of bone and bone marrow of the jaws.

2. Causes include extension of periapical or periodontal disease, fracture, surgery, and bacteremia.

3. Staphylococci and streptococci are most common infectious agents.

4. Pain, paresthesia, and exudation are typically present.

5. Radiographic changes (diffuse lucency) appear only after the inflammation has been present for an extended period.

6. Treatment—appropriate antibiotic and drainage of the lesion.

B. Chronic osteomyelitis.

1. Chronic osteomyelitis (chronic osteitis).

a. Chronic inflammation of bone and bone marrow of the jaws.

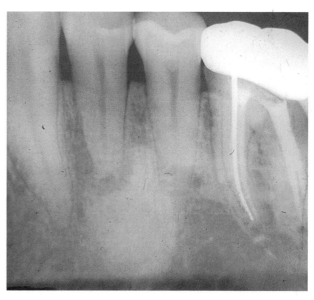

Figure 4-26 Focal sclerosing osteomyelitis. *(From Regezi JA, Scuibba JJ, Jordan RCK: Oral Pathology: Clinical Pathologic Correlations, ed 6. St. Louis, Saunders, 2012.)*

b. Mild to moderate pain and possibly an exudate.

c. Lucent or mottled radiographic pattern.

d. Treated with antibiotics and sequestrectomy.

2. Chronic osteomyelitis with proliferative periosteitis (Garré's osteomyelitis).

a. Form of chronic osteomyelitis that involves the periosteum.

b. Usually associated with carious molar in children.

c. Lucent or mottled radiographic pattern plus concentric periosteal layering.

d. Treated with tooth removal and antibiotics.

3. Focal sclerosing osteomyelitis (condensing osteitis) (Figure 4-26).

a. Bone sclerosis (opacity) resulting from low-grade inflammation, usually secondary to chronic pulpitis.

b. Asymptomatic and found on routine examination.

c. Treatment consists of determining and addressing the cause, and possibly endodontics.

4. Diffuse sclerosing osteomyelitis.

a. Bone sclerosis (opacity) resulting from low-grade inflammation, usually secondary to chronic pulpitis or periodontal disease.

b. Low-grade pain, swelling, or drainage may be present.

c. Jaw fracture and osteomyelitis are late complications secondary to densely sclerotic bone.

d. Treatment consists of determining and addressing the cause and probable use of antibiotics.

5. Bisphosphonate-related osteonecrosis of the jaws.

a. Characterized by exposed bone in maxillofacial region for longer than 8 weeks in a patient who has received a bisphosphonate medication.

b. Usual presenting symptom is jaw pain.

c. Tooth mobility, infection, sequestration, and pathologic fracture are potential outcomes.

d. Risk of development much greater with intravenous bisphosphonates as opposed to oral drugs, and osteonecrosis is more likely to develop in areas of oral trauma.

e. Treatment includes conservative local measures such as chlorhexidine rinses, antibiotic therapy, and conservative surgery.

1.18 Bone (Nonodontogenic) Lesions—Malignancies

Malignancies manifesting in bone include sarcomas, lymphomas or leukemias, and metastatic carcinomas. Numb lip, representing neoplastic invasion of nerve, is a frequent presenting symptom.

A. Osteosarcoma.
   1. Sarcoma in which new bone (osteoid) is formed.
   2. Cause is unknown, although an association with several specific genetic alterations has been detected.
   3. Clinical features.
      a. Pain, swelling, and paresthesia are typically present; PDL invasion results in uniform widening.
      b. Mean age of patients is 35 years (range, 10 to 85 years).
      c. Mandible affected more commonly than maxilla.
   4. Most jaw tumors are microscopically low-grade lesions.
   5. Treatment and prognosis.
      a. Treated with resection and usually neoadjuvant chemotherapy (preoperative) or adjuvant chemotherapy (postoperative).
      b. 5-year survival rate 25% to 40%.
      c. Prognosis better for mandibular tumors than for maxillary tumors.
      d. Initial radical surgery results in survival rate of 80%.
B. Chondrosarcoma.
   1. Rare sarcoma of the jaws in which cartilage is produced by tumor cells.
   2. Clinical features and treatment similar to osteosarcoma.
C. Ewing's sarcoma.
   1. Rare "round cell" malignant radiolucency of children.
   2. Aggressive multimodality therapy; fair prognosis.
D. Burkitt's lymphoma (see Box 4-11).
E. Metastatic carcinoma (Box 4-15).
   1. Pain, swelling, and especially paresthesia may occur.
   2. Ill-defined lucent-to-opaque radiographic changes are noted.
F. Multiple myeloma (see Box 4-11).

1.19 Hereditary Conditions

A genetic causation is known for many oral conditions. Some of these have already been outlined. Others are listed

---

> **Box 4-15**
>
> ### *Malignancies Most Commonly Metastatic to the Jaws*
>
> Adenocarcinoma of the *breast*
> Carcinoma of the *lung*
> Adenocarcinoma of the *prostate*
> Adenocarcinoma of the *colon*
> Carcinoma of the *kidney* (renal cell)

---

here, although many uncommon to rare hereditary syndromes are not included.

A. White sponge nevus.
   1. Autosomal dominant condition secondary to mutations of keratin 4 or 13.
   2. Results in asymptomatic white, spongy-appearing buccal mucosa bilaterally.
   3. Biopsy for diagnosis; no treatment necessary.
B. Epidermolysis bullosa.
   1. The term *epidermolysis bullosa* encompasses several genetic conditions and one acquired disease.
   2. Hereditary patterns range from autosomal dominant to autosomal recessive.
   3. Clinically common to all forms is the appearance of bullae from minor trauma (especially over elbows and knees).
   4. Oral lesions (blisters, scarring, and hypoplastic teeth) are characteristically seen in severe recessive form.
C. Hereditary hemorrhagic telangiectasia.
   1. Rare autosomal dominant condition in which telangiectatic vessels are seen in mucosa, skin, and occasionally viscera.
   2. Red macules or papules (telangiectasias) are an occasional source of bleeding.
   3. Epistaxis (nosebleed) is a frequent presenting sign; oral bleeding may occur.
D. Cleidocranial dysplasia.
   1. This autosomal dominant condition is manifested by many alterations, especially of teeth and bones.
   2. The most distinctive features include delayed tooth eruption and supernumerary teeth, hypoplastic or aplastic clavicles, cranial bossing, and hypertelorism.
E. Hereditary ectodermal dysplasia (Figure 4-27).
   1. X-linked recessive condition that results in partial or complete anodontia.
   2. Patients also have hypoplasia of other ectodermal structures, including hair, sweat glands, and nails.
F. Gardner's syndrome.
   1. Autosomal dominant disorder.
   2. Consists of intestinal polyposis, osteomas, skin lesions, impacted permanent and supernumerary teeth, and odontomas.
   3. Intestinal polyps have a very high rate of malignant conversion to colorectal carcinoma.

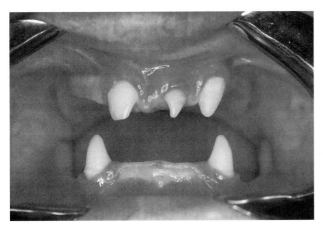

Figure 4-27 Hereditary ectodermal dysplasia. *(From Regezi JA, Scuibba JJ, Jordan RCK: Oral Pathology: Clinical Pathologic Correlations, ed 6. St. Louis, Saunders, 2012.)*

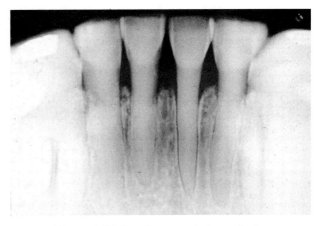

Figure 4-29 Dentinogenesis imperfecta.

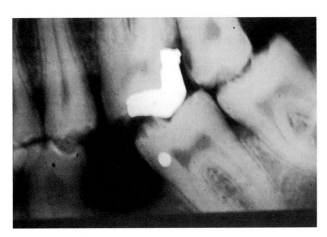

Figure 4-28 Amelogenesis imperfecta.

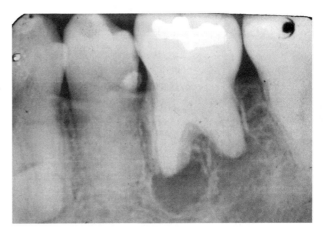

Figure 4-30 Dentin dysplasia.

G. Osteopetrosis (Albers-Schönberg disease, marble bone).
   1. Generalized bone condition that may be inherited as an autosomal dominant (less serious) or recessive trait (more serious).
   2. Lack of bone remodeling and resorption leads to bone sclerosis.
   3. Bone pain, blindness and deafness from sclerosis of ostia, anemia from sclerosis of marrow, and osteomyelitis secondary to diminished vascularity are seen.
H. Amelogenesis imperfecta (Figure 4-28).
   1. Rare group of hereditary conditions that affect enamel tissue intrinsically.
   2. All teeth of both dentitions are affected.
      a. Enamel is typically yellow in color, reduced in volume, and pitted.
      b. Dentin and pulps are normal.
      c. Although teeth are soft, there is no increase in caries rate.
      d. Represents a cosmetic problem that is treated with full crown coverage.

I. Dentinogenesis imperfecta (Figure 4-29).
   1. Autosomal dominant condition in which there is intrinsic alteration of dentin.
   2. All teeth of both dentitions are affected.
      a. Teeth have yellow or opalescent color.
      b. Extreme occlusal wear secondary to enamel fracture (poor dentin support).
      c. Short roots, bell-shaped crowns, and obliterated pulps.
      d. May be seen with osteogenesis imperfecta.
      e. Represents a cosmetic problem that is treated with full crown coverage.
J. Dentin dysplasia (Figure 4-30).
   1. Autosomal dominant condition in which there is intrinsic alteration of dentin.
   2. All teeth of both dentitions are affected.
      a. Teeth have normal color.
      b. Pulps are obliterated but may have residual spaces (chevrons).
      c. Roots are short and are surrounded by dental granulomas or cysts that may contribute to tooth loss.
      d. Teeth are not good candidates for restoration.

K. Regional odontodysplasia.
1. Dental abnormality of unknown cause; genetics, trauma, nutrition, and infection have been suggested.
2. A quadrant of teeth exhibit short roots, open apices, and enlarged pulp chambers.
3. The radiographic appearance of these teeth has suggested the term *ghost teeth*.
4. Teeth are usually extracted because of the poor quality of enamel and dentin.

2.0 Oral Radiology

Sanjay M. Mallya

The proper clinical use of ionizing radiation for optimal application to patient care requires knowledge and integration of radiologic concepts. This review follows a standard sequence similar to the textbook *Oral Radiology: Principles and Interpretation*, ed 7 (2013, Mosby, St. Louis) by White and Pharoah.

This review is not meant to be a comprehensive treatment of radiology, but rather a guide to study in preparing for the Radiology section of Part II of the National Board Dental Examination. Radiographic interpretation of oral disease is covered in the Pathology section of this review book. Students are referred to other sources, including the text by White and Pharoah, for more complete discussions in each area of radiology. This review is intended to help organize and integrate knowledge of concepts and facts. It also can help students identify areas requiring more concentrated study.

Outline of Review

2.1 Radiation Physics
2.2 Radiation Biology
2.3 Health Physics
2.4 X-Ray Film and Intensifying Screens
2.5 Projection Geometry
2.6 Processing X-Ray Film
2.7 Digital Imaging
2.8 Radiographic Quality Assurance and Infection Control
2.9 Intraoral Radiographic Examinations
2.10 Radiographic Anatomy
2.11 Radiographic Appearance of Caries
2.12 Radiographic Appearance of Periodontal Disease
2.13 Panoramic Imaging

2.1 Radiation Physics

A. Matter.
1. Generation, emission, and absorption of radiation occur at the subatomic level.
a. Electrons.
(1) Exist in orbitals around the nucleus and carry an electrical charge of −1.
b. Nucleus.
(1) Proton: charge of +1 and mass 1836 times the mass of the electron.
(2) Neutron: no charge and slightly heavier than the proton.
2. Ionization.
a. Occurs when an electrically neutral atom loses an electron and becomes a positive ion; the free electron is a negative ion.
B. Radiation.
1. Electromagnetic radiation.
a. Movement of energy through space as a combination of electrical and magnetic fields.
b. Quantum theory considers electromagnetic radiation as small bundles of energy called photons that travel at the speed of light and contain a specific amount of energy. Electromagnetic radiations comprise a spectrum of radiations with varying energy.
c. Wave theory considers these radiations to be propagated in the form of waves. Wavelength is inversely proportional to the photon energy—the shorter the wavelength, the higher the energy.
d. The spectrum of electromagnetic radiations includes gamma rays, x-rays, UV rays, visible light, infrared radiation (heat), microwaves, and radio waves, arranged in order of decreasing energies (or increasing wavelength). Gamma rays, x-rays, and UV radiation have sufficient energy to ionize biologic molecules and are referred to as *ionizing radiation*.
2. Particulate radiation.
a. Atomic nuclei or subatomic particles moving at high velocity.
b. Alpha and beta particles and electrons (cathode rays) are examples.
C. X-ray machines.
1. X-ray tube (Figure 4-31).
a. Cathode.
(1) Tungsten filament is the source of electrons within an x-ray tube.
(2) Molybdenum focusing cup electrostatically focuses electrons emitted by the incandescent filament into a narrow beam directed at a small area on the anode (focal spot).
b. Anode.
(1) Tungsten target.
(a) Converts kinetic energy of electrons generated from the filament into x-ray photons.
(b) Focal spot is an area on the target onto which the focusing cup directs electrons.
(c) As the size of the focal spot decreases, the sharpness of the radiographic image increases.
(2) Copper stem.
(a) Dissipates heat and reduces risk of target melting.

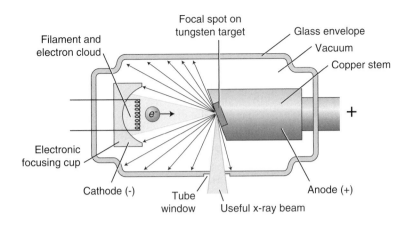

Figure 4-31 X-ray tube with major components labeled. *(From White SC, Pharoah MJ: Oral Radiology: Principles and Interpretation, ed 7. St. Louis, Mosby, 2014.)*

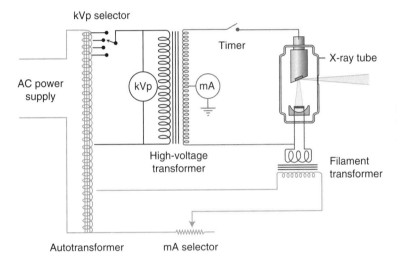

Figure 4-32 Dental x-ray machine circuitry with major components labeled. *(From White SC, Pharoah MJ: Oral Radiology: Principles and Interpretation, ed 7. St. Louis, Mosby, 2014.)*

2. Power supply (Figure 4-32).
   a. Heats x-ray tube filament.
      (1) Provides low-voltage current by use of a step-down transformer that reduces the voltage of the incoming alternating current.
      (2) Controlled by a milliamperage (mA) switch that regulates the temperature of the filament and the number of electrons emitted.
      (3) Tube current.
         (a) Flow of electrons through the tube from the filament to the anode and back to the filament.
         (b) The quantity of radiation produced by an x-ray tube is directly proportional to the tube current (mA) and the exposure time (s).
         (c) Controls the number of photons generated (intensity of the beam) but not the beam energy.
   b. High-voltage transformer generates high potential difference between the anode and the cathode.
      (1) The kVp control selects voltage from different levels on the autotransformer and applies it across the primary winding of the high-voltage transformer.
      (2) The high-voltage transformer increases voltage significantly and provides the high voltage required by the x-ray tube to accelerate electrons from the cathode to the anode and to generate x-rays.
      (3) Beam quality refers to the mean energy of an x-ray beam, which increases with increasing kVp.
      (4) The number of photons (beam intensity) also increases with increasing kVp.
      (5) Because line current is alternating (60 cycles/sec), the polarity of the x-ray tube alternates, and the x-ray beam is generated as a series of pulses.
   c. Time exposure (s).
      (1) The timer controls the length of time high voltage is applied to the tube and the time during which the tube current flows and x-rays are produced.
3. Producing x-rays.
   a. High-energy electrons produced by the filament interact with the tungsten atoms at the target resulting in an energy loss, which is converted to heat and x-ray photons.
   b. Bremsstrahlung radiation.

(1) Primary source of x-ray photons from the x-ray tube.

(2) Results from stopping or slowing of high-speed electrons at the target.

(a) An electron is attracted toward positively charged nuclei and loses velocity.

(b) Lost kinetic energy is given off in the form of new bremsstrahlung x-ray photons.

(c) Bremsstrahlung interactions generate x-ray photons with a continuous spectrum of energy.

c. Characteristic radiation.

(1) Results when electrons from the filament collide with and eject an inner orbital electron, which is replaced by an outer orbital electron and release of a photon of specific energy.

4. Factors controlling the x-ray beam.

a. Kilovoltage.

(1) kVp affects both the quality and the quantity of the x-ray photons.

(2) When the kVp increases, the total number of photons produced increases, and mean energy and maximum energy of the x-ray beam increase.

b. Milliamperage and exposure time.

(1) mA and s affect the quantity of the x-ray photons produced. Although they can be individually varied, their product (mAs) is used as the parameter to describe the x-ray beam.

(2) When the mAs increases, the total number of photons increases, but the mean and maximum energies of the x-ray beam are unchanged.

c. Filtration.

(1) Accomplished by placing an aluminum filter in the path of the beam.

(2) Reduces patient dose by preferentially removing lower energy (less-penetrating) photons from the beam.

(3) After filtration, the total number of photons decreases. However, because lower energy photons are preferentially removed, the mean energy of the x-ray beam increases.

(4) Governmental regulations require total filtration to be equal to the equivalent of 1.5 mm of aluminum for up to 70 kVp and 2.5 mm of aluminum for higher voltages.

d. Collimation.

(1) A collimator is a metallic barrier with an aperture to reduce the size of the x-ray beam and the volume of irradiated patient tissue.

(2) Dental x-ray beams are usually collimated to a circle 2.75 inches (7 cm) in diameter with the collimator typically built into open-ended aiming cylinders.

(3) Rectangular collimators further limit the size of the beam to just larger than the image receptor to reduce further unnecessary patient exposure.

e. Inverse square law.

(1) Intensity of the x-ray beam at a given point is inversely proportional to the square of the distance from the source.

(2) Changing the distance between the x-ray tube and the patient has a marked effect on beam intensity.

(3) This principle is also applied to operator protection, where the operator stands at a distance of at least 6 feet from the x-ray source to minimize the intensity of the x-ray photons.

D. Interactions of x-rays with matter.

1. Coherent scattering.

a. Occurs when a low-energy photon passes near an outer electron, the photon ceases to exist, and the excited electron returns to ground state, generating another photon with the same energy as in the incident beam.

b. Approximately 8% of interactions with photons in a dental x-ray beam.

2. Photoelectric absorption.

a. Occurs when a photon collides with a bound electron, which is ejected from its orbital, and the incident photon ceases to exist.

b. Frequency of photoelectric interaction is directly proportional to the third power of the atomic number of the absorber and contributes greatly to the differences in radiographic density of enamel, dentin, bone, and soft tissue on radiographs.

c. About 30% of interactions with photons in a dental x-ray beam.

3. Compton scattering.

a. Occurs when a photon interacts with an outer orbital electron, which recoils from the impact, and the incident photon is scattered in a new direction with lower energy.

b. About 62% of interactions with photons in a dental x-ray beam.

E. Dosimetry (Table 4-6).

1. Exposure.

a. Measure of radiation quantity; capacity of radiation to ionize air.

2. Absorbed dose.

a. Unit is gray (Gy), where 1 Gy equals 1 joule/kg.

3. Effective dose.

a. Used to estimate risk in humans.

b. Unit of effective dose is sievert (Sv).

4. Radioactivity.

a. Decay rate of radioactive material.

b. Unit is becquerel (Bq); 1 Bq equals 1 disintegration/sec.

2.2 Radiation Biology

A. Radiation biology is the study of the effects of ionizing radiation on living systems.

Table 4-6

Summary of Units and Quantities

QUANTITY	SYSTEME INTERNATIONAL D'UNITES UNIT	DEFINITION	TRADITIONAL UNIT	CONVERSION
Exposure	Air kerma (Gy)	Energy absorbed in air, 1 joule/kg	Roentgen (R)	1 Gy = 100 rad 1 rad = 0.01 Gy (1 cGy)
Absorbed dose	Gray (Gy)	Energy absorbed in tissue, 1 joule/kg	Rad	1 Gy = 100 rad 1 rad = 0.01 Gy (1 cGy)
Effective dose	Sievert (Sv)	Energy absorbed in tissue times tissue weighting factors, 1 joule/kg	—	—
Radioactivity	Becquerel (Bq)	For radioactive isotopes, 1 disintegration per second	Curie (Ci)	1 Bq = 2.7×10^{-11} Ci 1 Ci = 3.7×10^{10} Bq

Source: http://physics.nist.gov/cuu/units/units.html. Accessed Dec. 1, 2006.

1. Deterministic effects.
    a. There is a threshold below which a response is not seen.
    b. Severity of response is proportional to dose.
    c. Changes resulting from killing of many cells after moderate to high doses of radiation.
    d. Example: oral mucositis after radiation therapy.
2. Stochastic effects.
    a. There is no minimum threshold dose.
    b. Probability of response, rather than severity, is dose-dependent.
    c. Changes resulting from damage to DNA of single cells.
    d. Examples: radiation-induced cancer and heritable effects.
B. Radiation chemistry.
    1. Direct effect.
        a. Direct alteration of biologic molecules (carbohydrates, lipids, proteins, DNA) by ionizing radiation.
        b. Approximately one third of biologic effects of x-ray exposure result from direct effects.
    2. Indirect effects.
        a. Radiation effects mediated through water.
        b. Ionizing radiation converts water to hydrogen and hydroxyl free radicals (radiolysis of water), which alter biologic molecules.
        c. About two thirds of radiation-induced biologic damage results from indirect effects.
    3. Changes in biologic molecules.
        a. Nucleic acids.
            (1) Damage to the DNA molecule is the primary mechanism for radiation-induced cell death, mutation, and carcinogenesis.
C. Cellular radiation effects.
    1. Intracellular structures.
        a. Nucleus.
            (1) The nucleus is far more radiosensitive than cytoplasm, especially in dividing cells.
            (2) The sensitive site in the nucleus is DNA.
            (3) Chromosome changes serve as useful markers for radiation injury.
    2. Effects on cell kinetics.
        a. Mitotic delay.
            (1) Mitotic delay occurs after irradiation of dividing cells.
            (2) Severity is dose-dependent.
        b. Cell death.
            (1) Cell death is caused largely by damage to chromosomes, preventing successful mitosis.
            (2) Radiation also causes cell death by apoptosis.
        c. Recovery.
            (1) Cell recovery involves enzymatic repair of single-strand breaks of DNA.
            (2) Double-strand breaks (damage to both strands of DNA at the same site) is usually lethal to a cell.
    3. Radiosensitivity and cell type.
        a. Cells that are mitotically active and undifferentiated and have long mitotic futures (e.g., oral mucous membrane basal cells) are more radiosensitive than cells that no longer divide (e.g., neurons or striated muscle cells).
D. Radiation effects at the tissue and organ level.
    1. Short-term effects.
        a. Rapidly proliferating tissues (bone marrow, oral mucous membrane) are lost primarily by mitosis-linked death.
    2. Long-term effects.
        a. Long-term deterministic effects depend primarily on mitotic activity of the parenchymal cells and the extent of damage to fine vasculature.
E. Radiation effects on oral cavity.
    1. Rationale of radiotherapy.
        a. Irradiation often used to treat radiosensitive oral malignant tumors, usually squamous cell carcinomas.

b. Fractionation of total x-ray dose into multiple small doses provides greater tumor destruction than is possible with a large single dose.

2. Radiation effect on oral tissues.

a. Oral mucous membrane.

(1) Near the end of the second week of therapy, as basal epithelial cells die, the mucous membrane begins to show areas of redness and inflammation (mucositis).

(2) As mucous membrane breaks down, it forms a white-to-yellow pseudomembrane (desquamated epithelial layer).

(3) At the end of therapy, mucositis is most severe, discomfort is at the maximum, and food intake is difficult.

(4) Secondary yeast infection by *C. albicans* is a common complication and may require treatment.

(5) After radiation therapy is completed, mucosal healing begins and is usually complete by about 2 months.

(6) At later intervals (months to years), the mucous membrane becomes atrophic, thin, and relatively avascular, which complicates denture wearing.

b. Taste buds.

(1) Radiation therapy causes extensive degeneration of normal histologic architecture of taste buds and loss of taste acuity during the second or third week.

c. Salivary glands.

(1) Dose-dependent and progressive loss of salivary secretion usually seen in the first few weeks after initiation of radiotherapy.

(2) Mouth becomes dry (xerostomia) and tender, and swallowing becomes difficult and painful because residual saliva loses normal lubricating properties.

(3) Reduced salivary flow that persists beyond 1 year is unlikely to show significant recovery.

(4) Salivary changes have a profound influence on oral microflora, often leading to radiation caries.

d. Teeth.

(1) Irradiation of developing teeth with therapeutic doses severely retards tooth formation.

(2) Depending on the severity of the dose, aberrant formation or arrested root development may occur.

e. Radiation caries.

(1) Carious lesions result from changes in salivary glands and saliva, including reduced flow (resulting in xerostomia), decreased pH, reduced buffering capacity, and increased viscosity.

(2) Best restorative results are achieved from a combination of restorative dental procedures,

excellent oral hygiene, and topical applications of sodium fluoride.

f. Bone.

(1) Primary damage to mature bone results from radiation-induced damage to the vasculature of the periosteum and cortical bone, which are normally already sparse.

(2) After irradiation, normal marrow may be replaced with fatty marrow and fibrous connective tissue that becomes hypovascular, hypoxic, and hypocellular.

(3) Endosteum becomes atrophic, showing a lack of osteoblastic and osteoclastic activity, and some lacunae of compact bone are empty; this is an indication of necrosis.

(4) When these changes are so severe that bone death results, the condition is termed *osteoradionecrosis*; this is the most serious clinical complication that occurs in bone after irradiation.

(5) The decreased vascularity of the mandible renders it easily infected by microorganisms from the oral cavity.

(6) This infection may cause a nonhealing wound in irradiated bone that is difficult to treat and causes extensive bone loss.

(7) Osteoradionecrosis is more common in the mandible than in the maxilla because of richer vascular supply to the maxilla and because the mandible is more frequently irradiated.

F. Effects of whole-body irradiation.

1. When the whole body is exposed to low or moderate doses of radiation, characteristic changes (termed *acute radiation syndrome*) develop, which are quite different from changes seen when a relatively small volume of tissue is exposed.

2. Radiation effects on embryos and fetuses.

a. Prenatal irradiation may lead to death or specific developmental abnormalities, depending on the stage of development at the time of irradiation.

b. No effects on embryos or fetuses have been shown from low doses used in dental radiography.

G. Late somatic effects seen in years after exposure.

1. Carcinogenesis.

a. Radiation-induced cancer is a stochastic effect; that is, there is no threshold below which the effect does not occur.

b. The risk of developing cancer increases with increasing dose.

c. Radiation-induced cancers are not distinguishable from cancers produced by other causes.

d. Incidence of leukemia increases soon after exposure of bone marrow and returns nearly to baseline rates within 40 years.

e. Radiation-induced solid cancers, including in the thyroid, brain, and salivary glands, generally

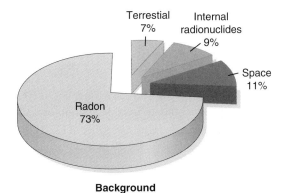

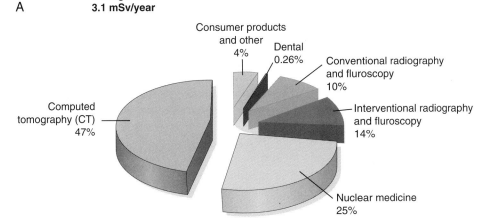

Figure 4-33 Distribution of ubiquitous background **(A)** and man-made **(B)** sources of radiation. The two sources contribute equally to the total average radiation exposure. Medical and dental diagnostic and therapeutic radiation is the major source of exposure to man-made radiation. *(From White SC, Pharoah MJ: Oral Radiology: Principles and Interpretation, ed 7. St. Louis, Mosby, 2014.)*

appear 10 or more years after exposure, and elevated risk remains for the patient's lifetime.

   f. Persons younger than 20 years old are more at risk for solid tumors and leukemias than adults.

2.3 Health Physics

A. Dentists must be prepared to discuss with patients the benefits and possible risks associated with x-rays and describe means to minimize these risks.

B. Sources of radiation exposure (Figure 4-33).

   1. The average annual exposure to individuals living in the United States is approximately 6.2 mSv. This includes exposure from ubiquitous background radiation and man-made radiation sources.

   2. Ubiquitous background radiation—contributes to approximately 3.1 mSv, accounting for 50% of radiation exposure of people living in the United States (Figure 4-33, *A*).

      a. Radon is the major contributor (73%) to background radiation exposure. Radon, a gas, is produced by radioactive decay of uranium in the soil.

      b. Other sources of background radiation exposure include terrestrial, internal radionuclides, and space radiation.

   3. Man-made sources of radiation—contribute to approximately 3.1 mSv, accounting for 50% of

radiation exposure of people living in the United States (Figure 4-33, *B*).

      a. Radiation exposure from medical or dental diagnostic and treatment procedures accounts for approximately 96% of man-made sources.

         (1) Computed tomography (CT) scans are the major contributor to medical radiation exposure, accounting for 47% of man-made sources.

         (2) Dental x-ray examinations are responsible for only 0.26% of man-made radiation exposure.

      b. Consumer and industrial products and sources —4%.

         (1) Include smoking, domestic water supplies, combustible fuels, dental porcelain, television receivers, pocket watches, smoke alarms, nuclear power, and airport inspection systems.

C. Exposure and dose in radiography.

   1. The goal of health physics is to prevent occurrence of deterministic effects and reduce the likelihood of stochastic effects by minimizing the exposure of office personnel and patients during radiographic examinations.

   2. This goal is accomplished by the philosophy that exposure should be *As Low As Reasonably Achievable* (ALARA).

3. Dose limits.
   a. Occupational exposure limit is 50 mSv of whole-body radiation exposure in 1 year.
      (1) Data from radiation monitoring services show that individuals occupationally exposed in operation of dental x-ray equipment typically receive an annual average of 0.2 mSv (0.4% of allowable limit).
   b. There are no dose limits for patients exposed in the course of dental and medical treatment.
4. Estimates of risk.
   a. Primary risk from dental radiography is radiation-induced cancer.
   b. Organs at risk include the thyroid gland, red bone marrow, and salivary glands.
   c. Although the risk involved with dental radiography is extremely small, no basis exists to assume that it is zero.
D. Methods of exposure and dose reduction.
   1. Patient selection.
      a. Dentists should exercise professional judgment to identify patients likely to benefit from diagnostic exposure. The American Dental Association has developed guidelines to help dentists to select patients for radiographic examination.
      b. Diagnostic radiography should be used only after clinical examination, consideration of the patient's history, and dental and general health needs.
   2. Conduct of examination.
      a. Use E/F-speed films or digital imaging for periapical and bite-wing examinations.
      b. Use rare-earth intensifying screens for panoramic and cephalometric radiography.
      c. Use an extended (16-inch) source-patient distance (focal spot-to-film distance) to reduce patient exposure and improve image clarity.
      d. Collimation—beam shape.
         (1) Rectangular collimation reduces patient exposure by more than 50% compared with round collimation.
      e. Leaded aprons and collars.
         (1) Leaded thyroid collars are recommended for individuals younger than 30 years old.
         (2) Leaded lap aprons are required in most states.
      f. Receptor/film-holders that align the collimated beam with the image receptor should be used.
      g. A kilovoltage range of 60 to 80 kVp is most suitable for dental radiographs.
      h. Exposure time.
         (1) Set mA value to highest possible value if variable.
         (2) Adjust exposure time to achieve optimum radiographic density.
         (3) Adjust exposure time to account for patient size and anatomic location.

   i. Operator protection.
      (1) The operatory should be arranged so that the operator can stand at least 6 feet from the patient and not in the path of the primary x-ray beam during exposure.
      (2) Ideally, the operator can leave the room or take a position behind a suitable barrier or wall during exposure.
      (3) The operator should never hold films in the patient's mouth.
      (4) Neither the operator nor the patient should hold the radiographic tube housing during exposure.
3. Processing film.
   a. Perform film processing under manufacturer-recommended time and temperature conditions.
   b. Use proper safelights.
4. View film-based and digital radiographs in a semi-darkened room to improve diagnosis.

2.4 X-Ray Film and Intensifying Screens

A. X-ray film.
   1. Composition.
      a. Emulsion.
         (1) Silver halide grains (primarily silver bromide) are sensitive to x-radiation and visible light; they are flat, tabular crystals in modern emulsions and are attached to base with a collagenous vehicle.
         (2) The smaller the crystals, the greater the image resolution.
      b. Base.
         (1) A flexible plastic film base supports the emulsion.
   2. Intraoral x-ray film.
      a. Identification dot—a raised dot impression in the corner of film used for film orientation.
   3. Screen film—film sensitive to visible light and placed between two intensifying screens when an exposure is made.
B. Intensifying screens.
   1. Intensifying screens are made of a base supporting material and a phosphor layer (usually rare-earth elements lanthanum and gadolinium).
   2. Phosphors incorporated into intensifying screens fluoresce in proportion to the x-ray energy absorbed.
   3. Use of intensifying screens results in substantial reduction in patient dose but decreased image resolution because of dispersion of light from the phosphors.
C. Image characteristics.
   1. Radiographic density—overall degree of darkening of exposed film.
      a. Measured as optical density of area of x-ray film.
         (1) Optical density $= \log_{10} \dfrac{Io}{It}$.

(2) Where *Io* is the intensity of incident light (e.g., from viewbox), and *It* is the intensity of light transmitted through the film.

(3) In a well-exposed and processed radiograph, the optical density of enamel is about 0.4; of dentin, about 1.0; and of soft tissue, about 2.0.

b. Increasing mA, kVp, or exposure time increases the number of photons reaching the film and increases the density of the radiograph.

c. Reducing the distance between the focal spot and the film also increases the film density.

d. The thicker the subject or the greater its density, the more the beam is attenuated, and the lighter the resultant image.

2. Radiographic contrast—range and number of densities on a radiograph.

a. Subject contrast is the range of characteristics of the subject that influences radiographic contrast.

b. Film contrast is the capacity of radiographic films to display differences in subject contrast, that is, variations in intensity of the remnant beam.

c. Scattered radiation results from photons that have interacted with the subject by Compton or coherent interactions, cause emission of photons that travel in directions other than that of primary beam, and cause an overall darkening of the image that results in loss of radiographic contrast.

3. Radiographic speed—amount of radiation required to produce an image of a standard density.

a. The fastest dental film currently available has a speed rating of F (preferred). Only films with a D or faster speed rating are appropriate for intraoral radiography.

4. Film latitude—measure of range of exposures that can be recorded on film.

a. A film optimized to display a wide latitude can record a subject with a wide range of subject contrast.

b. A film optimized to display a narrow latitude can distinguish objects with similar subject contrasts.

5. Radiographic noise—appearance of uneven density of a uniformly exposed radiographic film.

a. Radiographic mottle is uneven density resulting from the physical structure of the film or the intensifying screens.

6. Radiographic artifacts—defects caused by errors in film handling (e.g., fingerprints or bends in the film), errors in film processing (e.g., splashing developer or fixer on a film), or marks or scratches from rough handling.

7. Radiographic blurring.

a. Sharpness is the ability of a radiograph to define an edge precisely.

b. Resolution, or resolving power, is the ability of a radiograph to record separate structures that are close together.

c. Causes of increased radiographic blur.

(1) Increased size or decreased number of silver grains in film emulsion.

(2) Use of intensifying screens in extraoral radiography.

(3) Movement of film, subject, or x-ray source during exposure.

(4) Large focal spot or short source-to-object distance.

2.5 Projection Geometry

A. A radiograph is a two-dimensional representation of a three-dimensional object and is subject to distortion.

B. Image sharpness is improved by the following.

1. Use of as small an effective focal spot as is practical.

2. Increasing the distance between the focal spot and the object by using a long, open-ended cylinder.

3. Minimizing the distance between the object and the receptor.

C. Image size distortion (magnification) is minimized by the following.

1. Increasing focal spot-to-film distance.

2. Decreasing object-to-receptor distance.

D. Image shape distortion is minimized by the following.

1. Positioning the receptor parallel to the long axis of the object.

a. Foreshortening results from excessive vertical angulation when the x-ray beam is perpendicular to the receptor but not the tooth.

b. Elongation results when the x-ray beam is oriented at right angles to the object but not to the receptor.

2. Orienting the central ray perpendicular to the object and the receptor.

E. Paralleling and bisecting-angle techniques.

1. Bisecting-angle technique—the receptor is placed as close to the teeth as possible, and the central ray is directed perpendicular to an imaginary plane that bisects the angle between the teeth and the receptor.

2. Paralleling technique (preferred method for making intraoral radiographs)—the receptor is placed parallel with the long axis of the tooth, and the central ray is directed perpendicular to the long axis of the teeth and the receptor.

F. Object localization.

1. Two projections taken at right angles to each other.

2. Tube shift technique—"SLOB" (*Same Lingual, Opposite Buccal*).

a. If the tube is shifted and directed at a reference object (e.g., the apex of a tooth) from a more mesial angulation and the object in question also moves mesially with respect to the reference object, the object lies lingual to the reference object.

b. Alternatively, if the tube is shifted mesially and the object in question appears to move distally, it lies buccal to the reference object.

2.6 Processing X-Ray Film

A. When a beam of photons exposes an x-ray film, it chemically changes the photosensitive silver halide crystals in the film emulsion (a latent image). Exposed areas become radiolucent, whereas nonexposed areas become radiopaque.

B. The developing process converts a latent image into a visible radiographic image.

C. Formation of latent image.
   1. Silver halide crystals contain sensitivity sites that trap electrons generated when the emulsion is irradiated to produce crystals containing neutral silver atoms (latent image).

D. Processing solutions.
   1. Developer solution.
      a. Converts exposed silver halide crystals (with neutral silver atoms at each latent image site) into metallic silver grains that are seen as dark on a radiograph.
      b. Developers.
         (1) Phenidone is as the first electron donor that reduces silver ions to metallic silver at the latent image site.
         (2) Hydroquinone provides an electron to reduce oxidized phenidone back to its original active state so that it can continue to reduce silver halide grains to metallic silver.
   2. Rinsing.
      a. Dilutes the developer, slowing the development process.
      b. Removes the alkali activator, preventing neutralization of the acid fixer.
   3. Fixing solution.
      a. Dissolves and removes undeveloped silver halide crystals (without latent image sites) from the emulsion.
      b. Clearing agent.
         (1) Aqueous solution of ammonium thiosulfate ("hypo") that dissolves silver halide grains.
      c. Hardener.
         (1) Aluminum sulfate complexes with gelatin in the emulsion during fixing and prevents damage to gelatin during subsequent handling.
   4. Washing.
      a. After fixing, the processed film is washed in water to ensure removal of all thiosulfate ions and silver thiosulfate complexes that would stain the film if left.

E. Manual processing procedures.
   1. Replenish the developer and the fixer and stir the solutions.
   2. Mount films on hangers.
   3. Set timer—typically 5 minutes at 68°F. Table 4-7 shows effect of temperature on development time.

Table 4-7	
Development Times by Temperature	
TEMPERATURE (°F)	**DEVELOPMENT TIME (MINUTES)**
68	5
70	4.5
72	4
76	3
80	2.5

   4. Develop films for the indicated time.
   5. Rinse in running water for 30 seconds.
   6. Fix—place hanger and film in fixer solution for 10 minutes.
   7. Wash and dry—after fixation of films is complete, place the hanger in running water for at least 10 minutes to remove residual processing solutions.

F. Automatic film processing.
   1. Most automatic processors have an in-line arrangement of rollers.
   2. The primary function of rollers is to move the film through the developing solutions.
   3. The chemical compositions of the developer and fixer are modified to operate at higher temperatures than the temperatures used for manual processing and to meet requirements of rapid development, fixing, washing, and drying of automatic processing.
   4. It is important to maintain constituents of the developer and fixer carefully to preserve optimal sensitometric and physical properties of the film emulsion within the narrow limits imposed by the speed and temperature of automatic processing.
   5. As with manual processing, 8 oz. of fresh developer and fixer should be added per gallon of solution per day.

G. Safelighting.
   1. Use a Kodak GBX-2 safelight filter or equivalent with a 15-watt bulb at least 4 feet from the working surface.
   2. An ML-2 filter should not be used because it fogs panoramic film.
   3. A "penny test" checks for proper safelighting by determining whether an exposed film, covered with a penny in the darkroom, shows an image of the penny after processing. If so, it implies film fogging and light leaks or improper safelighting.

H. Common causes of faulty radiographs.
   1. Box 4-16 lists common causes of faulty radiographs.
   2. Mounting radiographs.
      a. The preferred method of positioning periapical and occlusal films in the film mount is to arrange them with the dot (bump) facing the viewer so that images of teeth are in anatomic position and have

Box 4-16

Common Problems in Film Exposure Development

Light Radiographs

Processing Errors

Underdevelopment (temperature too low; time too short; thermometer inaccurate)

Depleted developer solution

Diluted or contaminated developer

Excessive fixation

Underexposure

Insufficient milliamperage

Insufficient peak kilovoltage

Insufficient time

Film-source distance too great

Film packet reversed in mouth

Dark Radiographs

Processing Errors

Overdevelopment (temperature too high; time too long)

Developer concentration too high

Inadequate fixation

Accidental exposure to light before processing

Improper safelighting or light leaks

Overexposure

Excessive milliamperage

Excessive peak kilovoltage

Excessive exposure time

Film-source distance too short

Insufficient Contrast

Underdevelopment

Underexposure

Excessive peak kilovoltage

Excessive film fog

Film Fog

Improper safelighting (improper filter; excessive bulb wattage; inadequate distance between safelight and work surface; prolonged exposure to safelight)

Light leaks (cracked safelight filter; light from doors, vents, or other sources)

Overdevelopment

Contaminated solutions

Deteriorated film (stored at high temperature; stored at high humidity; exposed to radiation; outdated)

Dark Spots or Lines

Fingerprint contamination

Black wrapping paper sticking to film surface

Film in contact with tank or another film during fixation

Film contaminated with developer before processing

Excessive bending of film

Static discharge to film before processing

Excessive roller pressure during automatic processing

Dirty rollers in automatic processing

Light Spots

Film contaminated with fixer before processing

Film in contact with tank or another film during development

Excessive bending of film

Yellow or Brown Stains

Depleted developer

Depleted fixer

Insufficient washing

Contaminated solutions

Blurring

Movement of patient

Movement of x-ray tube head

Double exposure

Partial Images

Top of film not immersed in developing solution

Misalignment of x-ray tube head ("cone cut")

Emulsion Peel

Abrasion of image during processing

Excessive time in wash water

---

the same relationship to the viewer as when the viewer faces the patient, that is, with the right quadrants in the left side of the film mount and the left quadrants in the right side.

2.7 Digital Imaging

Digital imaging is becoming increasingly important in dental radiography. It is estimated that about 15% to 25% of dental offices use some form of digital imaging. It is most frequently used for intraoral radiography but also is available for panoramic and cephalometric imaging. Cone-beam CT imaging is exclusively digital.

A. Analog versus digital.
   1. Analog—continuous gray scale; a conventional film image.
   2. Digital.
      a. Gray scale divided into discrete number of values.
      b. Number of values is a power of 2; typically from 2^8 or 256 gray steps.

c. An 8-bit image has 256 gray levels, a 12-bit image (2^{12}) has 4096 gray levels.

d. Images are composed of many pixels (picture elements), each having a discrete gray level.

B. Digital detectors.
1. Charge-coupled device (CCD) and complementary metal oxide semiconductors (CMOS).
   a. Silicon sensor captures x-ray energy from exposure as a voltage potential.
   b. Silicon chip reads out voltage of each pixel.
   c. Usually connected to computer by a wire but may be wireless.
   d. Rapid display of image on monitor after exposure.
   e. Used for intraoral, panoramic, and cephalometric imaging.
2. Photostimulable phosphor plates (PSP).
   a. Plates made of barium fluorohalide with traces of europium.
   b. Plates capture and store x-ray energy from dental exposure.
   c. After exposure, the plates are placed into the reader where stored energy is released as fluorescence by laser.
   d. Reader measures released light from plate and forms image.
   e. Time to image display after plate is placed in reader varies from seconds to minutes.

C. Digital detector characteristics.
1. Contrast resolution.
   a. Ability to distinguish shades of gray.
   b. Limited by bit-depth of image capturing receptor.
   c. Usually displayed as an 8- to 12-bit image (256 to 4096 gray levels).
2. Spatial resolution.
   a. Ability to detect edges or separate two close points.
   b. For intraoral systems—film better than CCD and CMOS, both of which are better than PSP.
   c. For panoramic and cephalometric systems—film, CCD, and PSP all equivalent.
3. Detector latitude.
   a. Range of structures of varying density shown on image.
   b. PSP better than CCD and CMOS, which are better than film.
4. Detector sensitivity.
   a. Dose required to achieve standard gray level.
   b. Doses for CCD and CMOS about half of F-speed film.

D. Digital image display.
1. Image adjustment.
   a. Brightness and contrast—usually beneficial but may introduce artifacts, particularly in images with narrow latitude.
   b. Sharpening and smoothing—sometimes useful, but sharpening may introduce a grainy appearance, and smoothing may give a blurring effect.

Excessive image sharpening may also create artifacts at the edges of radiopaque restorations, which may be mistaken for recurrent caries.
2. Image analysis.
   a. Measurement—usually used for endodontics. Accuracy depends on calibration with known object.

2.8 Radiographic Quality Assurance and Infection Control

A. Radiographic quality assurance.
1. A quality assurance program in radiology is a series of procedures implemented to ensure optimal and consistent operation of each component in the imaging chain. When all components are functioning properly, the result is consistently high-quality radiographs made with low exposure to patients and office personnel. When a problem is identified, it is important to determine the probable source and take corrective action.
2. Daily tasks.
   a. Compare radiographs with reference film to reveal problems before they interfere with diagnostic quality of images.
   b. Record all errors in a retake log for films that must be reexposed.
   c. Replenish processing solutions.
   d. Check temperature of processing solutions.
3. Weekly tasks.
   a. Replace the processing solutions, clean the processing equipment and viewboxes, and review the retake log.
4. Monthly tasks.
   a. Clean the intensifying screens and rotate the film stock.
   b. Examine photostimulable phosphor plates for scratches.
   c. Inspect lead aprons and thyroid collars for cracks or tears.
5. Yearly task.
   a. Have the x-ray machine calibrated by a health physicist.
   b. Verify digital sensors with a quality assurance phantom.

B. Infection control.
1. The goal of an infection control program is to avoid cross-contamination among patients and between patients and operators.
2. Apply universal precautions.
   a. Universal precautions are infection control guidelines designed to protect workers from exposure to diseases spread by blood and certain body fluids. Under universal precautions, all human blood and saliva are treated as if known to be infectious for HIV and hepatitis B virus. The means employed to protect against cross-contamination are used universally, that is, for all individuals.
   b. Wear gloves during all radiographic procedures.

c. Disinfect and cover x-ray machine, working surfaces, chair, and apron.

d. Sterilize nondisposable instruments.

e. Use barrier-protected film (sensor) or a disposable container.

f. Prevent contamination of processing equipment.
  (1) Remove film from a packet without touching (contaminating) it.
  (2) Put on a clean pair of gloves, pick up the film packet by its color-coded end, and pull the tab upward and away from the packet to reveal the black paper tab wrapped over the end of the film.
  (3) Holding the film over a clean towel, carefully grasp the black paper tab that wraps the film and pull the film from the packet.
  (4) When the film is pulled from the packet, it falls from the paper wrapping onto the towel.
  (5) After opening all films, gather the contaminated packaging and container and discard them along with the contaminated gloves.

2.9 Intraoral Radiographic Examinations

A. Criteria of quality.
  1. Every radiographic examination should produce radiographs of optimal diagnostic quality, incorporating the following features.
    a. Complete areas of interest recorded on the image.
    b. Least possible amount of distortion.
    c. Optimal density and contrast to facilitate interpretation.
  2. It is unnecessary to retake a view that fails to open a contact or show a periapical region if the missing information is available on another view.
B. Periapical radiography.
  1. Paralleling technique (also called right-angle or long-cone technique).
    a. Film is supported parallel to the long axis of the teeth (Figure 4-34, *A*).
    b. The central ray of the x-ray beam is directed at right angles to the teeth and the film.
  2. Bisecting-angle technique.
    a. Position the film as close as possible to the lingual surface of the teeth, resting in the palate or in the floor of the mouth (Figure 4-34, *B*).
    b. Direct the central ray of the x-ray beam at right angles to an imaginary plane that bisects the film plane and the long axis of the teeth.
  3. Bite-wing examinations.
    a. Direct the central ray slightly downward through the contacts and include crowns of the maxillary and mandibular teeth and the alveolar crests.
C. Occlusal radiography.
  1. Displays a large segment of a dental arch.
  2. May include the palate or floor of the mouth and a reasonable extent of contiguous lateral structures.

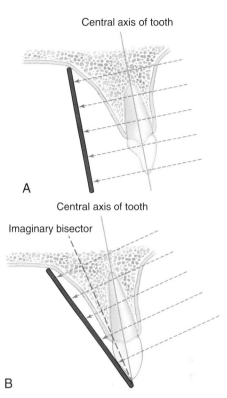

Figure 4-34 Intraoral radiographic techniques. **(A)** Paralleling technique illustrates parallelism between the long axis of the tooth and the receptor. The x-ray beam is directed perpendicular to each. **(B)** Bisecting angle technique illustrates that the receptor is positioned at an angle to the long axis of the tooth. The x-ray beam is directed perpendicular to the bisector of this angle. *(From White SC, Pharoah MJ: Oral Radiology: Principles and Interpretation, ed 7. St. Louis, Mosby, 2014.)*

D. Radiographic examination of children.
  1. Concern about radiation protection is most important for children because of their greater sensitivity to irradiation.
  2. The best way to reduce unnecessary exposure is for the dentist to make the minimal number of films required for each patient and to use thyroid shields.
E. Pregnancy.
  1. No incidences have been reported of damage to a fetus from dental radiography.
  2. Prudence suggests that radiographic examinations be kept to a minimum consistent with the mother's dental needs.
  3. With the low patient dose afforded by use of optimal radiation safety techniques, an intraoral or extraoral examination should be performed whenever a reasonable diagnostic requirement exists.

2.10 Radiographic Anatomy

A. Teeth (Figure 4-35).
  1. Enamel.
    a. The enamel cap characteristically appears more radiopaque than other tissues because it is the most dense naturally occurring substance in the body.

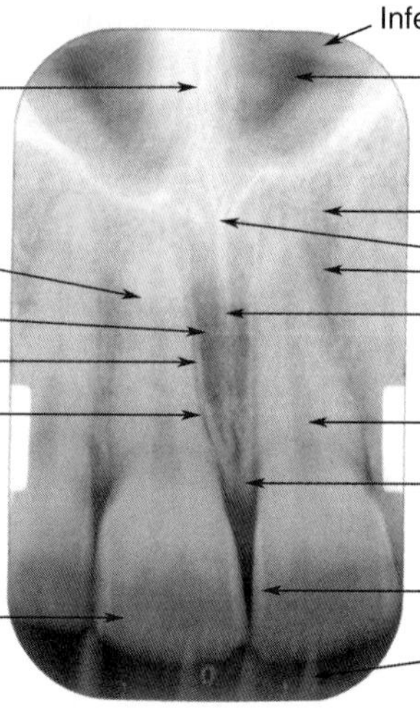

Figure 4-35 Periapical radiograph of the anterior maxilla with anatomic features identified.

Labels on radiograph: Inferior concha, Nasal fossa, Nasal septum, Cancellous bone, Anterior nasal spine, Lateral fossa, Tip of nose, Intermaxillary suture, Incisive foramen, Lamina dura, Pulp, Periodontal ligament space, Alveolar crest, Enamel, Dentin, Bite block

2. Dentin.
   a. Dentin is about 75% mineralized, and because of its lower mineral content, its radiographic appearance is roughly comparable to that of bone.
   b. Dentin is smooth and homogeneous on radiographs because of its uniform morphology.
   c. The junction between enamel and dentin appears as a distinct interface that separates these two structures.
3. Cementum.
   a. The thin layer of cementum on the root surface has a mineral content of approximately 50%.
   b. Cementum is not usually apparent radiographically because the contrast between it and dentin is so low, and the cementum layer is so thin.
4. Pulp.
   a. The pulp of normal teeth is composed of soft tissue and consequently appears radiolucent.
   b. At the apex of a developing tooth, the root pulp canal diverges, and the walls of the root rapidly taper to a knife-edge. When a tooth reaches maturity, pulpal walls in the apical region begin to constrict and finally come into close apposition.
   c. In normal, fully formed teeth, the root canal is usually apparent, extending to the apex of the root; an apical foramen is usually recognizable. The canal sometimes may appear constricted in the region of the apex and not discernible in the last millimeter or so of its length. In this case, the canal may occasionally exit on the side of the tooth, just short of the radiographic apex.
   d. Aging or trauma to a tooth (e.g., caries, a blow, restorations, attrition, erosion) also may stimulate dentin production, leading to a reduction in size of the pulp chamber and canals.
B. Supporting structures.
   1. Lamina dura.
      a. Tooth sockets are bounded by a thin radiopaque layer of dense bone. The name *lamina dura* ("hard

layer") is derived from its radiographic appearance.
      b. This layer is continuous with the shadow of cortical bone at the alveolar crest.
      c. Developmentally, the lamina dura is an extension of the lining of the bony crypt that surrounds each tooth during development.
      d. Small variations and disruptions in continuity of the lamina dura may represent superimpositions of trabecular pattern and small nutrient canals passing from mandibular bone to the PDL.
      e. The presence of an intact lamina dura around the apex of a tooth strongly suggests a vital pulp.
   2. Alveolar crest.
      a. The level of the alveolar crest is considered normal when it is not more than 2 mm from the cementoenamel junction (CEJ) of adjacent teeth.
   3. PDL space.
      a. The PDL appears as a radiolucent space between the tooth root and the lamina dura.
      b. The shape of a tooth creates the appearance of the PDL space. When an x-ray beam is directed so that two convexities of a root surface appear on a film, a double PDL space may be seen.
   4. Cancellous bone.
      a. Cancellous bone (also called *trabecular bone* or *spongiosa*) lies between the cortical plates in both jaws. The radiographic pattern of trabeculae normally shows considerable intrapatient and interpatient variability.
      b. To evaluate the trabecular pattern in a specific area, the practitioner should examine the trabecular distribution, size, and density and compare them throughout both jaws.
      c. If trabeculae are apparently absent (suggesting the presence of disease), it is often helpful to examine previous radiographs of the region in question.

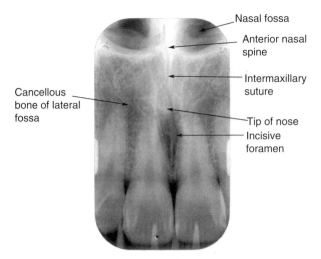

Figure 4-36 Periapical radiograph of the anterior maxilla with anatomic features identified.

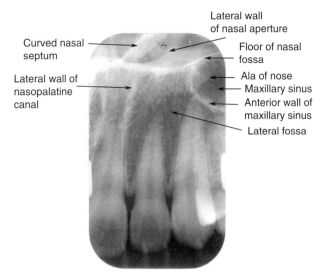

Figure 4-37 Periapical radiograph of the anterior maxilla with anatomic features identified.

d. If prior films are unavailable, it may be appropriate to expose another radiograph at a later time to monitor for evidence of changes.

5. Maxilla.

a. Intermaxillary suture (Figure 4-36 and see Figure 4-35).

(1) The intermaxillary suture (also called the *median suture*) appears on intraoral periapical radiographs as a thin radiolucent line in the midline.

b. Anterior nasal spine (see Figures 4-35 and 4-36).

(1) The anterior nasal spine is radiopaque and most frequently demonstrated on periapical radiographs of the maxillary central incisors in between and slightly above the root apices of the maxillary central incisors.

c. Nasal fossa (see Figures 4-35 and 4-36).

(1) On periapical radiographs of incisors, the inferior border of the fossa appears as a radiopaque line extending bilaterally away from the base of the anterior nasal spine.

d. Incisive foramen (see Figures 4-35 and 4-36).

(1) The incisive foramen (also called the *nasopalatine* or *anterior palatine foramen*) in the maxilla is the oral terminus of the nasopalatine canal.

(2) Its radiographic image is usually projected between the roots and in the region of the middle and apical thirds of the central incisors.

(3) The foramen varies markedly in its radiographic shape, size, and sharpness. It may appear smoothly symmetrical or irregular, with a well-demarcated or ill-defined border.

(4) The presence of an incisive canal cyst is suspected if the width of the foramen exceeds 1 cm, if enlargement can be demonstrated on successive radiographs, or if it appears to have

caused divergence of the roots of the central incisors.

(5) The lateral walls of the nasopalatine canal may be visualized as a pair of radiopaque lines running superiorly from the incisive foramen.

e. Lateral fossa (Figure 4-37 and see Figure 4-36).

(1) The lateral fossa (also called the *incisive fossa*) is a gentle radiolucent depression in the maxilla near the apex of the lateral incisor.

(2) The image is often misinterpreted as a pathologic condition. However, the presence an intact lamina dura around the root of the lateral incisor should direct attention to the anatomic nature of this radiolucency.

f. Nose (see Figures 4-35 through 4-37).

(1) The soft tissue of the tip of the nose is frequently seen in projections of the maxillary central and lateral incisors, superimposed over the roots of these teeth.

g. Maxillary sinus (Figures 4-38 and 4-39 and see Figure 4-37).

(1) The borders of the maxillary sinus appear on periapical radiographs as a thin, delicate, radiopaque line (actually a thin layer of cortical bone).

(2) In adults, the sinus is usually seen to extend from the distal aspect of the canine to the posterior wall of the maxilla above the tuberosity.

(3) Root apices may project anatomically into the floor of the sinus, causing small elevations or prominences. The thin layer of bone covering the root is seen as a fusion of the lamina dura and the floor of sinus. Rarely, defects may be present in the bony covering of the root apices in the sinus floor, and a periapical radiograph fails to show the lamina dura covering the apex.

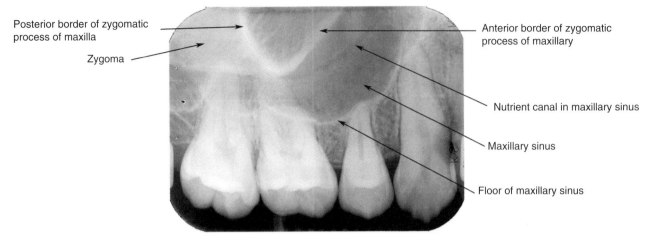

Posterior border of zygomatic process of maxilla

Zygoma

Anterior border of zygomatic process of maxillary

Nutrient canal in maxillary sinus

Maxillary sinus

Floor of maxillary sinus

Figure 4-38 Periapical radiograph of the posterior maxilla with anatomic features identified.

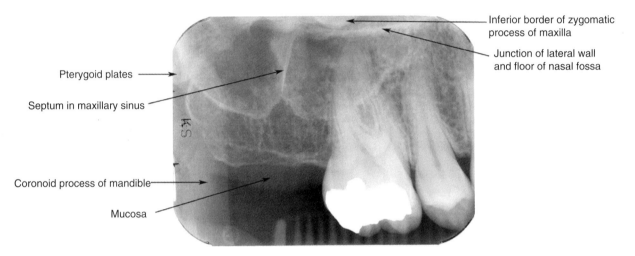

Inferior border of zygomatic process of maxilla

Junction of lateral wall and floor of nasal fossa

Pterygoid plates

Septum in maxillary sinus

Coronoid process of mandible

Mucosa

Figure 4-39 Periapical radiograph of the posterior maxilla with anatomic features identified.

(4) Often, one or several radiopaque lines traverse an image of the maxillary sinus. These septa represent folds of cortical bone projecting a few millimeters away from the floor and wall of the antrum.

h. Zygomatic process of maxilla (see Figures 4-38 and 4-39).
   (1) On periapical radiographs, the zygomatic process of the maxilla appears as a U-shaped radiopaque line with its open end directed superiorly. The enclosed rounded end is projected in the apical region of the first and second molars.

i. Zygoma (see Figure 4-38).
   (1) The inferior portion of the zygomatic bone may be seen extending posteriorly from the inferior border of the zygomatic process of the maxilla.
   (2) The zygoma can be identified as a uniform gray or white radiopacity over the apices of the molars.

j. Pterygoid plates (see Figure 4-39).
   (1) The medial and lateral pterygoid plates, when apparent, almost always cast a single radiopaque, homogeneous shadow without evidence of trabeculation posterior to the maxillary tuberosity.
   (2) The hamular process extends inferiorly from the medial pterygoid plate. It may exhibit trabeculae.

6. Mandible.
   a. Genial tubercles (Figure 4-40).
      (1) The genial tubercles are located on the lingual surface of the mandible slightly above the inferior border and in the midline.
      (2) They are well visualized on mandibular occlusal radiographs as one or more small projections.
      (3) Their appearance on periapical radiographs of the mandibular incisor region is variable; often they appear as a radiopacity (3 to 4 mm in

diameter) in the midline below the incisor roots.

(4) When genial tubercles are seen on periapical radiographs, it is often possible to see the lingual foramen.

b. Mental protuberance (see Figure 4-40).

(1) On periapical radiographs of the mandibular central incisors, the mental protuberance (ridge) may occasionally be seen as two thick radiopaque lines extending bilaterally forward and upward toward the midline.

c. Mental fossa (see Figure 4-40).

(1) The mental fossa is a radiolucent depression on the labial aspect of the mandible extending laterally from the midline and above the mental ridge.

d. Mental foramen (Figure 4-41).

(1) The mental foramen is usually seen near the apex of the second premolar.

(2) Its image is quite variable, and it may be identified only about half of the time because the opening of the mental canal is directed superiorly and posteriorly.

(3) It may be round, oblong, or irregular and partially or completely corticated.

(4) When the mental foramen is projected over one of the premolar apices, it may mimic periapical disease. Look carefully for the presence of an intact lamina dura to rule out periapical disease.

e. Mandibular canal (Figure 4-42).

(1) The radiographic image of the mandibular canal is a dark, linear shadow with thin, radiopaque superior and inferior borders cast by the layer of bone that bounds the canal.

(2) Sometimes the borders are seen only partially or not at all. This is more common in patients with osteopenia or osteoporosis.

f. Nutrient canals (see Figure 4-41).

(1) Nutrient canals carry a neurovascular bundle and appear as radiolucent lines of fairly uniform width. They are most often seen on mandibular periapical radiographs running vertically from the inferior dental canal directly to the apex of a tooth or into the interdental space between the mandibular incisors.

g. Mylohyoid ridge (see Figure 4-41).

(1) The mylohyoid ridge is a slightly irregular crest of bone on the lingual surface of the mandibular body.

(2) Its radiographic image runs diagonally downward and forward from the area of third molars to premolar region, at approximately the level of the apices of the posterior teeth.

h. Submandibular gland fossa (see Figure 4-41).

(1) On the lingual surface of the mandibular body, immediately below the mylohyoid ridge in the

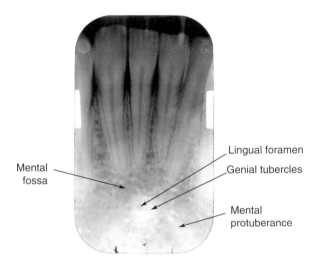

Figure 4-40 Periapical radiograph of the anterior mandible with anatomic features identified.

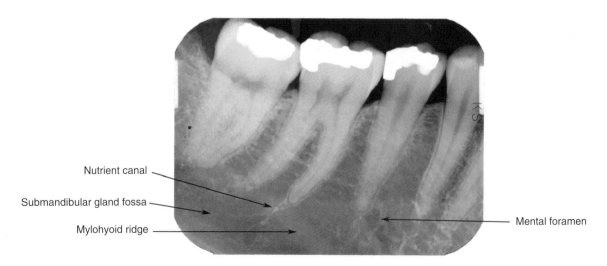

Figure 4-41 Periapical radiograph of the posterior mandible with anatomic features identified.

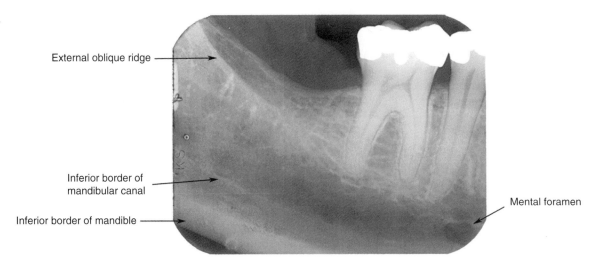

External oblique ridge

Inferior border of mandibular canal

Inferior border of mandible

Mental foramen

Figure 4-42 Periapical radiograph of the posterior mandible with anatomic features identified.

molar area, there is frequently a depression in the bone. This concavity accommodates the submandibular gland and often appears as a radiolucent area with a sparse, trabecular pattern characteristic of the region.

(2) Although the image may appear strikingly radiolucent (accentuated by the dense mylohyoid ridge and the inferior border of mandible), awareness of its possible presence should preclude its being confused with a bony lesion.

i. External oblique ridge (see Figure 4-42).

(1) The external oblique ridge is a continuation of the anterior border of the mandibular ramus.

(2) Characteristically, it is projected onto posterior periapical radiographs superior to the mylohyoid ridge, with which it runs an almost parallel course.

(3) It appears as a radiopaque line of varying width, density, and length, blending at its anterior end with the shadow of the alveolar bone.

j. Inferior border of mandible (see Figure 4-42).

(1) Occasionally, the inferior mandibular border is seen on periapical projections as a characteristically dense, broad radiopaque band of bone.

k. Coronoid process (see Figure 4-39).

(1) The image of the coronoid process of the mandible is frequently apparent on periapical radiographs of the maxillary molar region as a triangular radiopacity, with its apex directed superiorly and anteriorly, superimposed on the region of the third molar.

2.11 Radiographic Appearance of Caries

Caries requires the presence of bacteria and a diet containing fermentable carbohydrates. The mutans group of

streptococci plays a central role in the demineralization. The demineralized tooth surface, called the *carious lesion*, is not the disease but is a reflection of ongoing or past microbial activity in the plaque.

A. Use of intraoral radiographs.

1. Caries appears as a radiolucent zone.

2. Radiography is a valuable supplement to a thorough clinical examination of the teeth for detecting caries.

3. Clinical access to proximal tooth surfaces in contact is quite limited.

4. A radiographic examination can reveal carious lesions in occlusal and proximal surfaces that would otherwise remain undetected.

5. Bite-wing radiographs are the most useful radiographic examination for detecting interproximal caries.

B. Proximal surfaces.

1. The shape of the early radiolucent lesion in the enamel is classically a triangle with its broad base at the tooth surface.

2. When the demineralizing front reaches the dentinoenamel junction, it spreads along the junction, frequently forming the base of a second triangle with the apex directed toward the pulp chamber.

3. This triangle typically has a wider base than in the enamel and progresses toward the pulp along the direction of the dentinal tubules.

4. A lesion in proximal surfaces most commonly is found just apical to the contact point.

5. Various dental anomalies such as hypoplastic pits and concavities produced by wear can mimic the appearance of caries.

6. Approximately half of all proximal lesions in enamel cannot be detected by radiography.

C. Occlusal surfaces.
1. Carious lesions in children and adolescents most often occur on occlusal surfaces of posterior teeth.
2. The classic radiographic appearance of occlusal caries extending into the dentin is a broad-based, radiolucent zone, often beneath a fissure, with little or no apparent changes in the enamel.

D. Buccal and lingual surfaces.
1. Small caries on the buccal and lingual surfaces of teeth are usually round.
2. As they enlarge, they become elliptic or semilunar.
3. They often demonstrate sharp, well-defined borders.

E. Root surfaces.
1. Radiographs of proximal root surfaces may reveal lesions that have gone undetected clinically.
2. A pitfall in the detection of root lesions is that a surface may appear to be carious as a result of the cervical burnout phenomenon.
3. Caries may be distinguished from an intact surface primarily by the absence of an image of the root edge and by the appearance of a diffuse rounded inner border where the tooth substance has been lost.

F. Dental restorations.
1. A carious lesion developing at the margin of an existing restoration may be termed *secondary* or *recurrent caries.*
2. A lesion next to a restoration may be obscured by the radiopaque image of the restoration.
3. Liners without radiopaque fillers appear radiolucent and may resemble recurrent or residual caries.

2.12 Radiographic Appearance of Periodontal Disease

The most common disorders of the periodontium are gingivitis and periodontitis, which represent chronic infectious diseases. Essential components of these diseases are the presence of certain bacteria in plaque and the inflammatory host response. Gingivitis is a soft tissue inflammation involving the gingiva surrounding teeth. Periodontitis entails the loss of soft tissue attachment and supporting bone of the involved teeth.

A. Radiographs are especially helpful in the evaluation of the following points.
1. Amount of bone present.
2. Condition of the alveolar crests.
3. Bone loss in the furcation areas.
4. Width of the PDL space.
5. Local initiating factors that cause or intensify periodontal disease.
   a. Calculus.
   b. Poorly contoured or overextended restorations.
6. Root length and morphology and crown-to-root ratio.
7. Anatomic considerations.
   a. Position of the maxillary sinus in relation to a periodontal deformity.

8. A permanent record of the condition of the bone throughout the course of the disease.

B. Limitations of radiographs.
1. Radiographs provide a two-dimensional view of a three-dimensional situation.
2. Radiographs typically show less severe bone destruction than is actually present.
3. Radiographs do not demonstrate soft tissue-to-hard tissue relationships and provide no information about the depth of soft tissue pockets.
4. Bone level is often measured from the CEJ; however, this reference point is not valid in situations in which either overeruption or severe attrition with passive eruption exists.
5. For these reasons, although radiographs play an invaluable role in treatment planning, they must be used to supplement a careful clinical examination.

C. Normal anatomy.
1. The normal alveolar bone crest lies at a level approximately 0.5 to 2 mm below the level of the CEJs of adjacent teeth.
2. In the absence of disease, this bony junction between the alveolar crest and lamina dura of posterior teeth forms a sharp angle next to the tooth root.
3. The PDL space is often slightly wider around the cervical portion of the tooth root, especially in adolescents with erupting teeth.

D. Mild periodontitis.
1. The early lesions of adult periodontitis appear as areas of localized erosion of the interproximal alveolar bone crest.
2. The anterior regions show blunting of the alveolar crests and slight loss of alveolar bone height.
3. The posterior regions may also show a loss of the normally sharp angle between the lamina dura and alveolar crest.

E. Moderate periodontitis.
1. Horizontal bone loss.
   a. *Horizontal bone loss* is a term used to describe the radiographic appearance of loss in height of the alveolar bone around multiple teeth; the crest is still horizontal (i.e., parallel with the occlusal plane) but is positioned apically more than a few millimeters from the line of the CEJs.
   b. In horizontal bone loss, the crest of the buccal and lingual cortical plates and the intervening interdental bone have been resorbed.
2. Vertical osseous defects.
   a. The term *vertical* (or *angular*) *osseous defect* describes the types of bony lesions that are most commonly localized to one or two teeth.
   b. With these defects, the crest of the remaining alveolar bone typically displays an oblique angulation to the line of the CEJs in the area of involved teeth.

F. Severe periodontitis.
1. In severe adult periodontitis, the bone loss is so extensive that the remaining teeth show excessive mobility and drifting.
2. Extensive horizontal or vertical osseous defects may be present.
3. As with moderate bone loss, the lesions seen during surgery usually are more extensive than is suggested by the radiographs alone.
G. Multirooted teeth.
1. Progressive periodontal disease and its associated bone loss may extend into the furcations of multi-rooted teeth.
2. Widening of the PDL space at the apex of the inter-radicular bony crest of the furcation is strong evidence that the periodontal disease process involves the furcation.
3. The bony defect may involve either the buccal or the lingual cortical plate and extend under the roof of the furcation.
4. The most common route for furcation involvement of the maxillary permanent first molar is from the mesial side.
H. Periodontal abscess.
1. A periodontal abscess is a rapidly progressing, destructive lesion that usually originates in a deep soft tissue pocket.
2. If the lesion persists, a radiolucent region appears, often superimposed over the root of a tooth.
I. Differential diagnosis.
1. Most cases of bone loss around teeth are caused by periodontal diseases.
2. Squamous cell carcinoma of the alveolar process occasionally is treated as periodontal disease, resulting in a delay in diagnosis and treatment.
3. Any lesion of bone destruction that has ill-defined borders and a lack of peripheral bone response (sclerosis) should be viewed with suspicion.

2.13 Panoramic Imaging

A. Introduction and rationale.
1. Panoramic imaging is a technique for producing a single tomographic image of facial structures.
2. This is a curvilinear variant of conventional tomography based on the principle of reciprocal movement of an x-ray source and an image receptor around a central point or plane.
3. Principal advantages of panoramic images.
   a. Broad coverage of facial bones and teeth.
   b. Low patient radiation dose.
   c. Convenience of examination for the patient.
   d. Can be used in patients unable to open their mouths.
   e. Patients readily understand panoramic images; they are also a useful visual aid in patient education and case presentation.

f. Panoramic images are most useful clinically for diagnostic problems requiring broad coverage of the jaws.
4. The main disadvantage of panoramic radiology is that the image does not display the fine anatomic detail available on intraoral periapical radiographs.
B. Principles of panoramic image formation.
1. Image layer.
   a. The image layer is a three-dimensional curved zone or "focal trough" where structures lying within this layer are reasonably well defined on the final panoramic image. The structures seen on a panoramic image are primarily structures located within the image layer.
   b. Objects outside the image layer are blurred, magnified, or reduced in size and are sometimes distorted to the extent of not being recognizable. The shape of the image layer varies with the brand of equipment used.
2. Patient positioning and head alignment.
   a. Remove dental appliances, earrings, necklaces, hairpins, and any other metallic objects in the head and neck region.
   b. Align the occlusal plane so that it is lower anteriorly, angled 20 to 30 degrees below horizontal.
   c. Position patients with their backs and spines as erect as possible.
3. Image receptors.
   a. Intensifying screens are routinely used in panoramic radiography because they significantly reduce the amount of radiation required for properly exposing a radiograph.
   b. Several manufacturers have developed digital acquisition panoramic machines. The receptor on such a machine is either an array of CCDs or a film-sized PSP rather than film.
C. Interpreting the panoramic image.
1. Introduction.
   a. View the image as if you were looking at a patient, with the structures on the patient's right side positioned on your left (Figures 4-43 and 4-44).
   b. The image is presented to you in the same orientation as that of periapical and bite-wing images, making interpretation more comfortable.
2. Anatomic structures (see Figures 4-43 and 4-44).
3. Superimpositions and ghost images (see Figure 4-44).
   a. Many radiopaque objects out of the image layer superimpose on the image of normal anatomic structures. Such objects typically appear blurred and project either over the midline structures (as with cervical vertebrae) or onto the opposite side of the radiograph in reversed configuration and more cranially positioned than the real structure. These contralateral images are termed "ghost images," and they may obscure normal anatomy or be mistaken for pathology.

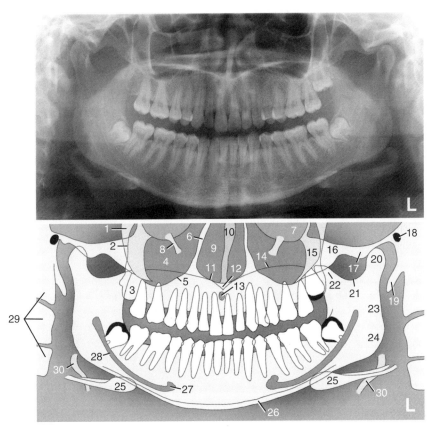

1. Pterygomaxillary fissure
2. Posterior border of maxilla
3. Maxillary tuberosity
4. Maxillary sinus
5. Floor of the maxillary sinus
6. Medial border of maxillary sinus/
   lateral border of the nasal cavity
7. Floor of the orbit
8. Infraorbital canal
9. Nasal cavity
10. Nasal septum
11. Floor of the nasal cavity
12. Anterior nasal spine
13. Incisive foramen
14. Hard palate/floor of the nasal cavity
15. Zygomatic process of the maxilla
16. Zygomatic arch
17. Articular eminence
18. External auditory meatus
19. Styloid process
20. Mandibular condyle
21. Sigmoid notch
22. Coronoid process
23. Posterior border of ramus
24. Angle of mandible
25. Hyoid bone
26. Inferior border of mandible
27. Mental foramen
28. Mandibular canal
29. Cervical vertebrae
30. Epiglottis

Figure 4-43 Panoramic radiograph with anatomic features identified. *(From White SC, Pharoah MJ: Oral Radiology: Principles and Interpretation, ed 7. St. Louis, Mosby, 2014.)*

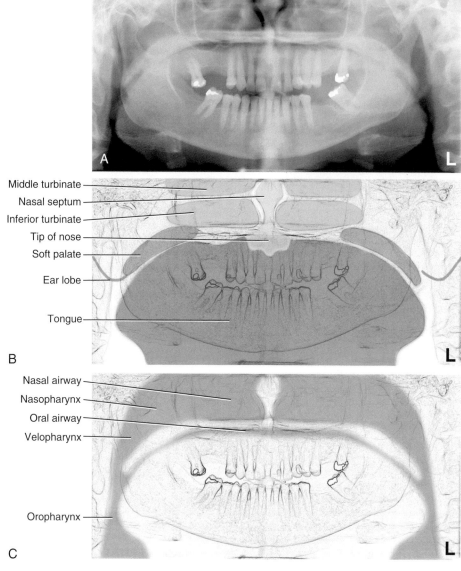

Figure 4-44 Panoramic radiograph **(A)** showing superimposed soft tissue structures **(B)** and airway space **(C)**. *(From White SC, Pharoah MJ: Oral Radiology: Principles and Interpretation, ed 7. St. Louis, Mosby, 2014.)*

Sample Questions

1. Acantholysis, resulting from desmosome weakening by autoantibodies directed against the protein desmoglein, is the disease mechanism attributed to which of the following?
   A. Epidermolysis bullosa
   B. Mucous membrane pemphigoid
   C. Pemphigus vulgaris
   D. Herpes simplex infections
   E. Herpangina

2. HPV has been found in all of the following lesions *except* one. Which one is the *exception*?
   A. Oral papillomas
   B. Verruca vulgaris of the oral mucosa
   C. Condyloma acuminatum
   D. Condyloma latum
   E. Focal epithelial hyperplasia

3. Intranuclear viral inclusions are seen in tissue specimens of which of the following?
   A. Solar cheilitis
   B. Minor aphthous ulcers
   C. Geographic tongue
   D. Hairy leukoplakia
   E. White sponge nevus

4. The odontogenic neoplasm, which is composed of loose, primitive-appearing connective tissue that resembles dental pulp, microscopically is known as _____.
   A. Odontoma
   B. Ameloblastoma
   C. Ameloblastic fibroma

D. Ameloblastic fibro-odontoma

E. Odontogenic myxoma

5. A biopsy specimen of the lower lip salivary glands showed replacement of parenchymal tissue by lymphocytes. The patient also had xerostomia and keratoconjunctivitis sicca. These findings are indicative of which of the following?

A. Lymphoma

B. Crohn's disease

C. Mumps

D. Sjögren's syndrome

E. Mucous extravasation phenomenon

6. A patient seeks help for recurrent palatal pain. She presents with multiple punctate ulcers in the hard palate that were preceded by tiny blisters. Her lesions typically heal in about 2 weeks and reappear during stressful times. She has _____.

A. Aphthous ulcers

B. Recurrent primary herpes

C. Recurrent secondary herpes

D. Erythema multiforme

E. Discoid lupus

7. Conservative surgical excision would be appropriate treatment and probably curative for which of the following?

A. Nodular fasciitis

B. Fibromatosis

C. Fibrosarcoma

D. Rhabdomyosarcoma

E. Adenoid cystic carcinoma

8. On a routine radiographic examination, a well-defined radiolucent lesion was seen in the body of the mandible of a 17-year-old boy. At the time of operation, it proved to be an empty cavity. What is this lesion?

A. Osteoporotic bone marrow

B. Aneurysmal bone cyst

C. Odontogenic keratocyst

D. Static bone cyst

E. Traumatic bone cyst

9. A 21-year-old woman went to her dentist because of facial asymmetry. This asymmetry had developed gradually over 3 years. The patient had no symptoms. A diffusely opaque lesion was found in her right maxilla. All laboratory tests (complete blood count, alkaline phosphatase, calcium) were within normal limits. A biopsy specimen was interpreted as a fibro-osseous lesion. This patient most likely has _____.

A. Cementoblastoma

B. Fibrous dysplasia

C. Cherubism

D. Osteosarcoma

E. Chronic osteomyelitis

10. A cutaneous maculopapulary rash of the head and neck preceded by small ulcers in the buccal mucosa would suggest which of the following?

A. Primary herpes simplex infection

B. Rubeola

C. Varicella

D. Primary syphilis

E. Actinomycosis

11. The idiopathic condition in which destructive inflammatory lesions featuring necrotizing vasculitis are seen in the lung, kidney, and upper respiratory tract is known as _____.

A. Epidermolysis bullosa

B. Stevens-Johnson syndrome

C. Sturge-Weber syndrome

D. Wegener's granulomatosis

E. Secondary syphilis

12. From the following list, select the jaw lesions or diseases that are characterized microscopically by the presence of conspicuous numbers of multinucleated giant cells. (Choose four.)

A. Central giant cell granuloma

B. Ossifying fibroma

C. Hyperparathyroidism

D. Calcifying epithelial odontogenic tumor

E. Aneurysmal bone cyst

F. Calcifying odontogenic cyst

G. Cherubism

13. For each clinical feature listed, select the most closely linked disease or lesion from the list provided.

A. Solitary, shallow, oval ulcer of buccal mucosa	1. Granular cell tumor
B. Bilateral, reticular white lines of buccal mucosa	2. Leukemia
C. Generalized enlargement of erythematous gingival tissues	3. Amalgam tattoo
D. Solitary nodular mass of the dorsal tongue	4. Aphthous ulcer
E. Darkly colored macule of attached gingiva	5. Mucous extravasation phenomenon
F. Fluctuant nodule of lower lip	6. Lichen planus

14. From the following list, select the systemic diseases in which patients may develop aphthous ulcers. (Choose three.)

A. Celiac sprue

B. Sarcoidosis

C. Amyloidosis

D. Behçet's syndrome

E. Crohn's disease

F. Neurofibromatosis

15. X-ray beam A is produced using 70 kVp, 7 mA, and 0.1 s. X-ray beam B is produced using 70 kVp, 10 mA, and 0.15 s. Which of the following statements are correct? (Choose two.)

A. Beam A has higher mean energy.

B. Beam B has higher mean energy.

C. Beam B has a higher number of x-ray photons.

D. The mean energies of the two beams are equal.

E. The maximum energy of the x-ray photons is higher for beam B.

16. Which of the following items influence the mean energy of an x-ray beam? (Choose two.)
    A. Kilovoltage
    B. Milliamperage
    C. Exposure time
    D. Amount of filtration
    E. Collimation
    F. Using a rotating anode

17. The function of the filament is to _____.
    A. Convert electrons into photons
    B. Convert photons into electrons
    C. Release photons
    D. Release electrons
    E. None of the above

18. The *most* radiosensitive of the following cells in terms of cell killing is the _____.
    A. Cardiomyocyte
    B. Basal epithelial cell
    C. Endothelial cell
    D. Neuron
    E. Polymorphonuclear leukocyte

19. For each of the numbered radiation effects, indicate whether the effects are stochastic or deterministic.
    A. Stochastic effect
    B. Deterministic effect
    ___ 1. Thyroid cancer
    ___ 2. Xerostomia
    ___ 3. Cataract formation
    ___ 4. Heritable effects
    ___ 5. Oral mucositis

20. Photoelectric interactions are highest in _____.
    A. Enamel
    B. Dentin
    C. Cementum
    D. Pulp

21. The photosensitive component of an x-ray film is _____.
    A. Silver halide crystals
    B. Sodium thiosulfate crystals
    C. Gelatin
    D. Rare earth elements

22. The effective dose from a limited cone-beam CT scan of the anterior maxilla is 20 µSv. The effective dose from a full-mouth radiographic examination (with round collimation and thyroid collar) is 120 µSv. Based on these data, which of the following statements is *true* regarding radiation-induced cancer risk?
    A. Risk from the full-mouth radiographic examination is higher.
    B. Risk from the CT scan is higher.
    C. Risk from both examinations is the same.
    D. Risks cannot be compared because they are different imaging modalities.

23. You are unsure of the location of an opaque mass seen over a molar root on a periapical view. A second view of the same region, made with the x-ray machine oriented more from the mesial, reveals that the object has moved mesially with respect to the molar roots on the first view. The location of the object is _____.
    A. Buccal to the roots
    B. Lingual to the roots
    C. In the same plane as the roots
    D. Unknown because information is insufficient to form an opinion

24. Cone-cutting results from _____.
    A. Too great a target-film distance
    B. Not selecting the proper kVp
    C. Not enough time exposure
    D. The x-ray machine being improperly aimed

25. If your film-based radiographs start coming out too light, it may be that the _____.
    A. Exposure time is too long
    B. Developer needs changing
    C. Developer is too hot
    D. Fixer needs changing
    E. Films are not sufficiently washed

26. If an unwrapped, nonprocessed x-ray film is exposed to normal light for just a second and then processed, it _____.
    A. May still be used but will be a little dark
    B. May still be used but will be a little light
    C. May still be used but will be brown
    D. Will be completely black
    E. Will be completely clear

27. To ensure high radiographic image quality, it is important to _____ daily.
    A. Check the temperature of the processing solutions
    B. Clean the processing equipment
    C. Clean the intensifying screens
    D. Calibrate the mA linearity

28. Radiographs of a pregnant patient _____.
    A. Should never be made
    B. Should be made only in the third trimester of pregnancy
    C. Should be made only with triple leaded aprons on the patient's lap
    D. Should be made when there is a specific need

29. Radiographic examination plays an important role in assessing periodontal disease. Intraoral radiographs permit assessment of several disease features related to periodontal disease. Which features from the following list cannot be assessed by radiographic examination? (Choose two.)
    A. Bone loss in the furcation areas
    B. Amount of bone present
    C. Crown-to-root ratio
    D. Depth of the soft tissue pocket
    E. Assessment of the three-dimensional nature of the vertical periodontal defect.

Orthodontics and Pediatric Dentistry

STEVEN J. LINDAUER, BHAVNA SHROFF,
ESER TUFEKCI, MARK TAYLOR

1.0 Orthodontics

This review summarizes key concepts important to orthodontic diagnosis and treatment. It is organized in a manner similar to standard textbooks on the subject, including *Contemporary Orthodontics*, ed 5, by Proffit et al, and *Textbook of Orthodontics*, ed 3, by Bishara (see References). This review is not meant to be an in-depth examination of all of the intricacies of orthodontics but rather to serve as a guide for further study. It should help students pinpoint areas where they require additional information, and the test questions that follow can help in this manner as well. Students can consult other sources, such as the aforementioned textbooks, for more detailed explanations of the material.

Outline of Review

1.1 Epidemiology of Malocclusion

Malocclusion is not a disease but a variation from what is considered ideal. It is difficult to estimate the prevalence of malocclusion in the population. Studies have focused instead on the prevalence of characteristics of malocclusion, such as the presence of incisor crowding, overjet (usually accompanying Angle class II malocclusions), reverse overjet or anterior crossbite (usually associated with Angle class III malocclusions), midline diastema, deep or open bite, and posterior crossbite. Various characteristics of malocclusion are seen more commonly at different ages and in different ethnic groups. It is important to note which characteristics are likely to change or improve naturally over time and distinguish them from others that may require treatment or intervention during development.

Prevalence

A. Crowding.
   1. Incisor crowding tends to increase in children as the permanent teeth erupt because permanent incisors require more space than their predecessors.
   2. Lower incisor crowding continues to worsen into adulthood.
   3. Nearly 15% of adolescents and adults have severely crowded incisors, suggesting that extraction of teeth would be necessary to create enough space to align them.
B. Angle classification (see 1.4, Orthodontic Diagnosis, for definitions).
   1. Overjet of greater than 5 mm, suggesting class II malocclusion, occurs in 23% of children, 15% of adolescents, and 13% of adults.
   2. Reverse overjet, suggesting class III malocclusion, is much less frequent than class II malocclusion in the U.S. population.
   3. Class II relationships are more common in whites of northern European descent.
   4. Class III relationships are more prevalent in Asian populations (2% to 5%).

5. Estimation of the percentage of the U.S. population that fall into Angle's four major classification groups.
   a. Class I normal occlusion: 30%.
   b. Class I malocclusion: 50% to 55%.
   c. Class II malocclusion: 15%.
   d. Class III malocclusion: approximately 1%.

1.2 Growth and Development

Theories of Growth Control

No single theory explains all of craniofacial growth control.

A. *Direct genetic control*—bone, as all other tissues, is directly under the control of genetics.
B. *Epigenetic growth control*—cartilage is the primary determinant of skeletal growth and indirectly controls the growth of bone. Cartilage grows and is then replaced by bone.
C. *Environmental growth control: the functional matrix theory*—growth of bone is influenced by adjacent soft tissues through environmental changes in forces exerted on the bones that stimulate their growth.

Endochondral versus Intramembranous Bone Formation

A. *Endochondral bone formation*—formed first in cartilage, then transformed into bone. Bones formed in this way are probably less susceptible to environmental influences during growth and are under more direct genetic control. The bones of the cranial base are endochondral.
B. *Intramembranous bone formation*—formed by secretion of bone matrix directly within connective tissues, without intermediate formation of cartilage. Growth of intramembranous bones is more influenced by the environmental forces around them. The cranial vault, maxilla, and mandible are examples of intramembranous bones.

Sites of Growth in the Craniofacial Complex

A. Cranial vault.
   1. Intramembranous bones that form without cartilaginous precursors.
   2. At birth, the bones are widely separated by loose connective tissues at the fontanelles. Apposition of bone along the edges of the fontanelles eliminates these open spaces, but the bones remain separated by the cranial sutures.
   3. As brain growth occurs, the cranial bones are pushed apart, and apposition of new bone occurs at the sutures.
   4. Remodeling also occurs with new bone added on the external surfaces and removed on the internal surfaces (periosteal apposition and endosteal resorption).

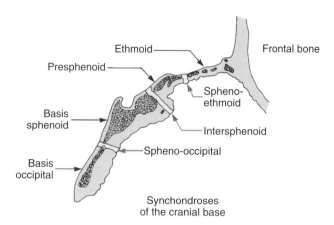

Figure 5-1 Diagrammatic representation of the synchondroses of the cranial base, showing the location of these important growth sites. *(From Proffit WR, Fields HW, Sarver DM: Contemporary Orthodontics, ed 5. St. Louis, Mosby, 2013.)*

B. Cranial base.
   1. Ethmoid, sphenoid, and occipital bones (Figure 5-1) at the base of the skull are formed initially in cartilage and later transformed into bone by endochondral ossification.
   2. As ossification occurs, three bands of cartilage remain, which are important growth centers called *synchondroses*: sphenoethmoid synchondrosis, intersphenoid synchondrosis, and sphenooccipital synchondrosis.
   3. Each synchondrosis acts like a two-sided epiphyseal plate with growing cartilage in the middle and bands of maturing cartilage cells extending in both directions that are eventually replaced by bone.
   4. These synchondroses eventually become inactive: the intersphenoid probably around age 3, the sphenoethmoid around age 7, and the sphenooccipital considerably later.
   5. Because they are endochondral bones, the bones making up the cranial base are minimally affected directly by growth of the brain.

C. Maxilla.
   1. Growth of the maxilla is intramembranous. Growth occurs at the sutures posterior and superior to the maxilla at its connections to the cranium and cranial base and by surface remodeling.
   2. The maxilla migrates downward and forward away from the cranial base (Figure 5-2) and undergoes significant surface remodeling (Figure 5-3).
   3. Surface remodeling includes resorption of bone anteriorly and apposition of bone inferiorly.
   4. Much of the anterior movement of the maxilla is negated by anterior resorption, and downward migration is augmented by inferior apposition of bone.
   5. As with all bones, interstitial growth within the mineralized mass of the maxilla is impossible; addition

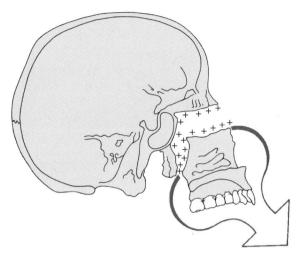

Figure 5-2 As growth of surrounding soft tissues translates the maxilla downward and forward, opening up space at its superior and posterior sutural attachments, new bone is added on both sides of the sutures. *(Redrawn from Enlow DH, Hans MG:* Essentials of Facial Growth. *Philadelphia, Saunders, 1996.)*

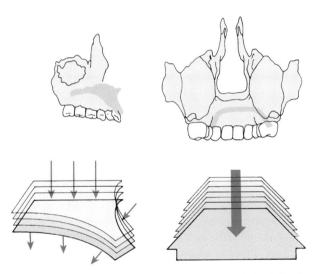

Figure 5-3 Remodeling of the palatal vault (which is also the floor of the nose) moves it in the same direction as it is being translated; bone is removed from the floor of the nose and added to the roof of the mouth. On the anterior surface, bone is removed, partially canceling the forward translation. As the vault moves downward, the same process of bone remodeling also widens it. *(Redrawn from Enlow DH, Hans MG:* Essentials of Facial Growth. *Philadelphia, Saunders, 1996.)*

of new bone can occur only at the surfaces. Increased space for the eruption of posterior teeth occurs by addition of bone posteriorly at the tuberosity as the maxilla migrates downward and forward.

D. Mandible.
1. Growth of the mandible is both endochondral and intramembranous.

2. Cartilage covers the surface of the mandibular condyle at the temporomandibular joint (TMJ). However, this cartilage does not grow independently similar to an epiphyseal plate or synchondrosis.
3. Cartilage is transformed into bone at the condyle as the mandible grows downward and forward, away from the cranial base. Surface apposition and resorption occurs in other areas of the mandible.
4. Most growth of the mandible occurs by new bone forming at the condyle and by resorption of the anterior part of the ramus with apposition posteriorly. Minor amounts of remodeling occur anteriorly and inferiorly.
5. Embryonic development.
   a. The mandible develops in the same area as the cartilage of the first pharyngeal arch: Meckel's cartilage. However, development of the mandible itself proceeds just lateral to Meckel's cartilage and is entirely intramembranous in nature.
   b. Meckel's cartilage disintegrates, and its remnants are transformed into a portion of two of the small bones of the middle ear (malleus and incus). Its perichondrium persists as the sphenomandibular ligament.
   c. Condylar cartilage develops independently and is initially separated by a gap from the body of the intramembranous mandible. It later fuses with the developing mandibular ramus.
6. As with the maxilla, interstitial growth within the mineralized mass of the mandible is impossible. Space for eruption of the posterior teeth occurs as the anterior portion of the ramus resorbs extensively. In a child with crowded teeth, it is unreasonable to expect that interstitial growth of the mandible will occur to create space within the body of the mandible to alleviate the crowding.
7. Extensive surface apposition occurs on the posterior surface of the ramus.
8. Mandibular growth rotation.
   a. As growth at the condyle facilitates movement of the mandible downward and forward, away from the cranial base, a gap is available between the maxilla and mandible in which the maxillary and mandibular teeth erupt.
   b. *Average closing rotation*—in most children, condylar growth exceeds molar eruption, and the mandible rotates slightly closed over time. This closing rotation, along with the downward and forward growth of the mandible itself, helps make the chin appear more prominent as children age. It also indicates that posterior face height increases more than anterior face height in most cases.
   c. *Severe closing rotation*—in some children, condylar growth greatly exceeds molar eruption, and the mandible rotates more substantially closed, leading

to development of a shorter face and a deeper anterior overbite tendency.

d. *Opening rotation*—rarely, condylar growth is less than molar eruption, and the mandible rotates open during growth. In these children, a long lower face and tendency for an anterior open bite develop.

Timing of Growth

A. Cephalocaudal gradient of growth.
1. In general, structures farther from the brain grow more and later.
2. In the third month of fetal development, the head takes up almost 50% of the total body length. By the time of birth, the trunk and limbs have grown so that the head is 30% of the body. In an adult, the head represents about 12% of the total height.
3. The mandible is farther from the brain than the maxilla and grows more and later.
B. Scammon's growth curves.
1. Neural tissues, including the brain, continue to grow rapidly after birth and reach near 100% adult size by about age 6 or 7.
2. Lymphoid tissues, including tonsils and adenoids, also grow quickly, reaching twice the adult size by about age 10, and then involute during the pubertal growth spurt to reach adult size.
3. Genital or reproductive tissues do not grow much until puberty and then rapidly increase to adult size corresponding to the time of the pubertal growth spurt.
4. General body tissues, including muscle and bone, grow rapidly after birth, then slow in growth during childhood, and then accelerate again at the same time as reproductive tissues proliferate.
5. Maxillary and mandibular growth (Figure 5-4).
a. The maxilla, located closer to the brain than the mandible, grows earlier and follows a pattern closer to that of neural tissues.
b. The mandible grows later and exhibits more characteristics of a growth spurt paralleling the pubertal growth spurt in body height.
C. Growth velocity curve (Figure 5-5).
1. The velocity curve shows that growth in height is very rapid after birth but decelerates quickly to a lower, more constant level in childhood.
2. Around puberty, growth accelerates again, reaching a pubertal growth peak before slowing and virtually stopping at maturity.
3. Predicting the timing of this growth spurt may be important for orthodontic treatment designed to take maximal advantage of growth changes.
D. Sex differences.
1. Girls reach their growth peak about 2 years earlier on average than boys. Average peak growth for girls is around age 12 and for boys is age 14.

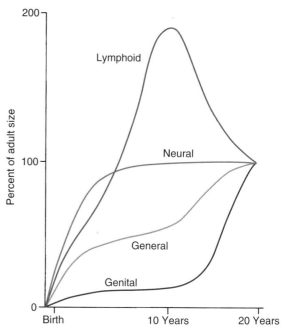

Figure 5-4 Growth curves for the maxilla and mandible shown against the background of Scammon's curves. Growth of the jaws is intermediate between the neural and general body curves, with the mandible following the general body curve more closely than the maxilla. The acceleration in general body growth at puberty, which affects the jaws, parallels the dramatic increase in development of the sexual organs. Lymphoid involution also occurs at this time. *(From Scammon RD: The measurement of the body in childhood. In: Harris JA, editor. The Measurement of Man. Minneapolis, University of Minnesota Press, 1930.)*

2. There is considerable individual variation in the timing of growth relative to chronologic age; early-maturing boys may reach peak growth before late-maturing girls.
3. Generally, the earlier the peak of growth, the shorter the duration of the growth spurt will be, and less overall growth occurs.
4. Girls generally start growth sooner, grow for a shorter amount of time, and grow less than boys.
E. Predictors.
1. Chronologic age is not a perfect predictor of when peak growth will occur (correlation about 0.8).
2. Basing growth predictions on dental age is even less reliable (correlation about 0.7). In other words, children whose teeth erupt early do not erupt early.
3. Physical growth status correlates well with skeletal age, which is determined by the relative level of maturation of the skeletal system.
a. A hand-wrist radiograph, revealing the ossification of the bones of the hand and wrist, is the standard for assessing skeletal development.
b. Another possibility is evaluating the development of the vertebral bones as visualized on a

cephalometric radiograph (cervical vertebral maturation).

c. It is also possible to plot increases in body height over time.

d. Successive cephalometric radiographs can be superimposed (usually using the stable cranial base structures) to determine when a growth spurt or termination of significant growth is occurring in an individual.

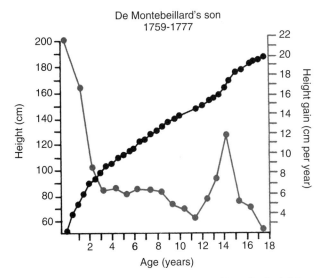

**De Montebeillard's son
1759-1777**

Figure 5-5 Growth can be plotted either in height or weight at any age or in the amount of change in any given interval. A curve such as the age line is called a *distance curve*, whereas the height line is a *velocity curve*. Plotting velocity rather than distance makes it easier to see when accelerations and decelerations in the rate of growth occurred. These data are for the growth of one individual, the son of a French aristocrat in the late eighteenth century, whose growth followed the typical pattern. Note the acceleration of growth at adolescence, which occurred for this individual at about age 14. *(Data from Scammon Amer F Phys Anthrop, 1927. IN Proffit WR, Fields HW, Sarver DM: Contemporary Orthodontics, ed 5, St Louis, Mosby, 2013.)*

4. Because sex hormones have a direct effect on endochondral bone growth, sexual development and growth in height are well correlated.

F. Directions of growth.

1. Growth in width of the jaws is generally completed before the adolescent growth spurt begins.

2. Growth in length of the jaws continues through the growth spurt.

3. Vertical growth continues longer.

Cleft Lip and Palate and Other Developmental Abnormalities

A. Incidence.

1. The most common craniofacial defect, second only to clubfoot in congenital deformities, is clefting of the lip or palate or both, occurring in 1 in 700 births.

B. Embryology.

1. Nearly all the tissues of the face and neck originate from ectoderm.

2. There are principal stages in craniofacial development. Some abnormalities in facial form and jaw relationships can be traced to malfunctions that occur during specific stages (Table 5-1).

3. Cleft lip occurs when there is a failure of fusion between the frontonasal (medial nasal) process and the maxillary process. This fusion includes the lip and alveolar ridge (the primary palate).

4. Closure of the secondary palate occurs about 2 weeks later, when the palatal shelves elevate and join together in a process that proceeds from anterior to posterior.

1.3 Development of Occlusion

A. Stages of normal dental development.

1. Gum pad stage.

a. Birth to about 6 to 7 months of age, ending with the eruption of the first incisor.

Table 5-1

Stages of Embryonic Craniofacial Development

STAGE	TIME (HUMANS, POSTFERTILIZATION)	RELATED SYNDROMES
Germ layer formation and initial organization of structures	Day 17	Fetal alcohol syndrome
Neural tube formation	Days 18-23	Anencephaly
Origin, migration, and interaction of cell populations	Days 19-28	Hemifacial microsomia, mandibulofacial dysostosis (Treacher-Collins syndrome), limb abnormalities

Formation of organ systems
  Primary palate
  Secondary palate
	
	Days 28-38
	Days 42-55
		
		Cleft lip and/or palate, other facial clefts
		Cleft palate

Final differentiation of tissues	Day 50–birth	Achondroplasia synostosis syndromes (Crouzon's, Apert's)

From Proffit WR, Fields HW, Sarver DM: *Contemporary Orthodontics*, ed 4. St. Louis, Mosby, 2007.

b. The future position of the teeth can be observed by the elevations and grooves present on the alveolar ridges.

2. Primary dentition stage.
   a. Starts with the eruption of the primary teeth and lasts until about 6 years of age, when the first permanent tooth erupts.
   b. The maxillary anterior primary teeth are about 75% of the size of their permanent successors.
   c. The mandibular anterior primary teeth are about 6 mm narrower mesiodistally on average than their successors.
   d. Overbite, defined as the vertical overlap of the mandibular teeth by the maxillary teeth, develops as teeth erupt. Overbite can be measured in millimeters, but it is preferable to measure it in percentages. Overbite normally varies from 10% to 40%.
   e. Open bite is lack of overbite. Open bite or reduced amount of overbite is not unusual in children during the primary dentition because of thumb- or finger-sucking habits.
   f. Overjet is the horizontal distance between the mandibular teeth and the maxillary teeth. Overjet normally ranges from 0 to 4 mm. Digit sucking habits also cause an increase in overjet.
   g. Spacing.
      (1) Children in the primary dentition often have generalized spacing between their teeth. The extra space helps accommodate the larger sized permanent teeth as they erupt. If a child lacks spacing or has crowding in the primary dentition, the permanent dentition will exhibit crowding.
      (2) Spacing is especially noticeable in two locations called the *primate spaces*—between the lateral incisor and canine in the maxilla and between the canine and first primary molar in the mandible.
   h. Crowding is uncommon in the primary dentition.
   i. Molar relationship.
      (1) *Flush terminal plane*—the distal aspects of the second deciduous maxillary and mandibular molars are at the same sagittal level.
      (2) *Mesial step*—the mandibular terminal plane is mesial to the maxillary terminal plane.
      (3) *Distal step*—the mandibular terminal plane is distal to the maxillary terminal plane.
      (4) By the age of 5, about 90% of children have a terminal plane relationship that is flush or with a 1-mm or greater mesial step.
      (5) The first permanent molar is guided along the terminal plane during eruption. The terminal plane relationship determines the molar classification in the mixed dentition.

3. Mixed dentition stage.
   a. Starts around age 6 with the eruption of the first permanent tooth.
   b. As each permanent tooth erupts, it is expected that its antimere (corresponding contralateral tooth) will erupt within 6 months.
   c. "Ugly duckling stage"—as the maxillary central incisors erupt, they move labially, and a temporary diastema is often present between them. This has been referred to as the "ugly duckling stage" of the mixed dentition. This is a normal stage of development but does not always occur. When the permanent canines erupt, their mesial movement will likely close the diastema if one is present and if it is 2 mm or less.
   d. The mandibular incisors erupt lingually to the primary incisors, and they move facially.
   e. A transient open bite may be observed as a result of partial eruption of anterior teeth. Under normal conditions, the open bite resolves with further tooth eruption.
   f. The molar relationship is described in the sagittal plane according to the Angle classification. The Angle classification system was introduced by Angle in 1907 and is based on the anterior-posterior relationship of the first mandibular molar to the maxillary permanent first molar.
      (1) Class I molar or normo-occlusion.
      (2) Class II molar or disto-occlusion.
      (3) Class III molar or mesio-occlusion.
   g. *Predicting molar relationship*—according to Bishara (2001), during the transition period from the primary to the mixed dentition, flush terminal plane develops into a class I in 56% of cases and into a class II in 44% of cases. Mesial step can transition into a class I or, much less commonly, a class III molar occlusion according to the initial severity.
   h. *Normal characteristics of the mixed dentition*—molar and canine relationships are class I; "leeway space" is present; well-aligned incisors or up to moderate crowding of the incisors; proximal contacts are tight.
   i. Leeway space.
      (1) The difference in mesiodistal size between the primary canine, primary first molar, and primary second molar and their permanent replacements. The leeway space is larger in the mandibular arch, averaging 2.5 mm per side. In the maxillary arch, the leeway space measures about 1.5 mm per side.
      (2) The leeway space can affect the eventual classification of the molar in the permanent dentition or may aid in resolution of crowding, or a combination of both.

4. Permanent dentition stage.
   a. Begins when the last primary tooth is lost.
   b. The maxillary teeth should overlap the mandibular teeth vertically and buccolingually.
   c. The arches have curvature in the sagittal plane (curve of Spee) and the frontal plane (curve of Wilson).
   d. Overbite is generally 10% to 20% but can vary up to 50%.
   e. Overjet should be 1 to 3 mm.
   f. The interarch relationship (also referred to as the *buccal occlusion*) should be class I molar, premolar, and canine.
   g. Permanent dentition relationships are fairly stable once established, with one notable exception: during the second to fourth decades of life, there is a tendency for anterior crowding to develop or worsen over time.

B. Dimensional changes in the dental arches.
   1. Width.
      a. The maxillary intercanine width increases by approximately 6 mm between the ages of 3 and 13. An additional increase of 1.7 mm occurs until age 45.
      b. The maxillary intermolar width in the primary dentition increases 2 mm between the ages of 3 and 5. The permanent intermolar width increases by 2.2 mm between the ages of 8 and 13 and decreases about 1 mm by age 45.
      c. Part of the increase in width of the maxillary arch is because the alveolar bone is divergent, and the width increases as growth and eruption occurs.
      d. The mandibular intercanine width increases by 3.7 mm from age 3 to 13. From age 13 to 45, the intercanine width decreases by 1.2 mm.
      e. The mandibular primary intermolar width increases by 1.5 mm between the ages of 3 and 5. The permanent molar width increases by 1 mm from age 8 to 13 and decreases by 1 mm by age 45.
   2. Length.
      a. Arch length is measured at the midline from a point midway between the central incisors to a tangent touching the distal surfaces of the second primary molars or the mesial surfaces of the first permanent molars.
      b. In the maxilla, there is a small decrease in arch length with age because the incisors become more upright.
      c. In the mandibular arch, a similar decrease in arch length is observed in the mixed and permanent dentition as a result of uprighting of the incisors and the loss of the leeway space.
   3. Circumference (perimeter).
      a. A measure of the amount of space available for the dentition.

   b. Measured from the distal aspect of the second primary molar (mesial aspect of the first permanent molar) on one side and around the arch to the distal aspect of the second primary molar on the other side.
   c. Mandibular arch circumference decreases significantly in the mixed to permanent dentition because of the mesial shift of the permanent molars into the leeway space, the mesial drift tendency of the posterior teeth in general, the slight amount of interproximal wear, and the lingual positioning of the incisors secondary to the differential growth of the maxilla (less) compared with the mandible (more).
   d. Maxillary arch circumference increases very slightly.

C. Sequence of eruption.
   1. Eruption is earlier by 5 months on average in females compared with males.
   2. Primary dentition.
      a. Primary teeth begin calcification between the third and fourth month in utero.
      b. The mandibular teeth usually start the calcification process before the maxillary teeth.
      c. At birth, no teeth are present in the newborn infant.
      d. Eruption of the first primary tooth starts at about 6 to 7 months of age, and new teeth continue to erupt until age 2 to 3.
      e. The typical sequence of eruption is *A-B-D-C-E*: the central incisor (A), the lateral incisor (B), the first primary molar (D), the canine (C), and the second primary molar (E).
   3. Permanent dentition.
      a. The permanent teeth begin calcification shortly after birth.
      b. The first permanent molar shows signs of calcification the second postnatal month, and the third permanent molar begins to calcify around age 8 to 9 years.
      c. Mandibular arch eruption sequence: first molar, central incisor, lateral incisor, canine, first premolar, second premolar, second molar, and third molar.
      d. Maxillary arch eruption sequence: first molar, central incisor, lateral incisor, first premolar, second premolar, canine, second molar, and third molar. In the maxillary arch, the eruption sequence in the posterior segments is frequently asymmetrical.

1.4 Orthodontic Diagnosis

The first step in orthodontic treatment planning is gathering the data required to make a diagnosis. The information comes from talking to the patient or parents or both, clinical examination, and diagnostic records.

A. Patient interview.
  1. Chief complaint—why treatment is desired.
  2. Medical and dental history.
    a. Although it is usually impossible to pinpoint a cause of malocclusion, it may be possible in a few cases when there is a history of early tooth loss, trauma, family history of a certain type of malocclusion, habits, or a developmental malformation.
    b. Medical problems that may affect orthodontic treatment, including susceptibility to periodontal disease, and medications that inhibit bone remodeling (bisphosphonates).
  3. Growth history.
  4. Social and behavioral assessment.
    a. Cooperation.
    b. Habits.
B. Clinical examination (oral and extraoral).
  1. Pathology—including caries and periodontal problems, oral hygiene.
  2. Function—mastication, jaw opening, TMJ, speech, functional shifts, interferences.
  3. Dental and occlusal characteristics.
    a. Intraarch.
      (1) Teeth present or missing.
      (2) Arch shape, symmetry.
      (3) Alignment—crowding, spacing, rotations.
        (a) Space analysis in the mixed dentition using radiographs or proportionality tables or both.
      (4) Tooth size analysis—tooth size discrepancies (Bolton, 1958).
    b. Interarch (in three dimensions)—discrepancies may be dental or skeletal in origin. For example, a patient with a class II interarch relationship may have a class I skeletal relationship (maxilla and mandible are in good relationship) or a class II skeletal relationship with the maxilla forward or the mandible back or both.
      (1) Anterior-posterior.
        (a) Angle classification.
          (i) *Class I normal occlusion*—mesiobuccal cusp of the maxillary first molar in the buccal groove of the mandibular first molar and intraarch relationships among teeth are correct.
          (ii) *Class I malocclusion*—mesiobuccal cusp of the maxillary first molar in the buccal groove of the mandibular first molar (but intraarch relationships are abnormal).
          (iii) *Class II*—mesiobuccal cusp of the maxillary first molar anterior to the buccal groove of the mandibular first molar.
            1. Division 1—maxillary incisors flared.

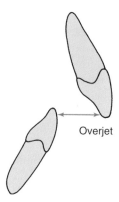

Figure 5-6 Overjet is defined as horizontal overlap of the incisors. Normally, the incisors are in contact, with the upper incisors ahead of the lower by only the thickness of the upper edges (i.e., 2- to 3-mm overjet is the normal relationship). If the lower incisors are in front of the upper incisors, the condition is called reverse overjet or anterior crossbite. *(From Proffit WR, Fields HW, Sarver DM:* Contemporary Orthodontics, *ed 5. St. Louis, Mosby, 2013.)*

            2. Division 2—maxillary incisors upright (laterals flared) and deep overbite.
          (iv) *Class III*—mesiobuccal cusp of the maxillary first molar posterior to the buccal groove of the mandibular first molar.
        (b) Overjet.
          (i) Excess overjet (usually with class II) (Figure 5-6).
          (ii) Reverse overjet (anterior crossbite—usually with class III).
      (2) Vertical (overbite)—normal (20% overbite), deep (>50% overbite), or open.
      (3) Width (transverse, posterior crossbite).
        (a) *Normal*—maxillary lingual cusp in mandibular fossa.
        (b) *Crossbite or lingual crossbite*—maxillary buccal cusp in mandibular fossa (Figure 5-7).
        (c) *Complete lingual crossbite*—whole maxillary tooth lingual to mandibular tooth.
        (d) *Complete buccal crossbite*—whole maxillary tooth buccal to mandibular tooth.
  4. Facial esthetics and proportions.
    a. Frontal examination.
      (1) Right-left symmetry and proportions ("rule of 5's").
      (2) Vertical proportions (vertical facial thirds).
      (3) *Lip posture (lip competence)*—with the teeth together and lips at rest, the lips should lightly touch or be slightly apart. A gap of more than 3 to 4 mm indicates lip incompetence because

b. There is a significant difference in esthetics and cephalometric values among racial and ethnic groups.

c. Cephalometric measures should be used to explain or support a diagnosis based on occlusal and esthetic characteristics, to help differentiate the underlying cause of an observed malocclusion. Individual cephalometric measures should not be used by themselves to make a diagnosis.

7. Other radiographic information.

a. Panoramic or full-mouth radiographs, or both, are necessary to evaluate locations and orientations of teeth, root parallelism, bone heights.

b. Periapical radiographs, especially of incisors, are recommended to document and follow signs of root resorption that may be present or induced during treatment.

c. Three-dimensional cone-beam computed tomography may be performed to locate unerupted or impacted teeth more precisely, evaluate skeletal asymmetry, assess craniofacial defects, or construct cephalometric or other radiographic images.

1.5 Treatment Planning

A. Development of a problem list.

1. Diseases or pathologic processes (systemic diseases, caries, periodontal concerns).

2. Factors contributing to or describing the malocclusion (e.g., dental crowding, anterior deep bite, class II interarch relationship, mandibular deficiency, long lower face, flat lips).

3. Cephalometric measures in themselves are usually not considered problems, but what they indicate may be (e.g., protrusive maxilla, small mandible, flared maxillary incisors, vertical growth tendency).

B. Prioritization of the problem list—listing the problems in order of priority is important because it helps when developing a systematic plan that addresses as many of the patient's problems as possible. The problems are not always addressed in their priority sequence during treatment.

1. Systemic diseases or pathology take top priority and usually need to be controlled before orthodontic treatment can begin.

2. Impacted teeth are usually a high priority.

3. Esthetic or occlusal problems may be next, depending on the severity, the patient's chief complaint, or other concerns.

4. Within occlusal problems, interarch relationships usually take priority over intraarch relationships (class II interarch relationship takes priority over mild anterior crowding). However, priority may vary depending on severity (e.g., severe crowding might take priority over mild anterior overbite).

5. Habits should also be considered.

6. Growth potential and growth tendencies should also be considered. (e.g., a class III growth tendency in someone who is already class III and with substantial growth remaining would be considered a problem.)

C. Development of treatment objectives—treatment objectives mirror problems and should be listed in priority order.

D. Evaluation of possible solutions—for each problem or objective, the possible solutions should be examined, and the appropriate option for a given patient should be chosen.

E. Compromises and other considerations.

1. The ideal is to achieve the best possible function, esthetics, and stability for each patient.

2. Often, the ideal goals cannot be met by a reasonable orthodontic plan. One goal may need to be sacrificed at the expense of achieving the best possible result for a given patient.

3. The relative risk/cost-benefit should be considered along with the patient's preferences. Not all patients want to incur the risks and costs of surgery to achieve the ideal result. Some patients may be at increased caries or periodontal risk, and objectives can be modified to decrease treatment time to reduce those risks.

4. Alternative treatment options should be presented to patients who can help make a decision on the best treatment, given various circumstances. Informed consent to treatment is important. Patients need to know and understand the relative risks and benefits.

1.6 Biology of Tooth Movement

A. Fundamental principles—biology of tooth movement refers to the orthodontic movement of a tooth within and through the alveolar bone. It results from the application of a force system to the tooth and the transduction of that mechanical signal into a biologic signal and a response.

1. A force system is applied at the crown of a tooth, and the mechanical signal is transmitted or transducted to the supporting structures of the tooth (bone and periodontal ligament [PDL]). For tooth movement, the force need not be continuous, but it is critical that the force be applied for a minimally acceptable period of time to elicit the biologic response necessary. The amount of force (heavy or light) determines the biologic pathway of tooth movement and the formation or lack of formation of a hyalinized zone with undermining resorption.

2. The PDL, a well-organized connective fibrous tissue, remodels significantly during orthodontic tooth movement. Under physiologic conditions, the PDL is rich in collagen fibers well organized to resist the forces of mastication.

3. *Pressure or compression side*—side toward which the tooth is moving. This is where bone resorption is

taking place. Resorption of the alveolus is primarily the result of osteoclastic activity. The osteoclast is a giant, multinucleated cell with a ruffled border. The resorption lacunae created are called *Howship's lacunae.*

4. *Tension side*—side opposite to the direction of the movement of the tooth. Apposition of bone occurs on this side. Areas of resorption may also undergo appositional remodeling if the tooth movement changes direction and the pressure side of the alveolus undergoes tension.

5. Different types of tooth movement are characterized by different patterns of stress distribution in the PDL and corresponding areas of bone resorption and bone apposition.

   a. *Intrusion*—when a tooth is intruded, the area of compression of the PDL is concentrated at the apex of the tooth.

   b. *Tipping*—during tipping, the crown and the apex move in opposite directions, creating two areas of compression: the cervical area on the side toward which the tooth is tipping and the apical region on the side opposite from which the tooth crown is moving. The tension areas are located on the opposite sides of where compression occurs.

   c. *Translation or bodily movement*—during bodily movement or translation, one side of the PDL experiences compression (the side toward which the tooth is moving), and the other side experiences tension.

B. Biologic control of orthodontic tooth movement.

1. During tooth movement, the tension and the compression occur in the PDL and at its two interfaces: with the bone on the alveolar side and with the cementum on the dental (tooth) side. Tension and compression also occur with physiologic tooth movements during functions such as mastication. Forces ranging from 1 to 50 kg (10 to 500 N) are experienced by the PDL during mastication, and the supporting apparatus of the tooth (alveolar bone and PDL) undergoes bone bending and compression and tension of the PDL.

2. When an orthodontic force is applied, two scenarios can develop depending on whether the force is heavy or light.

   a. *Heavy force*—the use of heavy orthodontic forces does not make tooth movement more efficient. It actually delays tooth movement by causing a lag period after the initial movement of the tooth within the PDL.

      (1) Initial period of tooth movement.

         (a) Bone bending and creation of a piezoelectric signal occurs in less than 1 second. The piezoelectric signal is characterized by a quick decay rate and the production of an equivalent signal of opposite direction when the force is released.

         (b) The PDL is compressed, and fluid is expressed from the area of compression, resulting in instant movement of the tooth within the PDL in 1 to 2 seconds.

         (c) As the fluids are expressed from the PDL, pain is felt as a result of the pressure applied within 5 seconds. The tooth is now compressed against the bone surface, and no further tooth movement occurs until undermining resorption takes place.

         (d) Undermining resorption occurs within the alveolar bone (in the marrow spaces) and moves toward the PDL area.

            (i) Appearance of osteoclastic cells in the bone marrow spaces is the first indication of undermining resorption.

            (ii) Undermining resorption can last 2 weeks to a few weeks. No tooth movement can occur until the undermining resorptive process is completed when heavy orthodontic forces are applied.

            (iii) The compressed PDL undergoes significant tissue changes. On the compression side, the hyalinized zone starts to develop (an area of the PDL that has lost all structural organization shows signs of necrosis and a lack of cellular activity).

            (iv) Hyalinization of the PDL occurs within hours of the application of a heavy force.

            (v) Cells from the surrounding bone marrow start to migrate into the area from the bone marrow spaces within 3 to 5 days, and undermining resorption simultaneously starts within the bone marrow spaces.

      (2) Secondary period of tooth movement (after undermining resorption).

         (a) The hyalinized PDL is in the process of healing.

         (b) Secondary tooth movement occurs after a lag period during which undermining resorption takes place.

   c. *Light force*—the use of light forces causes smooth, continuous tooth movement without formation of a significant hyalinized zone in the surrounding PDL. As a result, teeth subjected to light orthodontic forces start to move earlier and in a more physiologic way than teeth subjected to heavy forces.

      (1) Initial reaction includes partial compression of the blood vessels and a distortion of the PDL fibers.

(2) Within minutes, blood flow is altered, the oxygen tension changes, and prostaglandins and cytokines are released within the PDL.

(3) Metabolic changes, such as enzyme activity and chemical messengers that alter cellular activity, start to appear in this area of the PDL after a few hours. First messengers that have been suggested in the literature include hormones (parathyroid hormone and calcitonin), fibroblast distortion, substance P, some neurotransmitters, and prostaglandins.

(4) Within a few hours, as signal transduction starts in the PDL, the second messenger cyclic adenosine monophosphate levels increase.

(5) Cellular differentiation takes place in the PDL, and the coupling between osteoclast and osteoblast activities results in frontal resorption of the alveolus within a few days.

(6) The process of frontal resorption as seen with light force application allows a faster and more efficient biologic response than heavy forces and results in an earlier onset of tooth movement.

(7) Even when light forces are applied to a tooth, because the PDL itself is nonuniform and stresses created in the PDL vary depending on the location observed, it is likely that some areas along the tooth will experience some undermining resorption.

3. Deleterious effects of orthodontic forces.
   a. Mobility of teeth subjected to orthodontic forces.
      (1) Forces cause bone and PDL to undergo remodeling, and the PDL is temporarily widened.
      (2) Moderate mobility of the teeth occurs during tooth movement and resolves with the completion of therapy as long as there is no active periodontal disease.
      (3) If the tooth is in traumatic occlusion or the patient is grinding or clenching, the mobility is significantly increased, and there may be a need to adjust the occlusion or at least monitor it until the tooth does not have an occlusal interference.
   b. Pain.
      (1) Heavy orthodontic forces applied to a tooth can cause pain as soon as the PDL is initially compressed.
      (2) Typically, pain occurs within a few hours of the initiation of force application and lasts 2 to 4 days. The pain experienced after the application of heavy forces is due to the development of areas of ischemia or necrosis (hyalinization) in the PDL. These areas undergo remodeling, and the pain decreases until the next appliance activation.

      (3) The best way to decrease the pain during orthodontic tooth movement is to minimize the amount of force applied on the tooth.
      (4) Patients should be given acetaminophen (Tylenol) rather than aspirin or ibuprofen. Evidence indicates that the analgesic mechanism of action of acetaminophen does not completely overlap that of aspirin and ibuprofen. Acetaminophen may also have a more favorable adverse effect profile compared with aspirin and ibuprofen.
   c. Tissue inflammation.
      (1) Usually results from poor oral hygiene.
      (2) A less likely cause is an allergic reaction to latex or nickel. Nickel allergy occurs to some degree in about 20% of the general U.S. population, but its effects are not observed frequently in orthodontics. The onset of an allergic reaction primarily depends on the quality of the stainless steel used to fabricate the orthodontic appliances. Better quality stainless steel does not leak nickel in the oral environment.
   d. Effect on the pulp.
      (1) Symptoms ranging from mild pulpitis to loss of vitality are rare.
      (2) Loss of vitality is seen in teeth that have had a history of trauma or extensive restorations or in teeth that are moved with unusually heavy force or over long distances.
      (3) If the apex of a tooth is moved out of the alveolar bone, the blood supply can be potentially severed, and the tooth may lose vitality.
      (4) Teeth that have been successfully endodontically treated can be moved orthodontically without specific concerns. Endodontically treated teeth do not appear to be more prone to root resorption than vital teeth.
   e. Root resorption during orthodontic tooth movement.
      (1) Root resorption is a potential side effect of orthodontic therapy.
      (2) As the PDL experiences hyalinization in specific stress areas of compression, the adjacent cementum shows signs of resorption by clastic cells.
      (3) Heavy continuous forces have more potential to create root resorption than light forces.
      (4) The resorptive defect repairs, but its ability to do so is a function of its severity, size, and location on the root. Small defects repair easily to the initial contour of the root. Larger defects and specifically defects located at the apex do not repair to the contour of the tooth. In those cases, the length of the root is irreversibly reduced, and the root/crown ratio is modified.

(5) Occurrence and severity of root resorption are difficult to predict for a given individual. There are numerous risk factors for root resorption.

(a) Genetic factors—a patient with a family history of root resorption is more likely to experience it during orthodontic tooth movement. Susceptibility to root resorption seems to be of multifactorial polygenic inheritance.

(b) Heavier forces, certain types of tooth movement, and more movement of a tooth during treatment increase the potential for root resorption.

(c) Single-rooted teeth such as maxillary lateral incisors have a higher incidence of root resorption than multirooted teeth.

(d) Teeth subjected to trauma, bruxism, and heavy masticatory forces have a higher incidence of resorption.

(e) A tooth that had signs of root resorption before the initiation of treatment will likely to continue to resorb during orthodontic therapy.

(f) Movement of roots into the cortical plate of the bone.

(g) Asians are less at risk for root resorption than Hispanics or whites.

(6) Teeth with substantial root resorption but intact marginal peridontium do not experience any more mobility than unresorbed teeth. The longevity of teeth experiencing root resorption is not compromised as long as the supporting periodontium is healthy. The current standard of care for patients at risk for root resorption or presenting with root resorption at the onset of treatment includes the following.

(a) Use of light forces.

(b) Building periods of rest into treatment when wires are kept passive to allow for repair to occur.

(c) Taking periodic periapical radiographs to monitor the amount of resorption occurring.

(d) Detailed informed consent and good communication with the patient and parents and any referring providers.

C. Rapid acceleratory phenomenon.

1. It is possible to accelerate tooth movement by performing a surgical procedure involving tissue reflection and selective corticotomy cuts and perforations around teeth to be moved. Bone grafting is also often performed. This is followed by a period where tooth movement proceeds rapidly—termed the *rapid acceleratory phenomenon*.

1.7 Mechanical Principles in Tooth Movement

Physical laws of statics are applied to explain the force systems developed by orthodontic appliances. The biologic reaction to force systems results in orthodontic tooth movement.

A. Forces.

1. Forces are vectors and have direction and magnitude (e.g., a force directed mesially moves a tooth mesially).

2. Forces can act anywhere along their line of action (a pulling force is the same as a pushing force).

3. The point of force application also influences tooth movement.

4. A force acting through the center of resistance of a tooth can cause pure translation of the tooth in the direction of the force (Figure 5-11). Pure translation is movement of all points on the tooth in the same direction the same amount; there is no rotation. This is also called *bodily movement*.

5. For a free body floating in space, the center of resistance is coincident with the center of mass or gravity.

6. For a tooth, the location of the center of resistance depends on the size and shape of the tooth and the

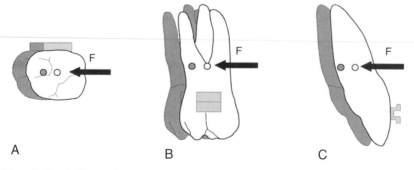

A   **B**   **C**

Figure 5-11 A-C, White circles indicate the center of resistance at the starting tooth position. Shaded circles show the center of resistance moved in the direction of the force. A force through the center of resistance causes all points of the tooth to move the same amount in the same direction. This type of movement is called *translation* or *bodily movement*. *(From Bishara SE:* Textbook of Orthodontics, *ed 3. Philadelphia, Saunders, 2001.)*

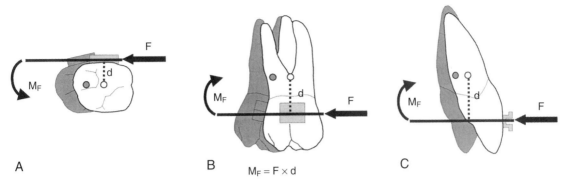

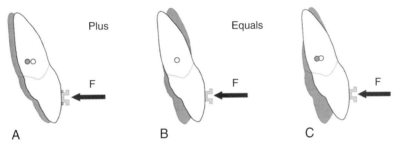

Figure 5-12 A-C, A force, applied at a bracket that does not act through the center of resistance, causes rotation of a tooth. This tendency to rotate is measured in moments and is called the *moment of the force (M$_F$)*. The magnitude of M$_F$ is measured as the magnitude of the force times the perpendicular distance from the line of force to the center of resistance (i.e., M$_F$ = F × d). Rotations are shown in the first **(A)**, second **(B)**, and third **(C)** order. *(From Bishara SE:* Textbook of Orthodontics, *ed 3. Philadelphia, Saunders, 2001.)*

Figure 5-13 A-C, Rotational movement caused by a force not acting through the center of resistance is best visualized as the simultaneous process of tooth translation. A, Moves the center of resistance in the direction of the force and tooth rotation. **B,** Around the center of resistance. **C,** The result is a combination of translation and rotation around the center of resistance. *(From Bishara SE:* Textbook of Orthodontics, *ed 3. Philadelphia, Saunders, 2001.)*

quality and level of the supporting structures (PDL and alveolar bone).

7. In a healthy tooth, the center of resistance is presumed to be about one half the distance from the alveolar crest to the root apex. This is about 10 mm from where an orthodontic bracket would be located on the crown of a tooth.

8. The center of resistance is more apical for a periodontally compromised tooth with loss of attachment.

B. Moments.
   1. A moment is defined as a tendency to rotate and may refer to rotation, tipping, or torque in orthodontics.
      a. Orders of tooth movement and rotation (Figure 5-12).
         (1) First order or rotation (in the occlusal view).
         (2) Second order or tipping (viewed from the buccal or lingual).
         (3) Third order or torque (viewed from the mesial or distal).
   2. If a force is applied at any point other than the center of resistance, in addition to moving the center of resistance in the direction of the force, a moment is created (Figure 5-13).

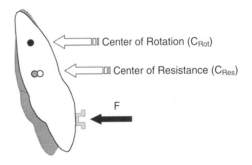

Figure 5-14 The center of rotation is an arbitrary point about which a body appears to have rotated as determined from its initial and final position. It is the result of the relative amounts of translation and rotation occurring during tooth movement. *(From Bishara SE:* Textbook of Orthodontics, *ed 3. Philadelphia, Saunders, 2001.)*

   3. The center of rotation is the mathematical point about which the tooth appears to have rotated after movement is complete (Figure 5-14).
   4. Increasing the magnitude of the force or applying the same force even farther from the center of resistance increases the tendency for rotation. The *magnitude of*

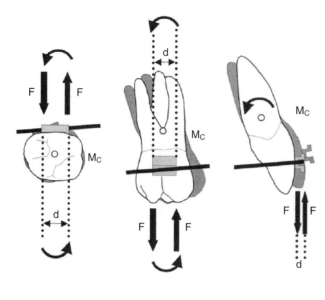

$$M_C = F \times d$$

Figure 5-15 Diagrammatic representation of couples in the first, second, and third order. The forces acting on the teeth are equal and opposite *(straight arrows)*. The rotational tendency *(curved arrows)* is called the *moment of the couple (M_c)*. The moment of the couple is measured as the magnitude of one of the forces *(F)* of the couple times the perpendicular distance between the two forces of the couple *(d)* (i.e., $M_C = F \times d$). *(From Bishara SE: Textbook of Orthodontics, ed 3. Philadelphia, Saunders, 2001.)*

a moment (M) is equal to the magnitude of the applied *force (F)* times the *distance (d)* of that force from the center of resistance (M = Fd).

C. Couples.
   1. A couple is two equal and opposite, noncollinear forces (Figure 5-15).
   2. A couple applied to a tooth produces pure rotation without translation.
   3. The tooth rotates about its center of resistance regardless of the point of application of the couple.
   4. The magnitude of the moment created by a couple depends on the force magnitude and distance between the forces (M = Fd).
   5. Couples are usually applied by engaging a wire in an edgewise bracket slot.
D. Equivalent force systems.
   1. Determining how a tooth will move can be calculated by expressing what the tooth will "feel" at the center of resistance secondary to force systems applied at the bracket. For example, a force at the bracket would cause the tooth to feel a force at the center of resistance plus a tendency to rotate, tip, or torque in the direction of the force.
E. Types of tooth movement.
   1. Pure rotation.
      a. When a couple is applied to a tooth, it rotates around its center of resistance.
      b. The center of rotation is at the center of resistance.
   2. Tipping (uncontrolled tipping).
      a. When a force is applied at the bracket, the center of resistance moves in the direction of the force, and the tooth crown tips in the direction of the force, whereas the apex moves in the opposite direction.
      b. The center of rotation is apical to the center of resistance.
      c. This is the easiest and fastest tooth movement to accomplish but often the least desirable.
   3. Crown movement (controlled tipping).
      a. A force is applied at the bracket; a small couple is also applied to partially negate the tipping of the crown caused by the force.
      b. The center of rotation is at the root apex.
      c. This is a slightly more difficult type of tooth movement and occurs more slowly.
   4. Pure translation (bodily movement).
      a. A force is applied at the bracket; a larger couple is also applied to exactly negate the tipping of the crown caused by the force.
      b. The center of rotation is so far apical to the tooth (at infinity) that the tooth translates without tipping.
      c. This is a difficult and slow type of tooth movement.
   5. Root movement.
      a. A force is applied at the bracket, and an even larger couple is applied to more than negate the tipping of the crown caused by the force. Only the root moves in the direction of the force.
      b. The center of rotation is at the crown of the tooth.
      c. This is the most difficult and slowest type of tooth movement.
F. Static equilibrium.
   1. All orthodontic appliances obey Newton's Third Law: for every action, there is an equal and opposite reaction.
   2. For each appliance, the sum of the forces and the sum of the moments acting on it sum to zero.
   3. It is impossible to design an appliance that defies this law of physics.
   4. Examples of types of appliances.
      a. Equal and opposite forces.
         (1) An elastic band or a coil spring stretched between two brackets produces equal and opposite forces (the sum of the forces equals zero).
      b. One-couple appliances.
         (1) Inserted into a bracket at one end and tied as a point contact at the other end.
         (2) A couple is produced only at the engaged end.
         (3) Equal and opposite forces (in a direction opposite to the couple at the engaged end)

are produced at the two attachment sites (Figure 5-16).

(4) The sum of the forces (equal and opposite) is zero. The sum of the moments (the couple created by the wire plus the oppositely directed couple produced by equal and opposite forces) is zero.

c. Two-couple appliances.

(1) Inserted into a bracket at both ends.

(2) Both a couple and a force are produced at each end.

(3) The magnitude of the couple is largest at the end closer to the bend in the wire (Figure 5-17) or at the bracket that is more severely angled in the case of a straight wire.

(4) The sum of the forces (equal and opposite) is zero. The sum of the moments (the couples created by the wire at each end plus the couple produced by the equal and opposite forces) is zero.

G. Anchorage—anchorage is defined as resistance to movement. Because forces applied to teeth are distributed along the root surface to activate cells in the PDL, the anchorage value of any tooth is roughly equivalent to its root surface area.

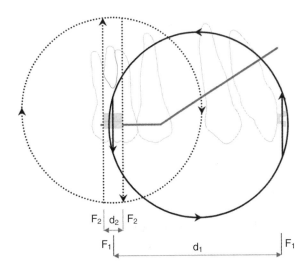

Figure 5-16 Equilibrium in a one-couple system. The first circle *(solid)* shows a passive intrusion arch. It is activated by tying it down anteriorly at the level of the bracket. This causes an intrusive force at the incisor and an extrusive force at the molar. This circle shows the direction of the couple associated with this extrusive and intrusive force. The second circle *(dotted)* shows a second couple at the molar bracket *(M_C)* that is equal and opposite in the direction to the first couple. *(From Bishara SE: Textbook of Orthodontics, ed 3. Philadelphia, Saunders, 2001.)*

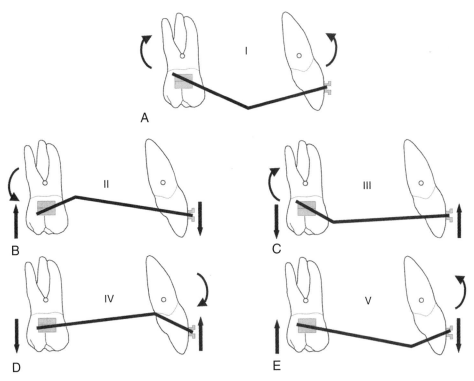

Figure 5-17 V bend couple. **A,** A centered V bend, which produces an equal and opposite couple and equal and opposite equilibrium forces that cancel each other out. **B-E,** The tooth with the greater M_C (greater angle of entry) and direction of rotation is shown with curved arrows. The associated equilibrium forces are shown with straight arrows. *(From Bishara SE:* Textbook of Orthodontics, *ed 3. Philadelphia, Saunders, 2001.)*

1. *Reciprocal tooth movement*—two equal anchorage value teeth or groups of teeth (units) are moved against each other and move the same amount toward or away from each other.

2. *Reinforced anchorage*—adding additional teeth to a unit to distribute the force over a greater area and slowing the movement of the anchor unit. Another method for reinforcing anchorage would be extraoral force, such as with headgear, with interarch elastics, or by using an implant (see later).

3. *Stationary anchorage*—the term *stationary* is used, although it is not an accurate name. Teeth meant to be the anchor are activated to undergo difficult, slow movements, such as bodily movement (translation) or root movement, which distribute forces dispersed over large areas of the PDL, whereas the reactive units undergo tipping, which occurs faster and more easily as a result of concentrated forces in the PDL.

4. *Cortical anchorage*—anchor teeth roots are moved into cortical bone, which resorbs more slowly than medullary bone. This is a controversial concept because root resorption would likely be increased as roots are forced into cortical bone.

5. *Implants for anchorage*—implants, including palatal implants, miniscrews or temporary anchorage devices, and bone plates, can serve as absolute anchorage for holding or moving teeth. A stable implant does not move because it has no PDL.

1.8 Orthodontic Materials

Orthodontic tooth movement is achieved by the forces that are exerted on the tooth by an archwire via brackets during orthodontic treatment. The forces transmitted to a tooth depend on the physical and mechanical properties of the wires used and the relationship between the brackets in which the wire is engaged. The faciolingual and occlusogingival dimensions of the edgewise bracket slot allow the use of wires with different cross-sectional shapes and sizes. The two bracket slot sizes most commonly used are 0.018 inch × 0.025 inch and 0.022 inch × 0.028 inch. The magnitude of the forces generated in the faciolingual and occlusogingival direction is partly dependent on the bracket slot size.

A. Wire material properties.

1. Stress-strain relationship—the mechanical behavior of a ductile orthodontic wire (e.g., stainless steel) in tensile loading may be analyzed in a force-deflection or stress-strain plot (Figures 5-18 and 5-19). *Stress (σ)* is the internal response of a wire to the application of external forces defined as *force (load) (F)* per *cross-sectional area (A)* ($\sigma = F/A$). *Strain (ε)* is the deformation or deflection of the archwire as a consequence of the stress and is defined as the *dimensional change (Δd)* divided by the *original dimension (d)* ($\varepsilon = \Delta d/d$).

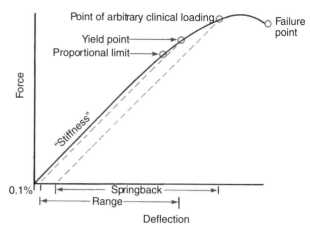

Figure 5-18 Typical force-deflection curve for an elastic material such as an orthodontic archwire. The stiffness of the material is given by the slope of the linear portion of the curve. The range is the distance along the x-axis to the point at which permanent deformation occurs (usually taken as the yield point, at which 0.1% permanent deformation has occurred). Clinically useful springback occurs if the wire is deflected beyond the yield point (as to the point indicated here as "arbitrary clinical loading"), but it no longer returns to its original shape. At the failure point, the wire breaks. *(From Proffit WR, Fields HW, Sarver DM: Contemporary Orthodontics, ed 5. St. Louis, Mosby, 2013.)*

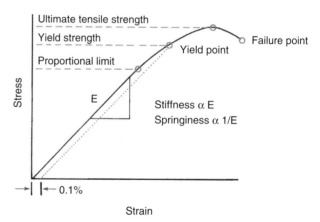

Figure 5-19 Stress and strain are internal characteristics that can be calculated from measurements of force and deflection, so the general shapes of force-deflection and stress-strain curves are similar. Three different points on a stress-strain diagram can be taken as representing the strength. The slope of the stress-strain curve, *E*, is the modulus of elasticity, to which stiffness and springiness are proportional. *(From Proffit WR, Fields HW, Sarver DM: Contemporary Orthodontics, ed 5. St. Louis, Mosby, 2013.)*

2. Ideal characteristics—an ideal orthodontic wire should have the following properties: high strength, low stiffness, high working range, and high formability. These important characteristics of wires depend on the alloy composition, the crystal structure of the metal, and the manufacturing process.

3. Wire properties—each of the major elastic properties (strength, stiffness, and range) is affected by a change

in the length and cross section of a wire (see Figure 5-18). Doubling the length of a wire decreases its strength by half, makes it eight times less stiff (or eight times springier), and gives it four times the range. Similarly, when the diameter of a wire is doubled, it becomes 8 times stronger and 16 times stiffer, and its working range is decreased by half.

4. Wire selection—for large orthodontic movements (usually during initial stages of orthodontic treatment), wires with a low load/deflection rate are desirable because they are able to provide constant low forces as the tooth moves and the appliance is deactivated. However, for minimal tooth movements such as in maximum anchorage extraction cases or during finishing, a high load/deflection rate is desirable. Several factors influence the load/deflection rate of an appliance.
   a. *Wire material*—the load/deflection rate is proportional to the modulus of elasticity of the material. Stainless steel exhibits the highest modulus of elasticity. The most flexible wire (wire with the lowest load/deflection rate) is made of a nickel titanium alloy.
   b. *Wire cross section*—the load/deflection rate varies directly with the fourth power of the diameter of a round wire and with the third power of the width of a rectangular wire.
   c. *Wire length*—the load/deflection rate varies inversely with the third power of the length of a wire segment. Increasing the interbracket distance by incorporating loops or helices into the archwire decreases the load/deflection rate.

B. Orthodontic archwire materials.
   1. Nickel-titanium—these wires offer two very important characteristics: a very low modulus of elasticity and an extremely wide working range.
   2. Beta titanium—these wires are frequently known as TMA (titanium-molybdenum alloy) wires. They have an intermediate modulus of elasticity (approximately half that of stainless steel and twice that of nickel titanium). They exhibit excellent resilience, which provides a wide working range. One drawback of these wires is their high coefficient of friction. They have high formability, which allows the clinician to bend the wires and incorporate stops or loops into them if desired. They can also be spot-welded.
   3. Stainless steel—stainless steel wires remain popular because of their good mechanical properties, excellent corrosion resistance, and low cost. The typical composition of stainless steel alloys used in orthodontics is 18% chromium and 8% nickel ("18-8"). Chromium gives this wire its corrosion resistance. When compared with nickel-titanium and beta titanium archwires, these wires exhibit the highest elastic modulus (stiffness) and lowest springback. They can be soldered and welded.

1.9 Orthodontic Appliances

A. Fixed appliances.

In modern orthodontic treatment, the straightwire (preadjusted edgewise) systems are the commercially available appliances most commonly used. In the original, standard edgewise appliance, the orientation of the bracket slot was at right angles to the long axis of the tooth, and the thickness of the bracket base was the same for all teeth. During treatment, bends were placed to position each tooth individually in the buccolingual direction (in-out, first-order bends), to provide proper angulation in the mesiodistal direction (second-order bends) and in the buccolingual direction (torquing or third-order bends). In the straightwire appliance system, this information is incorporated into the brackets for each individual tooth, eliminating or reducing the need for first-order, second-order, and third-order bends. These built-in adjustments (the "bracket prescription") in the bracket slots help to achieve the proper position of each individual tooth.

1. Preadjusted edgewise appliances (brackets with prescriptions) allow the following.
   a. *Rotational control*—by twin bracket wings or by the incorporation of rotational arms in a single-wing bracket system.
   b. *Horizontal control*—by varying the relative thickness of the bracket base for teeth of different thickness.
   c. *Mesiodistal tip control*—the slot of the bracket is angulated relative to the base of the bracket to provide the proper tipping movement for each tooth.
   d. *Torque*—the slot is angulated labiolingually to provide the proper root and crown movements.
      (1) Brackets.
         (a) *Metal brackets*—these brackets are made of stainless steel. Their disadvantage is the unesthetic appearance of the metal color.
         (b) *Ceramic brackets*—these brackets are made of monocrystalline or polycrystalline ceramics. Although highly esthetic, these brackets are prone to fracture during torsional and tipping activations. They exhibit increased frictional resistance to sliding mechanics. They may cause abrasion of opposing teeth.
         (c) *Self-ligating brackets*—a locking mechanism is incorporated into these bracket systems to hold the archwire in the slot. This mechanism eliminates the need for a ligature placement. It is purported that these systems shorten treatment time by reducing friction and because the wire is efficiently kept engaged in the bracket slot; however, these claims are controversial and generally unsubstantiated scientifically.

(2) Bands—in contemporary orthodontic treatment, all of the teeth (including molars) may be bonded. However, banding the molar teeth is preferred by many clinicians. Before banding, separators are placed between the teeth to create enough space to allow band fitting and subsequent cementation. Elastomeric or metal separators may be used.

(3) Bonding—brackets are attached to the enamel surfaces using bonding resins. Direct bonding is the direct attachment of orthodontic appliances to the etched teeth using either chemically cured or light-cured adhesives. Indirect bonding techniques involve first positioning the brackets on study casts with a water-soluble adhesive and then transferring them to the mouth with a custom tray for bonding to the teeth. The principal mechanism of attachment between the tooth surface and resin-bonding systems is the mechanical interlocking of the bonding agent onto the etched enamel.

(a) Bonding procedure.

(i) *Enamel prophylaxis with pumice*—this procedure removes the pellicle and enhances the wettability of the enamel surface for subsequent acid application.

(ii) *Enamel etching*—the most commonly used enamel etching agent is 37% phosphoric acid. Conventional acid-etching (two-step) creates a microporous enamel surface that increases the retention of the resin. The enamel surface is then conditioned with an application of a primer.

1. Self-etching primers (one-step) combine the conditioning and priming steps into a single treatment step. The advantage of self-etching primers is the reduced clinical chair time.

(iii) *Bracket positioning*—each bracket is placed in a position relative to teeth in the same arch to ensure proper relationships between the teeth at the completion of treatment. If a light-cured type of composite resin is used, once the bracket is positioned, the adhesive is cured using a light source such as halogen, plasma, or light-emitting diode (LED).

B. Appliances to modify the growth of the maxilla and the mandible—these appliances allow differential growth of the jaws. During adolescence, the mandible has more potential for growth than the maxilla. Whether an extraoral force (headgear) or a functional appliance is used to modify growth in class II patients, differential mandibular growth is expected with restraint of the maxilla. Growth modification is most successful in preadolescent children with good compliance and growth potential.

1. Headgear—headgear is used to modify growth of the maxilla, to distalize (retract) or protract maxillary teeth, or to reinforce anchorage. There are different types of headgear that can be used to achieve a desired effect. The type of headgear and desired force levels should be selected according to the specific treatment objectives for a patient. Headgear should be worn preferably 12 to 14 hours per day to achieve the goals. For orthopedic changes, a force level of 250*g* to 500*g* per side is recommended; for dental movements, 100*g* to 200*g* per side should be used. The success of headgear treatment depends on patient compliance.

a. *High-pull headgear*—commonly used in the treatment of preadolescent patients with class II malocclusions and increased vertical dimension, minimal overbite, and increased gingival exposure on smile. It consists of a high-pull headstrap and a standard facebow inserting into the headgear tubes of the maxillary first permanent molar attachments. The objectives are restriction of anterior and downward maxillary growth and molar distal movement, intrusion, and control of maxillary molar eruption.

b. *Cervical-pull headgear*—used to correct class II malocclusions with deep bite. It consists of a cervical neckstrap and a standard facebow inserting into the headgear tubes of the maxillary first permanent molar attachments. The objectives are to restrict anterior growth of the maxilla and to distalize and erupt maxillary molars. Because of the direction of the line of force, this appliance produces an extrusive and distal force on the maxillary first molars.

c. *J-hook headgear*—consists of a high-pull headstrap that attaches to two hooks on the anterior part of the maxillary archwire. This J-hook design delivers intrusive and posteriorly directed extraoral forces to the anterior maxilla. However, it is generally used to retract canines and incisors, rather than for orthopedic purposes.

d. *Protraction headgear (reverse-pull, facemask)*—used in patients with class III malocclusions where there is a maxillary deficiency. It is adjustable and consists of two pads that rest on the soft tissue in the forehead and chin region that are connected by a midline framework. A metal bar with hooks connected to the framework allows attachment of elastics to exert a downward and forward pull on the maxilla.

e. *Chin cup (chin cap)*—used to correct class III malocclusions (resulting from excessive mandibular growth) in young children by restraining or redirecting mandibular growth. It consists of a head-strap and a cup that fits on the patient's chin to exert superior and posterior forces that usually also cause opening rotation of the mandible.

2. Functional appliances—functional appliances hold the mandible in a protrusive position and transmit the forces created by the resulting stretch of the muscles and soft tissues to the dental and skeletal components to produce movement of teeth and modification of growth, most commonly to achieve correction of a class II malocclusion. Because most functional appliances are removable, patient compliance plays a major role in their success. Whether fixed or removable, these appliances restrain the maxilla and displace the mandible, while allowing the normal amount of mandibular growth potential to express itself.

   a. Herbst appliance—a fixed (or sometimes removable) functional appliance that consists of a piston and tube device that places the mandible in a forward position as the patient closes the mouth. It is usually cemented or bonded to the maxillary and mandibular dental arches. There is a tendency for the mandibular incisors to procline (flare) because of the forces that are indirectly delivered to these teeth.

   b. Activator—this was the first removable functional appliance developed. The name "activator" was given because of the belief that mandibular growth was activated to correct class II malocclusions. This term is generically used today to describe any functional appliance that is used for this purpose. It consists of an acrylic body that covers part of the palate and the lingual aspect of the mandibular alveolar ridge. A labial bow fits anterior to the maxillary incisors. On the acrylic adjacent to the maxillary posterior teeth, facets are cut to allow occlusal, distal, and buccal movement of these teeth. On the lingual aspect of the mandibular posterior teeth, facets allow occlusal and mesial movement. In addition to their effects on the growth of the mandible, these appliances can tip anterior teeth and control eruption of teeth in the vertical dimension.

   c. Bionator—this removable appliance is less bulky than the activator. It consists of lingual, horseshoe-shaped acrylic with a wire in the palatal area. Facets are introduced into the acrylic to guide the maxillary and mandibular posterior teeth and hold the mandible forward in a postured relationship. A labial bow is present anterior to the maxillary incisors, extending distally, to eliminate the pressure from the buccal musculature.

   d. Twin block appliance—this removable or cemented appliance has a two-part design. The interaction between the maxillary and mandibular parts controls how much the mandible is postured forward and how much the maxilla and mandible are separated in the vertical dimension. This appliance is supposedly more easily tolerated by patients because of its two-part design.

   e. Mandibular anterior repositioning appliance (MARA; Allesee Orthodontic Appliances, Sturtevant, Wisconsin)—consists of oversized stainless steel crowns on the maxillary and mandibular molars, elbows that insert into the tubes on the maxillary crowns, and arms that protrude from the mandibular crowns. Because of the design of the appliance, the lower arms interfere when the patient attempts to bite down, forcing the mandible to reposition forward into a class I relationship; this results in anterior force to the mandibular arch and posterior force to the maxillary arch.

C. Noncompliant appliances to correct class II malocclusions—because compliance is a major concern when treating class II malocclusions, fixed appliances not requiring patient cooperation have been developed. Their use is generally indicated in patients with full or cusp-to-cusp ("end-on") molar/canine relationships, mild to moderate crowding (0 to 6 mm), and a profile or other characteristics that do not support an extraction treatment plan.

   1. Pendulum appliance—the cemented appliance consists of an acrylic body to use the palate as anchorage with wire extensions to the maxillary premolars. Two springs extending from the posterior portion of the appliance are inserted into lingual molar attachments and are activated to distalize the molar teeth. If expansion of the maxilla is also needed, an expansion screw may be incorporated into the acrylic body in the midpalatal region. In this case, the appliance is called a Pendex.

   2. Forsus Fatigue Resistant Device (3M Unitek Orthodontic Products, Monrovia, California)—consists of bypass rod, push rod, ball pin, and stainless steel spring module (force module) for each side. This interarch force delivery system has been shown to be efficient in treating class II malocclusions with minimal compliance and breakage problems. It delivers forward, downward force to the anterior mandibular arch and backward, upward force to the posterior maxillary arch.

D. Aligners—clear, removable aligners, such as Invisalign (Align Technology, San Jose, California), can be used to align teeth. A series of trays are manufactured according to a prescription developed by the provider to be worn by the patient. Additional attachments are usually required to aid in specific tooth movements and for aligner retention. Control of tooth movement is not as precise as with fixed appliances. Patient cooperation is required for wearing the trays full-time.

E. Appliances to correct posterior crossbites—maxillary or palatal expansion appliances are used to correct transverse discrepancies by skeletal expansion of the maxilla or by dental expansion. If expansion is carried out at a rate of about 0.5 mm/day, it is called rapid palatal expansion/rapid maxillary expansion. Slow expansion is carried out at a much slower rate of 1 mm/week.

1. *Hyrax appliance (banded type)*—for skeletal expansion, this is the most commonly used type of rapid palatal expansion/rapid maxillary expansion appliance. It consists of a metal framework with an expansion screw. Bands are cemented on the maxillary first premolars and molars that are connected to the expansion screw by rigid wires. The screw is activated by at least 0.25 mm (one quarter turn) daily and may produce force levels of 100 N. The maxillary arch width is increased by opening the midpalatal suture. Expansion is usually continued until the lingual cusps of the maxillary posterior teeth come into contact with the lingual inclines of the buccal cusps of the mandibular posterior teeth. A diastema usually appears between the central incisors as the midpalatal suture separates. In a few weeks, this space closes spontaneously as a result of the pull of the supracrestal fibers. When active expansion is completed, retention for 3 to 6 months is recommended with the appliance in place. The result is a combination of skeletal and dental expansion. However, it is widely believed that the skeletal component is more significant than the dental component (minimal dental tipping).

2. *Haas appliance*—for skeletal expansion, this appliance consists of bands that are cemented on maxillary first premolars and first molars. Two acrylic pads with a midline jackscrew are connected to the rest of the appliance. The acrylic pads are in contact with the palatal mucosa. It is believed that contact with the palate allows forces from the appliance to be applied directly to the underlying hard and soft tissues, minimizing the amount of dental tipping and maximizing the skeletal effect. However, difficulty in maintaining hygiene and possible inflammation of the palate are considered disadvantages by some clinicians.

3. *Hawley-type removable appliance with a jackscrew*—for skeletal or dental expansion, this appliance may be used to correct mild posterior crossbites in children and young adolescents. Compliance and difficulty retaining the appliance in the mouth are potential disadvantages.

4. *Quad-helix* and *W-arch*—generally for dental expansion, these appliances consist of heavy stainless steel wire with four (quad-helix) or three (W-arch) helices that are incorporated to increase the range and flexibility. They may be fixed or removable. They may be used for symmetrical or asymmetrical expansion of the maxillary dental arch and for correcting rotated molars. Because of the tendency to cause buccal tipping of teeth, they are suggested for use in cases where only a small amount of expansion is needed or in young children for skeletal expansion before the sutures are well developed.

5. *Transpalatal arch*—for dental movement, this appliance consists of heavy wire that extends from one maxillary first molar along the contour of the palate to the maxillary first molar on the opposite side. The arch is adapted to the contour of the palate approximately 2 to 3 mm away from the tissue. This appliance is very versatile because it may be used for expansion or constriction of the intermolar width, for producing root movement of the first molars, for derotation of these teeth, and for anchorage reinforcement.

F. Appliances used in the mixed dentition.

1. *Nance appliance*—used as a space maintainer or for anchorage purposes. It has a heavy wire soldered to the palatal aspect of the maxillary first permanent molars and connected to an acrylic button located in the most superior and anterior part of the palatal vault.

2. *Lower lingual arch*—made of heavy orthodontic wire adapted to the lingual aspect of the mandibular incisors. It may be fixed or removable. Two "U" loops in the wire mesial to the first molars make it possible to adjust this appliance. The lingual arch may be used for anchorage reinforcement, as a holding arch for space maintenance, for expansion, and for increasing dental arch length.

3. *Lip bumper*—consists of a heavy wire inserted into the buccal tubes on the mandibular first permanent molars. The anterior portion lies about 2 to 3 mm away from the alveolar process and the mandibular incisors and usually carries a plastic or acrylic pad. It is used to control or increase the mandibular dental arch length, to upright mesially or lingually tipped mandibular molars, and to prevent the interposition of the lower lip between the maxillary and mandibular incisors. By removing the pressure of the buccal musculature on the teeth, it allows lateral and anterior dentoalveolar development. By transmitting the force from the lip to the mandibular first molars, it causes distal movement and tipping of the mandibular first molars.

G. Appliances used to control vertical incisor position.

1. *Intrusion arch*—this is an archwire used for deep bite correction in which extrusion at the molars and intrusion at the incisors takes place. This archwire is activated for incisor intrusion by placing tip-back bends mesial to the molar tubes.

2. *Extrusion arch*—this is an archwire used for open bite correction in which intrusion at the molars and extrusion at the incisors takes place.

H. Elastics—elastomeric bands are used to produce forces for tooth movement. There are different types of elastics based on their purpose, location, and orientation.

1. *Class I elastics (intramaxillary elastics)*—used for traction between teeth and groups of teeth within the same arch. During canine retraction, they may be used to facilitate sliding mechanics.

2. *Class II elastics (intermaxillary elastics)*—worn from a tooth located in the anterior part of the maxilla (usually from the maxillary permanent canine) to a tooth located in the posterior part of the mandible (usually to the mandibular permanent first molar). They are used to correct class II malocclusion, to reduce overbite by extruding the molar, to retract anterior maxillary teeth, and to minimize anchorage loss in the maxilla during maxillary incisor retraction.

3. *Class III elastics (intermaxillary elastics)*—worn from a tooth located in the posterior part of the maxilla (usually from the maxillary permanent first molar) to a tooth located in the anterior part of the mandible (usually to the mandibular permanent canine). They are used to aid in protraction of the maxillary posterior teeth, to improve the overjet in an edge-to-edge or anterior crossbite relationship, and to make use of intermaxillary anchorage during mandibular incisor retraction.

4. *Crossbite elastics*—these are worn from the palatal of one or more maxillary teeth to the buccal of one or more teeth in the mandible to help correct crossbites. In addition to the desired forces, they cause extrusion of the teeth and should be used with caution in patients with an open bite tendency and a long lower anterior facial height.

5. *Anterior diagonal elastics (midline elastics)*—these elastics are run from one side of the maxillary teeth to the other side of the mandibular teeth crossing the midline. They are used in the correction of noncoinciding maxillary and mandibular dental midlines.

1.10 Early Treatment

Early treatment is designed to alleviate or prevent moderately severe orthodontic problems or potential problems before the permanent dentition is completely erupted. Often, further comprehensive treatment is indicated when the permanent dentition has erupted, unless the problem is very minor and localized. Setting goals is very important in early treatment. The endpoint should be well defined to avoid lengthy treatment that extends into the permanent dentition. Retention is needed until the permanent teeth erupt, and such devices may interfere with eruption or lose retention as primary teeth exfoliate.

A. Crowded and irregular teeth—caused by lack of adequate space for alignment or interferences with normal eruption.

1. Space maintenance (in cases where primary teeth have been lost and space is otherwise adequate).
   a. Band and loop.
   b. Distal shoe (before eruption of a permanent molar).
   c. Lingual arch.
   d. Nance appliance (maxillary arch).

2. Space regaining (localized space loss)—indicated when space loss is minor (<3 mm).
   a. Removable appliance with finger springs to tip teeth distally.
   b. Headgear (for the maxillary arch).
   c. Activated lingual arch (for the mandibular arch).
   d. Lip bumper (for the mandibular arch).
   e. Limited fixed appliances.
      (1) Followed by placement of a space maintainer after space is regained.

3. Moderate crowding (<4 mm).
   a. Arch expansion (this is a controversial topic).
   b. Extraction of primary canines.
      (1) Borrows space until permanent teeth erupt.
      (2) Lingual arch necessary if mandibular primary canines are extracted because the permanent incisors will upright lingually and space will be lost.
   c. Flaring of incisors.
      (1) Fixed appliances.
      (2) Removable appliances.

4. Severe crowding (>4 mm).
   a. Arch expansion (this is a controversial topic).
   b. Serial extraction.
      (1) Timed extraction of primary and ultimately permanent teeth.
      (2) Usually reserved for large space discrepancies (>10 mm per arch).
      (3) Sequence of extractions.
         (a) Extraction of primary incisors, if necessary.
         (b) Extraction of primary canines to allow permanent incisors to erupt and align.
         (c) Extraction of primary first molars to encourage eruption of the permanent first premolar (ideally, before the permanent canine erupts).
         (d) Extraction of permanent first premolars to allow the permanent canine to erupt and align.
      (4) Increased overbite usually results as the incisors tip lingually into any excess space.
      (5) Comprehensive treatment is almost always required later to achieve ideal alignment, root positioning, ideal overbite, and closure of excess space.

B. Anterior spacing.
   1. Maxillary midline diastema less than 2 mm.
      a. Commonly present and self-correcting.
      b. "Ugly duckling" stage.

c. Large space may indicate supernumerary tooth or mesiodens or missing lateral incisors.

d. Treatment may be indicated if there is an esthetic concern or central incisors are inhibiting eruption of lateral incisors or canines.

2. Large maxillary midline diastema greater than 2 mm.

a. Not likely to close spontaneously.

b. Fixed appliances may be indicated.

c. Frenectomy after treatment if space reopens persistently or bunching of tissue is unresolved after space is closed.

3. Generalized spacing.

a. Postpone treatment unless there is an esthetic complaint.

b. If spacing of anterior teeth is accompanied by protrusion, fixed appliances are usually required to achieve bodily movement.

C. Eruption problems.

1. Overretained primary teeth.

a. Remove primary tooth to encourage eruption of permanent tooth.

2. Ankylosed primary teeth.

a. Usually resorb on their own.

b. Remove if they cause a delay in permanent tooth eruption or if permanent tooth eruption path is deflected.

c. If the successor is missing, an ankylosed primary tooth should be removed to decrease chances of a vertical alveolar defect.

3. *Ectopic eruption*—eruption of a tooth into an unexpected location or into an adjacent tooth.

a. Lateral incisors.

(1) May cause loss of adjacent primary canine.

(2) Usually indicates lack of sufficient space.

(3) If unilateral, may cause midline shift.

(4) Treat by extracting primary canines or space regaining.

b. Maxillary first molars.

(1) May erupt into second primary molar.

(2) Upright erupting molar.

c. Maxillary canines.

(1) May lead to canine impaction.

(2) May resorb adjacent lateral incisor.

(3) Extraction of primary canine is indicated.

D. Missing teeth—most commonly missing permanent teeth (excluding third molars).

1. Mandibular second premolars.

a. Maintaining primary second molars may be an option.

b. Some reduction in width of the primary second molars may be necessary to attain good posterior interdigitation.

c. Early extraction of primary second molars (at age 7 to 9) may be attempted to encourage closure of the space, but this is unpredictable, and later orthodontic treatment is likely to be needed.

2. Maxillary lateral incisors.

a. Substituting canine in lateral position is an option.

b. Retaining space for later replacement is an option.

c. The best choice may depend on occlusion and esthetic demands.

E. Occlusal relationship problems.

1. Posterior crossbites.

a. Unilateral crossbites are usually due to a mandibular shift.

b. If causing a shift, treatment should be initiated.

(1) Equilibration to eliminate shift.

(2) Maxillary expansion using fixed or removable appliance.

2. Anterior crossbites.

a. Differentiate skeletal from dental causes.

b. Skeletal may be due to deficient maxillary or excessive mandibular growth.

c. Dental is usually due to inadequate space. After space is created, the teeth can be moved forward with fixed or removable appliances with or without extraction of adjacent primary teeth.

3. Maxillary dental protrusion with spacing.

a. May be due to skeletal discrepancy.

b. May be due to finger or thumb sucking.

c. Treatment is indicated if esthetically objectionable or in danger of trauma.

d. A removable appliance can be used to upright teeth.

4. Deep bites.

a. Biteplates can be used to open the bite posteriorly and allow eruption of posterior teeth in patients with short lower face heights.

b. In patients requiring overbite correction by intrusion, this should be deferred until later comprehensive treatment because of inability to retain in the mixed dentition.

5. Oral habits and open bites.

a. Pacifiers and finger sucking may cause increased overjet, decreased overbite, and posterior crossbite.

b. If the habit stops before eruption of permanent incisors, most of the negative changes resolve spontaneously.

c. Most important is convincing a child that he or she wants to stop; otherwise, any treatment is likely to fail.

d. Any reminder is helpful—bandage on finger, habit appliance.

e. Reward system.

f. If an appliance is used, it should remain in place for about 6 months after the habit appears to have ceased.

g. Open bites that persist after the habit has ceased are likely to have a skeletal component and may need more complex treatment.

1.11 Growth Modification

Treatment of Skeletal Problems in Preadolescents

Timing of Growth Modification

Successful growth modification can occur only during periods of growth. Early modification often requires retreatment because unfavorable growth continues. Waiting until the permanent dentition erupts may be too late to modify growth, especially in girls (because they stop growing earlier than boys).

A. Treatment of mandibular deficiency (class II).
  1. Theoretically, headgear restrains maxillary growth forward, whereas functional appliances stimulate mandibular growth, but the distinction is less clear in practice.
  2. Timing should be when the mandible is growing actively, before peak adolescent growth.
  3. Functional appliances.
    a. Often accelerate or redirect mandibular growth, but a long-term increase in size does not seem to occur.
    b. Also put a restraining force on maxillary growth.
    c. Move the mandibular teeth anteriorly and the maxillary teeth posteriorly.
  4. Headgear.
    a. Puts a restraining force on maxillary growth and allows the mandible to grow normally to catch up.
    b. Puts posterior forces only on maxillary teeth, usually the first molars.
B. Treatment of vertical deficiency (short face).
  1. Cervical headgear has an extrusive force on the maxillary molar, which erupts.

2. Functional appliances allow eruption of upper and lower posterior teeth.
C. Treatment of vertical excess (long face).
  1. High-pull headgear to the molars inhibits eruption of maxillary posterior teeth.
  2. Functional appliance with bite blocks to block posterior eruption.
D. Treatment of maxillary deficiency.
  1. Transverse deficiency can be treated with expansion.
  2. Anterior-posterior deficiency (class III) can be treated with a facemask (protraction headgear, reverse-pull headgear) (Figure 5-20).
    a. Anterior force is placed on the maxilla.
    b. Encourages growth at the maxillary sutures.
    c. Often used after rapid expansion to disrupt the sutures.
    d. Ideal timing is earlier (8- to 9-year-olds) to encourage maxillary growth (because the maxilla grows earlier than the mandible).
E. Treatment of mandibular excess.
  1. Chin cup or chin cap therapy to restrain mandibular growth.
    a. Generally redirects mandibular growth downward rather than deterring growth.
    b. Contraindicated in long-face individuals.
F. Treatment of facial asymmetry.
  1. Facial asymmetry may be due to a congenital anomaly or an early condylar fracture.
  2. Asymmetrical functional appliances may be helpful.
  3. Early surgery may be indicated when asymmetry is progressively worsening.

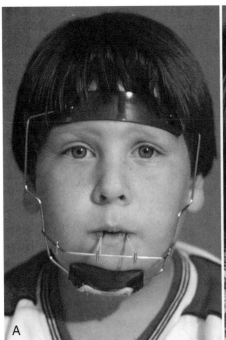 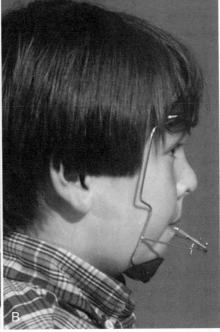

Figure 5-20 Delaire-type facemask. A, The facemask contacts the forehead and chin for anchorage and should be adjusted several millimeters away from the other soft tissues. **B,** Adjustment of the wire framework produces desired fit and direction of pull on the maxilla (usually downward for increased vertical facial development and patient comfort) when the elastics are placed from the mask to the splint. *(From Proffit WR, Fields HW, Sarver DM: Contemporary Orthodontics, ed 5. St. Louis, Mosby, 2013.)*

1.12 Comprehensive Treatment

A complete set of fixed appliances can be used when all permanent teeth have erupted.

A. Extraction versus nonextraction decisions.
   1. The need for extractions (usually first premolars) is usually dictated by the amount of crowding present. When space is needed, the arches can be expanded and anterior teeth flared forward but only to a limited degree because teeth require bony support. Expanding too much may be unstable and leave teeth in a periodontally compromised position. The alternative is creating space by extracting teeth.
   2. Another indication for extraction may be to camouflage a class II or class III malocclusion by extracting premolars in one arch only to achieve class I canines and a normal overjet and overbite. Upper premolars would be extracted to camouflage a class II; lower premolars would be extracted to camouflage a class III.
   3. There may be esthetic considerations to remove or not remove teeth because anterior tooth position affects lip fullness.
   4. Removing premolars and uprighting incisors generally increases overbite, whereas aligning moderately crowded teeth without extractions flares incisors and decreases overbite.
   5. Often the decision is not clear-cut, and various indications and contraindications should be considered.
   6. Indications for extraction.
      a. Large amount of dental crowding (arch length deficiency).
      b. Minimal overbite or open bite present.
      c. Flared incisors.
      d. Full (procumbent or protrusive) lips.
      e. Acute nasolabial angle.
      f. Anterior recession or minimal or thin attached gingiva.
      g. Camouflage of class II or class III relationship.
      h. Other missing or severely compromised teeth.
      i. Asymmetrical occlusion (unilateral class II or class III).
   7. Indications to avoid extraction.
      a. Minimal crowding or spacing present.
      b. Deep overbite.
      c. Upright incisors.
      d. Flat (recessive) lips.
      e. Obtuse nasolabial angle.

B. Stages of comprehensive treatment.
   1. Alignment—generally with light, flexible wires at first, followed by slightly stiffer wires.
   2. Overbite correction (leveling)—achieving overbite correction is necessary before molar correction and space closure because a deep overbite would prevent retraction (posterior movement) of the incisors to a normal overjet.

   a. Extrusion of posterior teeth may be favorable for patients with short lower face heights but is contraindicated in patients with long faces.
   b. Intrusion of anterior teeth, maxillary or mandibular depending on facial esthetics.
   c. Flaring of anterior teeth, especially in nonextraction treatment, may also decrease overbite.
   3. Correction of molar relationship.
      a. Growth modification.
      b. Interarch elastics.
      c. Distal movement of upper molars.
   4. Space closure.
      a. If molars have been moved to achieve a class I relationship or if teeth have been extracted, space closure is necessary.
      b. Depending on the amount of space that must be closed in each arch, the anchorage requirements may vary in each arch.
      c. Interarch elastics, extraoral force (headgear), or use of temporary anchorage devices may help in maintaining anchorage during space closure.
   5. Root correction.
      a. Especially when spaces have been closed, the teeth may have tipped into the extraction space, and roots need to be paralleled to improve stability and periodontal health.
      b. The incisors may have uprighted during retraction, and the roots may need to be torqued lingually.
   6. Detailing and finishing.
      a. *Intraarch*—final tooth positioning by rebracketing misbracketed teeth or by small bends in the wire to eliminate small discrepancies in all three dimensions: rotations, vertical relationships, and torque.
      b. *Interarch*—settling of the occlusion into a solid relationship can be accomplished using light wires or vertical elastics or by having the patient wear a positioner (a rubber or plastic appliance made with teeth reset into ideal position).
   7. Special considerations.
      a. *Tooth size discrepancies (Bolton discrepancy)*—smaller or larger teeth in one arch than the other can affect intercuspation and overjet present. Large teeth (most often mandibular second premolars) may require interproximal reduction (IPR) to reduce width. Small teeth (most often maxillary lateral incisors) may require buildups to fill space, or the discrepancy can be masked by IPR of lower incisors. Small discrepancies may be masked by tipping or torquing teeth to take up more space.
      b. *Unfavorable growth*—patients with anticipated unfavorable growth patterns, class II or class III, may be continued on headgear at night (e.g., to control further growth).

c. *Overtreatment*—anticipated rebound of anterior-posterior discrepancies (class II or III), crossbites, or rotations may be overcorrected in treatment in anticipation that they will rebound afterward to some degree.

d. *Supracrestal fiberotomy*—supracrestal gingival fibers exert some elastic force that may move teeth after treatment, especially rotations. Cutting these fibers has been shown to reduce significantly, but not fully eliminate, this tendency.

1.13 Retention

A. Purpose of retention.
1. Allow time for reorganization of the gingival and periodontal fibers.
   a. Significant reorganization of the PDL occurs in 3 to 4 months, and full-time retention is recommended for that time.
   b. Part-time retention after 4 months to about 12 months is recommended to allow more complete reorganization of the PDL. Long-term retention is often recommended.
2. Prevent soft tissue pressures from altering posttreatment tooth position.
3. Hold the new position of teeth until growth is completed.
   a. *Retention after class II correction*—relapse may occur, especially in patients who have worn class II elastics in treatment. There may also be unfavorable growth, and patients can wear a headgear or functional appliance on a limited basis.
   b. *Retention after class III treatment*—relapse may occur, especially because of continued mandibular growth.
   c. *Retention after overbite correction*—a retainer with acrylic lingual to the upper incisors usually blocks deepening of the bite.
   d. *Retention after open bite correction*—continuation of a finger-sucking habit (or a tongue thrust, although this is controversial) may intrude incisors or cause separation of posterior teeth, allowing them to erupt. In the absence of an obvious cause, open bite relapse usually occurs because of posterior tooth eruption rather than intrusion of incisors.
   e. *Retention after lower incisor alignment*—with or without growth, pressure from the lip may cause crowding of the lower incisors. There is little evidence that pressure from third molars causes incisor crowding. Late mandibular growth is a possible contributor to incisor crowding, even in patients who did not have orthodontic treatment.
   f. *Permanent retention* may be needed if the teeth have been placed in inherently unstable positions. Long-term retention is often recommended regardless.

B. Removable retainers.
1. Hawley retainer.
   a. Incorporates clasps for retention and an outer bow with adjustment loops.
   b. Acrylic on the palate can act as a potential biteplate to control overbite.
   c. The outer bow retains incisor position and rotations.
   d. Clasps or wires that cross the occlusion may wedge space open or prevent closure of spaces that remain or develop.
2. Wraparound retainer.
   a. Similar to a Hawley retainer but without wires that cross the occlusion.
3. Positioner.
   a. May be used as a finishing device and then as a retainer.
   b. Bulky and may not be tolerated well.
   c. Maintains interarch and intraarch relationships.
C. Fixed retainers.
1. Bonded flexible lingual wires attached to individual teeth or bonded rigid wires usually bonded to two teeth, especially between lower canines.
2. Maintain lower incisor position.
3. Hold diastema closed.
4. Maintain space for a pontic or implant.
5. Keep extraction spaces closed.
D. Active retainers.
1. For realignment of irregular teeth.
2. Irregular teeth are reset on a model, and the retainer is made to the new setup.
3. The retainer needs to have some flexibility to fit over the irregular teeth.
4. IPR may be required to allow space for teeth to rotate.

1.14 Adult Treatment and Interdisciplinary Treatment

Adult orthodontic treatment for the most part is identical to treatment of children with some differences.

A. *Psychological considerations*—usually self-motivated compared with children, whose motivation is often their parents'. Adults are generally more compliant and perform better oral hygiene. Appearance of the appliances may be a concern, and adults are more likely to request ceramic, lingual, or invisible braces (aligners).
1. *Periodontal improvement*—motivation may include a need to improve tooth positions for periodontal concerns.
2. *Restorative*—motivation may be to achieve a desired restoration or replacement of missing teeth.
3. *TMJ*—patients may be referred for orthodontic treatment to improve TMJ dysfunction. This is a highly controversial topic; orthodontic treatment is not considered a primary method for treating TMJ problems.

B. Periodontal aspects of adult treatment.
1. Any periodontal conditions should be stabilized before beginning orthodontic treatment.
2. Good oral hygiene must be maintained because gingivitis in adults may progress to periodontal disease; this is rarely the case in children.
3. Level and condition of attached gingiva must be monitored to prevent recession.
4. Patients with a history of periodontal disease must be monitored and be on a frequent maintenance schedule (every 2 to 4 months).
5. Steel ligatures retain less plaque than elastomeric ligatures.
6. Lower forces can be used on teeth with reduced support because the PDL area is reduced.
7. Closure of old extraction sites may be difficult because of remodeling and narrowing of the alveolar bone.
8. *Proper sequence for interdisciplinary treatment*—disease control (caries, periodontal disease); orthodontic tooth movement; definitive treatment (periodontal bone recontouring, final restorations such as crowns, bridges, implant restorations).

C. Lack of growth.
1. Because adults do not have the benefit of mandibular growth during treatment, all interarch corrections must be accomplished dentally or with surgery.
2. Without growth to supplement dental changes, overall treatment may proceed more slowly, although the tooth movement itself may proceed at the same rate.

1.15 Combined Surgical and Orthodontic Treatment

A. Indications—surgery is indicated when a problem is too severe for orthodontics alone (Figure 5-21). Growth modification in growing patients may allow some corrections that cannot be achieved in adults. Other considerations include functional limitations and esthetic goals, which may be indications for surgery even if orthodontic correction alone is possible.
B. Surgical procedures—any one or a combination of maxillary and mandibular procedures can be performed to correct a malocclusion and achieve good skeletal functional relationships with improved esthetics.
1. Anterior-posterior corrections.
a. Maxillary surgery.
(1) *Advancement (to correct a class III)*—Le Fort I downfracture of the maxilla mobilizes it so that it may be advanced.
(2) *Setback (to correct a class II)*—it is difficult or impossible to move the entire maxilla posteriorly; if desired, a premolar is usually extracted, and the anterior segment is moved posteriorly (segmental osteotomy).

b. Mandibular surgery.
(1) *Advancement (to correct a class II)*—bilateral sagittal split osteotomy (BSSO) of the ramus is the most preferred procedure. Paresthesia is a common side effect, usually disappearing in 2 to 6 months, but 20% to 25% of patients continue to have long-term alterations in sensation.
(2) *Setback (to correct a class III)*—BSSO can also be used to move the mandible posteriorly. Airway reduction leading to possible sleep apnea may limit use of mandibular setback procedures, so class III correction is often done by advancing the maxilla instead.
2. Vertical corrections.
a. Maxillary surgery.
(1) *Superior repositioning (to correct an open bite)*—Le Fort I is used to move the maxilla superiorly, allowing the mandible to autorotate closed to correct an open bite and shorten the face.
(2) *Inferior repositioning (to correct a deep bite)*—Positioning the maxilla downward would rotate the mandible open to reduce overbite and lengthen the face. This is one of the least stable surgical procedures.
b. Mandibular surgery.
(1) Surgical procedures in the mandible to rotate it closed (to correct an open bite) are not recommended because they cause downward rotation at the gonial angle and stretch the muscles of the pterygomandibular sling, causing instability.
(2) Anterior and downward rotation of the mandible (to correct a deep bite) can be accomplished with BSSO for patients with a deep bite and short lower face (tripoding).
3. Transverse corrections—for correction of crossbites, the maxilla can be expanded or constricted during a Le Fort I procedure. Changes in mandibular width are more difficult.
a. *Maxillary expansion*—can be accomplished surgically with positioning of the lateral segments in ideal position or as a surgically assisted rapid expansion where surgical cuts are made to free up the lateral segments. Expansion proceeds with a jackscrew device, as in adolescents.
b. *Maxillary constriction*—can be accomplished surgically with bone removed to allow for constriction of the lateral segments.
4. Genioplasty—the chin can be augmented to improve esthetic outcome using an osteotomy or by adding implant material. The sliding osteotomy is the preferred method and can be used to move the chin in all three dimensions. Reduction is generally the least predictable for esthetic changes.

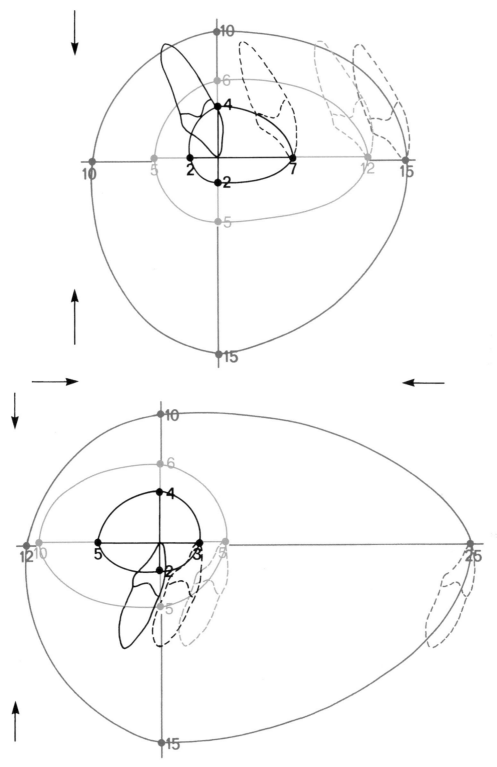

Figure 5-21 With the ideal position of the upper and lower incisors shown by the origin of the x-axis and y-axis, the envelope of discrepancy shows the amount of change that could be produced by orthodontic tooth movement alone (the inner envelope of each diagram), orthodontic tooth movement combined with growth modification (the middle envelope), and orthognathic surgery (the outer envelope). The possibilities for each treatment are not symmetrical with regard to the planes of space. There is more potential to retract than procline teeth and more potential for extrusion than intrusion. Because growth of the maxilla cannot be modified independently of the mandible, the growth modification envelope for the two jaws is the same. Surgery to move the lower jaw back has more potential than surgery to advance it. *(From Proffit WR, Fields HW, Sarver DM:* Contemporary Orthodontics, *ed 5. St. Louis, Mosby, 2013.)*

C. Timing of surgery.
1. Surgery is rarely performed before the adolescent growth spurt except in cases with significant psychological impact of a facial deformity. In those cases, the expectation is that the procedure may need to be redone later.
2. In cases with growth excess, such as a class III with excessive mandibular growth, surgery should be delayed until growth is complete. Otherwise, the mandible may continue to grow, and the class III relationship will return.
3. In cases with growth deficiency, such as a class II with a small mandible, surgery can be considered earlier.
4. Exceptions where early surgery is indicated include cases with congenital growth deficiencies or cases where growth is restricted because of mandibular ankylosis. In these cases, correction is required because progressive worsening of the growth deficiency occurs without it.
D. Sequencing of combined surgical-orthodontic treatment.
1. *Pretreatment considerations*—disease control and, especially, good gingival health and adequate attachment should be established before treatment begins. Unerupted or impacted third molars usually need to be removed well in advance (6 to ≥9 months) of surgery to allow good bone healing in the area.
2. Orthodontics is performed to align the teeth within each arch and remove compensations in the dentition that may mask the underlying skeletal discrepancy. For example, in class III patients, the lower incisors are often upright and the upper incisors are flared, giving the appearance of a minimal anterior crossbite. By flaring the lower incisors and uprighting the upper incisors, the crossbite is made more severe, allowing a more significant movement of the jaws to correct the discrepancy. Before surgery, models are taken to ensure that the occlusion will fit when surgery is performed.
3. Surgery is performed with the orthodontic appliances on. Rigid wires to stabilize the teeth are present in the appliances. The jaws are repositioned according to the planned correction and are held in place using rigid internal fixation or (rarely) intermaxillary wire fixation. A soft diet is required for 6 to 8 weeks after surgery.
4. The patient returns to continue orthodontics usually for about 6 months to detail the occlusion and finish.
5. Surgery first—this is a concept that encourages surgery earlier in the combined orthodontic-surgical treatment sequence to correct skeletal relationships early and take advantage of the rapid tooth movement (rapid acceleratory phenomenon) that occurs immediately after surgical intervention.

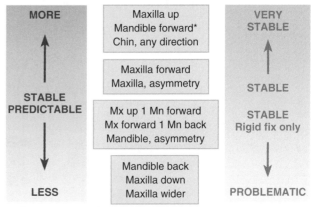

Figure 5-22 Hierarchy of stability. In this context, "very stable" means a greater than 90% chance of no significant postsurgical change; "stable" means a greater than 80% chance of no change, and major relapse is quite unlikely; "problematic" means some degree of relapse is more likely, and major relapse is possible. *(From Proffit WR, Fields HW, Sarver DM:* Contemporary Orthodontics, *ed 5. St. Louis, Mosby, 2013.)*

E. Maximizing skeletal movements.
1. In surgery to correct a class II occlusion, extraction of mandibular premolars with closure of that space would increase the overjet presurgically and allow a greater surgical movement of the jaws to correct the class II. This would be recommended for a patient needing maximal esthetic change, usually to bring the lower jaw forward.
2. In surgery to correct a class III occlusion, if maximizing skeletal movement were the goal to achieve desired esthetics, upper premolars might be extracted to make the anterior crossbite more severe presurgically.
F. Stability of orthognathic surgical procedures (Figure 5-22).

2.0 Pediatric Dentistry

Mark Taylor

Because pediatric dentistry is multidisciplinary in nature, this review encompasses a wide range of dentistry. However, pediatric dentistry is not the same as dentistry for adults. Children present the practitioner with a set of challenges, treatment decisions, and treatment that can be quite different from that of adults.

Given that pediatric dentistry involves all disciplines, it is impossible in a format of this kind to cover all topics. The intent of this section is to prepare the candidate for the National Board Dental Examination; it is not meant to be an all-inclusive review of pediatric dentistry. For more in-depth review, *McDonald and Avery's Dentistry for Children and Adolescents*, ed 9, by Dean, Avery, and McDonald, and *Pediatric Dentistry, Infancy Through Adolescence*, ed 5, by Casamassimo, Fields, McTigue, and Nowak, are excellent sources (see References).

Outline of Review

2.1 Development and Developmental Disturbances of the Teeth
2.2 Management of Child Behavior in the Dental Setting
2.3 Local Anesthesia and Nitrous Oxide Sedation for Children
2.4 Restorative Dentistry for Children
2.5 Pulp Treatment for Primary Teeth
2.6 Space Management in the Developing Dentition
2.7 Periodontal Problems in Children
2.8 Dental Trauma in Children
2.9 Miscellaneous Topics in Pediatric Dentistry

2.1 Development and Developmental Disturbances of the Teeth

Development of the Tooth

A. Initiation (bud stage).
  1. Week 6 of embryonic life.
  2. All primary teeth and permanent molars arise from the dental lamina.
  3. Permanent incisors, canines, and premolars arise from the primary predecessor.
  4. Failure of initiation results in congenitally missing teeth.
  5. Excessive budding results in supernumerary teeth (Figure 5-23).
B. Proliferation (cap stage).
  1. Peripheral cells of the cap form the inner and outer enamel epithelium.
  2. Failure in proliferation results in congenitally missing teeth.
  3. Excessive proliferation results in a cyst, odontoma, or supernumerary tooth, depending on amount of cell differentiation.
C. Histodifferentiation and morphodifferentiation (bell stage).
  1. Cells of dental papilla differentiate into odontoblasts.
  2. Cells of the inner enamel epithelium differentiate into ameloblasts.
  3. Failure in histodifferentiation results in structural abnormalities of the enamel and dentin (amelogenesis imperfecta, dentinogenesis imperfecta).
  4. Failure in morphodifferentiation results in size and shape abnormalities, such as peg lateral incisors and macrodontia (Figure 5-24).
D. Apposition.
  1. Ameloblasts and odontoblasts deposit a layerlike matrix.
  2. Disturbances in apposition result in incomplete tissue formation. For example, an intrusive injury to

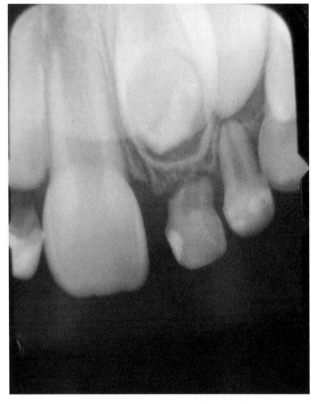

Figure 5-23 Supernumerary tooth obstructing eruption.

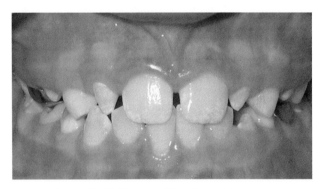

Figure 5-24 Peg maxillary lateral incisors.

a primary incisor may disrupt enamel apposition and result in an area of enamel hypoplasia.
E. Calcification.
  1. Enamel is composed of 96% inorganic material and 4% organic material and water.
  2. Calcification begins at cusp tips and incisal edges and proceeds cervically.
  3. Localized infection, trauma, and excessive systemic fluoride ingestion may cause hypocalcification.

Calcification and Eruption of the Dentition

A. Table 5-2 shows the approximate time calcification begins for primary teeth. The sequence of calcification of primary teeth is *A-D-B-C-E*, and all primary teeth begin calcification in utero.

Table 5-2

Approximate Calcification Start Times for Primary Teeth

TOOTH	CALCIFICATION
Central incisor (A)	14 weeks in utero
First molar (D)	15 weeks in utero
Lateral incisor (B)	16 weeks in utero
Canine (C)	17 weeks in utero
Second molar (E)	18 weeks in utero

Table 5-3

Eruption Times for Primary Teeth

	MAXILLA	MANDIBLE
Central incisor	10 months	8 months
Lateral incisor	11 months	13 months
Canine	19 months	20 months
First premolar	16 months	16 months
Second premolar	29 months	27 months

Table 5-4

Calcification Start Times for Permanent Teeth

	MAXILLA	MANDIBLE
First molar	Birth	Birth
Central incisor	3-4 months	3-4 months
Lateral incisor	10-12 months	3-4 months
Canine	4-5 months	4-5 months
First premolar	1.5 years	1.75 years
Second premolar	2 years	2.25 years
Second molar	2.5 years	2.75 years

Table 5-5

Approximate Calcification Start Times for Permanent Teeth

TIME	TEETH THAT BEGIN TO CALCIFY
Birth	First molars
6 months	Anterior teeth except maxillary laterals
12 months	Maxillary laterals
18 months	First premolars
24 months	Second premolars
30 months	Second molars

Table 5-6

Eruption Times (Years) of Permanent Teeth

TOOTH	MAXILLA	MANDIBLE
1	7-8	6-7
2	8-9	7-8
3	11-12	9-10
4	10-11	10-12
5	10-12	11-12
6	6-7	6-7
7	12-13	11-13
8	17-21	17-21

B. Eruption of primary teeth.
   1. Table 5-3 shows the approximate eruption times for primary teeth.
   2. Sequence is A-B-D-C-E.
   3. Teeth B, C, and D tend to erupt earlier in the maxilla.
   4. A 6-month variation in time of eruption is considered normal.
C. Calcification of permanent teeth.
   1. It is important to know the calcification times of permanent teeth because if the practitioner sees a pattern of hypoplasia or hypocalcification of the permanent teeth, the approximate timing of the cause can be determined. This information can aid the dentist in counseling parents in regard to anticipated enamel defects.
   2. Table 5-4 shows the average times at which calcification begins for permanent teeth.
   3. Because this table can be difficult to memorize, it is helpful to remember that a different group of teeth begin calcification every 6 months; this is only an approximation but is easier to remember (Table 5-5).
   4. Eruption of permanent teeth.
      a. Average eruption times are listed in Table 5-6.
      b. Eruption begins when the crown has completed calcification.
      c. Average numbers to know for eruption of teeth.
         (1) Typically, it takes 4 to 5 years for most crowns to complete formation except for first molars (3 years) and cuspids (6 years). This knowledge is important in determining the timing of enamel hypoplasia secondary to a systemic disturbance.
         (2) It takes approximately 10 years from start of calcification to root completion except for canines (13 years).
         (3) Teeth typically erupt through the bone with two thirds root formation.
         (4) Teeth typically erupt through the gingiva with three fourths root formation.
         (5) Interval between crown calcification and full interdigitation is about 5 years.

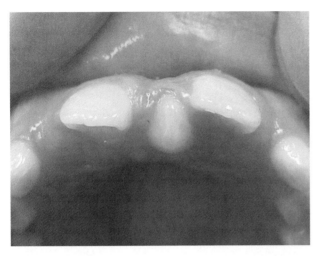

Figure 5-25 Rudimentary supernumerary, conical form.

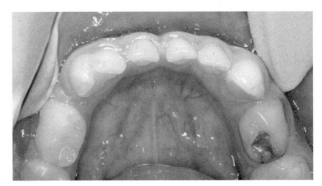

Figure 5-26 Fusion of primary lateral incisor and primary canine. There are nine discrete tooth entities.

(6) Eruption to root completion is approximately 3 years.

d. Sequence 6-1-2-4-5-3-7 is most common in the maxilla.

e. Sequence 6-1-2-3-4-5-7 is most common in the mandible.

Developmental Disturbances of the Teeth

A. Anomalies of number.

1. Supernumerary teeth (Figure 5-25).
   a. Male-to-female ratio is 2:1.
   b. Affect 3% of population.
   c. Most common supernumerary teeth are mesiodens, most of which are palatal.
   d. Classified as supplemental (has typical anatomy) or rudimentary (are conical, tuberculate, or molar-shaped).
   e. Supernumerary teeth may block normal eruption of permanent teeth. In such cases, consideration should be given to early removal to prevent impaction of the permanent teeth.

2. Congenital absence (hypodontia).
   a. Incidence 1.5% to 10%, excluding third molars.
   b. Most common congenitally missing tooth is the mandibular second premolar, followed by the lateral incisor, followed by the maxillary second premolar.
   c. Treatment options with congenital absence.
      (1) Congenital absence of premolar is commonly treated orthodontically if the patient would have normally required extraction treatment. In these cases, all spaces are closed. If the patient has excellent occlusion, normal overbite and overjet, and minimal or no crowding, the congenital absence may be treated prosthetically.
      (2) Congenital absence of lateral incisor may be treated by placing the canine in the lateral incisor position and then performing restorative lateralization of the permanent canines. Alternatively, the canines may be placed in their normal position and the lateral incisors replaced prosthetically.

B. Anomalies of size.

1. Microdontia and macrodontia.
   a. Microdontia is seen in ectodermal dysplasia, chondroectodermal dysplasia, hemifacial microsomia, and Down syndrome. Another example of microdontia is a "pegged" lateral incisor.
   b. Macrodontia is seen in facial hemihypertrophy and otodental syndrome.

2. Fusion (Figure 5-26).
   a. Fusion is the union of two primary or permanent teeth.
   b. More common in primary teeth.
   c. Fused teeth have two pulp chambers and two pulp canals.
   d. Almost always in anterior teeth.
   e. In addition to examining the root structure, the key to determining fusion is to count erupted teeth. Because fusion ordinarily occurs between two teeth, there is one less discrete tooth entity than normal. In other words, in a primary dentition, children have 10 discrete tooth entities per arch; in a patient with fusion, there are only 9 discrete tooth entities.

3. Gemination (Figure 5-27).
   a. Gemination is the division of a single tooth bud, resulting in a bifid crown.
   b. More common in primary teeth.
   c. Geminated teeth have a single pulp chamber.
      (1) Because gemination occurs on a single tooth, there is the normal complement of tooth masses.

C. Anomalies of shape.

1. Dens evaginatus.
   a. An extra cusp.
   b. Called talon cusps in incisors (Figure 5-28).
   c. Has enamel, dentin, and pulp; care must be taken with any operative procedure.

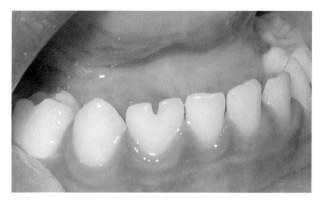

Figure 5-27 Gemination of a primary mandibular lateral incisor. This patient has the appropriate number of discrete tooth entities. There are three other primary incisors and a discrete primary canine present.

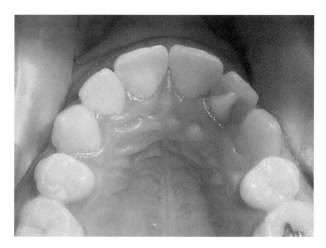

Figure 5-28 Talon cusp, lateral incisor.

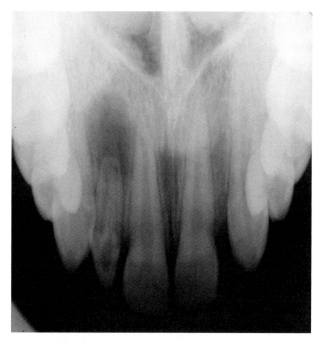

Figure 5-29 Dens in dente in a permanent peg lateral incisor. Also note the congenitally absent contralateral lateral incisor.

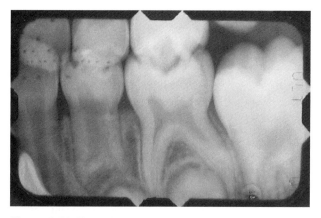

Figure 5-30 Taurodontism in the mandibular first primary molar.

2. Dens invaginatus (dens in dente) (Figure 5-29).
   a. Caused by invagination of the inner enamel epithelium.
   b. Has been termed "tooth within a tooth."
   c. Most common in permanent maxillary lateral incisors.
   d. If enamel and dentin are not formed correctly within the defect, a direct communication from the oral environment with pulp tissue can occur.
   e. Ideal treatment is preventive; a small restoration or sealant may be placed to prevent pulpal involvement.
3. Taurodontism (Figure 5-30).
   a. Characterized by vertically long pulp chambers and short roots.
   b. May be clinically significant if pulp therapy is required or during the exfoliation process.
4. Dilaceration.
   a. A dilacerated, or bent or twisted tooth, usually occurs as the result of an intrusive or displacement injury to a primary incisor. Because permanent

anterior teeth develop lingual to the primary predecessor, injuries to the anterior primary teeth may also displace or bend the developing permanent tooth.
   b. Dilaceration is also a consistent finding in congenital ichthyosis.
D. Anomalies of structure.
   1. Enamel hypoplasia.
      a. Hypoplasia refers to quantity deficiencies of enamel.
      b. May be due to environmental or genetic factors.
         (1) Environmental.
            (a) Systemic diseases, especially fevers, may cause disruption in the developmental process of the tooth.

(b) Fluorosis—occurs with excessive ingested fluoride.

(c) Nutritional deficiencies, particularly vitamins A, C, and D; calcium; and phosphorus.

(d) Neurologic defects, such as Sturge-Weber syndrome and cerebral palsy.

(e) Cleft lip and palate, radiotherapy and chemotherapy, nephrotic syndrome, lead poisoning, and rubella embryopathy all have been linked to hypoplasia.

(f) Local infection, trauma.

(2) Genetic—amelogenesis imperfecta (see "Amelogenesis imperfecta" further on).

2. Enamel hypocalcification.

a. Hypocalcification refers to quality deficiencies of enamel.

b. May be due to environmental or genetic factors.

(1) Environmental factors are the same as for hypoplasia.

(2) Genetic amelogenesis imperfecta, hypocalcified type—normal thickness of enamel but is poorly calcified and fractures easily.

3. Amelogenesis imperfecta.

a. Incidence of approximately 1 in 14,000.

b. The defect is related to the enamel only and is dependent on the developmental stage of the enamel.

c. Normal pulpal and root morphology.

d. Treatment depends on type and severity. Severe cases, especially in terms of quality of enamel, require full-coverage restorations. Veneers may be appropriate in some hypomaturation and hypoplastic types.

4. Dentinogenesis imperfecta.

a. Incidence approximately 1 in 8000.

b. Occurs during histodifferentiation stage.

c. Predentin matrix is defective resulting in amorphic, atubular dentin.

d. Primary and permanent teeth affected.

e. Teeth are reddish brown to gray opalescent color.

f. Roots are slender.

g. Pulp chambers and canals appear small or absent.

h. Enamel chips away easily.

i. Teeth can become severely abraded.

j. Treatment may include full-coverage crowns to prevent severe abrasion. Bonded veneers on anterior teeth have proven successful in some cases that are less severe.

5. Dentin dysplasia.

a. Primary and permanent teeth affected.

b. Types.

(1) Shields type 1.

(a) Normal crown anatomy.

(b) Color is closer to normal than in dentinogenesis imperfecta.

(c) Short, pointed roots.

(d) Absent pulp chambers and canals, primary and permanent teeth.

(e) Multiple periapical radiolucencies, primary and permanent teeth.

(2) Shields type 2.

(a) Primary teeth appear similar to dentinogenesis imperfecta.

(b) Permanent teeth have normal color, pulp stones, thistle tube–shaped pulp chambers with no periapical radiolucencies.

6. Other conditions affecting dentin.

a. Regional odontodysplasia.

b. Vitamin D–resistant rickets.

c. Hypoparathyroidism.

d. Pseudohypoparathyroidism.

2.2 Management of Child Behavior in the Dental Setting

A. Classification of behavior.

1. Cooperative.

a. Children with minimal apprehension and are communicative, comprehending, and willing.

b. These children respond well to behavior shaping.

2. Lacking cooperative ability.

a. Children who are deficient in comprehension or communication skills or both.

b. Examples are very young children (typically <3 years old) and children with certain disabilities.

3. Potentially cooperative.

a. Children who are capable of appropriate behaviors but are disruptive in the dental environment.

b. Types of potentially cooperative patients.

(1) Uncontrolled.

(a) Typically 3 to 6 years old.

(b) Characterized by a tantrum.

(2) Defiant.

(a) Can be all ages.

(b) Characterized by an "I don't want to" attitude in young children.

(c) Characterized by passive resistance in adolescents.

(3) Timid.

(a) Typically preschool and younger grade school–age children.

(b) Characterized by shielding behavior and hesitating behaviors. For example, children with shielding behavior may stand behind a parent in the reception area or may keep their hands close to their face and mouth.

(c) Timid children may deteriorate into uncontrolled behaviors, especially in the absence of proficient management techniques.

(4) Tense-cooperative.

(a) Typically older children (at least 7 years old).

(b) These children want to cooperate with the dentist and try to behave in an adult manner but are very nervous. These patients have also been termed "white knuckler" patients because they grip the arms of the dental chair so tightly.

(5) Whining.

(a) Whining behavior is usually continuous.

(b) Typically there is an absence of tears.

(c) This behavior is difficult to overcome in one dental visit.

B. Frankl behavioral rating scale.

1. Common behavioral scale used in pediatric dentistry.

2. Ratings.

a. Rating 1—definitely negative refusal of treatment; forceful crying, fearfulness, or any other overt evidence of extreme negativism.

b. Rating 2—negative reluctance to accept treatment; uncooperativeness; some evidence of negative attitude but not pronounced (sullen, withdrawn).

c. Rating 3—positive acceptance of treatment; cautious behavior at times; willingness to comply with the dentist, at times with reservation, but patient follows the dentist's directions cooperatively.

d. Rating 4—definitely positive good rapport with the dentist; interest in the dental procedures; laughter and enjoyment.

C. Variables influencing children's behavior in the dental environment.

1. Age.

a. Less than 2 years old—these children are typically lacking in cooperative ability.

b. 2 years old.

(1) There is a wide variance in ability to communicate in 2-year-olds.

(2) The dentist should use communication techniques such as Tell-Show-Do (TSD) because the child may have adequate communication skills and may be cooperative with a normal explanatory, friendly approach.

(3) It can be helpful to have the parent present because the 2-year-old may be unable to overcome anxiety resulting from separation from the parent.

c. 3 to 7 years old.

(1) Children in this age range are most often cooperative and willing to comply with dental procedures.

(2) Proper familiarization techniques and behavior-shaping strategies are valuable tools to influence children's behaviors positively in this age group.

d. 8 years old and older.

(1) As children get older, they normally try to control their apprehensions and anxieties to the best of their ability.

(2) If procedures prove to be stressful to these children, they may revert to undesirable behaviors.

(3) Proper familiarization techniques and behavior-shaping strategies are valuable tools to influence children's behaviors positively in this age group.

2. Maternal anxiety.

a. There is a high correlation between maternal anxiety and a child's negative behavior in the dental office.

b. This effect is greatest on children less than 4 years of age.

3. Past medical history.

a. Children who have had positive medical experiences are more likely to have positive dental experiences.

b. Children who have experienced pain during previous medical visits are more likely to exhibit negative behavior in the dental setting.

c. Previous surgery is correlated with negative behavior at a first visit.

4. Patient awareness of problems.

a. If a child thinks he or she has a dental problem, the child is more likely to exhibit negative behavior.

D. Functional inquiry.

1. Two goals of a functional inquiry.

a. Learn patient and parent concerns.

b. Estimate of cooperative ability.

2. Two methods.

a. Written questionnaire.

b. Direct interview.

3. Functional inquiry sample questions.

a. Reaction to past medical experiences?

b. Parental anxiety level?

c. Is the patient worried about the condition of his or her teeth?

d. How do you think the patient will react to an examination?

4. *Functional inquiry review of medical history*—these are questions on the medical history that can help the practitioner understand a child's potential behavior.

a. Attention-deficit/hyperactivity disorder (ADHD).

b. Learning disability.

c. Mental health disorder.

d. Drug or alcohol abuse.

e. Is this the child's first visit to the dentist? Is the child extremely nervous about dentistry?

f. Any difficult visits to a physician or hospital?

g. Child's hobbies or sports.

h. Parent or legal guardian comments.

i. Review patient's medications.

(1) Gives clues to potential behavior.

(2) Review adverse reactions; may alter behavior.

E. Behavior management techniques and strategies.
   1. Goal of treatment strategies.
      a. Perform quality dental care for the patient.
      b. Promote a positive patient attitude and confidence in self in the dental environment.
   2. Strategies before the appointment.
      a. Brochure or discussion with parent.
      b. DVD/video presentation.
      c. Brochures, DVDs, information on the office website.
      d. Modeling with siblings or parents.
   3. Behavior shaping.
      a. Definition—a procedure that slowly develops behavior by reinforcing successive approximations to a desired goal. For example, if the goal is to have a child patient open his or her mouth very wide, the dentist positively reinforces each effort on the part of the patient to open wide. If a child is asked to open his mouth for examination of the teeth and the child complies, but to a very limited degree, the dentist should give the child positive reinforcement. This response from the dentist is likely to cause the patient to open wider, which is followed again by positive reinforcement.
      b. Reinforcement of desired behavior may be verbal or nonverbal. Nonverbal reinforcement may consist of a pat on the shoulder, a smile, or a wink. Nonverbal reinforcers can be very effective.
      c. Reinforcement should be immediate and specific to the desirable behavior. Nonspecific reinforcement such as "You are a good boy" does not help shape the desired behaviors and becomes boring and meaningless to the patient after several times.
      d. TSD technique.
         (1) This is a behavioral management technique in which the dentist explains a procedure or a part of a procedure to the child patient using age-appropriate terminology (Tell), familiarizes the patient with the instruments and procedures by gentle demonstration (Show), then performs the procedure (Do).
         (2) Indications.
            (a) *Cooperative children*—these children should be introduced to dental procedures using TSD to maintain cooperative behavior.
            (b) *Children who are lacking cooperative ability*—some patients who initially may not seem to have cooperative ability may understand more than what an initial assessment reveals.
            (c) *Timid, tense-cooperative, and whining children*—familiarization with the various procedures can help children with initial anxieties to relax.
            (d) *Uncontrolled or defiant children*—when patients in these categories begin to listen and communicate, it is crucial for the practitioner to familiarize them with the various procedures.
   4. Aversive conditioning.
      a. *Definition*—a psychological strategy that uses some form of negative stimulus with the purpose of extinguishing or improving negative behavior.
      b. Purpose.
         (1) Establish better communication.
         (2) Gain control of behavior.
         (3) Protect the child from injury.
         (4) Eventually make the dental experience a pleasant one.
      c. Indications.
         (1) Normal children who are momentarily uncontrolled or defiant.
         (2) Usually 3 years old or older.
      d. Contraindications.
         (1) Patients who lack cooperative ability.
         (2) Younger than 3 years old.
         (3) Timid children.
         (4) Tense-cooperative children.
      e. Historically, aversive conditioning has been applied in various forms. A disapproving look may be construed as aversive conditioning. A method termed *voice control*, in which the dentist speaks to the child in firm tones, is considered a higher level of aversive conditioning. Hand-over-mouth exercise (HOME) is a technique in which the dentist places fingers or a hand over the patient's mouth in an effort to gain the attention of an uncontrolled patient.
         (1) Most pediatric dentistry graduate programs do not teach HOME as an acceptable behavior management technique.
         (2) Aversive conditioning should always be followed by positive reinforcement or praise for improved behaviors.
         (3) All pediatric dentistry programs teach that appropriate pharmacologic techniques (nitrous oxide, conscious sedation, general anesthesia) are acceptable.
         (4) Communication with parents before and after aversive conditioning is a necessity.
         (5) Using aversive conditioning can expose the dentist to liability. If the practitioner chooses to use aversive conditioning, informed parental consent should be obtained.
   5. Miscellaneous.
      a. *Appointment length*—studies are conflicting regarding the effect of appointment length on children's behavior in the dental environment.
      b. *Appointment time*—some dentists believe that morning appointments are better for preschool children because the patient is rested. However,

other dentists hold that children may be less active in the afternoon and more manageable. One study demonstrated no difference between morning and afternoon appointments.

c. There are two common methods for checking for cavities or trauma in a toddler.

   (1) The parent sits in the dental chair and cradles the child in his or her arms and helps restrain the patient's arms, if necessary. The dentist examines the patient with hands on both sides of the patient's head so head movement can be sensed and restricted, if necessary. The dental assistant is positioned on the opposite side of the chair from the dentist and can restrain the legs, if necessary.

   (2) In the second method, the parent and the dentist sit knee-to-knee. The patient's head rests on the dentist's thighs. The parent restrains the child's legs and the dental assistant can aid in restraining the patient's arms.

d. ADHD.

   (1) Basic information.

      (a) ADHD involves two sets of symptoms: inattention and a combination of hyperactive and impulsive behaviors.

      (b) ADHD usually manifests between the ages of 3 and 5, but manifestation varies widely.

      (c) Worldwide, 2% to 9.5% of all school-age children have ADHD.

      (d) Researchers have identified ADHD in every nation and culture they have studied.

      (e) Can persist into adulthood.

   (2) Common medications and examples of adverse reactions.

      (a) Methylphenidate (Concerta, Ritalin, Metadate): adverse effects include nausea, hypertension.

      (b) Atomoxetine (Strattera): adverse effects include hypertension, dry mouth, nausea.

      (c) Amphetamine/dextroamphetamine (Adderall): adverse effects include hypertension, headache, nausea, dry mouth.

   (3) Treatment modifications.

      (a) Depends on age and severity.

      (b) Shorter appointments.

      (c) Step-by-step verbal reinforcement.

e. Attire worn by the dental team.

   (1) Verification is inconclusive regarding the effect of the color and style of clothing and uniforms worn by the dental team on children's behavior. Other factors, such as parenting style and the ability of the dental team to communicate well with children, are much more important in determining the child's reaction to the dental environment.

Table 5-7

Common Local Anesthetics and Maximum Recommended Doses

ANESTHETIC	DURATION	MAXIMUM RECOMMENDED DOSE OF ANESTHETIC
2% lidocaine with 1:100,000 epinephrine	Pulpal: 60 min Soft tissue: 3-5 hr	4.4 mg/kg
3% mepivacaine	Pulpal: 20-40 min Soft tissue: 2-3 hr	4.4 mg/kg
4% prilocaine with 1:200,000 epinephrine	Pulpal: 60-90 min Soft tissue: 3-8 hr	4.4 mg/kg

2.3 Local Anesthesia and Nitrous Oxide Sedation for Children

A. Common local anesthetics and dosages.

1. The practitioner must know the maximum recommended dose of anesthetics used and then calculate, based on the patient's weight, the maximum number of cartridges.

2. The possibility for adverse reactions increases with concomitant use of sedative agents.

3. Table 5-7 shows three common local anesthetic solutions.

4. Calculation of maximum dose and cartridges—the *ADA/PDR Guide to Dental Therapeutics* indicates some cartridges contain 1.7 to 1.8 mL and others contain 1.8 mL depending on the anesthetic. Although many cartridges are labeled as 1.7 mL, the following calculations are based on cartridges that may contain up to 1.8 mL.

   a. Obtain the patient's weight in pounds and convert to kilograms by dividing by 2.2 (2.2 lb = 1.0 kg).

      (1) Example: (44-lb child)/(2.2 lb/kg) = 20 kg.

   b. Multiply weight in kilograms by the maximum recommended dose of local anesthetic to obtain the maximum milligram dosage.

      (1) Example: (20 kg) × (4.4 mg/kg lidocaine) = 88 mg.

   c. Calculate the number of milligrams per cartridge of anesthetic by multiplying the percent of local anesthetic times 10, then multiplying by the size of the cartridge, typically 1.8 mL.

      (1) Example: (2%) × (10) × (1.8) = 36 mg/cartridge.

   d. Divide the maximum milligram dosage (step 4b) by the number of milligrams per cartridge (step 4c) to obtain the maximum allowable cartridges of anesthetic.

      (1) Example: (88 mg maximum dose)/(36 mg/cartridge) = 2.44 cartridges.

B. Topical anesthetic.
   1. A good-tasting benzocaine topical anesthetic is recommended by authors of major pediatric dentistry texts.
      a. Benzocaine has a rapid onset.
      b. The mucosa is dried with gauze, and the topical anesthetic is applied for a minimum of 30 seconds.
   2. The usefulness of topical anesthetic in children is debated. Some authorities believe that placing topical anesthetic may cause more anxiety because the child has more time to anticipate the injection. In addition, the topical anesthetic can trigger a conditioned response because the injection always follows the topical application. However, most clinicians use a topical anesthetic.
C. Local anesthesia techniques for children.
   1. Mandibular primary molars.
      a. Innervation—inferior alveolar nerve.
      b. Inferior alveolar nerve block (mandibular block).
         (1) Indicated for deep caries, pulp therapy, and extractions.
         (2) In the primary dentition patient, the mandibular foramen is located lower than the plane of occlusion. Mandibular block injections for pediatric patients are made lower than what is done for adult patients.
         (3) About 1 mL of solution is deposited in the area of the mandibular foramen.
         (4) In the primary dentition, the syringe should bisect the primary molars on the opposite side of the injection.
      c. Lingual nerve block.
         (1) A small amount of anesthetic solution is deposited on insertion or withdrawal of the needle during administration of a mandibular block.
      d. Long buccal block.
         (1) A small amount of anesthetic solution is deposited in the mucobuccal fold distal to the most posterior tooth.
      e. Infiltration.
         (1) Some studies have shown that local infiltration anesthesia for primary molars is effective, especially for restorative procedures.
         (2) There is an increased probability for anesthesia failure using local infiltration for pulp therapy and extraction procedures.
   2. Mandibular primary anterior teeth.
      a. Innervation—inferior alveolar nerve.
      b. Infiltration.
         (1) Infiltration used alone in primary anterior teeth is effective for small carious lesions or extractions of mobile primary incisors.
      c. Inferior alveolar nerve block (mandibular block).
         (1) A mandibular block is used in cases that require regional anesthesia. Because some innervation of anterior teeth occurs from the opposite side across the midline, it is advisable to supplement a mandibular block with local infiltration anesthesia.
   3. Maxillary primary molars.
      a. Innervation—posterior superior alveolar nerve for permanent molars and the middle superior alveolar nerve for the mesiobuccal root of the first permanent molar and primary molars.
      b. Infiltration.
         (1) Local infiltration anesthesia is effective for first primary molars, owing to relatively thin overlying bone.
         (2) Local infiltration used alone for second primary molars is less effective because of the thickness of bone in the area.
      c. Posterior superior alveolar nerve block.
         (1) This block is used for second primary molars in conjunction with local infiltration anesthesia.
         (2) A posterior superior alveolar nerve block is used for the maxillary first permanent molar also, with a local infiltration applied for the mesiobuccal root.
   4. Maxillary primary anterior teeth.
      a. Innervation—anterior-superior alveolar branch of the maxillary nerve.
      b. Infiltration.
         (1) Local infiltration anesthesia is effective for maxillary anterior teeth.
         (2) The solution should be deposited close to the apex of the teeth to be anesthetized.
   5. Palatal tissues.
      a. Innervation—anterior palatine and nasal palatine nerves.
      b. Anesthesia for most restorative procedures or minor extractions can be accomplished by first depositing anesthetic via the free marginal gingiva. If needed, this can be supplemented by giving a palatal local infiltration injection in an area already blanched by anesthetic given previously.
      c. Surgical procedures may require anterior or nasal palatine nerve blocks. These injections are quite painful and are to be avoided if possible.
D. Complications of local anesthesia.
   1. Toxicity.
      a. The maximum dose of anesthetic should be calculated (see under "Common local anesthetics and dosages," earlier).
      b. Overdosage may cause central nervous system complications, such as dizziness, blurred vision, seizures, central nervous system depression, and death.
      c. Cardiac complications may include myocardial depression.

Table 5-8

Typical Pulse Rates, Blood Pressures, and Respiratory Rates in Children and Adults (Normal Patients)

	AGE 3	AGE 5	AGE 12	ADULT
Pulse (beats/min)	110	100	75	70
Systolic BP (mm Hg)	100	100	110	120
Diastolic BP (mm Hg)	60	65	70	75
Respiratory rate (breaths/min)	25	20+	20-	15

BP, Blood pressure.

2. Lip or cheek trauma.
  a. Because of the new sensation of being numb, some children either scratch their cheek or chew the lip or cheek area. Parents and patients should be warned of this possibility, and parents should supervise their children closely.
  b. Should the patient traumatize the cheek or lip, the parent should be reassured that these lesions almost always heal without complication. In addition, a description of the typical appearance (swelling, whitish yellow membrane) should be given to the parent, and the child should be seen at soon as possible in the office.
E. Nitrous oxide sedation for children.
  1. Physiologic differences between children and adults relative to nitrous oxide administration (Table 5-8).
    a. Basal metabolic activity is greater in children.
    b. Higher respiratory rate in children.
    c. Higher risk of airway obstruction in children because of narrower airway passages; large tonsils, adenoids, and tongue; and more oral secretions.
    d. Higher risk of desaturation in children because of less capability to expand on inspiration and less oxygen reserve.
    e. Heart rate is higher in children.
    f. Blood pressure is lower in children.
    g. Heart rate has a greater effect on blood pressure in children. For example, when there is a decrease in heart rate, blood pressure decreases relatively more in a child.
    h. Drug effects are more variable in children.
  2. The administration of nitrous oxide at levels less than 50% (with no combination with other sedative/narcotic/depressant agents) is considered to be minimal sedation. A minimally sedated patient may have temporary cognitive and coordination impairment, but heart and lung function is unimpaired. In addition, minimally sedated patients are able to communicate verbally.

3. Purpose of nitrous oxide sedation.
  a. Reduce fear, apprehension, or anxiety.
  b. Raise pain reaction threshold.
  c. Reduce fatigue.
  d. Enhance communication.
  e. Increase tolerance for longer appointments.
  f. Help in care of developmentally or physically challenged
  g. Decrease the gagging reflex.
4. Minimum alveolar concentration.
  a. Minimum alveolar concentration is a measure of potency. It is the concentration required to produce immobility in 50% of patients.
  b. Minimum alveolar concentration of nitrous oxide = 105%.
5. Four plateaus of stage I anesthesia (analgesia).
  a. *Paresthesia*—tingling of hands, feet.
  b. *Vasomotor*—warm sensations.
  c. *Drift*—euphoria, pupils centrally fixed, sensation of floating.
  d. *Dream*—eyes closed but open in response to questions, difficulty in speaking, jaw sags open.
6. Preparation of patient.
  a. Patient in reclined position.
  b. Use TSD.
  c. Describe sensations in advance.
  d. Adult-sized nasal hoods do not fit all children well. Smaller nasal hoods must be available for pediatric patients.
7. Technique basics.
  a. The bag is filled with oxygen, and the hood is placed on the patient's nose.
  b. The total flow rate is 4 to 6 L/min for most children. The practitioner can check the bag and make adjustments if necessary.
  c. The percentage of nitrous oxide is increased in 10% to 20% increments until the drift plateau is achieved and the patient is staring at the ceiling. The injection is given at this time.
  d. Maintenance dose during an operative procedure is typically about 30%.
  e. Nausea with or without vomiting is the most common complication with nitrous oxide use. This complication occurs with an excessive concentration of nitrous oxide or an excessively long procedure. Nitrous oxide levels should be reduced periodically during a procedure, especially after 30 minutes' duration.
  f. Patients must remain under observation while using nitrous oxide. The child's color, respiratory rate and rhythm, and responsiveness must be continually assessed.
8. Signs of saturation.
  a. Reminding child continuously to hold mouth open.
  b. No response to questions.

c. Agitation.

d. Sweating.

e. Nausea.

f. Unconsciousness.

9. *Diffusion hypoxia*—when nitrous oxide is discontinued, there is a high outpouring of nitrous oxide from the tissues into the lung. This can dilute available oxygen in the lungs. Although diffusion hypoxia is very rare (especially in normal, healthy individuals), patients should be given 100% oxygen for 3 to 5 minutes after a nitrous oxide procedure.

10. Contraindications of nitrous oxide sedation.

a. Patients with blocked eustachian tube, pneumothorax, pneumoperitoneum, sinusitis. Any rigid, noncompliant air space can lead to increased pressure with nitrous oxide use.

b. Pregnancy.

c. Significant emotional disturbances.

d. Patients with drug dependencies.

e. Some upper respiratory infections.

f. Patients being treated with bleomycin sulfate.

g. Methylenetetrahydrofolate reductase deficiency.

h. A physician consultation should be obtained for patients with significant medical conditions, such as obstructive pulmonary disease, congestive heart failure, and sickle cell disease. Also, patients with acute otitis media and tympanic membrane grafts should have a physician consultation before treatment.

2.4 Restorative Dentistry for Children

A. Anatomic differences in primary teeth compared with permanent teeth.

1. Primary teeth have thinner enamel.

2. The pulp chamber is relatively larger in primary teeth.

3. The pulp horns are closer to the surface of the tooth.

4. The enamel rods in the gingival third slope occlusally instead of cervically as in permanent teeth.

5. The crown is relatively shorter and has a greater constriction in the cervical region.

6. The interproximal contacts are broader and flatter than permanent teeth.

7. Enamel and dentin shades are generally whiter than permanent teeth.

8. The occlusal table is narrower on primary molars.

B. Basic principles in restoring primary molar teeth with amalgam.

1. Preparation depth is 0.5 mm into dentin; on primary molars, the depth of preparation is approximately 1.5 mm.

2. No. 330 and No. 245 burs are common for preparation of primary teeth. The No. 330 bur is 1.5 mm in length, and the No. 245 bur is 3.0 mm in length. These burs can aid the practitioner in establishing the proper depth of the preparation.

3. Rounded line angles decrease internal stresses in the restorative material and help prevent breakage with the smaller primary teeth.

4. Occlusal preparation extends into susceptible pits and fissures.

5. Buccal and lingual extensions for a class II preparation minimally break contact.

6. Buccal and lingual walls converge occlusally.

7. Gingival seat contact is broken.

8. Isthmus width is one third the intercuspal dimension.

C. Restoring primary molar teeth with composite.

1. Preparations may be more conservative than when using amalgam.

2. Preparation of class I restorations may be limited to the carious lesion if sealant is used as part of the restoration.

3. Some authors advocate more conservative class II preparations in which access to the interproximal lesion is gained through the marginal ridge or from the facial if the pits and fissures are not susceptible.

4. Preparation for a class II composite is similar to amalgam if caries exist occlusally and interproximally.

5. Composites are very technique-sensitive and are successful only if a dry field is maintained.

D. Posterior stainless steel crown preparation and adaptation.

1. Indications.

a. Teeth with extensive carious involvement.

b. Teeth with pulpectomy or pulpotomy treatment.

c. Malformed teeth.

d. Teeth with rampant caries.

e. Mesial lesions on first primary molars.

f. Ankylosed primary molars.

g. Young permanent molars as a semipermanent restoration.

h. Fractured teeth.

i. Teeth needed for abutments for appliances.

2. Contraindications.

a. If good esthetics are of primary importance.

b. Teeth nearing exfoliation.

c. Excessive crown loss resulting in lack of mechanical retention.

d. Space loss; if a neighboring tooth has tipped into the carious defect, adequate crown coverage may be impossible.

e. Caries extending cervically so that coverage of the defect becomes an issue.

f. As a permanent restoration in the permanent dentition.

E. Restoration of anterior primary teeth.

1. Incisors.

a. Small class III lesions may be restored with composite similarly to that of permanent incisors.

b. Compromised or involved incisal edge.

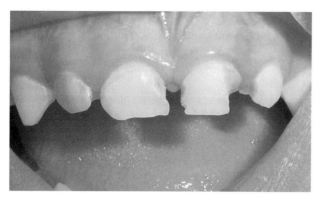

Figure 5-31 Composite crowns preoperatively.

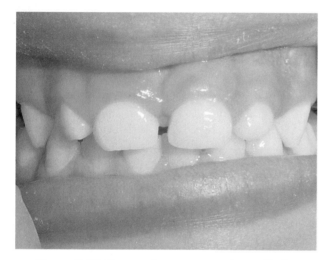

Figure 5-32 Composite crowns postoperatively.

(1) Some authors recommend a preparation that includes proximal reduction and labial or lingual dovetails in the cervical third.

(2) With significant incisal edge loss, a composite resin crown is a good choice if there is adequate tooth remaining for bonding and if esthetics is of primary importance (Figures 5-31 and 5-32).

(a) Preparation includes caries removal, mesial and distal IPR, and placing an undercut area approximately 1 mm incisal and following the free marginal gingiva. Preservation of enamel is important. An alternative preparation is to create a 1-mm cervical shoulder on the entire tooth.

(b) A celluloid crown form is trimmed and adapted to cover the cervical margins. At least one vent hole is created on the incisal edge to allow escape of excess composite.

(c) The crown form is filled with composite and seated.

(3) Primary incisors with extensive loss of tooth structure may require stainless steel crowns. Improved esthetics may be obtained in several ways.

(a) An open-face stainless steel crown can be created. The facial of the stainless steel crown is removed and is replaced by composite.

(b) Facings veneered to a stainless steel crown are available commercially or from some laboratories.

(c) Prefabricated zirconia anterior and posterior crowns are available. These crowns must fit passively because they do not flex the way stainless steel crowns do.

2. Primary canines.

a. The distal surface of primary canines is a common site for caries in caries-prone patients.

b. It is often necessary to place lingual, or sometimes labial, dovetails to aid in retention and placement of restorative material.

2.5 Pulp Treatment for Primary Teeth

A. *Treatment options.* The dentist has four treatment options if a primary tooth has pulp involvement. If the indications and contraindications for each of these procedures are known, the dentist may choose the treatment with the greatest efficacy.

1. Pulp capping.
2. Pulpotomy.
3. Pulpectomy.
4. Extraction.

B. General pulp therapy contraindications.

1. Pulp therapy is generally contraindicated in children who have serious illnesses. Extremely serious complications secondary to acute infection can arise should the pulp therapy fail.

2. Situations in which pulp therapy is contraindicated.

a. Patients susceptible to bacterial endocarditis.

b. Patients with leukemia.

c. Patients with nephritis.

d. Patients with cancer.

e. Patients with depressed polymorphonuclear leukocyte and granulocyte counts.

C. Important clinical signs.

1. *Mobility*—indicates loss of vitality if mobility is due to bone destruction, root destruction, or both. Vital pulpotomy technique is inappropriate.

2. *Swelling or fistula*—indicates necrotic pulp. Vital pulpotomy technique is inappropriate.

3. *Furcation radiolucency*—indicates necrotic pulp. Vital pulpotomy technique is inappropriate. Pulpectomy may be appropriate if the tooth does not demonstrate internal or external root resorption.

4. *Percussion or palpation sensitivity*—indicates at least advanced pulpal inflammation. Pulpotomy may not be advisable.

5. *Spontaneous pain*—indicates at least advanced pulpal inflammation. Other indicators should be used to

determine treatment of the tooth, but pulpotomy may not be advisable.

D. Pulp capping.
  1. Indirect pulp cap.
    a. Indications.
      (1) Symptom-free.
      (2) No radiologic evidence of pathosis.
      (3) Minimal caries in an area that, if caries were removed, would result in a pulp exposure.
    b. Procedure.
      (1) Caries removal, leaving caries that would expose the pulp.
      (2) Calcium hydroxide layer or base cement, or both.
      (3) Restoration of tooth.
      (4) Wait 6 to 8 weeks.
      (5) Reenter and remove remainder of caries. Some clinicians avoid this step and proceed with the restoration.
  2. Direct pulp cap.
    a. Indications.
      (1) Very small, pinpoint exposure only.
      (2) Noncarious exposure only.
      (3) Symptom-free.
      (4) Some authors are hesitant to recommend direct pulp caps on primary teeth because of a concern of internal root resorption.
    b. Procedure.
      (1) Calcium hydroxide layer.
      (2) Restoration of tooth.
E. Pulpotomy.
  1. Definition—coronal removal of vital pulp tissue.
  2. Indications.
    a. Vital primary tooth with carious or accidental exposure.
    b. Clinical signs of a normal pulp canal (e.g., no swelling, no draining fistulas, no pathologic mobility, no history of spontaneous pain, no pathologic radiographic radiolucencies).
    c. The tooth must be restorable. The dentist should think of restorability in terms of extent of decay and in terms of drift of adjacent teeth. For example, occasionally an adjacent tooth may tip into a carious defect, preventing an appropriate adaptation of a stainless steel crown (Figure 5-33).
  3. Procedure (Figures 5-34 to 5-36).
    a. Remove superficial and lateral decay.
    b. Remove roof of the chamber.
    c. Extirpate coronal pulp, No. 4 round bur, slow speed, light pressure.
    d. Dry cotton pellets to arrest pulpal hemorrhage.
    e. Formocresol application for 5 minutes; if hemorrhage cannot be controlled, consider pulpectomy or two-visit pulpotomy.
    f. Zinc oxide–eugenol (ZOE) buildup.
    g. Stainless steel crown coverage.

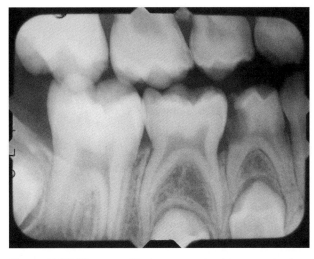

Figure 5-33 The mandibular second primary molar has tipped mesially into the carious lesion of the first primary molar. Obtaining a proper margin with a stainless steel crown would be very difficult.

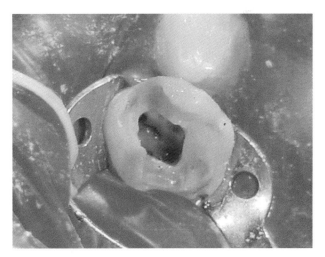

Figure 5-34 The coronal pulp tissue has been removed, and the remaining tissue has been treated.

  4. Evaluation—a successful pulpotomy is free from clinical and radiographic symptoms.
    a. Asymptomatic tooth.
    b. No mobility or fistulas.
    c. No furcation radiolucency.
    d. No internal or external root resorption.
    e. Success rate 70% to 97%.
  5. Medicaments.
    a. Formocresol.
      (1) Buckley's formocresol is the most commonly used medicament for pulpotomies on primary teeth.
      (2) 35% cresol, 19% formalin in aqueous glycerine.
      (3) Acts by direct contact.
      (4) A 20% solution produces equivalent results as full strength.

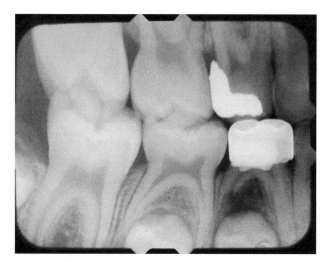

Figure 5-35 The pulpotomy on the mandibular first primary molar is failing. Note the furcation involvement and the external and internal root resorption. The failure may be related to the inadequate crown coverage on the distal aspect of the tooth.

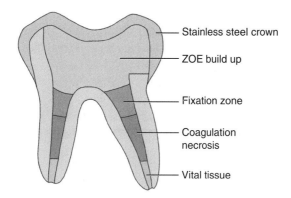

Figure 5-36 Pulp tissue zones in a formocresol pulpotomy. *ZOE,* Zinc oxide–eugenol

(5) Other medicaments have been studied or advocated because of a concern regarding possible toxic effects of formocresol.

b. Ferric sulfate.
   (1) Success rates comparable to formocresol.
   (2) Ferric sulfate is less toxic than formocresol.

c. Mineral trioxide aggregate.
   (1) Mineral trioxide aggregate pulpotomies generally show higher success rates than formocresol pulpotomies.

F. Pulpectomy.
   1. Definition—complete removal of all remaining pulp tissue.
   2. Indications.
      a. Necrotic or chronically inflamed, strategically located tooth with accessible canals.
      b. Essentially normal supporting bone.

3. Contraindications.
   a. Nonrestorable tooth.
   b. Internal or external root resorption.
   c. Teeth without accessible canals (commonly first primary molars).
   d. Significant bone loss.
4. Technique.
   a. Remove coronal pulp as for pulpotomy.
   b. Irrigate chamber gently with sodium hypochlorite or with sterile saline, and dry with cotton pellet.
   c. Carefully remove radicular pulp tissue with small file or barbed broach.
   d. Obtain test lengths 1 to 2 mm short of apex.
   e. Enlarge canal approximately three sizes.
   f. Wash frequently and carefully with sodium hypochlorite or sterile saline.
   g. Dry with paper points.
   h. Filling methods.
      (1) Pressure syringe.
         (a) Using a paper point or file, coat the walls of the canals with a creamy mix of ZOE.
         (b) Fill with creamy ZOE mix, starting 1 to 2 mm from the apex.
      (2) Condensation.
         (a) Coat the walls of the canals with creamy mix of ZOE.
         (b) Continue mixing ZOE to a condensable thickness, roll into points, and condense with small endodontic or amalgam pluggers.
5. Evaluation—a successful pulpectomy is free from clinical and radiographic symptoms.
   a. Asymptomatic tooth.
   b. No mobility or fistulas.
   c. No furcation radiolucency.
   d. No internal or external root resorption.

G. Decision-making tree—it is helpful to illustrate the decision-making process for pulp therapy in diagrammatic form (Figure 5-37).
   1. Furcation?
      a. If there is no furcation involvement, the tooth is likely vital, and a vital pulpotomy is generally appropriate if the tooth is restorable.
   2. First primary molar?
      a. If there is furcation involvement and the tooth is a first primary molar, an extraction should be strongly considered because of the difficulty of adequately removing diseased pulp tissue in this tooth.
   3. Restorable?
      a. The tooth must be restorable. The dentist should think of restorability in terms of extent of decay and in terms of drift of adjacent teeth. For example, occasionally an adjacent tooth may tip into a carious defect, preventing an appropriate adaptation of a stainless steel crown (see Figure 5-35). If

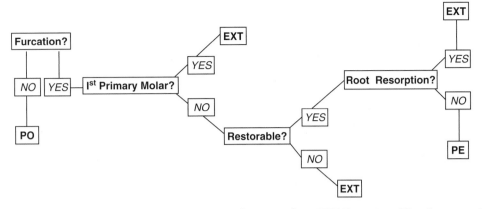

Figure 5-37 Decision-making tree for pulp therapy on primary molars. *EXT,* Extraction; *PE,* pulpectomy; *PO,* pulpotomy.

the tooth is not adequately restorable, it should be extracted.

4. Root resorption?

a. Generally, if a tooth has internal or external root resorption, it should be extracted. An exception to this rule is if the tooth is located strategically. For example, a second primary molar with mild to moderate root resorption on a 5-year-old patient may be considered for pulp treatment. The purpose of this treatment would be to maintain space until the first permanent molar erupts and then extract the primary molar and place a space maintainer. This strategy may avoid the need for a distal shoe space maintainer, making another space maintainer when the first permanent molar erupts.

2.6 Space Management in the Developing Dentition

A. Basic rules.

1. Eruption of anterior teeth should be reasonably symmetrical.

a. Extract contralateral primary tooth if there is a significant exfoliation asymmetry.

b. Exfoliation usually occurs during eruption of permanent incisors. A permanent incisor erupting may exfoliate the next, more distal primary tooth, which creates an asymmetry in exfoliation. This asymmetry can lead to significant midline deviations.

2. Primary dentition.

a. First primary molars—band-loop space maintainer (BLS) unilateral and bilateral loss.

b. Second primary molars—distal shoe or acrylic partial.

c. Incisors—consider esthetics and speech; use fixed or removable appliance.

3. Mixed dentition.

a. Primary mandibular canines—lower lingual holding arch (LLHA).

b. First primary molars—BLS unilateral or palatal holding arch (PHA) bilateral.

c. Second primary molars—PHA unilateral and bilateral.

B. Incisor loss.

1. Primary dentition.

a. Loss of a primary incisor in the primary dentition does not generally cause loss of overall arch circumference, as defined as the distance from the distal of the second primary molar, around the arch through the contact points, to the distal of the other second primary molar.

b. Loss of a primary incisor may result in localized space loss, especially if there was no interdental primary spacing before the loss.

c. Replacement of lost primary incisors is considered more for esthetics and possibly development of speech than for space maintenance. If the patient is not in the process of developing speech, placing an appliance is unnecessary if there is not an esthetic concern.

d. Partial dentures ("kiddie" partials).

(1) Removable.

(a) Posterior Adams clasps, "C" clasps, or ball clasps are placed for retention.

(b) The patient is usually at least 3 years old, and it is determined after consultation with parents that there is a reasonable expectation that the patient will tolerate wearing the appliance.

(2) Fixed (Figure 5-38).

(a) Orthodontic bands on second primary molars.

(b) 0.036-inch to 0.040-inch stainless steel wire is used.

(c) The replacement teeth are fixed to the wire.

(d) This appliance is intended mostly for patients younger than 3 years old or of questionable compliance in wearing a removable appliance.

e. Ectopic eruption.

(1) *Lingual eruption of permanent incisors—* characterized by a double row of teeth.

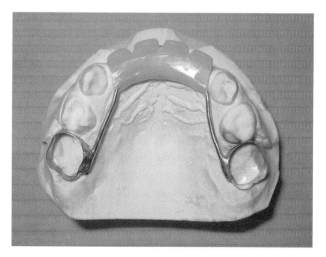

Figure 5-38 Fixed "kiddie" partial.

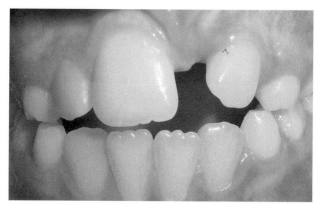

Figure 5-40 Space loss in permanent incisor region.

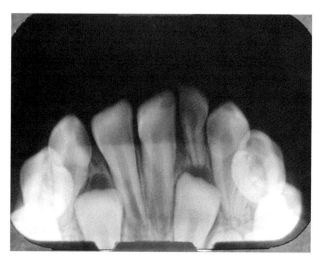

Figure 5-39 Ectopic eruption of mandibular permanent central incisors causing early exfoliation of a primary lateral incisor.

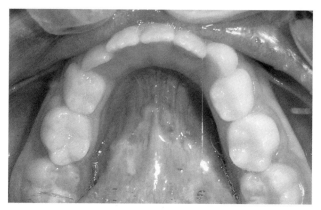

Figure 5-41 Mandibular midline is shifted to the left because of early loss of a primary canine.

      (a) This is a very common problem in the early mixed dentition.

      (b) If the primary incisor is very loose, no treatment is necessary initially. Most of these teeth exfoliate within a reasonable amount of time.

      (c) If the primary incisor is only moderately loose, extraction is usually the best option.

      (d) Erupting lingual incisors almost always move labially until they contact another tooth.

    (2) *Lateral ectopic eruption of permanent incisors*—characterized by early exfoliation of a primary lateral incisor (Figure 5-39).

      (a) Ectopic eruption of this type often results in a midline deviation.

      (b) With early detection, extraction of the remaining lateral incisor is the treatment

of choice so as to minimize a midline deviation.

  2. Permanent dentition.

    a. Loss of a permanent incisor.

      (1) Localized space loss can occur very quickly after loss of a permanent tooth (Figure 5-40). An appliance should be constructed and inserted as soon as possible after the tooth loss.

      (2) If localized space loss occurs, it may be treated with a removable appliance with finger springs or with fixed orthodontics.

C. Primary canine loss.

  1. Unilateral loss usually causes the following.

    a. Lingual collapse of permanent incisors.

    b. Loss of arch length.

    c. Increased overbite—after lingual collapse, the mandibular incisors erupt further, increasing overbite.

    d. Increased overjet secondary to lingual collapse of mandibular incisors.

    e. Midline deviation to the side of the canine loss (Figure 5-41).

  2. Bilateral loss usually causes the following.

    a. Lingual collapse of permanent incisors.

    b. Loss of arch length.

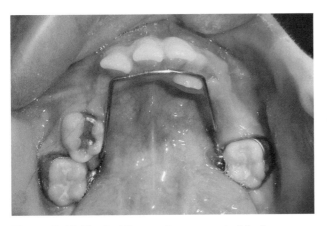

Figure 5-42 The holding arch was seated before eruption of the permanent lateral incisor, which erupted lingually.

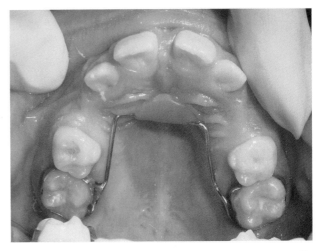

Figure 5-43 Nance holding arch features an acrylic button to aid in preventing mesial movement of maxillary posterior teeth.

     c. Increased overbite—after lingual collapse, the mandibular incisors erupt further, increasing overbite.

     d. Increased overjet secondary to lingual collapse of mandibular incisors.

  3. Appliances.

     a. Bilateral canine loss in a mixed dentition—LLHA.

     b. Unilateral canine loss in a mixed dentition.

       (1) Extract contralateral primary canine and place LLHA.

       (2) LLHA with a spur if a midline deviation has not occurred. A spur is a soldered extension from the main LLHA wire that engages the distal of the permanent lateral incisor, preventing distal drift.

D. Primary first molar loss.

  1. Primary dentition.

     a. Unilateral loss—BLS maintainer.

     b. Bilateral loss—BLS maintainer on both sides.

     c. Do not use LLHA until permanent incisors are erupted. Permanent incisors commonly erupt lingually and can be trapped by the appliance (Figure 5-42).

  2. Mixed dentition.

     a. Unilateral loss—BLS maintainer.

     b. Bilateral loss—LLHA or PHA, or Nance appliance (Figure 5-43).

E. Primary second molar loss.

  1. Reasons for space loss.

     a. Space loss as a result of early extraction.

     b. Space loss as a result of ectopically erupting first permanent molar.

  2. Unilateral loss.

     a. Primary dentition.

       (1) Distal shoe space maintainer.

         (a) A stainless steel crown is adapted to the first primary molar.

         (b) A 0.040-inch wire extends distally to the mesial of the unerupted first permanent molar.

         (c) A V-shaped extension is soldered to the wire, which is inserted gingivally and positioned mesial to the permanent first molar.

       (2) Acrylic partial denture.

         (a) This option may be indicated in children with multiple missing teeth (lack of abutment teeth) or medical conditions that contraindicate an appliance such as a distal shoe (e.g., a blood dyscrasia, a congenital heart defect, immunosuppression, diabetes).

         (b) The appliance is designed so that there is a mild amount of pressure applied by the acrylic on the alveolar ridge where the mesial of the unerupted first permanent molar would be. Often after extraction, the acrylic can be positioned mesial to the soft tissue contour of the first permanent molar.

     b. Mixed dentition.

       (1) Unilateral loss of a second primary molar in the mixed dentition usually requires a bilateral holding arch.

       (2) If a band and loop space maintainer is placed, there is no abutment tooth when the first primary molar exfoliates.

       (3) It is always important to consider the eruption/exfoliation sequence in planning space maintenance.

  3. Bilateral loss.

     a. Appliance choices.

       (1) Lingual holding arch (Figure 5-44).

       (2) PHA.

       (3) Nance holding arch.

       (4) Removable appliance.

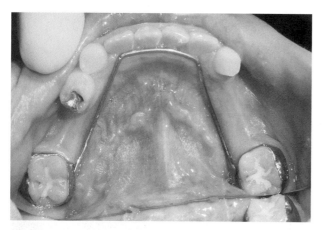

Figure 5-44 This lingual holding arch prevents posterior teeth from tipping mesially. The lingual holding arch can also be used to prevent lingual movement of incisors following premature primary canine loss.

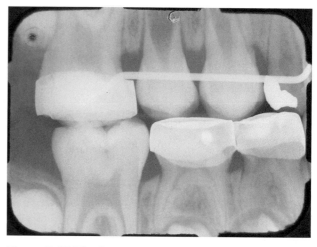

Figure 5-45 The first and second premolars erupted very early in this patient, who had extensive furcation involvement of the primary molars. There is approximately one third root development.

F. Factors to consider in planning for space maintenance.
 1. Amount of resorption of primary roots.
   a. If more than one fourth of the root remains owing to normal resorption, space maintenance is likely necessary.
   b. If less than one fourth of the root remains and if there is no bone left between the primary tooth and permanent tooth, space maintenance is likely unnecessary.
 2. Amount of bone covering the permanent tooth.
   a. If there is no bone remaining between the primary molar and permanent premolar and if the cusp tip of the permanent tooth is radiographically at the level of the furcation, no space maintenance is necessary.
   b. If bone is interposed between the primary molar and the permanent premolar, space maintenance is usually indicated.
   c. If there is bone destruction in the region of the primary molar furcation, it is possible that the permanent tooth may erupt very early, with less than three fourths root completion (Figure 5-45).
   d. If there is bone destruction in the region of the primary molar furcation, it is also possible that bone will form again, covering the permanent tooth.
   e. If the prediction of eruption of the permanent tooth is difficult, the dentist should use a space maintainer. Because space loss can occur very quickly, a space maintainer is often necessary, even if only for a few months' duration.
 3. Amount of root development.
   a. Eruptive movement begins on crown completion.
   b. The average tooth pierces the bone with two thirds root formation.

   c. The average tooth pierces the gingival tissue with three fourths root formation.
 4. Time elapsed since loss.
   a. Most space closure occurs within the first 6 months.
   b. Closure can occur in days.
   c. In the molar area, closure occurs essentially by tipping, not bodily movement of the tooth.
 5. Eruption of neighboring teeth.
   a. Active eruption of a neighboring tooth tends to increase amount of space loss. For example, if a second primary molar is removed during the eruption of the first permanent molar, more space loss will likely result.
 6. Patient's age.
   a. Chronologic age and average times of eruption are not important factors in planning space maintenance. The dentist should not use average times of eruption in treatment decisions.
   b. Teeth normally erupt through the gingiva with three fourths root development.
   c. "Rule of 7" for primary molars.
     (1) Eruption is delayed if loss of the primary molar occurs before age 7.
     (2) Eruption is accelerated if loss of the primary molar occurs after age 7. This does not mean that space maintenance is not needed after age 7. It only means that if a primary molar is lost after age 7, the permanent tooth on average tends to erupt faster that it ordinarily would.
 7. Delayed or deviant eruption.
   a. Ectopic permanent molars.
     (1) First permanent molars may become impacted under the distal aspect of the second primary molar (Figure 5-46).
     (2) More common in maxilla.

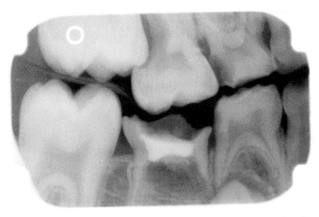

Figure 5-46 The maxillary first permanent molar is ectopically erupting under the distal aspect of the second primary molar.

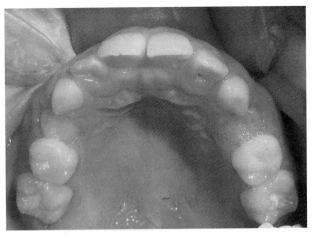

Figure 5-48 The maxillary first primary molars are ankylosed. These should be extracted before they become further submerged and are surgically more difficult. A space maintainer should be fabricated.

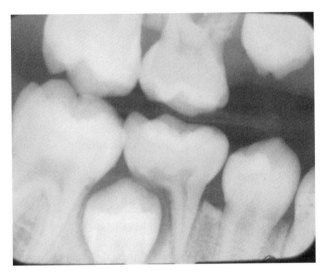

Figure 5-47 Distal eruption of a second bicuspid. After extraction of the second primary molar, the bicuspid usually uprights and erupts into a reasonably normal position.

(3) Varies in severity; if mild, some self-correct, or "jump."

(4) Treatment options.

    (a) Orthodontic separator.

    (b) Titanium clip separator.

    (c) Brass ligature wire.

    (d) Humphrey appliance.

    (e) Nance appliance and open coil spring.

b. Ectopic premolars.

  (1) Distal eruption (Figure 5-47).

    (a) This is most common in mandibular second premolars.

    (b) Resorbs the distal root of the second primary molar but not the mesial root.

    (c) Often requires extraction of the primary molar.

    (d) Space maintenance is necessary unless the cusp tip of the premolar is at the level of the floor of the pulp chamber of the primary molar and if, on extraction, the permanent tooth can be visualized.

  (2) Buccal or lingual eruption.

    (a) Buccal or lingual eruption of premolars is very common.

    (b) If the primary molar is not ready to exfoliate within a few weeks, extraction of the primary molar is the treatment of choice.

    (c) After extraction, the permanent premolar tends to move to a more normal position as long as there is adequate space for the tooth and the permanent tooth is only partially erupted.

c. Ankylosed primary molars.

  (1) Background.

    (a) Common: 1% (African-Americans) to 4% (whites).

    (b) Familial pattern.

    (c) Higher prevalence with congenitally absent premolars.

    (d) Usually begins after root resorption begins.

    (e) The change in occlusal height is due to the teeth other than the ankylosed teeth continuing normal eruption (Figure 5-48).

    (f) Ankylosis is progressive (i.e., the difference in occlusal height becomes greater with time). The practitioner must monitor the condition regularly.

  (2) Diagnosis.

    (a) Appearance—out of occlusion.

    (b) No mobility, even with advanced resorption.

(c) Hollow sound when tapped.
(d) Perhaps seen on radiograph—break in periodontal membrane.
  (3) Treatment.
    (a) Possibly, even probably, no treatment.
    (b) Observe for space loss and tipping of adjacent teeth.
    (c) If ankylosed tooth is below the normal height of contour of the interproximal surface of the adjacent tooth, extract and consider space maintenance.
    (d) As a temporary treatment, a stainless steel crown or composite bonding has been used to extend the existence of the ankylosed tooth.

8. Congenitally absent teeth.
  a. Incidence 1.5% to 10%, excluding third molars.
  b. If third molars are not included, the most common congenitally missing tooth is the mandibular second premolar, followed by the lateral incisor, followed by the maxillary second premolar.
  c. Treatment options with congenital absence.
    (1) Congenital absence of bicuspid is commonly treated orthodontically if the patient would have normally required extraction treatment. In these cases, all spaces are closed. If the patient has excellent occlusion, normal overbite and overjet, and minimal or no crowding, the congenital absence may be treated prosthetically.
    (2) Congenital absence of lateral incisor may be treated by placement of the canine in the lateral incisor position and restorative lateralization of the permanent canines. Alternatively, the canines may be placed in their normal position, and the lateral incisors may be replaced prosthetically.

2.7 Periodontal Problems in Children

A. Gingivitis.
  1. Very common in children.
  2. Treated with improved oral hygiene.
  3. Parental participation in oral hygiene is necessary in children younger than 8 years old because of the child's lack of manual dexterity.
  4. Parental supervision is often necessary in older children because of the child's lack of interest or understanding of consequences.
  5. Common conditions in children such as mouth breathing, crowded teeth, erupting teeth, and braces may further aggravate inflamed gingiva.
B. Puberty gingivitis.
  1. Prepubertal and pubertal period.
  2. Characterized by enlarged, bulbous interproximal gingival tissue on the labial aspects of the anterior teeth.

3. Treatment involves improvement in oral hygiene, removal of local irritants, and nutrition counseling.
C. Herpes simplex infection.
  1. Primary herpetic gingivostomatitis.
    a. Etiology—herpes simplex virus type 1.
    b. Usually affects children younger than 6 years.
    c. No previous exposure.
    d. Most primary infections are subclinical.
  2. Acute herpetic gingivostomatitis.
    a. Symptoms.
      (1) Liquid-filled yellow or white vesicles intraorally and periorally that rupture.
      (2) Ruptured vesicles are 1 to 3 mm in diameter with a pseudomembrane and have erythematous borders.
      (3) Location—mucous membrane, including tonsils, hard and soft palates, buccal mucosa, tongue, palate, gingiva.
      (4) Fever, malaise, lymphadenopathy.
      (5) Duration of 10 to 14 days.
    b. Treatment.
      (1) Topical anesthetics such as 0.5% dyclonine hydrochloride and viscous lidocaine.
      (2) Coating solutions such as diphenhydramine elixir and kaolin-pectin compound.
      (3) Topical acyclovir or penciclovir.
      (4) Analgesics such as acetaminophen and ibuprofen.
  3. Recurrent herpes simplex (cold sore or fever blister).
    a. Usually on the outside of the lips.
    b. Recurrence is frequently associated with emotional stress or local physical trauma.
    c. Treatment—systemic or topical antiviral medications.
D. Recurrent aphthous ulcer.
  1. Etiology unknown.
  2. Painful oval ulceration on unattached mucous membrane.
  3. Minor aphthae heal in 7 to 10 days.
  4. Treatment—topical antiinflammatory and analgesic agents.
E. Minimal attached gingiva and recession.
  1. A labial eruption path is the most common cause of inadequate attached gingiva.
    a. Sometimes orthodontic treatment may result in some increase of attached gingiva.
    b. Common treatment—free gingival graft.
  2. Other causes may be a high frenum attachment, high vestibule, self-inflicted injury, trauma, and use of smokeless tobacco.
F. Abnormal frenum attachment.
  1. Maxillary frenum.
    a. In the absence of recession, treatment of a heavy maxillary frenum with diastema is delayed until the permanent cuspids have erupted.

b. If the midline diastema has not closed, orthodontic closure is accomplished first, and a frenectomy is performed afterward.

  2. Lingual frenum (tongue tie).

   a. A patient is considered to have restricted tongue movement if the tongue cannot touch the maxillary alveolar process.

   b. With restricted tongue range of motion, children may be unable to develop proper speech sounds and surgery may be indicated in conjunction with speech therapy.

   c. Lingual frenum may also cause recession.

  3. Mandibular anterior frenum.

   a. A high mandibular anterior frenum may be associated with gingival recession.

   b. Frenectomy and gingival graft are common surgical treatments.

G. Periodontal disease in children.

  1. Aggressive periodontitis.

   a. Localized aggressive periodontitis in the permanent dentition—previously known as localized juvenile periodontitis.

    (1) Loss of attachment and bone on first permanent molars and permanent incisors.

    (2) Rapid loss of attachment.

    (3) Increased bacterial counts of *Aggregatibacter (Actinobacillus) actinomycetemcomitans.*

    (4) Most common in African-American children.

    (5) Treatment includes surgical intervention and antibiotics (metronidazole with or without amoxicillin, tetracycline).

   b. Generalized aggressive periodontitis.

    (1) Involvement of the entire dentition.

    (2) Significantly increased amount of plaque and calculus.

    (3) Treatment includes surgical intervention and antibiotics.

   c. *Localized aggressive periodontitis in the primary dentition*—previously known as localized prepubertal periodontitis.

    (1) Most common in the primary molar area.

    (2) Most common in African-American children.

    (3) Treatment includes débridement and antibiotics.

H. Acute necrotizing ulcerative gingivitis.

  1. Characteristics.

   a. Painful, bleeding gingival tissues.

   b. Blunting of interproximal papillae.

   c. Pseudomembrane on the marginal gingiva.

   d. Fetid breath.

   e. High fever.

  2. Caused by fusiform bacilli (spirochetes) and other anaerobes.

  3. Most common in teenagers and young adults.

  4. Responds well to débridement, oxidizing mouth rinses, and antibiotics.

2.8 Dental Trauma in Children

A. Etiology.

  1. Boys more commonly affected (male-to-female ratio 2:1).

  2. Maxillary anterior teeth most commonly affected.

  3. Children with increased overjet more commonly affected.

  4. Trauma to the primary dentition occurs in 30% of children.

  5. Trauma to the permanent dentition occurs in 22% of children by age 14.

B. Possible reactions of a tooth to trauma/

  1. Pulpal hyperemia—may lead to infarction and necrosis as a result of increased intrapulpal pressure.

  2. Internal hemorrhage.

   a. Capillary rupture secondary to increased pressure.

   b. Occurs within 2 to 3 weeks after trauma.

   c. May cause discoloration.

  3. Calcific metamorphosis (pulp canal obliteration).

   a. Partial obliteration of the pulp chamber and canal.

   b. These teeth normally remain vital.

   c. Yellow, opaque appearance.

  4. Internal resorption.

   a. Caused by osteoclastic action.

   b. "Pink spot" perforation may occur.

  5. Peripheral root resorption.

   a. Caused by damage of periodontal structures.

   b. Usually occurs in severe injuries with displacement of the tooth.

   c. Types.

    (1) *Surface*—normal PDL, small areas.

    (2) *Replacement*—ankylosis.

    (3) *Inflammatory*—granulation tissue, radiolucency.

  6. Pulpal necrosis.

   a. Caused by severing of apical vessels or prolonged hyperemia and strangulation.

   b. May not occur for several months.

  7. Ankylosis.

   a. Ankylosis can occur with PDL injury, which leads to inflammation and osteoclastic activity. This may cause fusion between bone and root surface.

   b. Clinically, occlusal or incisal surface of ankylosed tooth is gingival to adjacent teeth.

   c. During growth, eruption of normal teeth continues, but because ankylosed teeth are osseointegrated, these teeth appear to be sinking into the gingival tissue.

C. Consequences to permanent teeth with injury to the primary predecessor.

  1. Primary anterior teeth are positioned labial to their permanent successor. An injury that forces the root of the primary tooth into the developing permanent tooth may result in one of the following.

a. Hypocalcification and hypoplasia.

b. Reparative dentin.

c. Dilaceration (or bending of the permanent tooth).

D. Patient assessment—certain issues should be assessed for all trauma cases.

1. Medical history.

    a. Pay particular attention to the following.

        (1) Drug sensitivities.

        (2) Congenital or acquired cardiac problems.

        (3) Coagulation disorders.

        (4) Seizure disorders.

    b. Determine tetanus coverage.

        (1) Uncovered children—antitoxin (tetanus immune human globulin).

        (2) Children with previous but dated coverage—toxoid booster.

        (3) Active immunization.

            (a) Three injections of diphtheria, pertussis, and tetanus (DPT) vaccine during first year.

            (b) Booster at 1.5 and 3 years.

            (c) Booster at 6 years and then every 4 to 5 years.

    c. Neurologic assessment.

        (1) Obtain information regarding loss of consciousness.

            (a) Neck or head pain.

            (b) Numbness.

            (c) Amnesia.

            (d) Nausea/vomiting.

            (e) Drowsiness.

            (f) Blurred vision.

        (2) If in doubt regarding neurologic status, refer to an emergency medical facility.

2. Dental history questions.

    a. How did the trauma occur?

    b. When did the trauma occur?

    c. Where did the accident occur (school, home, athletic field)?

    d. Where in the craniofacial region did the trauma occur?

    e. Was there a previous injury to area?

    f. Was there previous treatment to area?

    g. Did the patient experience unconsciousness, headache, amnesia, or nausea?

    h. Is there a problem biting together in the normal manner?

3. Radiographs.

    a. X-ray injured tooth, adjacent teeth, and opposing teeth.

    b. Evaluate proximity of fracture to pulp.

    c. Estimate root development.

    d. Look for root and alveolar fractures.

    e. Note any periapical pathology.

    f. Note previous treatment.

    g. Typically, radiographs are indicated at 1-, 2-, and 6-month intervals after a traumatic incident.

4. Diagnostic tests.

    a. Electrical pulp tests and thermal tests may be unreliable in primary teeth.

    b. If a tooth is incompletely erupted or is being orthodontically treated, the tooth may be normal even if there is little sensitivity to electrical pulp testing.

5. General initial assessment of hard tissue injury.

    a. Check for crown fracture.

    b. Check for pulp exposures.

    c. Check for displaced or avulsed teeth.

    d. Check for mobility.

    e. Examine adjacent and opposing teeth for injury.

6. General follow-up assessment.

    a. Accomplished generally at 1, 2, and 6 months.

    b. Clinical examination.

        (1) Mobility.

        (2) Percussion sensitivity.

        (3) Discoloration and when discoloration began.

        (4) History of spontaneous pain.

        (5) Swelling or fistula.

        (6) Pulp testing.

    c. Radiologic examination.

        (1) External root resorption.

        (2) Internal root resorption.

        (3) PDL space.

        (4) Periapical radiolucencies.

        (5) Continued narrowing of pulp canal space.

            (a) Indicates vital pulp.

            (b) May lead to calcific metamorphosis.

        (6) Root fractures.

E. Treatment of traumatic injuries—all of the following require follow-up assessment as outlined under "General follow-up assessment."

1. Concussion and subluxation.

    a. Concussion is defined as an injury to the tooth without displacement or mobility. The PDL is inflamed and tender to percussion.

    b. Subluxation is defined as an injury to the tooth without displacement, but mobility is exhibited.

    c. Primary and permanent teeth.

        (1) Usually no treatment is immediately necessary.

        (2) Recommend soft diet.

        (3) Reinforce need for good oral hygiene.

        (4) Some authors recommend 0.12% chlorhexidine gluconate oral rinse or 3% hydrogen peroxide to aid healing.

        (5) Teeth with open apices are more likely to remain vital.

2. Intrusion.

    a. Primary teeth.

        (1) After an intrusive injury to an anterior primary tooth, the root of the primary tooth is likely

positioned closely to the labial of the permanent incisor.

(2) Unless it can be determined that the primary tooth is impinging on the permanent successor, intruded primary teeth are left alone in the hopes that they will spontaneously reerupt.

(3) These teeth should be reviewed, and radiographs should be obtained.

b. Permanent teeth (see Section 1, Endodontics).

3. Extrusion.

a. Primary teeth.

(1) The greater the distance from a normal position, the greater the chance for severing of the apical vasculature and pulpal necrosis. If a primary incisor is extruded greater than 3 mm, the tooth should likely be extracted.

(2) If the patient is seen before formation of a periapical blood clot, the tooth may be repositioned carefully and splinted for 7 to 14 days. Endodontic treatment should be initiated.

b. Permanent teeth (see Section 1, Endodontics).

4. Fracture through enamel only (primary and permanent teeth).

a. Smooth enamel.

b. Check vitality at 1, 2, and 6 months because of possible concussion injury.

5. Fracture through enamel and dentin (primary and permanent teeth).

a. Primary teeth.

(1) Smooth edges.

(2) Restore if necessary.

(a) Dentin/enamel bonding.

(b) Traditional strip crown for primary teeth.

(c) Incisal edge composite.

6. Fracture through enamel, dentin, and pulp.

a. Primary teeth.

(1) Pulpotomy for vital pulps.

(2) Pulpectomy for necrotic pulps, if there is not significant internal or external root resorption.

(3) Extraction is the treatment of choice if the tooth has internal or external root resorption.

b. Permanent teeth (see Section 1, Endodontics).

7. Avulsion.

a. Replanting primary teeth.

(1) Poor prognosis.

(a) Replantation could be considered if within 30 minutes of avulsion.

(b) Splint if necessary.

(c) Soft diet.

(d) Antibiotic prescription.

(e) Follow with primary endodontics.

(2) Space maintainer if endodontic treatment is impossible.

b. Replanting permanent teeth (see Section 1, Endodontics).

(1) Antibiotics after replantation.

(a) Not susceptible to tetracycline staining: doxycycline 4.4 mg/kg/day q 12h on day 1, 2.2 to 4.4 mg/kg/day for 7 days.

(b) Susceptible to tetracycline staining: penicillin V 25 to 50 mg/kg/day in three to four divided doses for 7 to 10 days.

(2) Endodontic treatment of replanted teeth (see Section 1, Endodontics).

8. Root fracture.

a. Primary teeth.

(1) Root fractures in primary teeth are rare, owing to the bone surrounding the teeth at that age being more malleable.

(2) If the root fracture is in the apical half, splinting may be unnecessary, especially if there is minimal mobility.

(3) If the root fracture is in the coronal half with increased mobility, either a rigid splint or extraction is the treatment of choice.

b. Permanent teeth (see Section 1, Endodontics).

9. Splinting.

a. Nonrigid splint for reimplantation and displacements.

(1) Bond 0.016-inch × 0.022-inch stainless steel orthodontic wire or 0.018-inch round stainless steel wire or monofilament nylon (20- to 30-lb test).

(2) 0.028-inch round stainless steel if three to four teeth are mobile.

(3) Titanium trauma splint.

(4) The wire must be passive (not cause pressure on the teeth).

(5) Use either composite or flowable composite.

(6) The splint should remain in place for 7 to 14 days.

(7) Long-term rigid splinting of replanted teeth increases risk of replacement root resorption (ankylosis).

2.9 Miscellaneous Topics in Pediatric Dentistry

A. Mouth guards.

1. Mouth guards are helpful in preventing the frequency and severity of dentoalveolar injuries.

2. Three main types of mouth guards.

a. Stock.

(1) Available at sporting goods stores.

(2) Are not custom-adapted to the teeth.

(3) Inexpensive.

b. Mouth-formed.

(1) Available at sporting goods stores.

(2) Two types.

(a) The boil and bite-type mouth guard is softened in hot water, then adapted to the teeth.

(b) The shell-type mouth guard has an outer shell that is firm and an inner liner that is made from ethyl methacrylate.
  c. Custom-fabricated.
    (1) Impression taken by the dentist.
    (2) Two types.
      (a) *Vacuum-formed*—mouth guard is adapted by heating the mouth guard material in a vacuum molding machine.
      (b) *Pressure-laminated*—has multiple layers of material and is subject to less distortion.
    (3) Mouth guard is trimmed and smoothed.
    (4) Custom mouth guards generally fit better and are worn more successfully by athletes.
  3. Mouth guards should be cleaned daily in cool water.
  4. Storage should be in plastic retainer cases.
B. Antibiotic prophylaxis for at-risk patients.
  1. A few cardiac conditions require antibiotic prophylaxis before rendering dental care that may cause a bacteremia. Because of the diversity of circumstances with each patient, it is recommended that the practitioner consult with the appropriate medical personnel if the complete medical status of the patient is not fully known.
  2. Cardiac conditions (important factors).
    a. Cardiac conditions that predispose to endocarditis.
    b. Dental procedures that may cause bacteremia (Table 5-9).
    c. American Heart Association prophylaxis recommendations.
  3. Compromised immunity.
    a. Patients with compromised immunity may have difficulty combating a bacteremia and require antibiotic prophylaxis.
    b. Because of the diversity of circumstances with each patient, it is recommended that the practitioner consult with the appropriate medical personnel if the complete medical status of the patient is not fully known.
    c. Partial list of conditions associated with compromised immunity.
      (1) Any immunodeficiency or immunosuppression.
      (2) Diabetes.
      (3) Organ transplantation.
      (4) Corticosteroid use.
      (5) Sickle cell anemia.
      (6) Neutropenia.
      (7) Lupus erythematosus.
      (8) Splenectomy.
      (9) Cancers.
  4. Shunts, indwelling vascular catheters, and other medical devices.
    a. Bacterial colonization may occur with various medical devices following bacteremia. Antibiotic premedication is indicated.

Table 5-9

Dental Procedures That May Cause Bacteremia

Endocarditis Prophylaxis Recommended—Likely Significant Bacteremia*

Dental extractions

Periodontal procedures including surgery, subgingival placement of antibiotic fibers or strips, scaling and root planing, probing, recall maintenance

Dental implant placement and reimplantation of avulsed teeth

Endodontic (root canal) instrumentation or surgery only beyond the apex

Initial placement of orthodontic bands but not brackets

Intraligamentary local anesthetic injections

Prophylactic cleaning of teeth or implants where bleeding is anticipated

Endocarditis Prophylaxis Not Recommended—Usually Insignificant Bacteremia

Restorative dentistry† (operative and prosthodontic) with or without retraction cord‡

Local anesthetic injections (nonintraligamentary)

Intracanal endodontic treatment; postplacement and buildup*

Placement of rubber dam*

Postoperative suture removal

Placement of removable prosthodontic or orthodontic appliances

Oral impressions‡

Fluoride treatments

Taking of oral radiographs

Orthodontic appliance adjustment

Shedding of primary teeth

In general, the presence of moderate to severe gingival inflammation may elevate these procedures to a higher risk of bacteremia

---

*Prophylaxis is recommended for patients with high and moderate cardiac risk as well as high-risk prosthesis conditions.

†This includes restoration of decayed teeth and replacement of missing teeth.

‡Clinical judgment may indicate antibiotic use in any circumstances that may create significant bleeding.

---

    b. Examples.
      (1) Vascular catheters.
      (2) Ventriculoarterial and ventriculovenous shunts used in hydrocephalus.
  5. Patients with prosthetic joints or other implanted devices require consultation with the child's physician regarding antibiotic prophylaxis.
C. Systemic fluoride supplementation.
  1. Systemic fluoride "rule of 6."
    a. If fluoride level is greater than 0.6 ppm, no supplemental systemic fluoride is indicated.
    b. If the patient is less than 6 months old, no supplemental systemic fluoride is indicated.
    c. If the patient is more than 16 years old, no supplemental systemic fluoride is indicated.
  2. Fluoride table (Table 5-10).

Table 5-10

Fluoride Supplementation Schedule Based on Fluoride Ion Level (ppm)

AGE	<0.3	0.3-0.6	>0.6
Birth–6 months	None	None	None
6 months–3 years	0.25 mg	None	None
3-6 years	0.50 mg	0.25 mg	None
6-16 years	1.0 mg	0.50 mg	None

D. Candidiasis (thrush, moniliasis).
  1. Caused by *Candida albicans*.
  2. Common in newborns or young children after antibiotic therapy.
E. Anticipatory guidance.
  1. Counseling patients and parents regarding the child's home oral health care that is age-appropriate and is focused on prevention.
  2. Subjects to discuss with parents.
    a. Oral hygiene.
    b. Oral development.
    c. Fluoride.
    d. Diet and nutrition.
    e. Oral habits.
    f. Trauma and injury prevention.
F. Digit-sucking habits.
  1. Very common up to age 3.
  2. Risk of malocclusion is a function of amount of time per day the habit is practiced, the duration of the habit in terms of weeks and months, and the intensity of the habit.
  3. Effects of digit-sucking.
    a. Increased overjet, owing to proclination of maxillary incisors and retroclination of mandibular incisors.
    b. Open anterior bite, owing to supereruption of posterior teeth.
    c. Posterior crossbite, owing to the tongue not being positioned between the maxillary alveolar processes and cheek constriction.
    d. Class II posterior occlusion with prolonged habits.
  4. Treatment.
    a. Traditionally, intervention by the dentist with appliance therapy is recommended at age 5 or 6 if the child has not stopped the digit-sucking habit. Some authors now recommend earlier intervention.
    b. Appliances.
      (1) Removable maxillary retainer with rounded stainless steel wire loops placed in the anterior palate region.
      (2) Fixed reminder appliance in which a stainless steel crib is placed in the anterior palate region (Figure 5-49).

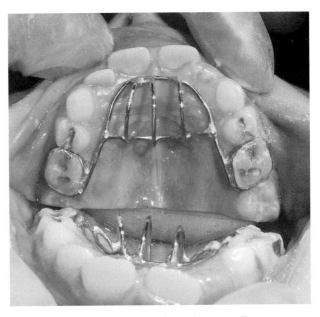

Figure 5-49 Fixed digit-sucking appliance.

      (3) "Bluegrass" appliance, which is a fixed appliance that features a six-sided plastic roller in the anterior palate region.
G. Teething.
  1. Symptoms that have been associated with teething include increased temperature, drooling, diarrhea, dehydration, and loss of appetite.
  2. Symptoms other than drooling and slight loss of appetite should be viewed with suspicion of a systemic disturbance.
  3. With any significant symptoms, the patient should be referred to a pediatrician. Serious complications can occur if the practitioner overlooks systemic disturbances by attributing them to teething.
  4. Teething symptoms may be reduced by using chilled teething rings. Some authors recommend using topical anesthetic and nonaspirin analgesics.
H. Natal and neonatal teeth.
  1. Natal teeth are teeth that are present at birth.
  2. Neonatal teeth are teeth that erupt in the first 30 days.
  3. Most natal and neonatal teeth are primary teeth (90%); very few are supernumerary teeth (10%). Most are mandibular incisors (85%).
  4. Treatment.
    a. Extract supernumeraries.
    b. Extract primary teeth if extremely mobile and there is danger of aspiration.
    c. If the tooth is causing ulceration on the ventral side of the tongue (Riga-Fede disease), the tooth may be smoothed or extracted.
    d. If the tooth is causing nursing difficulties, a breast pump or smoothing or extraction may be recommended.

I. Early childhood caries (ECC).
   1. *ECC definition by the American Academy of Pediatric Dentistry (AAPD)*—the presence of more than one decayed (noncavitated or cavitated), missing (owing to decay), or filled tooth surface in any primary tooth in a child younger than 6.
   2. Severe ECC.
      a. Younger than 3 years—any sign of smooth surface decay.
      b. Ages 3 to 5.
         (1) One or more cavitated, missing (owing to caries), or filled smooth surface in primary maxillary anterior teeth.
         (2) A decayed, missing, or filled surface (DMFS) score of greater than 4 (age 3), greater than 5 (age 4), or greater than 6 (age 5).
   3. Previously termed "baby bottle syndrome" or "nursing bottle caries."
   4. Typical presentation of "baby bottle syndrome."
      a. Caries are present on maxillary anterior teeth and primary molars.
      b. The mandibular incisors are unaffected because of the tongue covering these teeth during feeding.
      c. History often reveals that the child is consistently put to bed with a nursing bottle containing milk or a sugar-containing drink.
   5. AAPD recommendations.
      a. Infants should not be put to sleep with a bottle. Ad libitum nocturnal breast-feeding should be avoided after the first primary tooth begins to erupt.
      b. Parents should be encouraged to have infants drink from a cup as they approach their first birthday. Infants should be weaned from the bottle at 12 to 18 months of age.
      c. Repetitive consumption of any liquid containing fermentable carbohydrates from a bottle or no-spill training cup should be avoided.
      d. Oral hygiene measures should be implemented by the time of eruption of the first primary tooth.
      e. An oral health consultation visit within 6 months of eruption of the first tooth and no later than 12 months of age is recommended to educate parents and provide anticipatory guidance for prevention of dental disease.
      f. An attempt should be made to assess and decrease the mother's or primary caregiver's *Streptococcus mutans* levels to decrease the transmission of cariogenic bacteria and lessen the infant's or child's risk of developing ECC.
      g. In children younger than 2 with moderate to high caries risk, a smear of fluoridated toothpaste should be used. All children age 2 to 5 should use a pea-sized amount of fluoridated toothpaste.
J. Mixed dentition analysis.
   1. The purpose of this analysis is to predict, in the mixed dentition, the amount of crowding, or tooth size–arch length deficiency in the permanent dentition.
   2. Moyer's mixed dentition analysis.
      a. Basics.
         (1) The combined mesiodistal widths of the mandibular permanent incisors are used to predict the combined mesiodistal widths of the patient's buccal segment (cuspid–first bicuspid–second bicuspid).
         (2) Instruments—Boley gauge and study models.
         (3) Arch length is measured in segments.
            (a) *Anterior segment*—choose a midline point, measure from this point to the mesial of each primary canine, and sum.
            (b) *Posterior segments*—measure from the mesial of each primary canine to the mesial of the first permanent molar.
         (4) Measure mesiodistal diameter of the mandibular incisors and sum.
         (5) Predict permanent buccal segment tooth sizes by using the prediction chart.
         (6) Total the differences between arch lengths (space available) and tooth sizes to obtain amount of tooth size–arch length discrepancy.
         (7) The same procedure is used in the maxillary arch except that the predicted tooth sizes of the maxillary buccal segment are still calculated from the mandibular incisor measurement.
      b. Incisor region.
         (1) Measure mesiodistal diameter of the mandibular incisors and sum.
         (2) Measure the space available for mandibular incisors.
         (3) Subtract (1) from (2); a negative number indicates crowding in the incisor region.
         (4) In the example in Table 5-11, there is 3.2 mm of crowding in the anterior region.
      c. Buccal segment region.
         (1) Measure space available for 3-4-5 on each side of the arch.
         (2) Measure from the mesial of each primary cuspid to the mesial of the first permanent molar.

Table 5-11

Incisor Measurements (mm) for Mixed Dentition Analysis

	LEFT	INCISORS	RIGHT
Space available		19.8	
Tooth size		23.0	
Difference		−3.2	

(3) In the example in Table 5-12, there is 20.1 mm of space available for the mandibular left buccal segment and 19.5 mm of space available for the mandibular right buccal segment.

(4) Calculate the size of teeth 3-4-5 from prediction table (Table 5-13).

   (a) Find the total size of the mandibular permanent incisors in the top row.

   (b) The mandibular buccal segment (3-4-5) tooth size is 22.2 mm.

   (c) This tooth size is estimated at the 75th percentile, which essentially means that the teeth will be smaller than the predicted size in 75% of patients.

(5) Calculate tooth size–arch length differences in the buccal segments.

   (a) Subtract tooth size from space available on the patient's left and right buccal segments.

   (b) Negative numbers indicate crowding.

   (c) In the example in Table 5-14, there is 2.1 mm of crowding in the mandibular left buccal segment and 2.7 mm of crowding in the mandibular right buccal segment.

(6) To obtain the total amount of predicted crowding, add the three numbers in the difference row. In this example, there is 8.0 mm of predicted crowding in the mandibular arch.

(7) Allowance for late mesial shift of mandibular first permanent molars.

   (a) If the permanent molars are in an end-to-end relationship, they must shift mesially to achieve a class I molar occlusion.

   (b) This "late mesial shift" decreases available space because arch length is smaller.

   (c) Traditionally, −1.7 mm is added for each side that is in an end-to-end relationship.

   (d) In the example, if one side was in an end-to-end relationship, the total amount of crowding would be −9.7 mm.

3. Tanaka-Johnson analysis.

   a. Measurements of space available (arch length) are the same as for the Moyer analysis.

   b. Measurements of the permanent mandibular incisors are the same as for the Moyer analysis.

   c. Obtain the predicted tooth size for the mandibular buccal segment.

     (1) Divide the total tooth size of the mandibular incisors by 2.

     (2) Add 10.5 mm.

     (3) For example, if the total mesiodistal widths of the mandibular permanent incisors were 22.8 mm, the predicted buccal segment tooth size would be 21.9 mm ([22.8 mm/2] + 10.5 mm).

   d. Obtain the predicted tooth size for the maxillary buccal segment.

     (1) Divide the total tooth size of the mandibular incisors by 2.

     (2) Add 11.0 mm.

   e. The remaining calculations are similar to those for the Moyer analysis.

K. Child abuse and neglect.

   1. Dentists are mandated by law to report suspected child abuse or neglect. Proof of abuse or neglect is unnecessary.

Table 5-12

Incisor Measurements (mm) with Available Spaces for Teeth 3-4-5 for Mixed Dentition Analysis

	LEFT	INCISORS	RIGHT
Space available	20.1	19.8	19.5
Tooth size		23.0	
Difference		−3.2	

Table 5-14

*Mixed Dentition Analysis Summary**

	LEFT	INCISORS	RIGHT
Space available	20.1	19.8	19.5
Tooth size	22.2	23.0	22.2
Difference	−2.1	−3.2	−2.7

*Using data (in mm) from Tables 5-11 to 5-14 and minimum 75% tooth size from Table 5-13.

Table 5-13

Prediction of Available Space for Teeth 3-4-5 (Rows 2 and 3) Based on Incisor Tooth Size (Row 1) (mm)*

	19.5	20.0	20.5	21.0	21.5	22.0	22.5	23.0	23.5	24.0
Maximum 75%	20.6	20.9	21.2	21.5	21.8	22.0	22.3	**22.6**	22.9	23.1
Minimum 75%	20.1	20.4	20.7	21.0	21.3	21.6	21.9	**22.2**	22.5	22.8

*Note tooth size = 23.0 from Tables 5-11 and 5-12, with predicted available space in bold.

2. Failure to report suspected child abuse may result in significant legal ramifications for the dentist, including a fine, jail sentence, and civil liability.
3. Types.
   a. Physical.
      (1) Intentional, not accidental.
      (2) Common injuries include bruises, welts, lacerations, burns, and fractures.
      (3) 50% of physical abuse is in the craniofacial region.
      (4) 25% of physical abuse is in the oral region.
   b. Emotional.
      (1) Difficult to identify a causal link between parental behaviors and harm to the child.
      (2) Examples of emotional abuse include denial of affection, isolation, extreme threats, and corruption.
   c. Sexual.
      (1) Generally defined as activity of a sexual nature that is inappropriate for a parent-child relationship.
      (2) Examples of sexual abuse include any form of parent-child sexual activity, exhibitionism, and pornography.
   d. Neglect.
      (1) Generally defined as willful negligence to provide for the basic needs of a child, such as food, shelter, clothing, medical care, supervision, protection, and guidance.
      (2) Definition from the AAPD—"willful failure of parent or guardian to seek and follow through with treatment necessary to ensure a level of oral health essential for adequate function and freedom from pain and infection."
L. Pit and fissure sealants.
   1. Selection.
      a. Indications.
         (1) Deep pits and fissures.
         (2) Caries-free surface, although sealants placed on undetected incipient caries do not result in progressive lesions if the sealant remains intact.
      b. Contraindications.
         (1) Rampant caries.
         (2) Interproximal caries.
         (3) Well-coalesced grooves.
         (4) Inability to maintain a dry field.
   2. Technique.
      a. Cleaning.
         (1) It is agreed that it is necessary to have clean pits and fissures to have good retention; how this is accomplished varies among authors.
         (2) Methods.
            (a) Pumice prophylaxis with rubber cup or bristle brush.
            (b) Air polishing device.

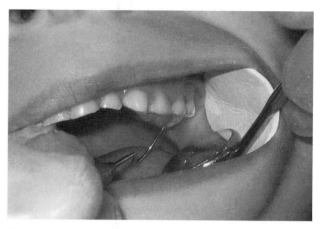

Figure 5-50 Dry angle usage to maintain a moisture-free field.

            (c) Toothbrush with pumice or toothpaste.
            (d) 3% hydrogen peroxide.
            (e) Enameloplasty.
      b. Isolation.
         (1) Rubber dam.
         (2) Cotton rolls or dry angles are used with high-volume evacuation (Figure 5-50).
      c. Acid etching.
         (1) 35% to 40% phosphoric acid is the most common etchant.
         (2) 20-second etching time for permanent teeth.
         (3) Etchant should not be rubbed into the tooth.
         (4) Some authors recommend longer etching times for primary teeth (approximately 30 seconds).
         (5) Wash for 30 seconds.
         (6) Dry with compressed air for 15 seconds.
         (7) If a frosty appearance is not achieved, repeat etching, washing, and drying.
      d. Placement.
         (1) Some authors recommend a bonding agent before sealant placement.
         (2) Ensure that sealant is placed in all occlusal, buccal, and lingual grooves.
         (3) Avoid excessive amount of sealant.
         (4) Polymerize sealant according to manufacturer's directions.
         (5) Check occlusion with articulating paper and adjust occlusion, if necessary.
   3. Resin-based sealants are most common and have superior retention compared with glass-ionomer–based sealants.
   4. The tag formation in the enamel is about 40 μm.
   5. Fluoride-containing sealants have similar retention rates as conventional sealants and show a 60% reduction of secondary caries.
   6. Any saliva contamination after isolation requires repeating the wash, dry, etch, wash, dry cycle.

References

Bishara WA: *Textbook of Orthodontics*, ed 3. Philadelphia, Saunders, 2001.

Bolton WA: Disharmony in tooth size and its relation to the analysis and treatment of malocclusion. *Am J Orthod* 28:113-130, 1958.

Casamassimo PS, et al: *Pediatric Dentistry, Infancy Through Adolescence*, ed 5. St. Louis, Mosby, 2012.

Ciancio SG, et al: *ADA Guide to Dental Therapeutics*, ed 5. Chicago, ADA, 2009.

Dean JA, Avery DR, McDonald RE: *McDonald and Avery's Dentistry for Children and Adolescents*, ed 9. St. Louis, Mosby, 2010.

Proffit WR, et al: *Contemporary Orthodontics*, ed 5. St. Louis, Mosby, 2013.

Sample Questions

1. Which of the following statements regarding crowding of the dentition is *true*?
   A. Crowding of the primary dentition usually resolves as the permanent teeth erupt.
   B. Spacing in the primary dentition usually indicates spacing will be present in the adult dentition.
   C. Approximately 15% of adolescents have crowding severe enough to consider extraction of permanent teeth as part of treatment.
   D. Lower incisor crowding is more common in African-American individuals than white individuals.

2. Bones of the cranial base include which of the following?
   A. Maxilla, mandible, and cranial vault
   B. Ethmoid, sphenoid, and occipital
   C. Palatal, nasal, and zygoma
   D. Frontal and parietal

3. According to Scammon's growth curves, which of the following tissues has a growth increase that can be used to help predict timing of the adolescent growth spurt?
   A. Neural tissues
   B. Lymphoid tissues
   C. Reproductive tissues

4. Children in the primary dentition most often present with a (an) _____.
   A. Increased overbite
   B. Decreased overbite
   C. Ideal overbite
   D. Significant open bite

5. An adult patient with a class II molar relationship and a cephalometric ANB angle of 2 degrees has which type of malocclusion?
   A. Class II dental malocclusion
   B. Class II skeletal malocclusion
   C. Class I dental malocclusion
   D. Class II skeletal malocclusion

6. Which of the following reactions is *least* likely to be observed during orthodontic treatment?
   A. Root resorption
   B. Devitalization of teeth that are moved
   C. Mobility of teeth that are moved
   D. Development of occlusal interferences

7. Doubling the force applied at the bracket of a tooth would have what effect on the moment affecting tooth movement?
   A. The moment would decrease by 50%
   B. The moment would not change
   C. The moment would double
   D. The moment would increase fourfold

8. Class II elastics are used by stretching an elastic between which of the two following points?
   A. From the posterior to the anterior within the maxillary arch
   B. From the posterior to the anterior within the mandibular arch
   C. From the posterior of the maxillary arch to the anterior of the mandibular arch
   D. From the posterior of the mandibular arch to the anterior of the maxillary arch

9. When class III elastics are used, the maxillary first molars _____.
   A. Move distally and intrude
   B. Move mesially and extrude
   C. Move mesially and intrude
   D. Move mesially only; there is no movement in the vertical direction

10. What is the usual order of extraction of teeth if serial extraction is chosen as the treatment to alleviate severe crowding?
    A. Primary second molars, primary first molars, permanent first premolars, primary canines
    B. Primary canines, primary first molars, permanent first premolars
    C. Primary first molars, primary second molars, primary canines
    D. Primary canines, permanent canines, primary first molars, permanent first premolars

11. A 7-year-old patient has a 4-mm maxillary midline diastema. Which of the following should be done?
    A. Brackets should be placed to close it.
    B. A radiograph should be taken to rule out the presence of a supernumerary tooth.
    C. Nothing should be done. It will close on its own.
    D. Nothing should be done. Treatment should be deferred until the rest of the permanent dentition erupts.

12. Reduction of overbite can be accomplished *most* readily by which of the following tooth movements?
    A. Intruding maxillary incisors
    B. Uprighting maxillary and mandibular incisors

C. Using a high-pull headgear to the maxillary molars

D. Using a lip bumper

13. Congenitally missing teeth are the result of failure in which stage of development?
    A. Initiation
    B. Morphodifferentiation
    C. Apposition
    D. Calcification

14. During an emergency dental visit in which a tooth is to be extracted because of extensive pulpal involvement, a moderately developmentally challenged 5-year-old child becomes physically combative. The parents are unable to calm the child. What should the dentist do?
    A. Discuss the situation with the parents.
    B. Force the nitrous oxide nosepiece over the child's mouth and nose.
    C. Use the hand over mouth exercise (HOME).
    D. Use a firm voice control.

15. Which of the following is the definition of conscious sedation?
    A. A minimally depressed level of consciousness that retains the patient's ability to maintain an airway independently and continuously and respond appropriately to physical stimulation or verbal command
    B. A significantly depressed level of consciousness in which the patient's ability to maintain an airway independently and continuously and respond appropriately to physical stimulation or verbal command is retained
    C. A minimally depressed level of consciousness in which the patient's ability to maintain an airway independently and continuously is retained

D. A significantly depressed level of consciousness in which the patient's ability to maintain an airway independently and continuously is retained

16. The enamel rods in the gingival third of primary teeth slope occlusally instead of cervically as in permanent teeth. The interproximal contacts of primary teeth are broader and flatter than the interproximal contacts of permanent teeth.
    A. The first statement is true, and the second statement is true.
    B. The first statement is true, and the second statement is false.
    C. The first statement is false, and the second statement is true.
    D. The first statement is false, and the second statement is false.

17. Formocresol has been shown to have a very good success rate when used as a medicament for pulpotomy procedures. Why is there continued interest to find another medicament that performs as well as or better than formocresol?
    A. Application of formocresol is a clinically time-consuming procedure.
    B. Formocresol is toxic, and there is the possibility of blood-borne spread to vital organs.
    C. It has been demonstrated that formocresol may cause spontaneous abortion.
    D. It has been demonstrated that formocresol may cause failure to develop adequate lung capacity in children.

18. The following teeth are erupted in an 8-year-old patient. What is the space maintenance of choice?

3	A	B	C	7	8	9	10	H	I		14
30	T	S	R	26	25	24	23	M	L	K	19

A. Band-loop space maintainer

B. Lower lingual holding arch

C. Nance holding arch

D. Distal shoe space maintainer

19. The mother of a 5-year-old patient is concerned about the child's thumb-sucking habit. On examination 6 months ago, the patient had a 5-mm overjet and a 3-mm anterior open bite. Today, the patient has a 10% overbite and a 3.5-mm overjet. The mother says that the child only sucks his thumb every night when falling to sleep. Which of the following is the best advice?
    A. Refer to a speech pathologist
    B. Recommend tongue thrust therapy
    C. Recommend a thumb-sucking appliance
    D. Counsel the parent regarding thumb sucking, and recall the patient in 3 months

20. Which of the following statements regarding orthodontic closure of a midline diastema in a patient with a heavy maxillary frenum is *true*?
    A. Orthodontic closure is accomplished before frenum surgery.
    B. Orthodontic closure is accomplished after frenum surgery.
    C. After orthodontic closure, frenum surgery is typically not indicated.
    D. After frenum surgery, orthodontic closure is typically not indicated.

21. In a 4-year-old patient, tooth E was traumatically intruded, and approximately 50% of the crown is visible clinically. What is the treatment of choice?
    A. Reposition and splint
    B. Reposition, splint, and primary endodontics
    C. Reposition, splint, and formocresol pulpotomy
    D. None of the above

22. In a 4-year-old patient, the maxillary right primary central incisor was traumatically avulsed 60 minutes ago. What is the treatment of choice?
    A. Replant, splint, and primary endodontics
    B. Replant, splint, and formocresol pulpotomy
    C. Replant, no splint, and primary endodontics
    D. None of the above

23. A young permanent incisor with an open apex has a pinpoint exposure as a result of a traumatic injury that occurred 24 hours previously. Which of the following is the *best* treatment?
    A. Place calcium hydroxide on the pinpoint exposure
    B. Open the pulp chamber to find healthy pulp tissue and perform a pulpotomy
    C. Initiate a calcium hydroxide pulpectomy
    D. Initiate conventional root canal treatment with gutta-percha

24. A permanent incisor with an open apex is extruded 4 mm following an injury 15 minutes ago. What is the treatment of choice?
    A. No immediate treatment; monitor closely for vitality
    B. Reposition, splint, and monitor closely for vitality
    C. Reposition, splint, and initiate calcium hydroxide pulpotomy
    D. Reposition, splint, and initiate calcium hydroxide pulpectomy

25. Which of the following is the *most* likely cause of pulpal necrosis after trauma to a tooth?
    A. Ankylosis
    B. Calcific metamorphosis
    C. Pulpal hyperemia
    D. Dilaceration

26. Order the sequence of events that occur when heavy orthodontic forces are placed on teeth.
    ____ A. The PDL experiences compression on the side toward which the tooth is moving
    ____ B. The alveolar bone experiences undermining resorption
    ____ C. The PDL undergoes hyalinization
    ____ D. Frontal resorption occurs at the surface of the alveolus

27. Which of the following orthodontic wire types would be the *best* choice for a patient with a known nickel allergy?
    A. Stainless steel
    B. Nickel titanium
    C. Beta titanium
    D. Multistranded cobalt chromium

28. The nature of the bond between the enamel and the resin used to attach an orthodontic bracket is _____.
    A. Chemical
    B. Mechanical
    C. Dependent on whether the resin used is light-cured or chemically cured
    D. Dependent on whether the surface preparation used is conventional etch or self-etch primer

29. In general, the width of the incisors in the primary dentition is smaller than the width of their successors in the permanent dentition. This is called the "leeway space" and provides room for eruption of the permanent incisors.
    A. Both statements are true.
    B. Both statements are false.
    C. The first statement is true, and the second statement is false.
    D. The first statement is false, and the second statement is true.

30. A wire with a low load/deflection rate is capable of generating constant forces that do not depend much on the amount of activation. Bending loops into an archwire reduces its load/deflection rate by increasing wire length.
    A. Both statements are true.
    B. Both statements are false.
    C. The first statement is true, and the second statement is false.
    D. The first statement is false, and the second statement is true.

31. Which of the following statements *best* describes the prognosis of a 12-year-old boy with moderate mandibular anterior crowding whose permanent dentition is fully erupted?
    A. Crowding is likely to improve as the arches expand during the adolescent growth spurt.
    B. Crowding is likely to improve as the mandible continues to grow anteriorly during the adolescent growth spurt.
    C. Crowding is likely to improve as resorption of the anterior portion of the ramus occurs over time.
    D. Crowding is not likely to improve over time.

32. Match the exhibited behavior of a child dental patient with the classification of potentially cooperative patient.

Exhibited Behavior	Classification
____ A. Gripping the arms of the chair very tightly	1. Timid
____ B. Patient says "I don't want to" and does not open the mouth	2. Defiant
____ C. Temper tantrum	3. Tense-cooperative
____ D. Shielding behavior	4. Uncontrolled

33. Order the four plateaus of stage I anesthesia (analgesia).

_____ A. Drift
_____ B. Paresthesia
_____ C. Dream
_____ D. Vasomotor

34. Which of the following are characteristics of primary tooth anatomy? (Choose three.)
   A. Occlusal table is wider
   B. Enamel is thinner
   C. Greater constriction at the cementoenamel junction
   D. Interproximal contacts are broader and flatter
   E. Enamel rods in gingival third slope cervically
   F. Pulp chamber is relatively smaller

35. Which of the following are likely contraindications for performing a pulpotomy on a primary molar? (Choose three.)
   A. A patient requiring infective endocarditis antibiotic premedication
   B. A 3-year-old patient
   C. Swelling associated with the tooth
   D. Furcation radiolucency
   E. Marginal ridge breakdown owing to extensive decay
   F. A patient with amelogenesis imperfecta
   G. A 5-year-old patient with a pinpoint carious pulp exposure

Patient Management

OSCAR AREVALO, MYRON ALLUKIAN, JR.,
MARCIA W. DEIBLER, CATHERINE FRANKL SARKIS

OUTLINE

1. Epidemiology
2. Prevention of Oral Diseases
3. Evaluation of Dental Literature
4. Infection Control
5. Materials and Equipment Safety
6. Dental Care Delivery Systems
7. Communication and Interpersonal Skills
8. Health Behavior Change
9. Anxiety and Pain Control
10. Professional Responsibilities and Liabilities

Charles-Edward Amory Winslow's (1877-1957) definition of *public health* is perhaps the most widely accepted and quoted. Winslow defined public health as "the science and art of preventing disease, prolonging life, and promoting physical health and efficiency through organized community efforts."

Today, a public health problem is defined as an issue that meets the following criteria:

- A condition or situation that is widespread and has an actual or potential cause of morbidity or mortality.
- There is a perception on the part of the public, government, or public health authorities that the condition is a public health problem.

Dental public health has been defined by the American Board of Dental Public Health as follows: "The science and art of preventing and controlling dental diseases and promoting dental health through organized community efforts. It is that form of dental practice which serves the community as a patient rather than the individual. It is concerned with the dental education of the public, with applied dental research, and with the administration of group dental care programs as well as the prevention and control of dental diseases on a community basis."

Material for this review is drawn from the texts *Dentistry, Dental Practice, and the Community*, ed 6, by Burt and Eklund; *Management of Pain & Anxiety in the Dental Office*, ed 5, by Dionne et al; *Jong's Community Dental Health*, ed 5, by Gluck and Morganstein; and *Wong's Essentials of Pediatric Nursing*, ed 7, by Wong et al. Please consult these texts and the other references included at the end of this review for more detailed information. All of the above-mentioned texts are listed in full in the References.

1.0 Epidemiology

Epidemiology is the study of the distribution and determinants of disease. In public health, groups of people are studied to answer questions about etiology of diseases, prevention, disease patterns, and allocation of resources.

A. Epidemiologic measures.
1. *DMFT/DMFS*—the conventional method of defining dental caries in a population is to measure either the number of teeth or the number of tooth surfaces that are decayed, missing, or filled as a result of caries. When this measure is applied to the permanent dentition, the acronyms DMFT and DMFS are used; when this measure is applied to the primary dentition, the acronyms *deft* and *defs* are used, with *e* indicating a carious primary tooth that is indicated for extraction. Measuring caries by affected surfaces (i.e., DMFS or DFS) is more precise than measuring caries by affected teeth.
   a. Problems associated with caries indices.
      (1) Not related to number of teeth at risk or age.
      (2) Can be invalid in older adults.
      (3) Preventive restorations.
      (4) Sealants.
2. *Gingival index (GI)*—the GI of Löe and Silness uses six indicator teeth or all erupted teeth. Scoring is on

The section editor acknowledges Bonnie Graham, JD, for her contributions as author of the section on Professional Responsibilities and Liabilities in the first edition of this book. Bonnie, who passed away in 2010, was a fabulous faculty, mentor, and surrogate mother to dozens of dental students.

a scale of 0 to 3, with 0 being normal and 3 being ulcerated tissue with a tendency toward spontaneous bleeding. The GI grades the gingiva on the mesial, distal, buccal, and lingual surfaces of the teeth. The GI has been used on selected teeth in the mouth as well as on all erupted teeth. The GI assigns grades by applying a four-category qualitative assessment (normal, mild, moderate, or severe inflammation) to four sites on each examined tooth. These values can be averaged to yield a score for the individual.

3. *Periodontal indices*—several indices have been developed in an attempt to provide a standardized method of measuring periodontal disease among groups of people in epidemiologic studies, most notably the periodontal index and the periodontal disease index. However, both of these indices have been criticized because they combine gingivitis and periodontitis measures into a common score. For this reason, these indices are not considered the best methods to measure periodontal disease.

   a. The Community Periodontal Index of Treatment Needs (CPITN), developed by the World Health Organization to summarize treatment needs, combines an assessment of gingival health, pocket depth, and the presence of supragingival and subgingival calculus. Proponents of the CPITN state that the CPITN allows for a rapid, simple, uniform method by which the average periodontal status and treatment needs of populations can be determined using minimal equipment. Critics of the CPITN, including the American Academy of Periodontology, argue that combining gingival health, pocket depth, and presence of calculus into one score is inconsistent with current approaches to describing periodontal disease and that failure of the CPITN to measure gingival recession leads to an inaccurate estimate of attachment loss.

4. *Simplified Oral Hygiene Index (OHI-S)*—the OHI-S sets forth a method of quantifying the amount of plaque and calculus in its two components, the debris index and the calculus index. These components are added to obtain a single score. The OHI-S has been widely used in surveys. It is quick and practical, although its lack of sensitivity makes it less useful in the individual patient than in a group.

B. Epidemiology of oral diseases.

1. *Caries*—a pathologic process of localized destruction of tooth tissues by microorganisms.

   a. *Caries in children*—important changes have occurred in the prevalence of dental caries in the United States. The prevalence of caries in the United States declined substantially from the early 1970s until the mid-1990s as a result of fluoridation, the use of fluorides, and other preventive measures. From the mid-1990s until the most recent (1999-2004) National Health and Nutrition Examination Survey (NHANES), among children 2 to 11 years old, this trend has reversed: a small but significant increase in primary decay was found. This trend reversal was more severe in younger children.

   b. *Early childhood caries (ECC)*—previously called "baby bottle tooth decay," ECC is caused by inappropriate feeding practices that result in progressive dental caries on the buccal and lingual surfaces of newly erupted primary maxillary anterior teeth of infants and toddlers. The current best estimate of ECC prevalence in the United States is approximately 5% nationwide. The U.S. Centers for Disease Control and Prevention (CDC) reported in 2005 that more than 28% of pre–school age children have experienced tooth decay. This figure suggests that more than 4 million children are affected nationwide—an increase of more than 600,000 additional preschoolers over a decade. However, the literature indicates important ECC prevalence difference across children of different race, ethnic, and socioeconomic backgrounds, with ethnic minority and lower socioeconomic status children being at greatest risk.

   c. *Coronal caries in adults*—the prevalence of coronal caries has declined in recent decades among U.S. adults. However, more than 90% of U.S. adults older than 20 years of age have at least one decayed or filled tooth. The prevalence of caries among dentate adults 20 years and older increases with age until 59 years old, after which it plateaus at approximately 30 decayed and filled surfaces. Data from U.S. national surveys of adults indicate that among dentate adults older than 20, the mean number of decayed and filled permanent teeth (DFT) was 8.0 and the mean decayed and filled permanent surfaces (DFS) was 20.9. Similarly, it has been determined that whites have significantly higher coronal DFS compared with nonwhites. For instance, according to data from NHANES 1999-2002, whites had a mean coronal DFS twice as high as African-Americans (i.e., 23.1 surfaces in whites versus 12.1 surfaces in African-Americans).

   d. *Root surface caries*—according to NHANES 1998-2002, approximately 18% of dentate adults older than 20 had root caries. Although the prevalence has decreased compared with previous national surveys, root surface caries is three times higher among adults 60 years and older compared with adults younger than 40. This prevalence is lower for whites compared with other racial groups.

2. *Periodontal diseases*—Loe defined periodontal disease as "a group of lesions affecting the tissues surrounding and supporting the teeth in their sockets." Most cases of periodontal disease can be classified as either gingivitis or periodontitis.

a. *Gingivitis*—the prevalence of gingivitis among school-age children has been reported to be 40% to 60%. National survey data suggest that the prevalence of gingivitis declines from its highest prevalence during the second and third decades and remains relatively constant after age 30. According to NHANES III, among the U.S. population 20 years and older, the prevalence of gingivitis was 53%.

b. *Chronic periodontitis*—chronic periodontitis is the most common form of periodontitis. The prevalence, extent, and severity increase with age. A study that used NHANES 2009-2010 data indicated that the total prevalence of periodontitis in adults 30 and older was 47.2%. This figure represents about 64.7 million adults 30 and older in the United States. According to the same study, periodontitis ranged from 24.4% in adults 30 to 34 to 70.1% in adults 65 and older.

3. *Oral cancer*—according to the National Cancer Institute, 41,380 (29,620 men and 11,760 women) new cases would be diagnosed and 7890 men and women would die of cancer of the oral cavity and pharynx in 2013. Most of these are epidermoid carcinomas and squamous cell carcinomas. Surveillance, Epidemiology, and End Results (SEER) data (2006-2010) indicate that the annual age-adjusted incidence of oral and pharyngeal cancer in the United States is 10.8 new cases per 100,000. These rates vary substantially by gender, with men showing an annual age-adjusted incidence rate of 16.2 per 100,000 compared with 6.2 per 100,000 for women. In the United States, oral cancer represents about 4% of all cancers and 2.2% of all cancer deaths. The incidence of oral and pharyngeal cancers increases with age and alcohol or tobacco use and is uncommon before age 40. The overall rate of new cases of disease has been stable in more recent years. However, there has been a more recent increase in cases of oropharyngeal cancer linked to infection with human papillomavirus.

Cancers of the lip and oral cavity account for approximately two thirds of all new oral and pharyngeal cancers, with the tongue being the most common site of incident cancers of the oral cavity. According to SEER, in 2006-2010, whites had a higher incidence of oral and pharyngeal cancers compared with other racial groups.

From 2006-2010, the median age at diagnosis of cancer of the oral cavity and pharynx was 62 years, and the median age at death was 67. Overall, the 5-year survival rate for oral and pharyngeal cancers is approximately 63%. However, survival rates vary considerably depending on gender and race. For instance, 5-year survival rates for white Americans is 64.7% compared with 44.5% for African-Americans.

Among African-Americans, the 5-year survival rates are 51.6% for women versus 42.9% for men. In 2010, approximately 275,193 individuals had a history of cancer of the oral cavity and pharynx—181,084 men and 94,109 women.

2.0 Prevention of Oral Diseases

A. Introduction.
1. Prevention is classified into three different levels.
   a. *Primary prevention*—prevents the disease before it occurs. This level includes health education, disease prevention, and health protection. Examples include community water fluoridation and sealants. Preventing a disease *before* it occurs is the most effective way to improve health and control costs.
   b. *Secondary prevention*—eliminates or reduces diseases *after* they occur. Examples include amalgam and composite restorations. This level requires more resources than primary prevention and is more costly.
   c. *Tertiary prevention*—limits a disability from a disease or rehabilitates an individual in later stages to restore tissues after the failure of secondary prevention; this is the most costly type of prevention for an individual. Examples include dentures, crowns, and bridges.
2. Prevention may be on a community or population basis or individual basis. Table 6-1 provides an overview of effective community and individual preventive measures for dental caries prevention. Only effective or evidence-based preventive measures should be used.
   a. On a community level, preventive measures may be implemented in a school, neighborhood, city, town, state, or nation. Prevention on a community level is usually the most cost-effective and most practical, because everyone in the target population benefits, such as in a school fluoride or sealant prevention program or a fluoridated community.
   b. On an individual basis, preventive measures may be implemented in a dental office or community setting. On an individual level in a dental office, the person needs to be motivated to seek out the service and have the ability to pay for the service. These requirements limit access to preventive services for some individuals.
B. Community-based and school-based prevention.
1. *Community water fluoridation*—the CDC has recognized community water fluoridation as "one of the ten great public health achievements of the twentieth century." Community water fluoridation refers to the adjustment of the concentration of fluoride of a community water supply for optimal oral health. The

Table 6-1

Effective Community and Individual Preventive Measures for Dental Caries Prevention

MEASURE	METHOD OF APPLICATION	TARGET	PERIOD OF USE
Community Programs			
Community water fluoridation	Systemic	Entire population	Lifetime
School water fluoridation	Systemic	Schoolchildren	School years
School fluoride tablet program	Systemic	Schoolchildren	Age 5-16 yr
School fluoride rinse program	Topical	Schoolchildren	Age 5-16 yr
School sealant program (professionally applied)	Topical	Schoolchildren	Age 6-8 and 12-14 yr
Individual Approach			
Prescribed fluoride tablets or drops	Systemic	Children	Age 6 mo–6 yr
Professionally applied fluoride treatment	Topical	Individual need	High-risk populations
Over-the-counter treatments	Topical	Individual need	High-risk populations
Fluoride toothpaste	Topical	Entire population	Lifetime
Professionally applied dental sealants	Topical	Children	Age 6-8 and 12-14 yr

From Gluck GM, Morganstein WM: Jong's Community Dental Health, ed 5. St. Louis, Mosby, 2002.

recommended level of fluoride for a community water supply in the United States ranges from 0.7 to 1.2 parts per million (ppm) of fluoride, depending on the mean maximum daily air temperature over a 5-year period. In the United States, most communities are fluoridated at approximately 1 ppm, which is equivalent to 1.0 mg of fluoride per liter of water. Based on epidemiologic studies of communities that were naturally fluoridated, community water fluoridation was first initiated as a clinical trial in 1945 in Grand Rapids, Michigan, on a trial basis.

In 2012, there were more than 210 million Americans living in fluoridated communities, or about 74% of the U.S. population living in areas with public water supplies. In 2011, the U.S. Department of Health and Human Services (DHHS) proposed decreasing the recommended levels of fluoride to 0.7 ppm because more recent data have shown that over time, water consumption is relatively the same regardless of the air temperature of a community. As of March 2014, this change has not been implemented, but it is expected to be in the near future. At 0.7 ppm or 1.0 ppm, fluoridated water is safe, odorless, colorless, and tasteless. Of all the measures used to prevent dental caries in the United States, water fluoridation is the most economical and cost-effective.

Fluoridation is considered the foundation for better oral health for a community. The effectiveness of fluoridation is well documented, and water fluoridation prevents tooth decay for people of all ages. Early studies demonstrated that fluoridation prevents 50% to 70% of caries in the permanent teeth of children. However, because of the widespread use

of many other fluoride-containing products now available, such as fluoride rinses, toothpastes, and professionally applied treatments, in the United States, the measurable effectiveness of community water fluoridation in the United States is about 20% to 40%. These fluoride products have an additive preventive benefit to fluoridation.

All health care providers have a responsibility to educate their patients about the safety and effectiveness of community water fluoridation, whether or not their community is fluoridated, in addition to other preventive measures.

2. *School water fluoridation*—school water fluoridation was developed and tested in the United States in the 1960s for use in rural schools with an independent water supply. Fluoridation of water supplies of individual schools is similar to community water fluoridation in that no direct action is required of beneficiaries other than direct consumption of or use of the water in food preparation. The major difference is that the recommended concentration for school water fluoridation is 4.5 times the concentration of fluoride recommended for community water supplies in the respective geographic area. The higher concentrations are recommended to compensate for part-time exposure because children spend only part of their time at school. Studies conducted on school fluoridation have shown that a 20% to 30% reduction in caries can be expected when children have consumed school water fluoridation for 12 years. The practicality of school water fluoridation is good when a community *does not* have a central water supply. All the children benefit with no individual effort required on the part of the recipient.

3. *Salt fluoridation*—in countries that do not have a safe public water supply or where community water fluoridation is not practical or feasible, community salt fluoridation may be used. Salt fluoridation is the controlled addition of fluoride during the manufacturing of salt for use by humans. Fluoride is added to salt products such as the salt used domestically, table salt, baker's salt, and salt distributed in bulk quantities to the food industry. The recommended fluoride concentration ranges from 200 to 350 mg of fluoride per 1 kg of salt, depending on the community's or country's circumstances. Community salt fluoridation has benefits similar to water fluoridation and can prevent dental caries by 33% to 66%. The combination of both salt fluoridation and water fluoridation in a community or country is not recommended. Salt fluoridation is not used in the United States.

4. *Fluoride supplements*—fluoride supplements are available only by prescription and are intended for use by children at risk for dental caries who live in nonfluoridated areas. For optimal benefits, use of fluoride supplements should begin when a child is 6 months old and be continued daily until the child is 16 years old. The need for taking fluoride supplements over an extended period of time makes dietary fluoride supplements less cost-effective than water fluoridation; fluoride supplements are considerably less practical as a widespread alternative to water fluoridation as a public health measure.

   Before prescribing any fluoride supplement, an accurate assessment of all potential sources of fluoride intake should be explored. Fluoridated water may be consumed from sources other than the home water supply, such as the workplace, school or day care, bottled water, filtered water, and from processed beverages and foods prepared with fluoridated water. If the daily intake of fluoride is insufficient, parents should be informed that small daily dosages are beneficial to a child's teeth.

   a. *Fluoride drops*—fluoride supplementation can best be accomplished initially by the use of fluoride drops. Around the age of 3, the drops can be replaced by chewable fluoride tablets or lozenges. For children in the first 3 years of life, studies show 47% less caries experience in the primary teeth and 43% less for 3- to 6-year-olds.

   b. *Tablets and lozenges*—another method for administering systemic fluoride is in school settings by the daily use of dietary fluoride supplements in the form of chewable tablets or lozenges. Supervised, self-administered use of fluoride tablets is a well-established regimen that has been used in the United States and abroad for more than 47 years. Lozenges and chewable fluoride tablets provide topical and systemic benefits. Studies conducted in the United States have shown that the daily use of fluoride tablets on school days provides up to a 30% reduction in new carious lesions.

   Because the daily compliance required for this regimen at home on an individual basis for 16 years may be more than most parents can achieve, this preventive method often is used in schools on a classroom basis. The daily consumption of fluoride tablets or lozenges in school settings is an excellent method to use in areas where the water is fluoride-deficient.

   See the Pedodontics section for fluoride supplementation chart.

   c. *Fluoride mouth rinse*—fluoride mouth rinse has been used in schools in the United States for approximately 4 decades, and it is the most popular school-based fluoride regimen in the United States. Fluoride rinse solutions are used to provide the tooth enamel surface with a constant supply of fluoride ions, which help remineralize initial carious lesions. This method is recommended only for children 6 years old or older because younger children may swallow the solution. For this reason, fluoride rinse solutions are not appropriate for the treatment of infants with ECC. The rinsing is generally supervised in classrooms by teachers or adult volunteers. This procedure is usually not used in schools in communities that have been fluoridated for 3 or more years.

   Numerous studies have demonstrated that dental caries can be prevented by approximately 25% to 28% by rinsing daily or weekly in school with dilute solutions of fluoride. Rinsing *weekly* with a 0.2% neutral sodium fluoride (NaF) solution requires fewer supplies and less time than *daily* rinsing with a 0.05% NaF solution

5. *Sealants*—a fissure sealant is a plastic, professionally applied material used to occlude the pits and fissures of teeth. The objective is to provide a physical barrier to the impaction of substrate for cariogenic bacteria in those crevices and to prevent caries from developing. Sealants are recommended for the first and second permanent molars for children at risk for dental caries. Sealants also can halt the carious process after it has begun and can be used as a form of prevention or treatment for incipient caries in pits and fissures.

   The use of fluorides is the best approach to preventing caries. However, fluoride is believed to be least effective on the occlusal or chewing tooth surfaces. Because most decay among school-age children occurs on the chewing surfaces, pit and fissure sealants are needed to provide nearly total caries prevention. The effectiveness of dental sealants on permanent first molars has been reported to be 71.3% for 5 years and 65% for 9 years after the initial application of the sealant.

6. *Topical fluoride*—the application of topical fluoride to the teeth increases tooth resistance to caries, especially on smooth surfaces. It is more effective for individuals at high risk for tooth decay. The fluoride can be delivered either brushed as a varnish or in a tray as a gel. Topical fluoride applications are not usually cost-effective in community-based or school-based prevention programs. Fluoride gels are discussed in the office-based preventive methods section.

   a. *Fluoride varnishes*—fluoride varnishes were accepted for use in the United States in 1994 and are used in place of topical fluoride solutions or gels when they are easier to apply. Fluoride varnish is considered a vehicle for holding fluoride in close contact with the tooth for a longer period of time, but it is not a substitute for dental fissure sealants. A theoretical advantage of varnishes over other methods of professional fluoride application is that varnishes are adhesive and should maximize fluoride contact with the tooth surface. Varnishes are a way of using high fluoride concentrations in small amounts of material.

   Tooth decay prevention by fluoride varnishes is expected to be similar to other topical fluorides. In primary teeth, the range is 18% to 25%. Fluoride varnishes may be especially useful to prevent root surface caries among the growing number of older adults who have gingival recession. In addition, fluoride varnishes may be especially practical for use with very young children, elderly adults, individuals with disabilities, and bed-bound patients who still have their own teeth. Fluoride varnishes are also used in programs to help prevent infant caries or ECC in high-risk children. Most states allow physicians to provide varnishes to at-risk children in their offices.

7. *Mouth guards*—mouth guards may be made for athletes as a community program in the schools or on an individual basis in the dental office. See Pedodontics section.

8. *Health education and health literacy.*

   a. Health education is necessary at all stages of designing, implementing, evaluating, and continuing oral health programs. The scope of health education may include educational interventions for children, parents, policy makers, or health care providers. Education of all relevant groups is a critical factor in the process to gain acceptance and use of preventive measures, although education alone cannot function as a method to prevent disease. Knowledge is a confidence-building element. Lacking appropriate knowledge, individuals can neither make nor be expected to make intelligent decisions about their oral health or, in the case of decision makers, for the oral health of their constituents.

   b. Health literacy is the capacity at which individuals obtain, process, and understand basic health information and services. It is an important skill for both patients and oral health professionals in preventing and managing diseases and for navigating the health care system to facilitate access.

C. Office-based preventive measures—office-based measures include sealants, topical fluoride, fluoride supplements, and health education. Sealants, supplements, and health education were discussed previously. Only topical fluoride gels and foams are discussed in this section.

   1. *Fluoride gels and foams*—the fluoride gel compounds that dental professionals routinely use in tray applications are highly concentrated. Careful attention is required for the technique, the amounts used, and the 4-minute exposure time. Fluoride gels and foams prevent tooth decay by about 26% on permanent teeth of children living in nonfluoridated communities. Professional gel tray applications have long been considered not to be cost-effective for public health programs, although they might be a reasonable approach for highly susceptible special groups in targeted initiatives.

   Since the early 1960s, acidulated phosphate fluoride (APF) has become the most widely used fluoride compound for professional application. APF has a pH of about 3.0 and was developed after experimental work showed that the topical uptake of fluoride by enamel was greater in an acidic environment. The agent has been tested in several concentrations, the most common being 1.23% fluoride, usually as NaF, in orthophosphoric acid. The material is nonirritating and nonstaining, tolerates the addition of flavorings, and is well accepted by patients.

   Procedures for the professional application of fluoride agents were originally developed on the assumption that the fluoride would form a fluorapatite in the crystalline structure of the enamel. A prophylactic treatment was considered mandatory before the application of the fluoride to maximize this reaction. Subsequent research showed that high-concentration fluoride, such as that in APF gels, tends to form a "calcium fluoride–like" material on the enamel surface and serves as a reservoir of fluoride that becomes available for remineralization when pH decreases. As a result of the formation of this calcium fluoride–like material, a prophylaxis before a professional fluoride application is unnecessary because it is no more beneficial than toothbrushing and flossing by the patient.

D. Home-based preventive methods—home-based methods include brushing, interdental cleaning, diet, fluoride gels, and fluoride mouth rinses (discussed previously).

1. *Brushing*—dental plaque has been depicted as the root cause of both caries and periodontal disease. Brushing is an individual approach for mechanical plaque removal and aids in removing the source of tooth decay.

   a. In terms of frequency of brushing to prevent periodontal disease, the limited existing information indicates that a thorough oral cleansing should be carried out at 24- to 48-hour intervals. Considering the time needed for plaque to mature bacteriologically, brushing after every meal is unnecessary to prevent gingivitis. But because toothbrushing with a fluoride toothpaste is also a major source of fluoride exposure for caries prevention, it is best carried out at least twice per day using a pea-sized amount of fluoride toothpaste to maintain oral health. Brushing in the morning and evening fits with most people's daily routines and should be the basis for education of the public and dental patients. For children younger than age 6, brushing with fluoridated toothpaste should be supervised by an adult to avoid unnecessary toothpaste ingestion.

2. *Interdental cleaning*—there is limited evidence that interdental cleaning, by floss or interdental brushes, reduces interdental gingivitis and plaque more than toothbrushing by itself. The rationale for supplementing toothbrushing with use of dental floss, interdental brushes, or wood points to clean below the contact areas is that even assiduous use of the toothbrush usually cannot penetrate these areas efficiently. Flossing does not prevent tooth decay but may be helpful for gingival health.

3. *Diet*—the precise cariogenicity of any food is not easily predicted. Controlling dental caries through diet modification is complex and has been only moderately successful. Adequate oral hygiene immediately after the ingestion of cariogenic foods and reducing the consumption of cariogenic food may be helpful in reducing the incidence of dental caries. When there is a general decline in the incidence of caries, there is a weaker association between sugar consumption and the incidence of caries, especially when there is an optimal concentration of fluoride in the drinking water. In general, it is more important to control the frequency of sugar consumption and whether it is consumed during daytime activity or immediately before bedtime and the length of time that residual food material, especially sticky sweets, remain in the mouth after eating. A diet that is generous in vegetables and fruits and is light in processed foods is recognized universally as compatible with general health and dental health.

4. *Fluoride gels*—fluoride gels for home use are available as additional measures to help achieve caries control. These gels contain either stannous fluoride (0.4%) or NaF (1.0%) and are formulated in a nonaqueous gel base that does not contain an abrasive system. Recommended use involves toothbrushing with gel (similar to using a dentifrice), allowing the gel to remain in the oral cavity for 4 minutes, and then expectorating thoroughly. Fluoride gels for home use are an adjunct to the use of professional, topical fluoride application and fluoride dentifrices as a collective means of achieving caries control in patients who are especially prone to caries formation.

3.0 Evaluation of Dental Literature

A. *Types of studies*—epidemiologic studies can be organized into three categories: descriptive, analytical, and experimental.

1. *Descriptive epidemiology*—descriptive epidemiology is used to quantify disease status in the community. However, for disease quantification to be descriptive of a group, it must be seen in proportion to it. The major parameters of interest are prevalence and incidence.

   a. *Prevalence*—indicates what proportion of a given population is affected by a condition at a given point in time. It is expressed as percentage and ranges from 0% to 100% (e.g., the prevalence of periodontal disease among 100,000 adolescents was 5%).

$$\text{Prevalence} = \frac{\text{Number of people with the disease}}{\text{Total number of people at risk}}$$

   b. *Incidence*—indicates the number of new cases that are expected to occur within a population over a period of time (e.g., the incidence of people dying of oral cancer is 10% per year in men 55 to 59 in our community).

$$\text{Incidence} = \frac{\text{Number of new cases of the disease}}{\text{Total number of people at risk}}$$

2. *Analytical epidemiology*—also called *observational epidemiology*, analytical epidemiology is used to determine the etiology of a disease. The researcher tries to establish a causal relationship between the factors and disease. Three study designs are commonly used: cross-sectional study, case-control study, and cohort study (prospective and retrospective).

   a. *Cross-sectional study*—study in which the health conditions in a group of people who are, or are assumed to be, a sample of a particular population (a cross section) is assessed at *one time*. Consider the hypothesis that drinking alcohol increases the risk of developing oral cancer. If researchers chose to conduct a cross-sectional study to explore this hypothesis, they might examine a group of men who drink alcohol and compare the occurrence of oral cancer among men who are not alcohol drinkers. The researchers could then determine whether there is an association between the presence of oral cancer and alcohol. Although this study is relatively quick and inexpensive, its potential to contribute to a judgment of causation is limited because it cannot determine whether the outcome (in this case, oral cancer) occurred before the men started drinking or if it developed as a result of some other cause (e.g., metastasis).

b. *Case-control study*—people with a condition ("cases") are compared with people without it ("controls") but who are similar in other characteristics. Hypothesized causal exposures are sought in the past medical records of the participants. If the researchers had chosen to conduct a case-control study to explore the same hypothesis, subjects would have been split into two groups—subjects with oral cancer and subjects without it, based on examinations. To search for an association with alcohol drinking, a history before the occurrence of oral cancer would be sought (e.g., through past medical records). The case-control study could establish a temporal relationship between the exposure and disease of interest, in this case, a history of alcohol drinking before the appearance of oral cancer.

c. Cohort study.

   (1) *Prospective cohort study*—a general population is followed through time to see who develops the disease, and the various exposure factors that affected the group are evaluated. In this case, the investigators choose or define a sample of subjects who do not yet have the outcome of interest, such as oral cancer. The investigators measure risk factors in each subject (e.g., habits) that may predict the subsequent outcome. They follow these subjects with periodic surveys or examinations to detect the outcome or outcomes of interest. Following the group over a period of time, the investigators describe the prevalence of outcomes (e.g., oral cancer) in the cohort. They then compare the prevalence of the disease in men who drink alcohol with the prevalence of men who do not drink.

   (2) *Retrospective cohort study*—used to evaluate the effect that a specific exposure has had on a population (e.g., occupational hazards). Investigators choose or define a sample of subjects who had the outcome of interest. They measure risk factors in each subject that may have predicted the subsequent outcome.

3. *Experimental epidemiology*—experimental epidemiology is used primarily in intervention studies. When etiology has been established, the researchers try to determine the effectiveness of a particular program

of prevention or therapy. There are two types: clinical trials and community trials.

a. *Clinical trials*—Clinical trials attempt to evaluate the effects of a treatment. A clinical trial aims to isolate one factor (e.g., a new drug) and examine its contribution to a patient's health by holding all other factors as constant as possible. Well-designed clinical trials use a double-blind design in which neither the subject nor the investigator knows to which group a subject belongs. This design helps prevent the potential for a biased interpretation of treatment effect (better or worse) that might occur if either the investigator or the subject knew to which treatment group (i.e., placebo or experimental agent) a subject belonged. Clinical trials compare the incidence of disease and side effects between the groups in the study to draw inferences about the safety and efficacy of the treatment or treatments under investigation.

b. *Community trials*—in a community trial, the group as a whole is studied rather than the individuals in it. The more similar the communities, the more valid the results. A known example of a community trial was the 1945 Newburgh-Kingston water fluoridation trial. In this study, NaF was added to the water of Newburgh, New York, and DMFT was compared with Kingston, New York, which was nonfluoridated.

B. Components of a scientific article—following is the standard format of most of the scientific research that appears in journals.

1. *Title*—the title of the study briefly indicates the topic and the focus of the study. The text of the title should reflect or indicate the central question being posed.

2. *Abstract*—the purpose of the abstract is to allow the reader to determine quickly whether the study is of interest. The abstract, which usually appears at the head of the article and is often reproduced in the literature database, summarizes the background and focus of the study, the population sampled or objects studied, and the experimental design. It also includes a brief statement of the findings and the conclusions. In addition, the abstract may include key words that allow the study to be indexed in the database.

3. *Introduction, literature review, and hypothesis*—in the introduction, the researcher attempts to educate the reader regarding the importance and the history of the problem. Past controversies are summarized, and the question is clarified. In the literature review, the researcher provides a summary of the field to date. It is the obligation of the researcher to make the reader aware of the relevant past research and findings; to define the key issues, variables, and questions involved; and to create a context and rationale for the current study. The theory being tested is stated, and the rival hypotheses are reviewed. Finally, the

researcher clearly states the research question or the hypotheses being tested.

4. *Methods*—the methods section organizes the research article and allows the reader to assess the validity of the study and the reliability of the measures. The reader should be provided with specific and detailed information regarding how the study was conducted. From this description, the reader should be able to replicate the study. This section, combined with the results section, provides the reader an opportunity to develop an independent understanding of what this research study has found and to evaluate the legitimacy of the conclusions offered by the author at the conclusion of the report. Although the author may be tempted to interpret or extend the study findings in the discussion and conclusion sections, the reader should be able to develop an independent conclusion after reviewing the methods and results section. The methods section usually includes four subsections:

   a. *Sampling strategy*—provides a description of the sampling strategy, the sample size, and the methods for assigning samples to conditions.

   b. *Measurement strategies and measurement instruments*—how the variables are measured determines exactly what is being studied. Although the variables studied are discussed in the abstract, the introduction, and the conclusion, the actual definitions of the variables are stated in the measurement strategy.

   c. *Experimental design*—describes operationally the study design in a step-by-step sequence. The description should be sufficiently detailed so that the reader is able to replicate the study.

   d. *Statistical analytical procedures*—the proposed strategy for quantifying, evaluating, and analyzing the results is presented along with the actual statistical procedures proposed. In the discussion, the experimenter describes how the appropriate sample size was determined (level of *power* chosen and *effect size* criteria). The proposed statistical analytical procedures are specified, and the chosen *statistical significance* level is stated.

5. *Results*—in the results section, the researcher describes the specific findings and actual outcomes of the project. The findings are reported clearly and descriptively but are not interpreted. Tables, charts, and graphs, where appropriate, are used to support the narrative, which provides a qualitative and quantitative descriptive and inferential statistical review. Subject characteristics are described, and the outcomes from the measurements of the dependent variable are reported. The experimenter provides, where relevant, such statistics as statistical significance, correlation, risk ratio, and effect size. After reporting the results of the test of the hypotheses, the experimenter also provides the results of any secondary analyses undertaken, additional observations, and related findings. This "post hoc" analysis may provide important cues for future studies and explorations of the topic.

6. *Discussion*—after the results are presented, the experimenter interprets and explains the results obtained. In this section, the researcher attempts to "make sense" of the findings. The first step in this discussion is to review the hypothesis and theory in the light of the findings. When the study is concerned with products or epidemiologic investigations, inferences are drawn about the material or the population, and an evaluation is made of the assumptions that led to the original study.

   Although such findings as "statistical significance" may be reported, it is also interesting for the researcher to speculate on the effects of the methodology, unanticipated characteristics of the subjects or of the conditions, and possible limitations of the theory. Although many readers rely on reports of statistical significance to determine the value of a study, commentaries in statistical and research methodology journals have criticized this approach in favor of an approach that emphasizes "effect size" and "variance analysis."

   Because research seldom genuinely "proves" or "disproves" a hypothesis, the discussion is likely to focus on the level of statistical support for the theory and the additional information provided by the secondary, or *post hoc*, analysis of the data. Also, the "lab notebook" (incidental and general observations) can be used to "shed light" on the research findings. Perhaps the subjects did not comply with the experimental protocol, or perhaps the subjects were influenced by external conditions. The discussion session is an opportunity for the researcher to editorialize and dialogue with the reader and to propose different ways to conceptualize the outcome data and to reconceptualize the theory.

7. *Summary and conclusions*—at the end of the article, the researcher provides a summary and interpretation of the study findings and attempts to draw conclusions related to the original theory and study question. Often, the commentary editorializes and goes beyond the actual findings to use the analysis as a basis for speculation and suggestions for future research. These speculations may go far beyond the actual findings of the study.

8. *References and bibliography*—accurate primary references are provided to the reader so that it is possible to pursue the problem further and to learn more. Where established research design methodologies, instruments, observation guidelines, and statistical techniques are used, their source in the literature should be provided so that the reader can verify and follow up what is asserted. Studies and formal reviews

should be documented so that the reader can draw an independent conclusion as to their content and findings.

C. Basic statistics—a basic understanding of general biostatistics principles provides the foundation for the important skill of critically interpreting new information as it becomes available in the scientific literature and via presentations.

1. *Statistics* can be defined as the practice, study, or result of the application of mathematical functions to collections of data to summarize or extrapolate that data. *Biostatistics* is the science of statistics applied to the analysis of biologic or medical data. The subject of statistics can be divided into *descriptive statistics*, or describing data, and *analytical statistics*, or drawing conclusions from data.

2. *Frequency distributions*—the distribution of measurements may take various different forms. Some more common situations are described next. Let us assume that each of these distributions represents the times required by a group of 100 dental students to complete a restorative dentistry final examination. The time limit to complete the examination was 1 hour.

   a. *Normal distribution*—a substantial number of naturally occurring phenomena are approximately distributed according to the symmetrical, bell-shaped, or normal distribution as shown in Figure 6-1. For this particular group of students, there was one clear average time. About as many finished faster than average as finished slower than average, and we have a bell-shaped distribution as a result.

   b. *Skewed distribution*—asymmetrical frequency distributions are skewed distributions. Positively skewed (to the right) distributions and negatively skewed (to the left) distributions can be identified by the location of the tail of the curve (not by the location of the hump—a very common error). Positively skewed distributions have a relatively large number of low scores and a small number of very high scores (Figure 6-2), whereas negatively skewed distributions have a large number of high scores and a relatively small number of low scores. For this particular group of students, we ended up with positively skewed (right-skewed) distribution. A relatively large number of students completed the examination in a short time, whereas a small number of students completed the examination toward the end of the time.

   c. *Bimodal distribution*—a peak in a distribution is called a mode. When a distribution has two peaks (Figure 6-3), it is called a bimodal distribution.

3. Measures of central tendency.

   a. *Mean*—the mean or average is the value obtained by adding all the measurements and dividing by the number of measurements. For example, for

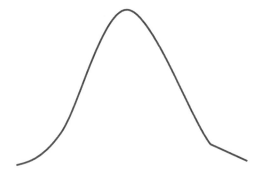

Figure 6-1 Normal distribution.

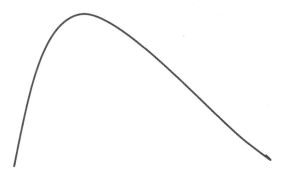

Figure 6-2 Positive skewed distribution.

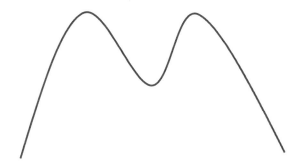

Figure 6-3 Bimodal distribution.

the following series of observations (21, 23, 29, 20, 18, 22, 14), the mean would be calculated as follows.

(1) Add up the observations.

$$21+23+29+20+18+22+14 = 147$$

(2) Divide the result from (1) by the number of measurements.

$$147/7 = 21$$

b. *Median*—the median is the middle measurement in a set of data where half the data are above and half the data are below the number. To find the median, two steps must be followed:

(1) Sort the observations in order of magnitude.

$$14, 18, 20, 21, 22, 23, 29$$

(2) Find the middle number.

$$14, 18, 20, \mathbf{21}, 22, 23, 29$$

c. *Mode*—the mode is the most frequent measurement in a set of data.

$$0, 1, 1, 2, 2, 3, 4$$

$$\mathbf{1, 2}$$

In this particular example, we have two measurements, 1 and 2, which are the most frequent. We have two modes.

4. Measures of dispersion.
   a. *Range*—the range is the simplest measure of variability. It is the difference between the highest and lowest values in the distribution. For example in the distribution

$$5, 20, 21, 21, 22, 23, 29$$

the range is

$$29 - 5 = 24$$

   b. *Variance (s^2)*—the variance is a method of ascertaining the way individual values are located around the mean. The larger the variance, the more widely the data items are spread about the mean value. A variance of zero indicates no spread at all (i.e., all the scores have the same value). Mathematically, it is defined as the sum of the squares of the deviations about the sample mean divided by one less than the total number of items. For instance, let us calculate the variance for the following series of observations.

$$21, 23, 29, 20, 18, 22, 14$$

   (1) Determine the mean, or 21, as calculated above.
   (2) Subtract the mean from every item in the distribution, square the difference, and add the results.

$$(21-21)^2 + (23-21)^2 + (29-21)^2 + (20-21)^2 +$$
$$(18-21)^2 + (22-21)^2 + (14-21)^2 = 128$$

   (3) Divide the result by the number of items in the distribution minus 1.

$$128/(7-1) = 21.33$$

The variance (s^2) = 21.33.

   c. *Standard deviation*—the standard deviation measures the typical or average deviation from the mean. Mathematically, the standard deviation is equal to the square root of the variance (s^2). Using the same distribution as used in the previous example, our standard deviation is equal to the square root of 21.33, or 4.62.

The mean is measured in the same units as the data items, but variance is measured in squared units. To overcome this, the square root of the variance is generally used as a measure of spread in preference to variance itself.

5. Inferential statistics.
   a. *Statistical significance*—the *p* value is the final arithmetic answer that is calculated by a statistical test of a hypothesis (H_0, called the *null hypothesis*). Its magnitude informs the researcher as to the validity of the H_0, that is, whether to accept or reject the H_0 as worth keeping. The *p* value is crucial for drawing the proper conclusions about a set of data. What numerical value of *p* should be used as the dividing line for acceptance or rejection of the H_0? Here is the decision rule for the observed value of *p* and the decision regarding the H_0:

$$\text{If } p < .05, \text{ reject the } H_0.$$
$$\text{If } p > .05, \text{ accept the } H_0.$$

   If the observed probability is less than or equal to .05 (5%), the null hypothesis is rejected (i.e., the observed outcome is judged to be incompatible with the notion of "no difference" or "no effect"), and the alternative hypothesis is adopted. In this case, the results are said to be "statistically significant." If the observed probability is greater than 0.05 (5%), the decision is to accept the null hypothesis, and the results are called "not statistically significant" or simply NS—the notation often used in tables.

   b. *Correlation/correlation coefficient (r)*—the correlation coefficient quantifies the relationship between variables (x and y) (Figure 6-4). *r* takes on values from −1 to +1 where

$$r = \text{x and y increase in the same direction}$$
$$-r = \text{x and y vary in opposite directions}$$

   c. *Multiple regression*—a multiple regression provides a mathematical model of linear relationship

Example of Correlation (r) = 0.87

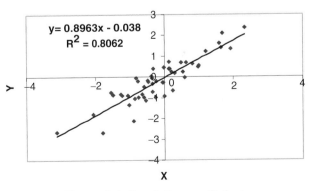

y= 0.8963x - 0.038
$R^2 = 0.8062$

Figure 6-4 Correlation coefficient.

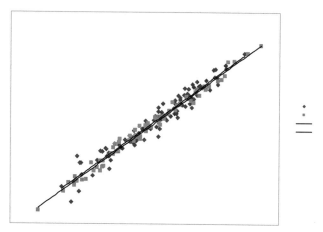

Figure 6-5 Multiple regression.

Table 6-2			
Caries Status			
WATER FLUORIDATED	**CARIES-FREE**	**NOT CARIES-FREE**	**TOTAL**
Yes	310	190	500
No	200	300	500
Total	510	490	1000

between a dependent (i.e., an outcome variable) and two or more independent or predictor variables (Figure 6-5).

d. *Chi-square (χ^2) test*—the chi-square test measures the association between two categorical variables. It is used for the comparison of groups when the data are expressed as counts or proportions. For example, an investigator might wish to compare the proportion of caries-free children living in a district whose water supply is fluoridated with the proportion of caries-free children living in a non-fluoridated district. In each district, the investigator would count the number of caries-free and non–caries-free children. The research question involves two categorical variables: caries status of the child (caries-free or not) and fluoridation status of the district (yes or no) (Table 6-2).

e. *t-test*—the t-test is used to analyze the statistical difference between two means. It provides the researcher with the statistical difference between treatment and control groups or groups receiving treatment A versus treatment B.

f. *Analysis of variance (ANOVA) test*—the ANOVA test analyzes whether or not the means of several groups are equal and generalizes a t-test to more than two groups.

6. *Biostatistics in decision making*—decision making frequently involves using quantitative data or tests of various kinds. Any health care practitioner using a diagnostic test wants to know how good the test is. To evaluate the quality of a diagnostic test, it is necessary, at a minimum, to know its validity, reliability, sensitivity, and specificity.

a. *Validity*—the validity of a test is the extent to which it actually tests what it claims to test (i.e., how closely its results correspond to the real state of affairs). The validity of a test is determined by its ability to show which individuals have the disease in question and which do not. Numerically, the validity of a test is determined by comparison with an accepted or gold standard that is known to be totally correct. To be really valid, a test should be highly sensitive, specific, and unbiased.

b. *Reliability*—reliability is equal to the repeatability and reproducibility of a test (i.e., the level of agreement between repeated measurements of the same variable). A reliable test would produce very similar results when used to measure a variable at different times.

c. *Sensitivity*—sensitivity is defined as the percent of persons *with* the disease who are correctly classified as having the disease (those who have the disease).

$$\text{Sensitivity} = \frac{\text{TP}}{\text{TP} + \text{FN}} \times 100\%$$

(1) True positive (TP)—those who have the disease.

(2) False negative (FN)—those who are incorrectly classified as *not* having the disease (i.e., missed diagnosis).

(3) The sensitivity of a test is its ability to detect people who do have the disease; it is the percentage of the people with the disease who are correctly detected or classified. A test that is always positive for individuals with disease (identifying every individual with the disease) has a sensitivity of 100%. A test that is insensitive leads to missed diagnoses (false-negative results), whereas a sensitive test produces few false-negative results.

d. *Specificity*—specificity is defined as the percent of persons *without* the disease who are correctly classified as not having the disease (those who do not have the disease).

$$\text{Specificity} = \frac{\text{TN}}{\text{TN} + \text{FP}} \times 100\%$$

(1) True negative (TN)—those who do not have the disease.

(2) False positive (FP)—those who do not have the disease but are identified by the test.

(3) The specificity of a test is its ability to detect people who do not have the disease. A test that is always negative for healthy individuals

Table 6-3

Sensitivity and Specificity of Diagnostic Tests

TEST RESULT	DISEASE	NO DISEASE
Positive	True positives	False positives
Negative	False negatives	True negatives

(identifying every person without disease) has a specificity of 100%. A test that is low in specificity leads to many false-positive diagnoses, whereas a test that is highly specific produces few false-positive results (Table 6-3).

4.0 Infection Control

A. *Diseases and routes of transmission*—dental professionals are at risk for any orally transmissible disease from the blood or saliva of the patients they treat. The transmissible diseases of greatest concern to the dental professional are hepatitis B virus (HBV), HIV, hepatitis C virus (HCV), and tuberculosis. However, the list of transmissible diseases is more widely encompassing. Each of these diseases is discussed in terms of etiology, diagnosis, risk of transmission, and recommendations for prevention.
  1. *Routes of transmission*—the route of transmission is the process by which a pathogen is transferred to a susceptible host.
    a. *Direct contact*—transmits infection by person-to-person contact.
    b. *Indirect contact*—the spread of infection by an inanimate object (i.e., by person → object → person).
    c. *Droplets or aerosols*—the spread of disease through the air by droplets that contain pathogens.
    d. *Parenteral contact*—the transmission of pathogenic microorganisms by piercing the skin (intravenously, subcutaneously, intramuscularly) through an accidental or intentional stick with a needle or other sharp instrument that is contaminated with blood or other body fluid.
  2. Transmissible diseases.
    a. HBV.
      (1) *Etiology*—the disease is produced by a highly infective virus known as the Dane particle. This intact virus consists of an inner core antigen (hepatitis B core antigen) and an outer coat surface antigen (hepatitis B surface antigen).
      (2) *Risk of transmission*—30% after percutaneous injury from an *infected* patient. The disease can be transmitted by 1×10^{-8} mL of blood.
      (3) *Diagnosis*—HBV is diagnosed based on a physical examination, medical history, and blood tests. HBV blood tests include hepatitis B antigens and antibodies and hepatitis B viral DNA (HBV DNA), which detects genetic material (DNA) from the HBV.
      (4) *Prevention*—a vaccine to immunize recipients against HBV is available. Three doses are given to confer immunity: an initial dose, a second dose 1 month later, and a third dose 6 months after the first. Because HBV is highly infectious, all dental personnel should be vaccinated against HBV. The mainstay of postexposure prophylaxis is hepatitis B vaccine, but hepatitis B immune globulin is recommended in certain circumstances in addition to vaccine for added protection.
    b. HCV.
      (1) *Etiology*—the disease is caused by HCV, a single-stranded RNA virus that appears to have cytopathic activity.
      (2) *Risk of transmission*—approximately 1.8% (range, 0% to 10%) after a needle-stick or sharps exposure.
      (3) *Diagnosis*—HCV is diagnosed based on a thorough medical history and physical examination to determine the symptoms and the likelihood of exposure to HCV and blood tests. The HCV test detects antibodies or genetic material (RNA) of the virus that causes hepatitis.
      (4) *Prevention*—no vaccine or postexposure prophylaxis is available; prevention is vital. Compared with HBV, HCV is less transmissible after a single exposure. The average risk of infection after a needle-stick injury is approximately 1.8%. This figure falls between risk estimates of HBV and HIV transmission.
    c. HIV.
      (1) *Etiology*—HIV is caused by an RNA virus.
      (2) *Risk of transmission*—0.3% from percutaneous exposures and 0.09% for mucous membrane exposures (less for skin contacts).
      (3) *Diagnosis*—HIV is diagnosed when antibodies to HIV are detected in the blood. The two primary blood tests used to detect HIV antibodies are enzyme-linked immunosorbent assay (ELISA) and Western blot assay, which is used to confirm the results of a positive ELISA test. HIV is diagnosed only after *two or more positive ELISA tests* are confirmed by a positive Western blot assay.
      (4) *Prevention*—no vaccine is available; use of standard infection control procedures is crucial. Postexposure prophylaxis consists of antiviral drugs similar to drugs given to patients with AIDS.

d. *Mycobacterium tuberculosis.*
   (1) *Etiology*—tuberculosis is caused by *M. tuberculosis*, a slow-growing bacterium that thrives in areas of the body that are rich in blood and oxygen, such as the lungs (although it may occur in almost any part of the body).
   (2) *Risk of transmission*—the most common mode of transmission of tuberculosis is inhalation of infected droplet nuclei. In some other parts of the world, bovine tuberculosis, which is carried by unpasteurized milk and other dairy products from tuberculous cattle, is more prevalent. A rare mode of transmission is by infected urine, especially for young children using the same toilet facilities.
   (3) *Diagnosis*—pulmonary tuberculosis is diagnosed based on a medical history and physical examination. In addition, some tests include sputum cultures, chest x-rays (if a person had a positive tuberculin skin test or an uncertain reaction to the tuberculin skin test because of a weakened immune system).
   (4) *Prevention*—patient medical histories should include questions on tuberculosis. Patients with suggestive symptoms should be referred for medical evaluation. These individuals should not remain in the dental office any longer than is required for a referral, and they should wear masks and be instructed to cover their mouths and noses when coughing or sneezing. Elective dental treatment should be deferred until a physician confirms that the patient does not have infectious tuberculosis. If urgent care is required, such care should be rendered in a facility that can provide tuberculosis isolation. Dental health care workers providing care in these circumstances should use respiratory protection. Dental health care workers symptomatic for tuberculosis should be evaluated and should not return to the workplace until a diagnosis of tuberculosis has been excluded or until they are receiving therapy and determined to be noninfectious.
B. *Barrier techniques*—barrier techniques provide a physical barrier between the body and microorganisms. They prevent microorganisms from contaminating the body and surfaces in the operatory and should be used wherever the potential exists for contacting blood, blood-contaminated saliva, or mucous membranes.
   1. Personal protective equipment (PPE).
      a. *Gloves*—one must wear gloves whenever touching anything that is contaminated with potentially infectious body fluids.
      b. *Masks*—it is recommended that a new mask be worn for each patient and that masks be changed routinely at least once every hour and more often in the presence of heavy aerosol contamination.
      c. *Protective glasses*—protective glasses protect eyes from spatter, splash, or metal chips from crown/amalgam restoration that have the potential for creating projectiles. During dental procedures, large particles of debris and saliva can be ejected toward the provider's face. These particles can contain large concentrations of bacteria and can physically damage the eyes. Protective eyewear is indicated not only to prevent physical injury but also to prevent infection. Protective glasses that give the best protection have both top and side shields, and some models are made to fit over regular corrective glasses.
      d. *Gowns*—protective clothing such as reusable or disposable gowns, laboratory coats, or uniforms should be worn when clothing is likely to be soiled with blood or other body fluids. Protective clothing should be changed at least daily or as soon as it becomes visibly soiled. Protective garments should be removed before oral health care providers leave areas of the facility used for laboratory or patient care activities.
   2. *Surface covers*—an effective cover must be impermeable to water. A material manufactured and advertised as a surface barrier should be accompanied by evidence of the impermeable nature of the product. Impervious-backed paper, aluminum foil, or plastic covers should be used to protect items and surfaces that may become contaminated by blood or saliva during use and that are difficult or impossible to clean or disinfect. Between patients, the coverings should be removed (with gloved hands), discarded, and replaced with clean materials (after gloves are removed and hands are washed).
C. *Occupational Safety and Health Administration (OSHA)*—OSHA is responsible for establishing standards for safe and healthy working conditions for all employees and regulating maintenance of these standards. These standards require all employers to provide to all employees "a workplace that is free from recognized hazards that are causing or likely to cause death or serious physical harm." OSHA is concerned with regulated waste within the office.
   1. OSHA blood-borne pathogens standard.
      a. The OSHA blood-borne pathogens standard sets forth the specific requirements OSHA believes can prevent the transmission of blood-borne diseases to employees. The blood-borne pathogens standard is highly comprehensive and detailed. It includes exposure determinations; an exposure control plan; engineering and work practice controls; and training of employees assisting or providing direct care as well as employees who clean operatories, instruments, and gowns.

b. The dental facility must have an exposure control plan designated to eliminate or minimize employees' exposure to blood-borne diseases. The plan sets forth the office's policy and protocols to protect employees from these diseases. Included in this plan are exposure determination, schedule of implementation, methods of compliance, training program, and use of PPE.

    (1) *Exposure determination*—every employee's daily activities are evaluated to determine whether he or she is exposed during specific duties.

    (2) *Schedule of implementation*—the dental facility must schedule in writing the various parts of the exposure control plan.

    (3) *Methods of compliance.*

        (a) *Standard infection control precautions*—the same infection control procedures are used for all patients.

        (b) *Engineering controls*—this section of the plan describes the devices, instruments, and materials used to prevent blood-borne pathogen exposure. Some examples include use of sharps containers and recappers.

        (c) *Practice controls*—policies and procedures, such handwashing for employees and when to change gloves.

    (4) *Training program*—employees in the dental facility must be provided with initial training and annual retraining. Records of the curriculum and attendance must be kept in the office. The training must be at a level that is understandable by the employees and provided on paid time at the dental office.

    (5) *Use of PPE*—PPE must be provided by the employer to all exposed employees (described previously under "Barrier Techniques").

1. *Immunization (hepatitis B vaccination)*—HBV vaccine must be offered to all exposed dental workers. The vaccine must be free to the worker. At the time of employment, each person should be asked to provide documentation of previous immunizations. A review of this documentation indicates which immunizations are needed, saving valuable time and emotional stresses in the event that exposure occurs on the job.

2. *Exposure incident and follow-up*—an exposure incident a specific occupational incident involving the eye, mouth, or other mucous membrane; nonintact skin; or parenteral contact with blood or other potentially infectious material, including saliva. The most common example is an injury from a contaminated sharp. After a report of an exposure incident, the employer must make immediately available, at no cost to the employee, a confidential medical evaluation and follow-up.

D. *Sterilization*—sterilization is basically absence of all life forms. The limiting requirement and basic criterion for sterilization is the destruction of high numbers of bacterial and mycotic spores because these are the most heat-resistant microbial forms. A basic guideline of effective clinical infection control is: *do not disinfect when you can sterilize.* Sterilization is the most important component of an infection control program.

By custom, the term *disinfection* is reserved for chemicals applied to inanimate surfaces, whereas *antiseptic* is used for antimicrobial agents that are applied to living tissues. A major distinction between high-level disinfection and sterilization is the ability of sterilization to kill spores of spore-forming bacteria (*Bacillus* and *Clostridium*). *Bacillus* spores are the benchmark organisms for sterilization. If a process kills *Bacillus* spores, it will also kill easier-to-kill bacteria, fungi, viruses, and protozoa.

1. Sterilization process.

    a. *Autoclaving*—the proper time and temperature for autoclaving is 250°F (121°C) for 15 to 20 minutes, which yields 15 lb pressure of steam, or 270°F (134°C) for a minimum of 3 minutes, which yields 30 lb pressure of steam. Moist heat destroys bacteria by denaturation of the high-protein-containing bacteria. There are two methods to ensure that the sterilization process is being performed properly: biologic monitors and process indicators.

        (1) *Biologic monitors*—also referred to as "spore tests." The process consists of placing into the autoclave bacterial spores on strips or in envelopes along with a normal instrument load. If the autoclave is working properly, the autoclave reaches the temperature and pressure required to kill the spores. Spore testing must be conducted weekly.

        (2) *Process indicators*—indicators change color, which shows that a normal load has reached a given temperature. However, this method demonstrates only that certain physical conditions have been reached. This method does not show that the microorganisms have been eliminated. Although process indicators are helpful, they do not replace biologic monitors.

    b. *Dry-heat sterilization*—dry-heat sterilization requires high heat for a specific period of time. This method requires a higher temperature (320°F [160°C]) and longer time (1 to 2 hours) than steam autoclaving. Because of the high temperatures, *only glass or metal objects can be sterilized by dry heat.*

    c. *Ethylene oxide (Chemiclave)*—ethylene oxide is a chemical widely used in the health care industry to sterilize medical devices. Ethylene oxide gas uses relatively low temperatures for sterilization. Using a heated unit, sterilization can be achieved in 2 to 3 hours at 120°F (48.9°C). However, a lengthy aeration time must follow each cycle.

d. *Chemical (cold) sterilization*—chemical sterilization is used for instruments and other items that are heat-sensitive or when methods that require heat are unavailable. Items are sterilized by soaking them in a particular chemical solution followed by rinsing them in sterile water. It takes 10 hours to kill bacterial spores in an instrument placed in a 2% solution of glutaraldehyde.

(1) Just immersing dental instruments in cold disinfectants would not destroy spores or the hepatitis viruses (they are resistant to physical and chemical agents).

2. *Disinfection*—disinfection is a process in which an antimicrobial agent destroys (germicide) or avoids the growth of (microbiostatic) pathogenic microorganisms. Disinfectants should be able to kill *M. tuberculosis*; this is the benchmark organism for disinfectants. Spores are not destroyed in this process. The term *disinfectant* is reserved for chemicals applied to inanimate surfaces (e.g., laboratory tops, counter tops, headrests, light handles).

3. *Antisepsis*—antiseptics are chemical agents similar to disinfectants, but they may be applied safely to living tissue. Alcohol is the most commonly used antiseptic to reduce the number of pathogenic microorganisms on the skin surface.

E. *Disposal of contaminated waste*—waste in the dental office must be disposed of according to state, local, and federal guidelines and requirements. The U.S. Environmental Protection Agency (EPA) regulates the transportation of waste from the dental office (e.g., biohazard waste, mercury, x-ray fixer). Following are the three general categories of waste produced in a dental office and the general guidelines for disposal.

1. *Sharps*—include scalpel blades, syringes, injection needles, and burs. Most states require special collection and storage of contaminated sharps. Treatment rooms must have sharps containers that must be collected by biohazard waste firms.

2. *Infectious waste*—includes materials contaminated with blood or bloody saliva, such as extracted teeth, gauzes, gloves, and gowns. These materials must be collected separately and disposed of by licensed waste firms.

3. *Noninfectious waste*—includes elements such as plastic covers and cups, patient bibs, and others. There are no guidelines for their disposal.

5.0 Materials and Equipment Safety

A. *Mercury hygiene*—dental health care workers can be exposed to mercury through direct skin contact with mercury or through the exposure to potential sources of mercury vapors.

1. Recommendations by the American Dental Association (ADA) Council on Scientific Affairs.

a. Train all personnel involved in the handling of mercury and dental amalgam regarding the potential hazards of mercury vapor and the need for good mercury hygiene practices.

b. Work in well-ventilated work areas, with fresh air exchanges and outside exhaust. Air-conditioning filters should be replaced periodically if the work areas are air-conditioned.

c. Use proper work area design to facilitate spill containment and cleanup. Floor coverings should be nonabsorbent, seamless, and easy to clean. The ADA Council on Scientific Affairs does not recommend the use of carpeting in operatories.

d. Periodically check the operatory's atmosphere for mercury vapor. This may be done by using dosimeter badges or through the use of mercury vapor analyzers. The current OSHA standard for mercury is 0.1 mg per cubic meter of air averaged over an 8-hour work shift.

e. Use high-volume evacuation systems (equipped with traps or filters) when finishing or removing amalgam.

f. Small mercury spills can be cleaned up safely using commercially available mercury cleanup kits and by following your state's recommendations (e.g., in Michigan, the Michigan Department of Environmental Quality's table *Management of Mercury Spills*). Cleanup of large mercury spills requires the use of an experienced environmental contractor specialized in toxic spill cleanup.

B. Environmental contaminants.

1. *Gases*—hazardous gases or vapors (e.g., nitrous oxide) should be vented directly to the outside air or should be collected from the air using scrubbing devices to protect individuals within the office and to prevent contamination of other local air systems.

2. *Airborne particles*—rotary instrumentation is capable of creating airborne contaminants from bacterial residents in the water spray system and microbes present in saliva, tissues, blood, and fine debris from teeth and plaque. These airborne contaminants could be present as spatter, mist, and aerosols. Spatter consists of large, visible particles (≥50 μm) that fall within 3 feet of the patient's mouth, coating the face and outer garments of the dental provider. Spatter is considered a potential route of infection for dental health care workers by blood-borne pathogens. Mist consists of droplets that approach or exceed 50 μm. Mist tends to settle from the air after 10 to 15 minutes. Mists produced by the cough of a patient with unrecognized active pulmonary or pharyngeal tuberculosis are likely to transmit the infection. Aerosols are

invisible particles that range in size from 5 to 50 μm and can remain floating in the air for hours. Although there is no scientific evidence that aerosols can transmit either HBV or HIV, it is acknowledged that aerosols may carry agents of respiratory infections borne by the patient.

   a. Use of PPE is required to prevent contamination from airborne particles. In addition, to help reduce exposure to airborne particles, adequate air circulation should be maintained and masks worn until personnel leave the operatory or air exchange has occurred in the room.

3. *Mercury*—dental amalgam waste can be recycled to help prevent the release of mercury to the environment. Although the contribution of dental amalgam to overall mercury pollution is negligible, the ADA has developed Best Management Practices for Amalgam Waste. These practices include using precapsulated alloys; recycling waste amalgam; using chair-side traps, vacuum pump filters, and amalgam separators; recycling extracted teeth that contain amalgam; and using appropriate line cleaners.

C. Operatory equipment.

1. *Noise control*—sources of noise in the dental office that can be potentially damaging to hearing are high-speed and low-speed handpieces, high-speed suction, ultrasonic instruments and cleaners, vibrators and other mixing devices, and model trimmers. The degree of risk to the dental health care worker depends on different factors, including the intensity or loudness (decibels [dB]), frequency (cycles per second [cps]), and duration (time) of the noise as well as personal susceptibility.

   Noise-induced hearing loss develops slowly over time and is caused by any exposure regularly exceeding a daily average of 90 dB. Protective measures are recommended when the noise level reaches 85 dB with frequency ranges from 300 to 4800 cps. Protection is mandatory in areas where the level transiently reaches 95 dB.

2. *Photopolymerization units and lasers*—dental personnel and patients should be protected from high-intensity visible light using colored plastic shields (attached to the fiberoptic tip). Special precautions are required when using a laser. Laser light can be inadvertently reflected from many surfaces in the dental operatory. The operatory should be closed, and appropriate signs are needed to indicate the presence of laser equipment. Eye protection is required for the operator, assistant, and patient to protect against reflected laser light.

3. *Waterlines*—the CDC recommends that coolant water used in nonsurgical dental procedures meet EPA regulatory standards for drinking water, which is less than or equal to 500 colony-forming units (cfu) of heterotrophic bacteria per milliliter (mL) of water.

Since 1995, owing to technologic improvements, water delivered to patients during nonsurgical dental procedures consistently contained no more than 200 cfu/mL of aerobic mesophilic heterotrophic bacteria at any point in time in the unfiltered output of the dental unit.

In 2012, the ADA Council on Scientific Affairs issued a new statement on dental unit waterlines. The specific recommendations are to employ one or more available commercial devices and procedures designed to treat, filter, and improve the quality of water. Commercially available options at the present time include the use of independent water reservoirs, chemical treatment regimens, source water treatment systems, daily draining and air purging regimens, and point of use filters. Previous CDC recommendations that dental waterlines be flushed at the beginning of the clinic day to reduce the microbial load is no longer recommended because studies have demonstrated that this practice does not affect biofilm in the waterlines or reliably improve the quality of water used during dental treatment.

D. *Hazardous chemicals*—the OSHA hazard communication standard requires employees to receive training about the risks of using hazardous chemicals and the safety precautions required when handling them. Employees must be trained in identification of hazardous chemicals and PPE to be used for each chemical. This training must occur within 30 days of employment or before the employee uses any chemicals and annually thereafter. Just as with the blood-borne pathogen standard, a written plan identifying employee training and detailing specific control measures used in the workplace must be compiled for hazardous chemicals. Penalties can be imposed on the employer if the office is not in compliance.

1. *Material safety data sheets (MSDSs)*—each office must have a material safety data manual that is alphabetized, indexed, and available to all employees. These manuals can be in hard copy or on a computer. The manual contains the MSDSs. These sheets come from the material manufacturer. If MSDSs are unavailable, the employer or a designated employee must request them from the manufacturer.

   a. The National Fire Protection Association color and number method is used to identify information about various hazardous chemicals easily on the MSDSs and product labels. The color and number method is used to signify a warning to employees using the chemicals.

      (1) Blue identifies the health hazard.

      (2) Red identifies the fire hazard.

      (3) Yellow identifies the reactivity or stability of a chemical.

      (4) White identifies the required PPE when using this chemical.

b. The level of risk for each category is indicated by the use of numbers 0 through 4. The higher the number, the greater the danger.

6.0 Dental Care Delivery Systems

In this section, we review third-party reimbursement, the managed dental care concept, delivery models, quality assurance principles, and the relationship of government and public health.

A. *Third-party reimbursement*—third-party reimbursement is a system in which a provider of coverage contracts to pay for some of the patient's dental treatment. Following are the major forms of third-party reimbursement currently in use.

1. *Usual, customary, and reasonable (UCR)*—under UCR, reimbursement is based on the dentist's usual charge, unless the charge exceeds certain parameters. For example, the plan pays the dentist fee unless the fee exceeds 80% of the charges for that service in a given geographic area. To determine UCR fees, dentists usually must become participating providers with a plan and agree to file their fees periodically.

2. *Table of allowances*—in this type of reimbursement, the third-party payer generally determines what fees it is willing to pay for each procedure. Participating dentists agree to charge plan members these prenegotiated fees as payment in full, or the plan may allow the dentist to engage in balance billing. Balance billing involves charging the patient any difference between what the plan agrees to pay and the dentist's UCR fees.

3. *Fee schedules*—a fee schedule is a list of fees established or agreed to by a dentist for the delivery of specific dental services. A fee schedule usually represents payment in full, whereas a table of allowances might not. With a fee schedule, the dentist must accept the listed amount as payment in full and not charge the patient anything. Fee schedules are sometimes established by public programs, such as Medicaid in many states.

4. *Reduced fee for service*—reduced fee for service is most commonly associated with preferred provider organization (PPO) plans, which are discussed later. Under reduced fee for service, participating dentists agree to provide care for fees usually lower than other dentists in a particular geographic area. Although PPO dental plans generally provide partial payment for care received from a nonparticipating dentist, the patient becomes responsible for the difference between the dentist's charge and the amount paid by the plan.

5. *Capitation*—under capitation, the dentist is paid a fixed amount (usually on a monthly basis) directly by the capitation plan. For this periodic per capita payment, the dentist agrees to provide specified dental services for patients who present and who are assigned to the dentist by the capitation plan. The dentist bears most of the financial risk for the treatment promised under the plan. For the dentist, such plans allow for predictable income for budgeting purposes, an influx of new patients (with potential referrals), and little processing of claims. The dentist can also control the type and frequency of services provided.

B. *Dental managed care*—dental managed care is a comprehensive approach to the provision of quality oral health care that combines clinical preventive, restorative, and emergency dental services and administrative procedures to provide timely access to primary dental care and other medically necessary dental services in a cost-effective manner.

1. *Dental health maintenance organization (D-HMO)*—D-HMO is the type of plan most commonly associated with dental managed care. This type of plan is also called a capitation dental plan, which derives from the payment mechanism. Dentists are paid on a per capita basis at a fixed (usually monthly) rate for each individual or family. The dentist is paid regardless of the number or types of services provided or the number of beneficiaries seen. Dentists are individually at risk in D-HMOs: if the value of services exceeds payments, it is the dentist's loss; however, if payment exceeds value, the dentist gains financially.

2. *Dental preferred provider organization (D-PPO)*—D-PPO is an arrangement between a plan and a panel of providers whereby the providers agree to accept certain payments (usually less than their usual fees) in anticipation of a higher volume of patients. This higher volume of patients results from a benefit structure that gives the subscriber a financial incentive to use providers from the panel. These incentives typically come in the form of reduced cost-sharing or richer benefits.

3. *Dental individual practice association (D-IPA)*—D-IPA is basically a hybrid D-HMO, a delivery system that combines the risk sharing of an HMO with fee-for-service reimbursement. D-IPAs may be owned and operated by participating dentists who sign a contract agreeing to certain conditions, including quality assurance, utilization review, and risk sharing. Dentists are collectively at risk, as opposed to in D-HMOs, where they are individually at risk. The dentist is paid on a fee-for-service basis and is at risk if payout exceeds premiums. If this occurs, either fees may be reduced, or the dentist may not receive payment for treatment beyond a certain amount. D-IPAs usually have an open invitation to all dentists in an area to join. It usually needs capitalization from its member dentists, accounting for the risk sharing,

and may allow for dentist input in plan and benefit design.

C. *Delivery models*—dental managed care plans can be designed with different delivery models, which include the staff model, the network model, and the closed model.

1. *Staff model*—the staff model usually has one or more dental offices that use salaried staff dentists. This model is found in many of the capitation plans. It may be a closed panel (offering services for its own beneficiaries) or a contracted dental office (providing services for one or more purchasers).

2. *Network model*—the network model uses multiple dental offices in various locations and is the most common method of delivering dental benefits in managed dental care. The administrator usually contracts with private dental offices that are principally fee-for-service practices. These offices may be limited to a specific geographic area or may be widespread over several states.

3. *Closed model*—in the closed model, also known as the exclusive provider organization, the beneficiaries have a limited choice of offices where they can go to obtain dental care. If they go to offices not included in the panel, they receive no benefits. This model is often used in a D-HMO or PPO plan.

D. *Quality assessment and quality assurance*—although people use the terms *quality assessment* and *quality assurance* as synonyms, they describe different concepts.

1. Quality assessment measures the quality of care provided in a particular setting, whereas quality assurance measures the quality of care and the implementation of any necessary changes either to maintain or to improve the quality of care rendered.

2. Quality assessment is limited to the assessment of whether or not standards of quality have been met, whereas quality assurance includes the additional dimension of action to take the necessary corrective steps to improve the situation in the future. Several concepts relate to quality assurance.

   a. Structure—layout and equipment of the facility.

   b. Process—actual services that the dentist and dental hygienist perform for the patient and how well they perform.

   c. Outcome—the change in health status that occurs as a result of the care delivered.

E. *Role of the government in public health*—The DHHS is the principal agency of the U.S. government for protecting the health of all Americans and providing essential human services, especially for citizens who are least able to help themselves. The following DHHS health agencies are involved with the delivery, funding, and research aspects of oral health.

1. *Administration for Children and Families (ACF)*—the ACF is responsible for federal programs that promote the economic and social well-being of families, children, individuals, and communities and is responsible for the Head Start program, which provides educational, social, medical, dental, nutritional, and mental health services to preschool children from low-income families.

2. *Centers for Medicare and Medicaid Services (CMS)*—CMS administers the Medicare and Medicaid programs, which provide health care to about one in every four Americans. Medicare provides health insurance for more than 43 million elderly and disabled Americans. Medicare does not cover dental care except when dental services are directly related to the treatment of a medical condition (e.g., extraction of teeth before radiation therapy for cancer).

   a. CMS is responsible for the oversight of the federal portion of the Medicaid program, a joint federal-state program that provides health coverage for approximately 55 million low-income Americans, including parents and children, people with disabilities, and elderly adults. Federal Medicaid laws mandate that states offer comprehensive dental services to children under the Early Periodic Screening Diagnostic and Treatment (EPSDT) program. States are required to provide dental examinations to children no later than age 3 and to treat comprehensively any oral problems identified. EPSDT also requires states to take action to ensure that children can truly access care. These actions include provision of information, transportation, and scheduling assistance. Medicaid adult dental coverage is optional, and states vary widely in the dental benefits made available to adults.

   b. CMS also administers the Children's Health Insurance Program (CHIP) through approved state plans (S-CHIP). S-CHIP provides health coverage to nearly 8 million children in families whose incomes are too high to qualify for Medicaid but who cannot afford private insurance. Dental coverage is not a requirement of the S-CHIP program. However, when it was created as part of the Balanced Budget Act of 1997, 49 of the 50 states chose to offer dental coverage as part of their S-CHIP programs and to provide relatively comprehensive benefits. Although not as broad as the Medicaid EPSDT program, coverage under most S-CHIP programs includes basic preventive, diagnostic, and restorative services.

   c. The Affordable Care Act (ACA), currently under implementation, contains a variety of initiatives that relate to oral health, including coverage and access, prevention, oral health infrastructure and surveillance, and the dental health workforce. ACA expands Medicaid coverage to 133% of the federal poverty level with an enhanced federal matching rate and extends CHIP until 2019. Oral health services were included as part of the pediatric essential health benefits.

3. *Health Resources and Services Administration (HRSA)*—HRSA provides access to essential health care services for people who have low incomes, are uninsured, or live in rural areas or urban neighborhoods where health care is scarce. Through its different bureaus, HRSA administers a variety of programs to improve oral health, including funding for prevention and fluoridation, and provides loan repayment to health professionals who work in underserved areas through the National Health Service Corps. HRSA also provides grants to migrant and community health centers to render comprehensive health care, including dental services, to the poor and migrants. Through the Ryan White CARE Act, HRSA funds dental care programs for people who are HIV-positive or have AIDS. HRSA-funded dental programs provided care to more than 4 million patients in fiscal year 2010.

4. *CDC*—the CDC provides a system of health surveillance to monitor and prevent disease outbreaks (including bioterrorism), to implement disease prevention strategies, and to maintain national health statistics. The Division of Oral Health has the responsibility for supporting state and local oral disease prevention programs, promoting oral health nationally, and fostering applied research to enhance oral disease prevention. Among the oral health–related activities of the CDC are dental infection control, community water fluoridation, oral health surveillance, oral and pharyngeal cancer and tobacco-related issues, and support for state oral health programs.

5. *U.S. Food and Drug Administration (FDA)*—the FDA is responsible for protecting the health of the nation against impure and unsafe foods, drugs, cosmetics, and other potential hazards.

6. *Indian Health Service (IHS)*—the IHS focuses on the goal of raising the health status of American Indians and Alaska Natives. The IHS supports a comprehensive health services delivery system of hospitals, health centers, school health centers, health stations, and urban Indian health centers to provide services to nearly 2.1 million American Indians and Alaska Natives of 566 federally recognized tribes. In 2013, more than 3.7 million dental services were delivered through IHS programs.

7. *National Institutes of Health (NIH)*—the NIH is the world's premier medical research organization, supporting more than 44,000 research and training grant projects nationwide. Among its institutes and centers is the National Institute of Dental and Craniofacial Research (NIDCR), which supports and conducts basic, clinical, and epidemiologic research.

8. *Agency for Healthcare Research and Quality (AHRQ)*—the AHRQ supports research on health care systems, health care quality and cost issues, access to health care, and effectiveness of medical treatments. It provides evidence-based information on health care outcomes and quality of care.

7.0 Communication and Interpersonal Skills

A. Listening and nonverbal communication.
1. *Listening* is an active process that involves the reception and selection of auditory information, the generalization and interpretation of the information, and the reconstruction of what was heard. Listening is fundamental to quality clinician-patient communication, with the goal of engaging, facilitating, and encouraging the patient to speak openly and feel comfortable with the health care provider. Strong listening skills also contribute to accuracy in diagnosis, collaborative treatment planning, and patient satisfaction.
  a. Listening techniques.
    (1) *Preparation*—preparing to listen by setting aside appropriate time for discussion, free from distraction. This preparation serves to build rapport, increase one's ability to anticipate the patient's actions and responses accurately, and improve patient adherence and satisfaction.
    (2) *Paraphrasing*—repeating, in one's own words, what someone has said. Paraphrasing serves to confirm one's understanding, validate a patient's feelings, convey interest in the patient's experience (building rapport), and highlight important points.
    (3) *Reflection*—hearing the patient's verbal message, interpreting the meaning of this communication, and conveying this interpreted meaning to the patient in an effort to ensure understanding.
    (4) *Acknowledging*—continually conveying attentiveness and interest through verbal and nonverbal means, including leaning forward, maintaining good eye contact, facing the patient, asking questions, summarizing points and concerns, nodding, smiling, and maintaining close proximity.
    (5) *Interpretation*—identifying the underlying reason for a communication. Interpretation serves to build rapport, increase patient trust and comfort with disclosure, and raise issues for discussion that may be important but with which the patient may be uncomfortable in initiating dialogue.

2. *Nonverbal communication*—involves the expression or reception of meaning through nonverbal means (e.g., facial expressions, gestures, eye contact, interpersonal distance, dress, touch, vocal tone, rate and rhythm of speech).
   a. Nonverbal communication may take the place of, modify, or regulate the flow of a verbal message and express emotion and interest.
   b. Characteristics of nonverbal communication.
      (1) *Continuous*—one can continually monitor a patient's nonverbal communication, even when not engaged in verbal exchange. One also can convey empathy and other messages to patients through nonverbal means.
      (2) *Automatic*—it often occurs on a semiconscious or precognitive level, allowing for additional insight into a patient's emotional experience; attention to a patient's nonverbal communication is important to understanding their experience and identifying and addressing concerns or discomfort.
      (3) *Informative*—the reception of nonverbal information can contribute to an understanding of patient emotions when a patient lacks the awareness of or ability to describe them, adding to a rich, multidimensional perspective of a patient's experience.
3. *Rapport* is a mutual sense of trust and openness between individuals that, if neglected, compromises communication.
   a. Rapport is reciprocal; patients are more likely to respect a clinician's beliefs and opinions if the clinicians is willing to listen to and respect theirs.
   b. Strategies for building rapport include greeting each patient by name; maintaining good eye contact; smiling; asking about a patient's interests (e.g., work or school, family); and disclosing some personal information, as appropriate.
4. *Empathy* is the active interest in and effort to understand another's perspective.
   a. Characteristics of empathy.
      (1) Understanding the patient's situation: for example, "How would I feel if I were he?".
      (2) Reflecting that understanding back to the patient: for example, "What can I say to him to let him know that I understand how he must feel?".
   b. A clinician who effectively conveys empathy builds rapport and trust, elicits and addresses the patient's feelings that have the potential to interfere with treatment, assists the patient in assuming responsibility for his or her feelings, accepts the patient's feelings as real and important, and remains objective and nonjudgmental.
   c. Empathy is of the utmost importance because a patient who feels understood is more likely to

disclose important information fully and accurately, feel confident in and adhere to the provider's treatment recommendations, and feel satisfied with the care provided.
5. To facilitate good communication, care must be taken in *verbal communication.*
   a. Using the following techniques requires caution in carefully constructing the verbal message.
      (1) *Presuming*—assuming a patient's thoughts or feelings may undermine rapport; alternatively, ask rather than presume.
      (2) *Overassertive communication*—verbal communication often is driven by strong emotion or the belief that one's perspective is the correct or only perspective; alternatively, clearly explain your impressions and recommendations, respecting any concerns or differing views a patient may have and taking the time to evaluate and discuss differing views or treatment options.
      (3) *Reliance on technical jargon and abstract or vague communication*—these may cause confusion and undermine rapport; alternatively, be simple, specific, and direct.
      (4) *Giving advice*—can interfere with patient adherence and patient decision-making responsibility; alternatively, provide information and education to the patient so that he or she may make an informed decision.
      (5) *Providing reassurance*—providing inappropriate reassurance (e.g., telling a patient everything will be fine) can backfire and result in compromised rapport and trust; alternatively, provide accurate information, discuss any patient concerns or questions fully, and offer support.
6. *Professionalism* is an essential component of the clinician-patient relationship.
   a. Professionalism is characterized by confidence; care; warmth; and appropriate ethical, professional behavior.
   b. Professionalism in communication may be conveyed in numerous ways, including leaning forward, maintaining eye contact, using facilitative nonverbal communication (e.g., smiling, nodding), maintaining a relaxed posture, exhibiting appropriate facial expressions, conveying respect and interest, and practicing ethically.

B. Clinical interviewing.
   1. *Clinical interviewing* is an art of communication that serves many functions.
      a. It allows a clinician to collect vital health history information.
      b. It serves to establish ground rules regarding communication (e.g., the level of formality or informality, how a patient may express emotion, how a

clinician is likely to respond, what is acceptable self-disclosure and what is not).

    c. It provides insight into a patient's response style and attitudes regarding their understanding of dental health and hygiene and toward illness and other health problems.

    d. It assesses the patient's perceived needs (e.g., their presenting problem).

    e. It assess the patient's values, what is important to the patient (e.g., a bright smile, straight teeth).

2. Numerous interviewing techniques are useful in eliciting important health information and facilitating communication.

    a. *Open-ended questions*—the use of open-ended questions invites a patient to express what he or she feels is important, strengthening rapport (e.g., "What brings you in today?").

        (1) In general, it is preferable to begin an interview in an unstructured manner and progress to a more structured format. This approach provides patients with an opportunity to express what is important to them in seeking the clinician's services.

    b. *Closed questions*—direct questions may be used to provide more guidance for a response or to elicit specific information (e.g., "Have you ever required premedication for a dental examination?").

        (1) Too many closed questions in succession can lead to patient disengagement.

    c. *Closed questions with options*—open questions that restrict potential answers by providing options (e.g., "So, what are you hoping to accomplish—reduce the need for future intervention or find a quick and inexpensive option?").

    d. *Leading questions*—leading questions direct the patient to respond in specific way (e.g., "That didn't hurt, did it?").

        (1) Leading questions are not recommended because they may easily undermine trust and rapport.

    e. *Probing*—probing allows a clinician to gather additional information regarding a particular topic without leading the patient toward a particular response (e.g., "Tell me more about the discomfort you've been experiencing in your left lower teeth.").

    f. *Laundry list questions*—these questions ask a patient to respond from a list of given choices (e.g., "Is the pain sharp, dull, constant, or throbbing?").

    g. *Summarizing*—chaining together a set of reflections. The clinician hears the patient's communication, interprets its meaning, and conveys a brief summary of one's understanding of what was said. Summarizing a patient's communication conveys understanding and concern in addition to encouraging further comment (e.g., "I understand that your denture has been quite uncomfortable for you and that it feels as though it is irritating your upper gum.").

    h. *Transitioning*—acknowledging the importance of a patient's communication and shifting to a new topic of discussion.

    i. *Silence*—the use of a silent pause in communication encourages the patient to speak.

    j. *Verbal and nonverbal facilitation*—these facilitative gestures and brief comments convey interest and warmth in addition to encouraging further comment (e.g., head nodding, or "I see.").

    k. *Empathy*—see earlier discussion of empathy under "Listening and nonverbal communication."

    l. *Observation*—commenting on a patient's behavior, especially that which is inconsistent with the patient's verbal communication, may encourage the patient to discuss a topic with which he or she may be uncomfortable but that may be important to treatment (e.g., "You seem uncomfortable when I mention the use of local anesthetic.").

C. Treatment planning.

1. *Treatment planning* is a joint agreement between the clinician and patient regarding shared decision making and collaboration.

    a. If a treatment plan is not acceptable to both the patient and the clinician, it is likely to fail, even if the treatment selected is the treatment of choice for a particular presenting problem.

2. Treatment plans involve many elements.

    a. Presentation of diagnosis.

        (1) It is important to be clear, use language free of technical jargon, and use illustrative methods (e.g., radiographs, pictures, drawings) to ensure that the patient fully understands the nature and origins of the presenting problem.

        (2) A clinician should be sensitive when relaying information that may be difficult to hear and with which to cope (e.g., presenting indications of oral cancer).

    b. Proposal of treatment approach.

        (1) The clinician presents treatment alternatives to the patient in descending order of desirability (e.g., treatment of choice, option 2, option 3, no treatment, referral).

        (2) Be sure to present only options that are consistent with your standard of care and that would be acceptable to you.

    c. Presentation of potential treatment benefits, hazards, and patient responsibilities.

        (1) Provide a comprehensive review of potential benefits and hazards and patient responsibilities in language that may be easily understood by the patient.

    d. Verify patient comprehension.

        (1) To verify patient understanding, ask the patient what his or her understanding is of the

treatment options. The clinician listens to the patient convey his or her understanding in his or her own words and corrects or clarifies any information as needed.

   e. Discussion.

     (1) It is important to provide an opportunity for patients to ask questions about the treatment alternatives and to allow sufficient time for discussion. As comprehension and comfort increase, satisfaction and adherence increase as well.

   f. Treatment decision.

     (1) Although a clinician may have a preferred treatment approach, the decision is ultimately the patient's.

     (2) Use caution in giving advice. When a patient takes responsibility for choosing his or her treatment, adherence, follow-up care, and satisfaction are improved.

     (3) Support the patient in his or her decision by providing encouragement.

   g. Document.

     (1) It is important to document the completion of each step of the treatment planning process.

  3. Patient education is an important component of treatment planning as well as throughout treatment.

   a. A patient who is well informed is more likely to adhere to treatment and follow-up and report satisfaction with services.

8.0 Health Behavior Change

A. Health behavior change is an intrinsically motivated change that happens outside of the dental office in the everyday settings of patients' lives.

B. Clinicians may approach the topic of health behavior change in ways that may serve to facilitate the desired behavior.

  1. The clinical environment is important to how influential information is received.

  2. The ability to convey empathy is critical in influencing health behavior change.

  3. Clinicians may facilitate the consideration of health behavior change by eliciting a rationale for change from the patient through thoughtful questioning regarding how or why the patient might change.

  4. Patient ambivalence is a normal part of the process of behavior change.

  5. It is important to have a flexible approach to communicating throughout the process.

C. *Stages of change model*—transtheoretical model (Prochaska & DiClemente, 1986).

  1. People change their behavior when they are ready to change.

  2. The behavioral change process occurs in several stages.

   a. Precontemplation—an individual is not considering a behavior change.

   b. Contemplation—an individual begins to consider a behavior change.

   c. Preparation—preparing to take steps to change (often expresses a desire to change a behavior).

   d. Action—an individual is engaged in taking action toward behavior change (often requires support for his or her efforts).

   e. Maintenance—an individual attempts to maintain a changed behavior.

D. Behavior change theory.

  1. *Social cognitive theory.*

   a. Behavioral motivation is influenced by cognitive factors and the social environment. Important tenets of this model are the following.

     (1) The notion of self-efficacy (one's perception of himself or herself as being effective).

     (2) Behavioral modeling (learning a behavior from models in the environment).

     (3) Social reinforcement (positive social consequences).

   b. This model is often used to illustrate the effectiveness of oral health care education. For example, demonstrating good oral health care (e.g., toothbrushing) for a patient; allowing the patient to practice the skill, supervised or unsupervised (providing confidence-building mastery experiences); and praising the patient for good work tend to lead to improved oral self-care.

  2. *Health belief model* (Rosenstock, 1966).

   a. Behavioral motivation (i.e., the likelihood one will engage in a particular behavior, such as preventive oral hygiene) is influenced by several factors.

     (1) Perceived susceptibility (to disease or problem).

     (2) Severity of the consequences.

     (3) Perceived costs and benefits (of engaging in the behavior).

     (4) Cues to action (external or internal stimuli that serve as prompts to engage or not engage in the behavior).

   b. This model is often used to predict the likelihood of a behavior or behavior change and to assess the need for behavioral intervention to assist in the change process.

   c. For example, this model asserts that a person is more likely to engage in good preventive oral health care if the patient believes he or she is susceptible to oral health problems; the consequences of not performing these health behaviors could be significant; as a result, taking the time to care for one's teeth to have healthy teeth is preferable to a lack of care leading to oral health problems; and there are cues in the environment to encourage the behavior (e.g., the individual owns a toothbrush, floss).

3. Theory of planned behavior.

 a. The best predictor of patient behavior is the individual's intention to perform the behavior which is influenced by several factors.

  (1) Attitudes regarding the behavior.

  (2) Perceived social norms regarding the behavior.

  (3) Degree to which the individual perceived the behavior to be within his or her control.

4. Self-determination theory.

 a. Theory regarding origin of motivation consisting of four assumptions about intrinsic motivation that must be met.

  (1) Competence—perceived ability to achieve desired outcome.

  (2) Autonomy—perception of oneself as being responsible for or in control of behavior change.

  (3) Relatedness—individual seeks interactions with others.

  (4) If the first three assumptions are not met, there will be decreased motivation and other difficulties.

5. *Cultural factors*—in our increasingly diverse communities, it is important to consider cultural factors in health care (e.g., access to and use of care, preventive care, diagnosis, treatment planning, clinician-patient communication).

E. Foundations for behavior change.

 1. *Health behavior* can be understood in terms of *cognitive behavioral theory*—as a complex interaction between one's thoughts, one's feelings, and one's behavior. Each interacts with and influences the other, resulting in behavior and behavioral patterns.

 2. *Behavior theory (ABC model)*—the occurrence of a particular behavior can be understood as a complex interaction between an antecedent (A), a facilitating factor to a behavior; a behavior itself (B); and the consequences of a behavior (C). This is referred to as behavior theory or the ABC model.

  a. For example, when an individual experiences discomfort because of particulate lodged between two teeth (A), the individual may choose to floss (B) and, as a result, experience a sense of relief (C).

 3. *Classical conditioning (also known as respondent or pavlovian conditioning)*—a neutral stimulus (one that is not associated with a particular response) is paired with an unconditioned stimulus (US), one that naturally elicits a particular response (UR). After many pairings, the conditioned stimulus (CS) elicits a conditioned response (CR), which is essentially a weaker form of the UR, without the presence of the US.

  a. For example, a dentist gives a painful injection (US), and the patient experiences anxiety and becomes upset (UR). Given that this scenario occurs many times, eventually the presence of a dentist alone (CS), without the presence of an injection (US), can elicit some degree of anxiety and feeling upset (CR).

  b. If such an associative learning response occurs (CR), it can be extinguished through a process known as *classical extinction*, in which the response is not reinforced.

  (1) For example, if on many occasions the anxiety-provoking dentist gives injections that are not painful, the response, anxiety and feeling upset, may no longer occur (may be suppressed) in response to the mere presence of the dentist.

4. *Operant conditioning*—a behavior is followed by a particular consequence (reinforcement or punishment), and the frequency of the behavior increases or decreases as a result.

 a. *Positive reinforcement*—a positive consequence that increases a desired behavior (e.g., receiving verbal praise or a tangible reward may increase the frequency of toothbrushing).

 b. *Negative reinforcement*—the removal of a negative stimulus that increases a desired behavior (e.g., the repair of a cavity should relieve a patient's toothache, which may increase the frequency of toothbrushing).

 c. *Positive punishment*—a negative consequence that decreases an undesirable behavior (e.g., giving a child an extra chore to do in response to his or her failure to brush his or her teeth may decrease the frequency of toothbrushing neglect). This is also known as *aversive conditioning*.

 d. *Negative punishment*—the removal of a positive stimulus to decrease an undesirable behavior (e.g., decreasing a child's weekly allowance from $3 to $1 may decrease the frequency of toothbrushing neglect).

  (1) Research supports the greater efficacy of reinforcement over punishment because the use of punishment has several disadvantages: it often results in the avoidance of the punisher; it can elicit negative emotions; and it fails to teach an alternative, more desirable behavior.

 e. *Operant extinction*—the removal of reinforcers to decrease a behavior.

  (1) For example, a young patient learns that if she cries at the dentist's office, her mother gives her much-needed attention and terminates the dental appointment. Asking the mother to refrain from providing this attention and allowing the dentist to continue communicating with the child for the remainder of the scheduled appointment is likely over time to decrease the crying behavior. However, the behavior may first appear to increase (*extinction burst*) before it decreases.

5. *Observational learning (modeling)* (Bandura, 1962)—the acquisition and performance of a skill through observation of another engaging in the task. This is most effective when the model is an individual the person views as similar (e.g., age, gender). This technique may be particularly useful if used in the context of asking an anxious or uncooperative child to observe his or her cooperative sibling.

C. Strategies for behavior change.

1. "OARS" in communication—*o*pen questions, *a*ffirmations, *r*eflective listening, *s*ummarizing (see Section 7.0, Communication and Interpersonal Skills).

2. *Assessment*—to create and implement an effective strategy for behavior change, one must first assess the behavior. Behavior assessment should include the following.

   a. *Identify the problem*—define the problem and determine its origin.

   b. *Consider motivation.*

   c. *Consider readiness*—a patient may be willing to change a behavior, but the present time may not be the ideal time to commit to such an endeavor (e.g., current life circumstances causing increased stress, sleep deprivation, decreased time to devote to such a task).

   d. *Consider willingness to change.*

   e. *Consider ability to change*—consider existing self-management skills, social support, current life stressors, and locus of control.

      (1) *Internal locus of control*—a tendency to attribute events to internal forces (internally motivated; e.g., "I failed my exam because I didn't study as much as I should have."). These individuals tend to be more motivated and successful at behavior change.

      (2) *External locus of control*—a tendency to attribute events to external forces (externally motivated; e.g., "I failed my examination because the test was unfair.").

   f. *Collect baseline data*—answer the question, "What is the target behavior frequency currently?" This allows you to establish a starting point for comparison later to determine whether the intervention is successful.

      (1) *Event and time sampling*—ask the patient to record each time the behavior occurs over a predetermined period of time. Charts or counters may be helpful in counting and recording the data.

      (2) In the case of a child, ask a parent to observe and record the behavior of the child.

      (3) Be aware of the potential for a *self-monitoring bias*, in which the target behavior tends to improve simply as a result of self-monitoring. Although it may appear as though the behavior is immediately improving without intervention, this effect is often short-lived, and the behavior returns to baseline within weeks.

   g. As the intervention is implemented, continually reassess the behavior to monitor for progress, provide reinforcement for behavior change, and determine whether the intervention is successful or whether it requires alteration.

      (1) Consider using charts to monitor progress because they provide visual positive reinforcement for behavior change.

      (2) Be sure to create reachable goals.

3. *Behavioral strategies*—all behavioral strategies may be conceptualized using the ABC model. Behavior change (B) can be successfully accomplished by altering either an immediate antecedent (A) or an immediate consequence (C). By altering A or B, a learning experience is created that shapes behavior. (For additional behavioral strategies, see Section 9.0, Anxiety and Pain Control.)

   a. *Altering antecedents and stimulus control*—changing one's routine by placing a behavior cue can increase the frequency of a behavior (e.g., keeping dental floss on the nightstand may serve as a daily reminder to floss). The removal of a behavior cue, in the case of a goal to decrease a behavior, can also be a useful strategy (e.g., someone who always smokes a cigarette in his or her favorite chair on the porch may remove the chair from the porch, making it less likely that person will engage in the behavior).

   b. *Shaping (stimulus-response theory)*—recognition and reinforcement of successive approximations of a behavior; in other words, creating small, doable steps, followed by praise for successfully completing these steps, toward achieving a target behavior.

      (1) This is a useful technique because the most common reason for failure in behavior change is setting unrealistic goals and expectations, leading to failure and decreased motivation.

      (2) When using shaping, begin slowly, with an easily accomplished task, and use positive reinforcement at each step.

   c. *The Premack principle*—making a behavior that has a higher probability of being performed contingent on (used as reinforcement) the performance of a less frequent behavior may increase the performance of the less frequent behavior (e.g., making reading a child's evening bedtime story contingent on toothbrushing).

   d. *Altering consequences*—altering the immediate consequences, such as in the use of a reward system (providing positive reinforcement) following a behavior, may alter future performance of the behavior (see point e).

e. *Providing feedback*—providing praise regarding work toward a specific goal. Visual aids (e.g., the use of charts, diagrams, records, logs) can be very useful in demonstrating success.

f. *Extinction*—identifying the positive consequences or reinforcements that maintain a behavior and ceasing or withholding these reinforcements or consequences (e.g., requiring a patient who regularly presents 20 minutes late to appointments to reschedule for another time, rather than see the patient when he or she arrives late each visit).

g. *Incompatible behavior and stimulus control*—the use of an incompatible behavior to decrease the frequency of an undesirable behavior (e.g., instructing an individual to put on a pair of gloves each time the individual feels compelled to bite his or her fingernails).

h. *Observational learning*—see Section 9.0, Anxiety and Pain Control.

4. *Cognitive strategies*—influencing one's behavior (and emotional response) through the use of reasoning or thought-provoking strategies. (For additional cognitive strategies, see Section 9.0, Anxiety and Pain Control.)

a. Establishing rapport.

b. Maintaining good communication.

c. *Motivational interviewing* (Miller & Rollnick, 2012)—a person-centered counseling style to assist in the resolution of ambivalence and help move toward behavior change. The "spirit of motivational interviewing" is a compassionate, accepting, collaborative process in which there is shared decision making and in which the patient's autonomy is honored in using a patient's strengths to elicit motivation to change. The process involves connecting behavioral goals to a patient's beliefs, values, and concerns. Motivational interviewing involves four processes.

(1) *Engaging*—forming a relationship with the patient.

(2) *Focusing*—exploring the patient's motivation to change behavior as well as the patient's values and goals in treatment and the meaning of these values and goals in his or her life.

(3) *Evoking*—eliciting from the client his or her own motivation to move toward change.

  (a) Strategies include discussing disadvantages of remaining in current behavior pattern, discussing advantages of change, exploring personal strengths that may contribute to change, and exploring intention to change.

(4) *Planning*—exploring how one might move toward change.

  (a) Ambivalence is a normal part of the change process.

(b) *Sustain talk*—patient's communication favors remaining in current behavior pattern.

(c) *Change talk*—patient's communication favors change or movement toward change.

(d) *Commitment talk*—patient's communication expresses a readiness, ability, and willingness to change behavior.

9.0 Anxiety and Pain Control

A. Stress and dental anxiety.

1. *Anxiety*—a subjective experience involving cognition, emotion, behavior, and physiologic arousal. Stress is a perceived threat to one's well-being. It is subjective in that each individual appraises each potentially stressful event in terms of its *familiarity*, *predictability*, *controllability*, and *imminence* and arrives at a conclusion regarding how anxiety-provoking he or she believes the situation to be.

2. Clinicians should be familiar with presenting symptoms of anxiety so that they may adequately recognize any potential anxiety response before it occurs.

3. It is essential that dental professionals be familiar with some *brief interventions* and *management strategies* for the treatment of anxiety to facilitate best a successful dental experience for an anxious patient. Effectively using these skills is likely to result in increased treatment compliance and patient follow-up, better quality of care, and better current and future dental experiences for both the patient and the clinician.

a. Provide the patient with a sense of control.

(1) *Provide information*—let patients know what to expect. Research indicates that negatively anticipated events are less stressful when they are *predictable* (e.g., tell patients what they will likely feel, see, smell, and taste; inform them of procedure length and keep them informed of progress; use the *Tell-Show-Do method*, particularly with children; offer patients mirrors for them to observe; offer patients choices when appropriate).

(2) *Use hand signals*—agree on a way in which the patient can express anxiety (e.g., raising a hand), which will serve as a signal for the clinician to break temporarily to allow the patient to regain coping.

(3) *Time structuring*—using a timing mechanism (e.g., an egg timer, a clock, counting to a certain number, singing a certain song) to encourage a behavior by increasing one's sense of control and expectations. This technique is particularly useful with children, who do not yet have a well-developed time sense, or an anxious

patient who cannot easily tolerate parts of a procedure (e.g., drilling).

b. *Acknowledge the patient's experience.* Demonstrate an understanding of how anxious or uncomfortable the patient feels and how important the patient's comfort is to you, the clinician.

c. *Use brief cognitive-behavioral interventions*, based on cognitive-behavioral therapy, which posits that thoughts, feelings, and behaviors are interrelated and influence one another; intervening in one of these areas can produce change in the remaining two areas.

   (1) *Diaphragmatic (paced) breathing and relaxation*—educate the patient regarding the relaxing benefits of deep breathing. Demonstrate this technique. Practice four to five breaths with the patient. Remind the patient to use these skills during the visit and to practice the skill at home.

   (2) *Progressive muscle relaxation*—a technique that involves systematically tensing and relaxing certain muscle groups, directing the patient to attend to the differences in sensation between tension and relaxation.

   (3) *Guided imagery*—a procedure in which a patient uses diaphragmatic breathing skills while imagining a pleasant scene of his or her choosing, evoking all senses.

   (4) *Hypnosis*—a technique involving attentional focus, paced breathing, and relaxation.

   (5) *Behavioral rehearsals*—providing a patient with the opportunity to practice coping strategies (e.g., diaphragmatic breathing) while experiencing a simulated procedure or part of a procedure.

   (6) *Systematic desensitization*—exposing a patient to items from a collaboratively constructed hierarchy of slowly increasing anxiety-provoking stimuli (related to the target fear) while using relaxation skills.

   (7) *Cognitive coping (reframing)*—assisting patients in changing their thinking about something to a more adaptive or realistic thinking style (e.g., helping the patient to change his or her thought from "I can't do this" to "This may be difficult for me, but I can manage this. I did okay last time.").

   (8) *Use praise*—demonstrate progress; set realistic expectations. Ask patients to practice coping skills at home and when in the office.

   (9) *Distraction*—giving the patient a competitive attentional focus can be useful (e.g., listening to music, watching a video).

4. Continually assess level of anxiety throughout treatment using a *subjective unit of distress scale*, asking patients to rate their level of anxiety from 0 (none at all) to 10 (the highest he or she had ever experienced) (e.g., "How anxious are you feeling now?").

5. Although most of the procedures listed previously may be used with children (with adaptation for developmental level), there are special considerations in pediatric anxiety.

a. Additional anxiety management strategies for children.

   (1) *Structure choices*—for example, plain or fruit-flavored dental floss.

   (2) *Tell-Show-Do*—explain, demonstrate, and allow the child to learn and understand what will be happening before proceeding.

   (3) Use *specific direction* and *specific feedback* (e.g., "I need you to open your mouth as widely as you can." "That's good the way you're opening your mouth for me. Keep up the good work.").

   (4) Teach simple *coping strategies* (e.g., deep breathing, counting to a specified number).

   (5) Use *praise.*

   (6) *Reward* good behavior.

   (7) Use *hand signals.*

   (8) Consider inviting a parent into the room for *support.*

   (9) Provide positive experiences by choosing to do simple, less anxiety-provoking procedures first.

B. Dental pain (Milgrom, 2001; Milgrom et al, 1995).

1. *Gate-control theory*—a dorsal spinal gating mechanism can control (by opening or closing, or partially closing) the flow of signals from noxious stimuli (i.e., stimuli that cause pain) from the periphery to the brain. The flow is varied according to what signals are received from the brain and may be influenced by inhibitory agents, competitive stimuli, or signals (e.g., cold, hot, emotions, expectations, memories, cultural attitudes).

a. This theory does not account for cognitive or emotional factors.

2. Pain is a complex phenomenon involving cognition, emotions, beliefs, expectations, and past experiences. Fear and anxiety and pain are interrelated. A fear response to a stressor initially causes a release of endorphins from the pituitary, resulting in an analgesic effect. However, ultimately, pain thresholds are reduced, and anxious patients are more likely to report pain or discomfort for many reasons (e.g., hypervigilance, muscle tension, cognitive misattribution of danger, conditioning, catastrophic thinking, perceived lack of control). In addressing patient pain, clinicians must attend to both pain and anxiety.

3. As with anxiety, a goal of minimizing pain and increasing the patient's coping skills is essential as well as *ongoing pain assessment.*

a. Clinicians may inquire about pain level through the use of the *subjective units of distress scale* (see following text) and *pulp vitality testers.*

4. The behavioral (nonpharmacologic) management of patient pain may be useful in the control of mild to moderate pain and an effective supplement to pharmacologic strategies.

5. Although most of the procedures listed previously may be used with children (with adaptation for developmental level), there are special considerations in pediatric pain.

   a. Research indicates that dentists consistently underestimate the pain experiences of children.

   b. Factors influencing pediatric dental pain include age (behavior, level of understanding, and self-report differ according to developmental level), perceived level of control, past experiences, expectations, and family or cultural norms and beliefs.

   c. *Ongoing assessment*—in addition to the subjective units of distress scale and pulp vitality testers, use of the Wong-Baker Faces Pain Rating Scale may be particularly useful with children. Because children do not have the cognitive and emotional maturity and verbal ability of adults, it is especially important to use observation skills in assessing a child's pain (facial expressions, verbal responses, behavior or motor responses, physiologic arousal).

   d. Additional pain management strategies for children (in addition to those used with adults, when developmentally appropriate and in addition to anxiety management strategies; see "Stress and Dental Anxiety," earlier).

      (1) When possible, use short and simple procedures. If multiple procedures are indicated, choose the simplest and least invasive procedure first.

      (2) When possible, use procedures that do not involve injections or handpieces.

      (3) Foster an environment of support and learning.

      (4) Introduce patients to tools, procedures, and sensations in a systematic manner.

      (5) Use Tell-Show-Do, graded exposure, and explanation.

      (6) Use age-appropriate language.

      (7) Structure time.

      (8) Give choices when possible and appropriate.

      (9) Use hand signals, and immediately respond to signal of discomfort.

      (10) Use distraction when appropriate (e.g., storytelling, imagery, hypnosis, breathing exercises). Distraction is less effective and not ideal for children who are extremely anxious and hypervigilant.

      (11) Provide information and offer hand mirrors to observe.

Refer to Section 5, Orthodontics and Pediatric Dentistry, for additional discussion of this topic.

10.0 Professional Responsibilities and Liabilities

A. *Ethical principles*—the *principles of ethics* guide the dentist's decision making in practice. Five fundamental principles form the foundation of the ADA *Principles of Ethics and Code of Professional Conduct*: patient autonomy, nonmaleficence, beneficence, justice, and veracity.

   1. Section 1. Principle: Patient Autonomy ("self-governance"). The dentist has a duty to respect the patient's rights to self-determination and confidentiality.

   2. Section 2. Principle: Nonmaleficence ("do no harm"). The dentist has a duty to refrain from harming the patient.

   3. Section 3. Principle: Beneficence ("do good"). The dentist has a duty to promote the patient's welfare.

   4. Section 4. Principle: Justice ("fairness"). The dentist has a duty to treat people fairly.

   5. Section 5. Principle: Veracity ("truthfulness"). The dentist has a duty to communicate truthfully.

B. *Informed consent*—consent and informed consent are two separate and distinct legal theories. Except where the patient's condition (e.g., an emergency) justifies the performance of a procedure or the rendering of a service, the patient's consent to treatment is required, even if the unauthorized procedure is skillfully performed and is beneficial to the patient.

   1. *Background*—the doctrine of informed consent emerged during the 1950s. It is based on the ethical principle of patient autonomy, and it requires that the patient be informed of any information that would affect a reasonable person's decision making, including the nature of a procedure explained in understandable terms, potential benefits and risks of the procedure or service, and costs of the procedure. Failure to do so invalidates the consent.

      Some courts have determined that in a situation in which a patient is mentally and physically able to consult about his or her condition, in the absence of an emergency, the patient's informed consent is a prerequisite to tests, treatment, intrusive procedures, or surgery. If a procedure is done without an informed consent, the dentist may be held accountable for assault and battery, which may not be covered by professional liability insurance. A technical assault and battery makes the dentist liable for any resulting injuries, regardless of whether the treatment was appropriate and not negligently administered. The duty to apprise a patient of the nature of the procedure is limited to the doctor performing the procedure for which consent is being obtained.

   2. Informed consent consists of the *information* that a doctor is required to share with the patient and the

consent that the doctor is required to obtain from the patient.

  a. Required informational elements for informed consent.

    (1) Explanation of the procedure in understandable terms.

    (2) Reasons for the procedure and the benefits and risks of the procedure and anticipated outcome.

    (3) Any alternatives and their risks and benefits, including no treatment at all.

    (4) The costs of the procedure and the alternatives.

  b. Required elements for consent.

    (1) Consent must be voluntary and not coerced.

    (2) Information and consent must be given in a language that the patient understands.

    (3) The patient must be given an opportunity to ask questions, and the doctor must be available to answer any patient questions.

    (4) Only the patient or the patient's legal guardian can authorize treatment decisions.

    (5) Make sure to check state regulations, which often outline who must obtain consent from the patient and whether it must be in writing or signed.

3. Any doubt as to the necessity of obtaining consent should be resolved in favor of procuring the consent.

4. *Emancipated minors*—in negligence law, a sliding scale is in effect. From ages 1 through 7, a child is considered an infant and is not responsible for his actions (i.e., cannot be contributorily or comparatively negligent, cannot assume a risk). From ages 8 through 14, the child is judged on a sliding scale of competence, depending on the sophistication of the child and the activity he or she is involved in (e.g., a 12-year-old driving a boat would be considered more responsible for his actions than an 8-year-old on a bicycle). Finally, from age 15 on, minors are considered totally responsible for their own actions (e.g., a 16-year-old driving a car is held to the same standard as all drivers, regardless of experience). Minors younger than 18 can give implied consent but not actual consent (i.e., they can get on the ride at the amusement park, but they cannot sign a release). The exception is the case of emancipated minors.

    A conscious, mentally competent patient younger than 18 may give consent to his or her own medical treatment, counseling, or testing if he or she is emancipated, married, a parent, pregnant, or in an emergency situation. An emancipated minor can also consent to treatment of his or her child.

5. *Exceptions*—in an emergency situation where immediate treatment is required to preserve life or limb or alleviate severe pain, and the patient or legally responsible party is not unable to give consent, the doctor may proceed without it. The factual basis of the emergency must be carefully recorded by the doctor in the patient's chart. Before treatment, documented efforts should be made to contact the appropriate consenting party.

C. *Risk management and risk avoidance*—risk management is a concept derived from industry wherein one identifies areas possibly exposing one to liability; weighs the risks against the benefits; and controls that exposure by monitoring, insuring, or eliminating the dangerous activity. It is basically a two-pronged attack where one is alerted to possible dangers and then handles incidents by immediate action. This heightened awareness and early warning system allow the practitioner to be prepared if and when a lawsuit is filed. It also provides a sound basis for determining whether to defend or settle the lawsuit. In addition to learning to identify potential exposures to liability, the second part of risk management is knowing what to do when something bad happens.

1. Documentation is an essential part of risk management. In the eyes of many courts, "If it is not written down, it did not happen," meaning that significant events should be written down and that the courts will not rely on memory, several years after the fact, particularly in cases of medical malpractice. Medical records must be thorough, consistent, and complete. They should include not only actual visits but also missed visits and other evidence of noncompliance.

2. To reduce liability for the physical facility, regular logs that detail inspections, maintenance, and phone calls reporting problems can provide evidence that things are being handled properly.

3. Another type of documentation is an incident report, which is completed when something happens. An incident report should be objective; this is no time to point fingers, as in "As usual, Tom did not bother to turn on the lights."

4. All documentation is discoverable; that is, the counsel for an injured party is entitled to all writings concerning the problem, including any handwritten notes.

5. Objectivity also requires that you do not create facts. Write down what you actually saw, not what somebody tells you. For example, "Patient found on floor" is an objective statement. "Patient slipped on spilled Coke" is not, unless you actually saw it. The problem is that if you state, "Patient slipped on spilled Coke," you may have created a liability situation.

  a. If possible, physically view the accident scene and document what you found—spilled Coke or water, or a clean, dry floor? Pools of slush or a clean, sanded sidewalk? Did you actually see the injured party or just hear about it? What happened to the injured party? Did an ambulance come, did a friend provide a ride, was he ambulatory, was he seen by a doctor, and so forth.

b. Your writings are discoverable; do not write anything you do not want read aloud in court. For example, do not characterize the patient using insulting remarks; instead, detail the behavior, as in "Patient was loud and aggressive, argumentative, refused to listen to office staff."

6. When an incident occurs, your insurance company should be put on notice. If you wait until you are actually sued, and you had prior notice, the insurance company may refuse to provide coverage.

7. Once you have written something, do not go back and change it when a lawsuit is filed. If you have second thoughts, provide an addendum. *Never* change anything you wrote. If you make a legitimate mistake, draw a single line through the error (so it can still be read), mark "error," and initial and date it.

D. *Documentation*—the primary weapon against a possible lawsuit is appropriate and adequate documentation. If you have been sued, it is your only defense. As stated earlier, according to some judges, if it is not written down, it did not happen.

1. *Be specific.* Write facts only, not opinions; describe observations, findings, and assessments. Generalizations are confusing, as in "Patient doing well" (compared with "Patient no longer experiencing pain on tooth No. 3"). What is your evidence? What have you observed?

2. *Be objective.* Avoid personal characterizations ("Patient uncooperative"). Instead, state specific behavior, such as "Refuses to eat, take medication, stop smoking," which implies noncompliance. Do not create facts; do not state, "Fractured mandible; patient punched by husband," unless you saw it. Instead, state, "Patient presents with fractured mandible; states husband hit her." If your information comes from the patient, always preface it with "Patient states:" Otherwise, you have created a fact that you cannot back up if you are called to testify.

3. *Be complete.* Take special care in documenting patient education and home care.

4. *Be timely.* Make all entries promptly.

5. *Be readable.* Write legibly; you may have to rely on your notes years later, and both you and your attorney must be able to read them. Make continuous entries in the chart; avoid gaps in time or treatment. Stay with traditional forms and abbreviations. Make certain entries are consistent and avoid contradictions.

6. *The integrity of the chart is your top priority and must be preserved.* Make corrections or alterations according to approved procedures:

a. If you realize your mistake at the time you are writing the note, draw a single line through the error so it is still readable. Write the correction and indicate the date, time, and your initials.

b. If you realize the error at a later time, write an addendum after the last note that was written in the chart. This is important because anyone subsequently reviewing the chart may already have read the existing note and will be unaware that the content of the note changed unless you reference this in an addendum.

(1) *Never* erase, white-out, or otherwise obliterate anything that was written in the chart. A plaintiff's attorney can say the obliterated material says anything he or she wishes.

(2) *Never* change so much as a comma once a lawsuit has been filed; the plaintiff probably already has a copy of the chart, and your alterations can be enough to lose the suit. Tampering or changing the record with self-serving intent can be disastrous.

7. *Never make or sign an entry for someone else* or have another make or sign an entry for you.

8. *Countersign carefully.* Never countersign an entry without reading it and, if necessary, checking the accuracy. You become as responsible as the person who originally signed.

9. *Do not complain, belittle, criticize, or blame others in your documentation.* It can provide the plaintiff with ammunition.

10. *Document informed consent in your progress notes*, in addition to having the patient sign an informed consent form. Document discussion, evidencing patient's understanding.

11. *Your chart may be read in court.* Avoid derogatory, insulting, or unprofessional remarks that you would be embarrassed to explain in front of judge and jury.

E. *Statute of limitations*—the statute of limitations varies from state to state, and there are two basic rules that states follow: the occurrence rule and the discovery rule. The occurrence rule allows for the statute of limitations to start to run when the possible injury or malpractice occurred. The discovery rule allows for the statute of limitations to run when the patient discovers or should have discovered the injury or malpractice. The type of rule followed by the state affects the minimum time required for patient record retention. Ethically, you should advise a patient when you have done something wrong because it is the right thing to do; legally, you should advise a patient because that will document the time of discovery and the statute will begin to run. In cases of minors, parents can sue immediately; however, the minor may have additional time after the age of 18 to bring suit on his or her own behalf; if you have a pediatric practice, you may have to retain your records longer.

F. *Confidentiality*—the original record is your custodial property and, by law, must be retained by you. *Copies* of charts and x-rays may be provided to patient or attorney with signed authorization by the patient (and you can charge copying fees). The chart is confidential and should not be discussed with anyone without authorization from the patient.

G. Witnesses.

1. *Expert testimony*—to prove an allegation of malpractice, the plaintiff must produce an expert who will testify to the existing standard of care in the profession and how it was breached by the defendant. The expert must be qualified by virtue of training, experience, and credentials, and the defense has the right to provide its own expert to rebut the plaintiff's expert. The expert can have *general* expertise in the field, such as a general dentist, or have *special* expertise, such as an oral surgeon or orthodontist. An expert witness appears voluntarily and attests to the expert's best medical judgment and opinion "to a reasonable medical certainty." Usually experts charge an hourly rate, including record review and preparation time. In some states, there is no limit on expert witness fees except that such fees should be "reasonable." As a witness, your fee arrangement cannot be contingent on the outcome of the litigation. When the expert witness is asked about compensation, he or she should not be flustered. The proper response is, "I am being paid for my expertise, training, experience, and time."

2. *Fact witnesses*—a fact witness is someone with first-hand knowledge of the facts of the case. He or she can testify only about first-hand knowledge and is not allowed to offer an opinion about treatment provided. A fact witness is usually subpoenaed and must appear; the individual cannot charge for his or her services; rather, the witness receives a statutory sum depending on the jurisdiction where he or she is appearing.

   a. Some courts have held that a fact witness who has treated a patient cannot testify against that patient's interests; that is, he or she may not give an opinion detrimental to the patient's case and must testify only to the facts in an objective fashion.

Bibliography

ADA Council on Scientific Affairs: Dental mercury hygiene recommendations. *J Am Dent Assoc* 134:1498, 2003.

American Dental Association: *ADA Principles of Ethics and Code of Professional Conduct.* Chicago, ADA, 2005.

American Dental Association: *ADA Principles of Ethics and Code of Professional Conduct.* Chicago, ADA, 2013.

Bandura A: *Social Learning Through Imitation.* Lincoln, NE, University of Nebraska Press, 1962.

Burt BA, Eklund SA: *Dentistry, Dental Practice, and the Community,* ed 6. St. Louis, Mosby, 2005.

Chambers DW, Abrams RG: *Dental Communication.* Sonoma, CA, Ohana Group, 1992.

Dionne RA, et al: *Management of Pain & Anxiety in the Dental Office,* ed 5. St. Louis, Mosby, 2002.

Gluck GM, Morganstein WM: *Jong's Community Dental Health,* ed 5. St. Louis, Mosby, 2003.

Mayes DS: *Dental Benefits: A Guide to Dental PPOs, HMOs and Other Managed Plans.* Brookfield, WI, International Foundation of Employee Benefit Plans, 2002.

Milgrom P, Weinstein P, Getz T: *Treating Fearful Dental Patients: A Patient Management Handbook.* Seattle, University of Washington, 1995.

Miller WR, Healher N, editors: *Treating Addictive Behaviors.* New York, Plenum Press, 1986.

Miller WR, Rollnick S: *Motivational Interviewing: Preparing People for Change,* ed 2. New York, Guilford Press, 2002.

Miller WR, Rollnick S: *Motivational Interviewing: Helping People Change,* ed 3. New York, Guilford Press, 2012.

Ost L, Skarat E: *Cognitive Behaviour Therapy for Dental Phobia and Anxiety.* New York, Wiley-Blackwell, 2013.

Prochaska JO, DiClemente CO: Toward a comprehensive model of change. In: Miller WR, Heather N, editors: *Addictive Behaviors: Processes of Change.* New York, Plenum Press, 1986, pp 3-7.

Ramseier C, Suvan J: *Health Behavior Change in the Dental Practice.* New York, Wiley-Blackwell, 2010.

Rosenstock IM: Why people use health services, *Milbank Memorial Fund Q* 44:94, 1966.

Selye H: The general adaptation syndrome and the diseases of adaptation. *J Clin Endocrinol* 6:117, 1946.

Weinstein P, Getz T, Milgrom P: *Oral Self-Care: Strategies for Preventative Dentistry.* Seattle, University of Washington, 1991.

Weintraub JA, Douglas CW, Gillings DB: *Biostats Data Analysis for Dental Health Care Professionals.* Chapel Hill, NC, CAVCO Publications, 1985.

Wong DL, et al: *Wong's Essentials of Pediatric Nursing,* ed 7. St. Louis, Mosby, 2005.

Sample Questions

1. Which of the following is *not* a process in motivational interviewing?
   A. Focusing
   B. Analyzing
   C. Evoking
   D. Engaging
   E. Planning

2. Which behavior change theory emphasizes the importance of self-efficacy and behavioral modeling and reinforcement?
   A. Cognitive behavioral theory
   B. Self-determination theory
   C. Social cognitive theory
   D. Classical conditioning
   E. Motivational interviewing

3. A patient is conflicted about wearing a night guard, despite your recommendations to prevent further

damage from bruxism. The patient states, "I have so much going on right now that I just don't think I'm going to be able to wear it consistently like I should." This is an example of:

A. Resistance

B. Sustain talk

C. Commitment talk

D. Back talk

E. Change talk

4. Informed consent requires that the patient be advised of all of the following *except* one. Which one is the *exception*?

A. Benefits of the procedure

B. Risks of the procedure

C. Description of the procedure using technical terms

D. Cost of the procedure

5. From the following list, select the ethical principles found in the ADA *Principles of Ethics and Code of Professional Conduct*. (Choose all that apply.)

A. Tolerance

B. Compassion

C. Beneficence

D. Integrity

E. Veracity

F. Competence

6. From the following list, select the elements required for a patient to give consent to treatment. (Choose all that apply.)

A. Patient must be able to pay.

B. Patient must voluntarily agree to treatment.

C. Patient must be given the opportunity to ask questions.

D. Patient must be a minor.

E. Patient must be experiencing an emergency.

F. Patient's family must agree.

7. Risk management includes all of the following *except* one. Which one is the *exception*?

A. Weighing the risks and benefits in practice

B. Monitoring risky activity

C. Exposing oneself to liability

D. Eliminating dangerous activity.

8. From the following list, select the items that support appropriate and adequate documentation of the patient record. (Choose all that apply.)

A. Include specific facts

B. Include personal characterizations

C. Include criticism of patient's behavior

D. Include complete documentation of contact with patient

E. Include abbreviations

F. Include timely entries and avoid gaps in time

9. The first time you perform a complicated dental procedure, you feel uncomfortable and nervous. At one point, you even think for a moment that you will be unable to complete the procedure. However, you stay with it, and near the end of the procedure you feel much better. Which concept does this scenario *best* exemplify?

A. Covert conditioning

B. Systematic desensitization

C. Habituation

D. Cognitive restructuring

E. Psychoeducation

10. During a previous dental visit, you assisted a patient by generating his statement, "Even if there is some pain, it will be brief. I have ways to cope and I've done well using them." The patient will remind himself of this during future dental procedures. This patient's statement exemplifies which of the following strategies?

A. Rational response

B. Self-efficacy induction

C. Relaxation statement

D. Imagery

E. Systematic desensitization

11. In clinical practice, you frequently encounter young patients who are nervous about seeing the dentist. Knowing which factors are important influences on young patients' comfort, consider which of the following will help your patients to feel more comfortable?

A. Inviting a parent into the operatory for support

B. Placing toys and children's books in the waiting room

C. Hanging child-friendly décor in the operatory

D. Talking to the child about his or her interests before beginning your work

E. All of the above

12. Dental intervention studies suggest that educating patients regarding dental care (patient education) is more effective than behavioral modification (behavioral intervention) in increasing compliance.

A. True

B. False

C. Sometimes

D. Both are equally effective

E. Cannot be determined

13. Which technique is typically *not* useful in treating an anxious patient?

A. Using less structure in establishing rapport

B. Reassuring the patient by telling the patient not to worry

C. Providing reasons before asking for sensitive information

D. Using empathy

E. Making expectations clear

14. The *most* common site for cancers in the oral cavity is _____.

A. Lip

B. Soft palate

C. Hard palate

D. Tongue

E. Tonsils

15. The *most* effective method to prevent caries on the occlusal surfaces among school-age children is _____.

A. Sealants

B. Community water fluoridation

C. School dietary fluoride

D. School fluoride mouth rinse

E. School fluoridation

16. Neither the subject nor the investigator knows to which group a subject belongs in which type of study design?

A. Matching studies

B. Randomized

C. Double-blind

D. Single-blind

E. None of the above

17. The _____ of a scientific article provides the reader with detailed information regarding the study design.

A. Introduction

B. Background

C. Literature review

D. Methods

E. Abstract

18. The variance for data set A is 25 and for data set B is 9. We can conclude _____.

A. There are more items in data set A than data set B

B. The mean of data set B is smaller than the mean of data set A

C. The items in data set A are more widely spread about the mean value than the items in data set B

D. The standard deviation for data set B is larger than the standard deviation for data set A

E. None of the above

19. What route of transmission of infectious disease is a needle-stick injury?

A. Direct contact

B. Indirect contact

C. Accidental contact

D. Parenteral contact

E. Droplets

20. Which of the following statements regarding recommendations for the use of masks is *true*?

A. Masks should be used whenever aerosols or spatter may be generated.

B. A new mask should be worn for each patient.

C. Masks should be changed at least once every hour.

D. Masks should be changed more frequently in the presence of heavy aerosol contamination.

E. All of the above

21. _____ refers specifically to the process in which an antimicrobial agent destroys (germicide) or inhibits the growth of (microbiostatic) pathogenic microorganisms on inanimate surfaces.

A. Antisepsis

B. Microbacterial control

C. Sterilization

D. Disinfection

E. Asepsis

22. Which of the following biologic tests is used to check the effectiveness of the sterilization process?

A. Spore test

B. Total bacterial count test

C. Aseptic test

D. EPA test

E. Disinfection test

23. Which of the following guidelines are for disinfectants used in dental practice?

A. Have an EPA registration number

B. Kill *Mycobacterium tuberculosis*

C. Have an ADA seal of approval

D. Must be used according to guidelines

E. All of the above

24. Which of the following statements about MSDSs is correct?

A. Employees have the right to know about on-the-job hazards.

B. MSDSs help to protect employees.

C. MSDSs contain information on hazardous materials, substance, and wastes.

D. MSDSs describe chemical hazards and how to work with chemicals safely.

E. All of the above

25. Some dental plans allow the dentist to charge the patient any difference between what the plan agrees to pay and the dentist's UCR (usual, customary, reasonable) fees. This arrangement is called _____.

A. Payment differential

B. Balance billing

C. Prospective reimbursement

D. Managed care

E. None of the above

26. Which of the following is true for the fluoride in fluoridated water?

A. It is odorless

B. It is colorless

C. It is tasteless

D. A and B

E. All of the above

27. Approximately how many people in United States live in a fluoridated community?

A. 80 million

B. 124 million

C. 180 million

D. 204 million

E. 262 million

28. What percentage of the U.S. population on public water supplies lives in a fluoridated community?

A. 26%

B. 37%

C. 55%

D. 74%

E. 85%

29. Fluoridation prevents tooth decay for what age group?

    A. 1 to 12 years

    B. 13 to 20 years

    C. 1 to 20 years

    D. All ages

    E. None of the above

30. Which one of the following is an effective community prevention program?

    A. Brushing twice a day

    B. Flossing once a day

    C. A and B

    D. School sealant programs

    E. Regular dental checkups

31. Which of the following is *not* an effective community prevention program?

    A. School fluoride rinse programs

    B. School sealant programs

    C. School fluoridation

    D. Community water fluoridation

    E. Flossing daily

32. What is the recommended level of fluoride for community water fluoridation?

    A. 1.2 to 2.2 ppm

    B. 0.7 to 1.2 ppm

    C. 0.2 to 2.2 ppm

    D. 2 to 4 ppm

    E. 7 to 12 ppm

33. What is the *most* cost-effective and practical measure to prevent tooth decay?

    A. School fluoride mouth rinse programs

    B. School fluoride tablet programs

    C. Brushing and flossing daily

    D. Community water fluoridation

    E. School sealant programs

34. Fluoride supplementation for a 2-year-old child who lives in a nonfluoridated community can best be accomplished by initially prescribing _____.

    A. Fluoride tablets

    B. Fluoride lozenges

    C. Fluoride drops

    D. Fluoride mouth rinses

    E. Fluoride toothpaste

35. An amalgam restoration is considered _____.

    A. Primary prevention

    B. Secondary prevention

    C. Tertiary prevention

    D. Both primary and secondary prevention

    E. Both primary and tertiary prevention

36. Who is responsible for educating the public on the safety and effectiveness of community water fluoridation?

    A. Hygienists

    B. Nurses

    C. Physicians

    D. Dentists

    E. All of the above

37. Which one of the following statements is *true*?

    A. Fluoride mouth rinses have been used in schools in the United States for about a decade.

    B. Fluoride varnish is a method of administering systemic fluoride.

    C. Sealants can halt the carious process after it has begun.

    D. Sealants are recommended for the first and second premolars.

    E. The use of sealants is the best approach for preventing dental caries.

Periodontics

KAREN NOVAK

NIKOLA ANGELOV

OUTLINE

1. Diagnosis
2. Etiology
3. Pathogenesis
4. Treatment Planning
5. Prognosis
6. Therapy
7. Prevention and Maintenance

The following sections help the reader review the process of diagnosis, treatment, and prevention while understanding the etiology and pathogenesis of the various periodontal conditions and how this may impact the ultimate prognosis for the patient. This review covers the topics outlined in the 2013 Specifications for the National Board Dental Examination, Part II. The information in this review is from *Carranza's Clinical Periodontology*, ed 10 and 11 (St. Louis, Saunders, 2006, 2012), by Newman et al, and from published literature.

Periodontal disease describes a group of inflammatory conditions that affect the supporting structures of the teeth or periodontium. The initiation, development, diagnosis, and subsequent treatment of periodontal disease follow a well-documented sequence (Figure 7-1). Microbial plaque is generally considered to be the initiating factor in periodontal disease. When plaque accumulates on tooth and gingival surfaces, it instigates the development of an inflammatory response in the periodontal tissues. The nature and duration of the inflammatory response are critical to the clinical outcome. If the inflammatory response is sufficient to control the challenge from plaque without destruction of periodontal ligament (PDL) or alveolar bone, the clinical condition is termed *gingivitis*. If there is destruction of PDL and alveolar bone, the condition is termed *periodontitis*. The fundamental diagnosis of gingivitis or periodontitis affects treatment. With gingivitis, there is no destruction of the periodontium, and treatment should be focused on removing plaque and controlling inflammation. In periodontitis, the removal of plaque and control of inflammation may be supplemented with attempts to repair or regenerate the lost periodontal tissues and correct any anatomic deformities that may have resulted from the disease process.

1.0 Diagnosis

A. Components of an accurate diagnosis of the extent and severity of periodontal disease.
1. Medical history, including any serious familial conditions of parents or siblings such as diabetes or cardiovascular disease, and history of tobacco use.
2. Dental history, including current and prior family history of periodontal disease.
3. Full-mouth series of periapical radiographs for assessment of alveolar bone levels.
4. Examination of the head, neck, oral cavity, and lymph nodes for any pathology.
5. Oral and radiographic examination of the periodontal structures for the presence of plaque and calculus (assessment of the patient's level of home care); inflammation (redness, swelling, bleeding on probing); and destruction of the periodontal tissues (probing pocket depths, clinical attachment levels, alveolar bone loss, tooth mobility, furcation involvement).
6. Notes should be made of areas of suppuration, abscess formation, minimal width of attached gingival (subtract pocket depth from width of gingiva), obvious recession, and areas of trauma from occlusion.
7. Examination of the teeth for dental caries, developmental defects, anomalies of tooth form, wasting, areas of hypersensitivity, and proximal contact relationships.

The section editors acknowledge Dr. M. John Novak for his previous contributions as author and editor of this section.

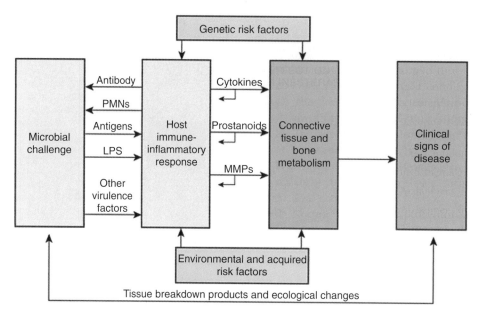

Figure 7-1 Schematic illustration of the pathogenesis of periodontitis. The microbial challenge presented by subgingival plaque bacteria results in an upregulated host immune-inflammatory response in the periodontal tissues that is characterized by the dysregulated and increased production of inflammatory cytokines (e.g., interleukins and tumor necrosis factor-α); prostanoids (e.g., prostaglandin E_2); and enzymes, including the matrix metalloproteinases (*MMPs*). These upregulated proinflammatory mediators are responsible for most periodontal tissue breakdown that occurs, including alveolar bone resorption via activation of osteoclasts. Over time, these changes result in the clinical signs of periodontal disease developing. The process is modified by environmental factors, such as smoking, and by genetic susceptibility. *LPS*, Lipopolysaccharide; *PMNs*, polymorphonuclear leukocytes. (*Modified from Page RC, Kornman KS: The pathogenesis of human periodontitis: an introduction. Periodontol 2000 14:9, 1997.*)

a. *Erosion (sometimes called corrosion)*—usually in the cervical area of facial surface of tooth; may be caused by acid beverages or citrus fruits.

b. *Abrasion*—loss of tooth substance by mechanical wear. Horizontal toothbrushing (scrubbing) with an abrasive dentifrice is the most common cause.

c. *Attrition*—occlusal wear resulting from functional contacts with opposing teeth; results in wear facets on the occlusal surfaces of teeth; may be due to functional or parafunctional habits.

d. *Abfraction*—occlusal loading resulting in tooth flexure, mechanical microfractures, and tooth substance loss in the cervical area; may appear similar to erosion.

e. *Hypersensitivity*—as a result of exposure of dentinal tubules in root surfaces to thermal changes following recession and removal of cementum by toothbrushing, dietary acids, root decay, or professional treatment such as scaling and root planing.

B. Periodontal examination.

1. *Probing pocket depth* (distance from the gingival margin to the base of the pocket detected with the periodontal probe, which can be classified as gingival, suprabony, and intrabony) (Figure 7-2); *clinical attachment loss* (distance from the cementoenamel junction [CEJ] to the base of the pocket detected with a periodontal probe); and *bleeding on probing* (measure of inflammation in the periodontal tissues)

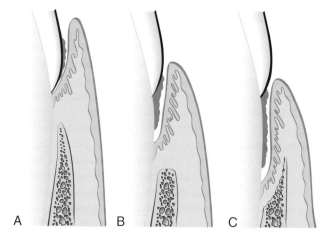

Figure 7-2 Different types of periodontal pockets. **A,** Gingival pocket. There is no destruction of the supporting periodontal tissues. **B,** Suprabony pocket. The base of the pocket is coronal to the level of the underlying bone. Bone loss is horizontal. **C,** Intrabony pocket. The base of the pocket is apical to the level of the adjacent bone. Bone loss is vertical. (*From Newman MG, et al: Carranza's Clinical Periodontology, ed 12. St. Louis, Saunders, 2015.*)

are the most objective periodontal measures and enable the clinician to differentiate between health, gingivitis, and periodontitis.

2. Additional measures include *gingival recession* (exposure of the root surface because of an apical shift in

the position of the gingival margin). Recession is measured from the CEJ to the crest of the gingival margin and is associated with attachment loss. Recession may be enhanced by trauma from toothbrushing, teeth that are positioned or have been moved buccally with orthodontics, or teeth that are large compared with the width of the periodontal supporting tissues.

3. *Alveolar bone loss* is frequently used as a measure of periodontal disease from examination of x-rays. This is not a reliable measure of periodontal disease because there is considerable variability in the normal height of the alveolar bone. Bone loss on x-rays should be evaluated in combination with probing pocket depth and clinical attachment loss to provide an accurate measure of a patient's periodontal status. Bone loss may be described as *horizontal* or *vertical*. Vertical defects can be classified by the number of bony walls they have remaining.

4. *Suppuration* is an important measure of the inflammatory response to periodontal infection because it is due to the presence of large numbers of neutrophils in the periodontal pocket. Suppuration from the pocket may be seen during periodontal probing or by palpation of the pocket wall. These areas should be aggressively treated to reduce the microbial challenge. Suppuration may be seen frequently in patients with severe disease or patients who have a systemic condition that alters the ability of the host to deal with infection.

5. *Mobility assessment*—increases in tooth mobility may be due to a loss of periodontal support, excessive occlusal forces, or a combination of both. Mobility is usually measured by placing an instrument on the buccal surface and an instrument on the lingual/palatal surface and moving the tooth buccolingually. Mobility can be measured in many ways but is assessed based on the ease and extent of tooth movement.
   a. Grade I—slightly more than normal.
   b. Grade II—moderately more than normal.
   c. Grade III—severe mobility faciolingually or mesiodistally (or both), combined with vertical displacement (the tooth can be depressed in the socket).

6. *Furcation assessment*—the complex anatomy of the furcation makes this a difficult area to treat and maintain.
   a. Classification of furcation involvements.
      (1) Grade I—incipient.
      (2) Grade II—cul-de-sac with definite horizontal component.
      (3) Grade III—complete bone loss in the furcation.
      (4) Grade IV—complete bone loss in the furcation and recession of the gingival tissues resulting in a furcation opening that is clinically visible.

   b. *Factors involved*—factors that can predispose a tooth to furcation involvement include short root trunk length, short roots, and narrow interradicular dimension. The presence of cervical enamel projections into the furcation also can be a predisposing factor.
   c. *Probing*—furcations in mandibular molars are probed from the buccal/facial and from the lingual. Furcations in maxillary molars are probed from the mesial (mesial furcation between mesiobuccal and palatal roots), buccal (buccal furcation between the two buccal roots), and distal (distal furcation between distobuccal and palatal roots).

C. Radiographic assessment.
   1. *Bone loss on traditional x-rays*—the average distance from the CEJ to the crest of the alveolar bone in health is approximately 2 mm. The normal angulation of the crest of the alveolar bone is parallel to a line joining the CEJs of adjacent teeth. A horizontal pattern of bone loss occurs parallel to this line. Angular bone loss is usually created when bone is lost on one tooth surface at a greater rate and greater extent than on an adjacent tooth surface. A full-mouth series of periapical radiographs is recommended to visualize all proximal root surfaces and bone levels.
   2. *Digital and subtraction radiography*—digital radiography allows for computerized images to be stored and corrected for exposure. Digital radiography may reduce exposure to radiation compared with traditional x-rays. Using serial x-rays of teeth and bone taken at the same location and angulation, changes in bone density can be observed using a computerized technique known as *subtraction radiography*. Changes in bone density may be associated with disease progression.
   3. *Cone beam computed tomography (CBCT)*—CBCT provides an accurate three-dimensional image of teeth and supporting structures, including bony defects. CBCT is an advanced imaging technique that is currently used primarily for patients requiring implant therapy.

D. Summarizing clinical findings—using the information described previously, the clinician can now diagnose one of the following conditions (Box 7-1).
   1. Periodontal health—no inflammation and no loss of clinical attachment and alveolar bone.
   2. Gingival disease—gingival inflammation with *no loss* of clinical attachment and alveolar bone.
   3. Periodontitis—periodontal inflammation that has extended into the PDL and alveolar bone, resulting in loss of clinical attachment and alveolar bone; usually accompanied by increased probing pocket depths, although deep pockets may not be present if recession of the gingival margin occurs at the same rate as attachment loss.

Classification of Periodontal Diseases and Conditions

Gingival Diseases

Plaque-induced gingival diseases*
Non–plaque-induced gingival lesions

Chronic Periodontitis†

Localized
Generalized

Aggressive Periodontitis

Localized
Generalized

Periodontitis as a Manifestation of Systemic Diseases

Necrotizing Periodontal Diseases

Necrotizing ulcerative gingivitis
Necrotizing ulcerative periodontitis

Abscesses of the Periodontium

Gingival abscess
Periodontal abscess
Pericoronal abscess

Periodontitis Associated with Endodontic Lesions

Endodontic-periodontal lesion
Periodontal-endodontic lesion
Combined lesion

Developmental or Acquired Deformities and Conditions

Localized tooth-related factors that predispose to
  plaque-induced gingival diseases or periodontitis
Mucogingival deformities and conditions around teeth
Mucogingival deformities and conditions on edentulous
  ridges
Occlusal trauma

Data from Armitage GC: Development of a classification system for periodontal diseases and conditions. *Ann Periodontol* 4:1, 1999.

*These diseases may occur on a periodontium with no attachment loss or on a periodontium with attachment loss that is stable and not progressing.

†Chronic periodontitis can be further classified based on extent and severity. As a general guide, extent can be characterized as localized (<30% of sites involved) or generalized (>30% of sites involved). Severity can be characterized based on the amount of clinical attachment loss (CAL) as follows: *slight* = 1 or 2 mm CAL; *moderate* = 3 or 4 mm CAL; and *severe* ≥ 5 mm CAL.

4. Necrotizing ulcerative gingivitis or periodontitis—usually accompanied by necrotic ulceration of the marginal gingival tissues, bleeding, pain, and fetid breath; may sometimes be accompanied by fever, malaise, and lymphadenopathy.
5. Periodontal abscesses.
6. Periodontitis associated with endodontic lesions.

E. Clinical features of gingivitis.
  1. *Overview*—gingivitis is frequently associated with changes in *color*, *contour*, and *consistency* that are due to changes in the levels of inflammation. Color changes are due to increases in blood flow; contour changes are due to increases in inflammatory exudates or edema within the gingival tissues; and consistency changes are due to levels of inflammation or fibrosis that frequently occurs when gingivitis is long-standing and chronic. Gingival bleeding is also a characteristic of gingivitis and can occur spontaneously, during mastication, during toothbrushing, or during periodontal probing. Gingivitis is usually characterized as gingival inflammation in the absence of clinical attachment loss. More recently, gingivitis also has been described in cases of gingival inflammation around teeth that have been successfully treated for periodontitis but have developed gingival inflammation with no additional attachment loss as a result of poor home care.
  2. *Plaque-induced gingivitis*—the most common form of gingivitis is the result of an interaction between plaque bacteria and the tissues and inflammatory cells of the host. The severity and duration of the response can be altered by local and systemic factors that can affect plaque formation and retention and the host response.
    a. *Gingival diseases modified by systemic factors*—systemic factors that alter the magnitude or duration of the host response affect the clinical appearance of gingivitis. Examples include endocrine changes during puberty, pregnancy, and diabetes. Blood dyscrasias (e.g., leukemia) may affect the immune response through their effects on white blood cells.
    b. *Gingival diseases modified by medications*—examples of medications that can cause gingival enlargement are phenytoin; immunosuppressive drugs such as cyclosporine; calcium channel blockers such as nifedipine, verapamil, and diltiazem; sodium valproate; and oral contraceptives.
    c. *Gingival diseases modified by malnutrition*—except for the effects of vitamin C deficiency (scurvy), there is little information on the effects of malnutrition.
  3. *Non–plaque-induced gingival conditions.*
    a. Gingival conditions, although uncommon, can occur in response to specific infections, including sexually transmitted infections (*Neisseria gonorrhoeae, Treponema pallidum*), viral infections (herpesviruses), and fungal infections (*Candida*).

b. Gingival conditions may also be hereditary (hereditary gingival fibromatosis) or the result of allergies to common foods, restorative materials, toothpastes or mouth rinses, and chewing gum.

c. Traumatic lesions can be *factitious* (unintentionally produced), *iatrogenic* (trauma-induced by a dentist or health professional), or *accidental* (damage through burns from hot foods and drinks).

d. Foreign body reactions can also occur to restorative materials, such as amalgam and polishing paste, when introduced into the gingival tissues.

F. Clinical features of periodontitis—periodontitis is defined as an inflammatory disease of the supporting tissues of the teeth caused by specific microorganisms or groups of specific microorganisms resulting in progressive destruction of the PDL and alveolar bone with pocket formation, recession, or both. The clinical feature that distinguishes periodontitis from gingivitis is the presence of clinically detectable attachment loss. The most common forms of periodontitis and their distinguishing characteristics are listed in Box 7-2.

1. *Necrotizing periodontal diseases*—the clinical appearance of necrotizing diseases is unique among periodontal diseases because of the characteristic ulceration and necrosis of the marginal gingiva. The gingiva may be covered by a yellowish white or grayish slough or pseudomembrane and have blunting of the papillae, bleeding on provocation or spontaneous bleeding, pain, and fetid breath. The disease may manifest as *necrotizing ulcerative gingivitis* (no attachment loss) or *necrotizing ulcerative periodontitis* (with attachment and bone loss). Predisposing factors may be stress, smoking, and immunosuppression such as seen with HIV infection.

2. *Abscesses of the periodontium*—a localized purulent infection defined by its tissue of origin, *gingival abscess* or *periodontal abscess*. Frequent causes are impaction of food, such as fish bones or popcorn, into the periodontal tissues. An abscess may also be caused by suppuration from a periodontal pocket being unable to discharge through the pocket into the mouth and draining into the periodontal supporting tissues, causing swelling and possible pain.

3. *Periodontitis associated with endodontic lesions*—these may be *endodontic-periodontal lesions* (pulpal necrosis leading to periodontal problems as pus drains through the PDL), *periodontal-endodontic lesions* (bacterial infection from a periodontal pocket spreads to the pulp causing pulpal necrosis), or a *combined lesion* (pulpal and periodontal necrosis occurring together) (Figure 7-3). If there is evidence of pulpal disease and periodontal involvement, the endodontic treatment should be completed first.

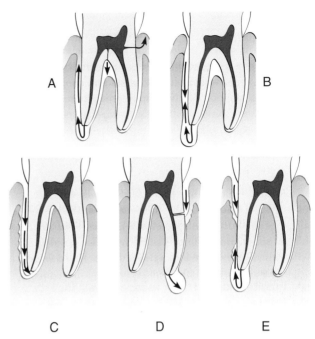

Figure 7-3 Diagrammatic representation of different types of endoperiodontal problems. **A,** Originally an endodontic problem, with fistulization from the apex and along the root to the gingiva. Pulpal infection can also spread through accessory canals to the gingiva or the furcation. **B,** Long-standing periapical lesion draining through the PDL can become secondarily complicated, leading to a retrograde periodontitis. **C,** Periodontal pocket can deepen to the apex and secondarily involve the pulp. **D,** Periodontal pocket can infect the pulp through a lateral canal, which can result in a periapical lesion. **E,** Two independent lesions, periapical and marginal, can coexist and eventually fuse with each other. *(Redrawn and modified from Simon JH, Glick DH, Frank AL: The relationship of endodontic-periodontic lesions. J Periodontol 43:202, 1972.)*

2.0 Etiology

A. Periodontal microbiology—dental plaque is considered the initiator of the periodontal disease process through its ability to promote an inflammatory response in the periodontal tissues, which may lead to destruction of those same tissues. Dental plaque is a complex biofilm that, if left intact, is resistant to antimicrobial agents such as antibiotics. Mechanical débridement is necessary to disrupt the biofilm. The composition of plaque is considered important in the inflammatory process, and specific microorganisms have been more frequently associated with this disease process than others.

1. Dental plaque composition.

a. Supragingival.

(1) Tooth associated—gram-positive cocci and short rods.

(2) Mature outer surface of plaque—gram-negative rods and filaments and spirochetes.

Box 7-2

Periodontitis

The disease periodontitis can be subclassified into the following three major types based on clinical, radiographic, historical, and laboratory characteristics.

Chronic Periodontitis

The following characteristics are common to patients with chronic periodontitis:

- Prevalent in adults but can occur in children.
- Amount of destruction consistent with local factors.
- Associated with a variable microbial pattern.
- Subgingival calculus frequently found.
- Slow to moderate rate of progression with possible periods of rapid progression.
- Possibly modified by or associated with the following:
  - Systemic diseases such as diabetes mellitus and HIV infection.
  - Local factors predisposing to periodontitis.
  - Environmental factors such as cigarette smoking and emotional stress.

Chronic periodontitis may be further subclassified into localized and generalized forms and characterized as slight, moderate, or severe based on the common features described above and the following specific features:

- Localized form: <30% of sites involved.
- Generalized form: >30% of sites involved.
- Slight: 1 to 2 mm CAL.
- Moderate: 3 to 4 mm CAL.
- Severe: ≥5 mm CAL.

Aggressive Periodontitis

The following characteristics are common to patients with aggressive periodontitis:

- Otherwise clinically healthy patient.
- Rapid attachment loss and bone destruction.
- Amount of microbial deposits inconsistent with disease severity.
- Familial aggregation of diseased individuals.

The following characteristics are common but not universal:

- Diseased sites infected with Aggregatibacter (formerly *Actinobacillus*) *actinomycetemcomitans*.
- Abnormalities in phagocyte function.

- Hyperresponsive macrophages, producing increased PGE_2 and IL-1β.
- In some cases, self-arresting disease progression.

Aggressive periodontitis may be further classified into localized and generalized forms based on the common features described above and the following specific features:

Localized Form
- Circumpubertal onset of disease.
- Localized first molar or incisor disease with proximal attachment loss on at least two permanent teeth, one of which is a first molar.
- Robust serum antibody response to infecting agents.

Generalized Form
- Usually affecting persons <30 years old (but may be older).
- Generalized proximal attachment loss affecting at least three teeth other than first molars and incisors.
- Pronounced episodic nature of periodontal destruction.
- Poor serum antibody response to infecting agents.

Periodontitis as a Manifestation of Systemic Diseases

Periodontitis may be observed as a manifestation of the following systemic diseases:

1. Hematologic disorders
   a. Acquired neutropenia
   b. Leukemias
   c. Other
2. Genetic disorders
   a. Familial and cyclic neutropenia
   b. Down syndrome
   c. Leukocyte adhesion deficiency syndromes
   d. Papillon-Lefèvre syndrome
   e. Chédiak-Higashi syndrome
   f. Histiocytosis syndromes
   g. Glycogen storage disease
   h. Infantile genetic agranulocytosis
   i. Cohen syndrome
   j. Ehlers-Danlos syndrome (types IV and VIII autosomal dominant)
   k. Hypophosphatasia
   l. Other
3. Not otherwise specified

Data from Flemmig TF: Periodontitis. *Ann Periodontol* 4:32, 1999; Kinane DF: Periodontitis modified by systemic factors. *Ann Periodontol* 4:54, 1999; and Tonetti MS, Mombelli A: Early-onset periodontitis. *Ann Periodontol* 4:39, 1999.

CAL, Clinical attachment loss; *IL-1β,* interleukin-1β; *PGE₂,* prostaglandin E₂.

b. Subgingival.
  (1) Cervical region.
    (a) Tooth associated—gram-positive rods and cocci.
    (b) Tissue associated—gram-negative rods and cocci, filaments, flagellated rods and spirochetes.
  (2) Deeper in sulcus or pocket.
    (a) Tooth associated—gram-negative rods.
    (b) Tissue associated—gram-negative rods and cocci, filaments, flagellated rods and spirochetes.
c. The major organic constituents of the plaque biofilm are polysaccharides, proteins, glycoproteins, and lipids. The major inorganic constituents are calcium and phosphorus with trace amounts of sodium, potassium, and fluoride. Saliva is the main source of inorganic components in supragingival plaque, whereas components in subgingival plaque are derived primarily from the gingival crevicular fluid.

B. Dental plaque formation—plaque formation can be divided into three phases.
1. The first phase is formation of the *pellicle*, which occurs within seconds after the tooth surface is cleaned. The pellicle consists of glycoproteins (mucins), proline-rich proteins, phosphoproteins (e.g., statherin), histidine-rich proteins, enzymes (e.g., amylase), and other molecules that serve as attachment sites for bacteria.
2. The second phase is the initial *adhesion and attachment of bacteria.* The initial adhesion is reversible and is mediated through van der Waals and electrostatic forces. After initial adhesion, a firm attachment is established that is dependent on specific bacterial adhesin molecules and host pellicle receptor interactions.
3. The third phase is *colonization and plaque maturation.* This occurs when the firmly attached, primary colonizing bacteria provide new receptors for attachment of other bacteria ("coadhesion"). The aggregated bacteria start growing, resulting in the formation of microcolonies and the development of a mature biofilm.
4. *Phases of specific bacteria*—there is a sequential nature to the deposition of bacteria on the tooth surface.
  a. *Streptococcus* and *Actinomyces* species are early or primary colonizers.
  b. Late (secondary) colonizers include *Prevotella intermedia, Prevotella loescheii, Capnocytophaga* species, *Campylobacter* species, *Porphyromonas gingivalis, Treponema* species, and *Aggregatibacter actinomycetemcomitans.*
  c. *Fusobacterium nucleatum* serves as an important middle or bridging microorganism because of its ability to coaggregate (cell-to-cell recognition of genetically distinct partner cell types) with both early colonizers and other secondary colonizers.

C. Dental plaque as a complex bacterial biofilm.
1. *Overview*—dental plaque is a biofilm composed of microcolonies encased in a polysaccharide matrix. Fluid-filled channels run through the plaque mass, permitting the passage of nutrients. Bacteria growing in a biofilm are more resistant to antimicrobials than bacteria grown in a planktonic, or free-swimming, form. Bacteria grown in biofilms communicate with each other through *quorum sensing.* Quorum sensing is important in the regulation of expression of specific genes and in controlling the microbial species in the biofilm (encouraging the growth of species of benefit to the biofilm and discouraging the growth of competitors).
2. *Maturation*—as the biofilm matures, there is a shift from a predominance of facultative, gram-positive microorganisms to gram-negative, anaerobic microorganisms.
3. *Complexes*—results of DNA-DNA hybridization studies ("checkerboard" analyses) have led to the identification of complexes of periodontal microorganisms that were given color designations.
  a. The so-called red complex (*P. gingivalis, Tannerella forsythia,* and *Treponema denticola*) is associated with bleeding on probing and deeper pockets.
  b. The presence of so-called orange complex microorganisms (*Fusobacterium* species, *Prevotella* species, and *Campylobacter* species) precedes the presence of the red complex, supporting the sequential nature of plaque formation and maturation.
  c. The existence of complexes of species in plaque also is a reflection of bacterial interdependency within the biofilm.

D. Factors influencing dental plaque biofilm formation—factors that can influence the rate of dental plaque biofilm formation between individuals include clinical wettability of the tooth surface, saliva-induced aggregation of oral bacteria, salivary flow conditions, diet, chewing fibrous food, smoking, tongue and palate brushing, stability of bacteria in the saliva, chemical composition of the pellicle, and retention depth of the dentogingival area. Plaque formation also varies by area of the mouth, tooth surface, and presence or absence of inflammation.

E. Characteristics of bacteria found in the dental plaque biofilm—gram-positive early colonizers use sugars as an energy source and saliva as a carbon source. Anaerobic microorganisms that predominate in mature plaque are asaccharolytic and use amino acids and small peptides as energy sources. Bacterial enzymes that degrade host proteins may be important in the acquisition of these amino acids and small peptides. Endotoxin is a constituent of gram-negative microorganisms that is an important initiator of the inflammatory host response.

F. Plaque hypotheses in the initiation of periodontal disease.

1. The *nonspecific plaque hypothesis* states that periodontal disease results from the elaboration of noxious products by the plaque biomass, indicating that the quantity of plaque is of most importance in the initiation of disease. This hypothesis is contradicted by the finding that some patients with little plaque have severe periodontitis.

2. The *specific plaque hypothesis* states that the pathogenic potential of plaque depends on the presence of, or increasing numbers of, specific microorganisms. As a result, many years have been spent trying to identify the specific pathogens associated with disease.

3. The *ecologic plaque hypothesis* states that putative periodontal pathogens are present in both healthy and diseased sites. A change in the pocket environment (e.g., a change in the nutrient status) is the primary cause for the overgrowth of the putative pathogens (Figure 7-4).

G. Microbiology of specific periodontal diseases.

1. *Periodontal health*—the microflora associated with periodontal health is primarily composed of gram-positive facultative cocci and rods. These microorganisms are primarily of the genera *Streptococcus* and *Actinomyces*.

2. *Gingivitis*—the microflora associated with gingivitis was assessed in a classic model system referred to as *experimental gingivitis*. In this model, periodontal health is established by professional cleaning and personal oral hygiene measures. This is followed by a 21-day period of abstinence from all oral hygiene measures. The initial microbiota is composed of gram-positive rods and cocci and gram-negative cocci. In the transition to gingivitis, gram-negative rods and filaments appear, followed by spirochetal and motile microorganisms.

3. *Chronic periodontitis*—the microflora of chronic periodontitis is composed predominantly of gram-negative, anaerobic species. The species often include *P. gingivalis*, *T. forsythia*, *P. intermedia*, *Campylobacter rectus*, *Eikenella corrodens*, *F. nucleatum*, *A. actinomycetemcomitans*, *Peptostreptococcus micros*, *Treponema* species, and *Eubacterium* species. There also is evidence that the herpesvirus microorganisms, Epstein-Barr virus 1 and human cytomegalovirus, are associated with chronic periodontitis and the presence of *P. gingivalis*, *T. forsythia*, *P. intermedia*, and *T. denticola*.

4. *Aggressive periodontitis*—*A. actinomycetemcomitans* is generally accepted as the primary etiologic agent of localized aggressive periodontitis. Other associated microorganisms include *P. gingivalis*, *E. corrodens*, *C. rectus*, *F. nucleatum*, *B. capillus*, *Eubacterium brachy*, *Capnocytophaga* species, and spirochetes. Generalized aggressive periodontitis is primarily associated with *P. gingivalis*, *P. intermedia*, *T. forsythia*, and *Treponema* species.

5. *Necrotizing diseases*—high levels of *P. intermedia*, spirochetes, and *Fusobacterium* species are found in necrotizing periodontal diseases.

6. *Periodontal abscesses*—microorganisms associated with abscesses of the periodontium include *F. nucleatum*, *P. intermedia*, *P. gingivalis*, *P. micros*, and *T. forsythia*.

7. *Dental implants*—healthy sulci around dental implants are characterized by a predominance of coccoid, aerobic species with a low number of gram-negative anaerobic species. In contrast, the pockets associated with periimplantitis are colonized by high proportions of anaerobic gram-negative rods, motile microorganisms, and spirochetes. They also may be colonized by other species such as *Pseudomonas*

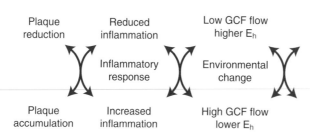

Figure 7-4 Ecologic plaque hypothesis in relation to periodontal diseases: gingivitis and periodontitis. Accumulation of plaque causes inflammation of adjacent tissues (gingivitis) and other environmental changes that favor the growth of gram-negative anaerobes and proteolytic species, including periodontopathogens. The increased proportions of such species results in destruction of periodontal tissues (i.e., periodontitis). *Eh*, Redox-potential; *GCF*, gingival crevicular fluid; *gram +ve*, gram-positive; *gram −ve*, gram-negative. (*Adapted from Marsh PD: Microbial ecology of dental plaque and its significance in health and disease. Adv Dent Res 8:263, 1994.*)

aeruginosa, Candida albicans, and *Staphylococcus* species.

H. Virulence factors of periodontopathogens—virulence factors (molecules that contribute to disease) of periodontal microorganisms can be classified into factors that promote colonization (fimbriae or pili); factors that promote host tissue destruction (extracellular proteolytic enzymes, specifically *P. gingivalis* gingipains and *A. actinomycetemcomitans* collagenase); factors that help the bacterium to evade the host immune response (extracellular capsule); molecules that degrade host immune cells (e.g., the *A. actinomycetemcomitans* leukotoxin); molecules that bind or degrade complement components; and molecules that promote invasion of host cells. Characteristics and select virulence factors of specific periodontal pathogens include the following.

1. *A. actinomycetemcomitans* is a nonmotile, gram-negative straight or curved rod. There are five serotypes based on polysaccharide composition. It grows as smooth, white, nonhemolytic colonies on blood agar plates. It is capnophilic, meaning it grows well in a carbon dioxide environment (5% to 10%). It is most closely associated with localized aggressive periodontitis. Specific virulence factors include the following.
   a. A leukotoxin that kills human neutrophils, monocytes, and some lymphocytes.
   b. Lipopolysaccharide.
   c. Collagenase.
   d. A protease that cleaves IgG.

2. *T. forsythia* is a nonmotile, gram-negative pleomorphic rod. It grows slowly only under anaerobic conditions and requires specific growth factors such as *N*-acetylmuramic acid. Specific virulence factors include proteolytic enzymes that cleave immunoglobulins and complement components. It is a member of the red complex of bacteria.

3. *Porphyromonas gingivalis* is a nonmotile, gram-negative pleomorphic rod. It grows anaerobically and becomes darkly pigmented on blood agar plates. It also can invade epithelial and endothelial cells. It is most closely associated with chronic periodontitis and is a member of the red complex of bacteria. Specific virulence factors include the following.
   a. Fimbriae important in adherence.
   b. Presence of a capsule.
   c. Proteases that cleave immunoglobulins and complement components.
   d. Proteases that cleave other tissue-associated host proteins (gingipains).
   e. Collagenase.
   f. A hemolysin.

4. *P. intermedia* and *Prevotella nigrescens* are nonmotile, gram-negative, rods. They grow anaerobically and become darkly pigmented when grown on blood agar plates. *P. intermedia* is most closely associated with

pregnancy gingivitis and necrotizing periodontal diseases.

5. *C. rectus* is a motile, gram-negative rod that has a polar flagellum. It grows anaerobically and grows as a pigmented colony when sulfide is added to the medium.

6. *F. nucleatum* is a nonmotile, gram-negative bacillus that has pointed ends. It grows anaerobically. Specific virulence properties include induction of apoptotic cell death in mononuclear and polymorphonuclear cells and release of tissue-damaging substances from leukocytes. *F. nucleatum* can be found in both healthy and diseased patients. *F. nucleatum* is considered to be an important bridging microorganism between early and late colonizers of dental plaque.

7. *Spirochetes* are motile, gram-negative spiral microorganisms. The spirochetes most often associated with periodontal diseases include *T. denticola, T. vincentii,* and *T. socranskii.* They are difficult to grow and require strict anaerobic conditions. Specific pathogenic properties include penetration of epithelium and connective tissue and production of proteolytic enzymes that can degrade collagen and destroy immunoglobulins and complement factors. Oral treponemes are closely associated with necrotizing periodontal diseases. *T. denticola* is a red complex bacterium.

8. *P. micros* and *Eubacterium* species are both gram-positive, anaerobic microorganisms. *P. micros* is a coccus; *Eubacterium* species are small, pleomorphic rods.

I. Local factors that may promote the accumulation and retention of plaque microorganisms and lead to periodontal disease—although bacterial plaque is the primary etiologic factor for the initiation of periodontal disease, other factors that may contribute to gingival inflammation include calculus, malocclusion, faulty restorations, complications associated with orthodontic therapy, self-inflicted injuries, use of tobacco, and radiation therapy.

1. *Calculus is mineralized bacterial plaque.* It forms on natural teeth and on prosthetic devices. Precipitation of mineral salts into soft plaque usually starts within 1 to 14 days of plaque formation. The initiation of calcification and rate of calculus formation vary among individuals, within an individual, and for individual teeth. Calculus can be classified as supragingival and subgingival.
   a. *Supragingival calculus* is often white in color, unless stained by food and tobacco products. Inorganic components, calcium phosphate (75%), calcium carbonate (3%), and traces of magnesium phosphate and other metals, account for 70% to 90% of supragingival calculus. Most of the inorganic component of calculus is crystalline in structure. The main crystal forms are

hydroxyapatite (58%), magnesium whitlockite (21%), octacalcium phosphate (12%), and brushite (9%). Saliva is the primary source of substances important in the mineralization of supragingival calculus. Because of the proximity of Wharton's, Bartholin's, and Stensen's ducts, supragingival calculus commonly forms on the lingual surfaces of mandibular anterior teeth and buccal surfaces of maxillary molars.

b. *Subgingival calculus* is often dark as a result of exposure to gingival crevicular fluid. The composition is similar to supragingival calculus. However, the components important in mineralization are derived from the gingival crevicular fluid rather than saliva.

c. The organic component of calculus is composed of a mixture of protein-polysaccharide complexes, desquamated epithelial cells, leukocytes, and microorganisms.

d. Calculus attachment occurs through four mechanisms.

   (1) Attachment via organic pellicle on enamel.

   (2) Mechanical locking into surface irregularities.

   (3) Close adaptation of calculus undersurface depressions to cementum.

   (4) Penetration into cementum.

e. Plaque becomes mineralized by two proposed mechanisms.

   (1) A local increase in the degree of saturation of calcium and phosphate ions, potentially secondary to an increase in pH of saliva and binding of calcium and phosphate ions into colloidal proteins in saliva, which ultimately leads to a precipitation of calcium phosphate salts.

   (2) The induction of small foci of calcification secondary to the presence of seeding agents such as the intercellular matrix of plaque. This second mechanism is known as the *epitactic concept* or *heterogeneous nucleation*. Mineralization starts extracellularly around both gram-positive and gram-negative microorganisms, although *Bacterionema* and *Veillonella* species can form intracellular hydroxyapatite crystals.

f. *Calculus deposits can be detected visually or with an explorer.* Drying calculus with air improves the ability to see it visually. Calculus located on interproximal surfaces (supragingival and subgingival) frequently can be seen radiographically.

g. Although calculus does not serve as a mechanical irritant to the gingival tissues, it is always covered with a layer of bacterial plaque. This bacterial plaque serves as the primary irritant.

2. *Materia alba* is a concentration of microorganisms, salivary proteins and lipids, desquamated epithelial cells, and leukocytes that is less adherent than dental plaque. Materia alba generally can be easily displaced with water spray or irrigation. The presence of bacteria may lead to materia alba serving as an irritant to gingival tissues.

3. *Stains* on the teeth do not contribute to gingival inflammation and are primarily an esthetic concern.

4. *Malocclusion*, manifest as irregular alignment of the teeth, may create plaque retentive areas and make plaque removal more difficult. Roots of teeth that are prominent in the arch or that are associated with frenum attachments often exhibit gingival recession. Mesial drift or extrusion associated with failure to replace missing teeth may result in occlusal problems that contribute to food impaction and plaque retention.

5. *Faulty restorations*, manifest by overhanging margins, rough surfaces, open margins, open contacts, and overcontoured crowns, may create an environment conducive to plaque retention. This is especially detrimental when the faulty restoration is located subgingivally, where a niche is created for the growth of disease-associated microorganisms and plaque removal is difficult.

6. *Subgingival margins*, even when not faulty, are associated with plaque accumulation, gingival inflammation, and deeper pockets. Well-contoured supragingival margins have little detrimental effect on the periodontium.

7. *Removable partial dentures* may result in increased mobility of abutment teeth and increased plaque accumulation.

8. *Orthodontic therapy* has been shown to increase plaque retention and to result in increases in the numbers of *Prevotella melaninogenica*, *P. intermedia*, and *Actinomyces odontolyticus*. It also can lead to direct damage of gingival tissues and the creation of excessive forces on the periodontium. These factors may be most important in adult patients undergoing orthodontic therapy. In all cases, periodontal health should be established before initiating orthodontic therapy.

9. *Self-inflicted injuries*, such as improper toothbrushing, improper use of toothpicks, application of fingernail pressure against gingival tissues, and application of caustic agents against the gingival tissues (e.g., aspirin) can damage gingival tissues.

10. Wearing *oral jewelry* in the tongue or lip also can result in recession, pocket formation, and bone loss.

11. An *aggressive horizontal brushing* technique can cause abrasions of the gingiva and tooth structure. This damage is enhanced if the patient also uses an abrasive dentifrice or uses an electronic toothbrush improperly. Gingival recession and root surface exposure can be sequelae of these habits.

3.0 Pathogenesis

The pathogenesis (genesis of pathologic change; the cellular events and reactions and other pathologic mechanisms occurring in the development of disease) of periodontal diseases is the result of a complex interaction between plaque microorganisms and the host response to the presence of microorganisms on tooth and gingival tissues. As outlined in Figure 7-1, microbial plaque is considered to be the initiator of the disease process because it serves as a challenge to the host and host tissues (periodontal tissues). How the host responds to the plaque challenge determines the severity and extent of the tissue damage associated with that response.

A. *Periodontal health*—in periodontal health, there is insufficient plaque challenge to elicit an inflammatory response that is clinically visible as a change in color, contour, or consistency of the gingival tissues. When clinically healthy periodontal tissues are viewed by histology, there is usually some degree of gingival inflammation as evidenced by the presence of neutrophils. Perfect periodontal health is nearly impossible to achieve because of the inability to remove plaque completely from tooth and gingival surfaces. The lack of plaque challenge can be due to several reasons.
  1. Minimal amounts of plaque present because of excellent oral hygiene.
  2. A plaque that is made up primarily of gram-positive bacteria that do not promote a discernible host response.
  3. A combination of both characteristics.

B. *Gingivitis*—pathologic changes observed in gingivitis are characterized by changes in color, contour, and consistency of the gingival tissues that are frequently associated with increased redness, swelling, and bleeding on probing. These clinical and histologic changes are due to the presence of an increased inflammatory response that extends into and destroys cells and matrices of the gingival tissues but does not result in destruction of PDL and bone. *The pathology associated with gingivitis is completely reversible with the removal of plaque and the resolution of the inflammation.*

C. *Periodontitis*—pathologic changes in periodontitis are the same as changes that occur in gingivitis except that the inflammation and tissue destruction extend from the gingival tissues into the PDL and alveolar bone, resulting in an irreversible destruction of periodontal tissues. The extent and severity of periodontal destruction reflects the extent and severity of the inflammatory process. The extent and severity of the inflammatory response can be influenced by several factors.
  1. The failure to remove plaque from tooth and gingival surfaces, resulting in a chronic challenge to the host.
  2. Environmental or genetic factors that may enhance the host response to the plaque challenge, resulting in an increase in the extent and severity of periodontal tissue damage.
  3. A combination of these factors.

D. Characteristics of the host response in periodontal disease.
  1. Cells of the host response.
    a. *Overview*—neutrophils, monocytes/macrophages, mast cells, and dendritic cells are considered to be cells of the innate immune response that is with us and protects us from birth. Lymphocytes are considered part of the *specific immune response*, and these cells develop antigen-specific responses throughout life. T cells, B cells, and plasma cells are the major cells of the specific response.
    b. *Polymorphonuclear neutrophils (PMNs; polymorphonuclear leukocytes)*—PMNs migrate from the blood vessels of the subepithelial vascular plexus into the periodontal pocket where they interact with plaque microorganisms (Figure 7-5). The primary role of PMNs is to protect the body from infection through phagocytosis and bacterial killing. However, they are also considered to be an important cell in the destruction of the periodontal tissues through the release of destructive molecules, such as matrix metalloproteinases (MMPs), lysosomal enzymes, cytokines, and reactive oxygen species (ROS). PMNs move from blood vessels toward sites of infection by a process of directed locomotion (*chemotaxis*) along a gradient of powerful *chemotaxins* such as C5a, IL-8, LtB$_4$, and the bacterial protein N-fMLP. PMNs are capable of internalizing microorganisms by a process of *phagocytosis* and, once internalized, they can kill and digest the microorganisms using a powerful mixture of oxygen radicals (H$_2$O$_2$, O$_2^-$) and granule enzymes (myeloperoxidase) that form the biologic equivalent of commercial bleach. Abnormalities in neutrophil function (Chédiak-Higashi syndrome, Papillon-Lefèvre syndrome, leukocyte adhesion deficiency) and numbers (neutropenia, agranulocytosis) make the host more susceptible to infection (Table 7-1).
    c. *Monocytes/macrophages*—monocytes are also part of the leukocyte family but live much longer in the tissues than neutrophils. They are responsible for ingesting antigens (e.g., bacteria) and presenting them to the cells of the specific immune response. They are also very important in regulating the immune response through the release of chemical signals called *cytokines*. Fixed macrophages and histiocytes are present in the gingival connective tissue as part of the reticuloendothelial system.
    d. *Mast cells* are important in immediate inflammation and are responsible for creating vascular permeability and dilation. They are important cells in anaphylaxis and allergic responses.

A. Chemotaxis

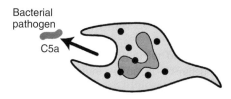

B. Initiate Phagocytosis

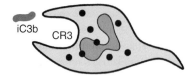

C. Oxygen Reduction

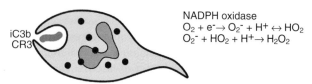

NADPH oxidase
$O_2 + e^- \rightarrow O_2^- + H^+ \leftrightarrow HO_2$
$O_2^- + HO_2 + H^+ \rightarrow H_2O_2$

D. Killing

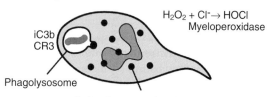

$H_2O_2 + Cl^- \rightarrow HOCl$
Myeloperoxidase

Defensins, neutral serine proteases, bactericidal/permeability increasing protein, LL37, lysozyme

Figure 7-5 After neutrophils exit the blood, they must kill the offending pathogens. This process consists of overlapping steps, as illustrated in this diagram. **A,** *Chemotaxis* refers to directed motility that enables the leukocyte to locate its target. C5a is a chemotaxin, which may be generated by any target that activates complement. **B,** *Phagocytosis* also requires the interaction of receptors with a few ligands. The diagram illustrates the important interaction between the opsonin iC3b, which coats an offending particle or cell, and the opsonic receptor CR3. **C,** *Oxygen reduction* requires the presence of oxygen and a certain oxidation-reduction (redox) potential, both of which can vary in the gingival crevice. The formation of several oxygen metabolites can kill some bacteria. **D,** *Killing* involves several processes. First, phagocytosis traps the microorganism in the stringent environment of the phagosome. Second, the phagosome and lysosomes (granules) fuse to form the phagolysosome. In this step, all the toxic compounds of the lysosome (e.g., defensins, neutral serine proteases) are dumped into the phagolysosome. Third, myeloperoxidase in the phagolysosome can convert hydrogen peroxide (*H₂O₂*) to hypochlorous acid (*HOCl*). *(From Newman MG, et al: Carranza's Clinical Periodontology, ed 12, St. Louis, Saunders, 2015.)*

e. *Dendritic cells* are distributed throughout the tissues and are important in antigen processing and presentation to cells of the specific immune response. Dendritic cells and macrophages express pattern recognition receptors that interact with microbe-associated molecular patterns on microorganisms to initiate immune responses. These types of innate immune responses provide immediate protection from microbial infection. Signaling pathways activated by pattern recognition receptors generally upregulate cytokine secretion and lead to enhanced signaling of the adaptive immune response.

f. *Lymphocytes*—the predominant lymphocytes are B cells and T cells. B cells differentiate into plasma cells and are responsible for the production of antibodies. T cells (derived from the thymus) fall into two major groups: T helper cells (CD4 cells), which help in the production of antigen-specific antibodies by B cells and plasma cells, and T cytotoxic cells (CD8 cells), which are important in controlling intracellular antigens such as bacteria, fungi, and viruses. Natural killer (NK) cells are T cells that can recognize and kill tumor and virally infected cells.

2. *Controlling the bacterial challenge*—neutrophils (PMNs) are the most important cells involved in controlling the bacterial challenge. They migrate from blood vessels under the gingival epithelium (subepithelial vascular plexus), into the periodontal pocket, where they form a barrier to protect the body from periodontal bacteria. They phagocytose and kill bacteria and release large quantities of oxygen radicals and enzymes (myeloperoxidase, lysozyme, collagenase) into the extracellular environment where they can damage host tissues.

3. *Tissue destruction in periodontal disease*—periodontal cells and tissues are destroyed by cells and proteins of the immune response. MMPs are considered the most important proteinases involved in the destruction of periodontal tissues. They are produced by most cells of the periodontal tissues, but PMNs produce large quantities of MMP-8 (collagenase) that is responsible for destroying collagen of the periodontal connective tissues and PDL (Table 7-2). MMPs are inhibited by tetracycline class antibiotics. Subantimicrobial formulations of doxycycline exploit this property, and doxycycline has been licensed as a systemic adjunctive drug for treating periodontitis. Oxygen radicals (superoxide and hydrogen peroxide) produced by inflammatory cells (PMNs and macrophages) are also toxic to cells of the periodontium having a direct effect on cell functions and DNA.

4. *Cytokines* are important signaling molecules released from cells. The cytokine IL-1 is important in bone

Table 7-1

Systemic Neutrophil Abnormalities Associated with Aggressive Periodontitis

CONDITION	NEUTROPHIL ABNORMALITY	PERIODONTAL MANIFESTATIONS
Neutropenia, agranulocytosis	Decreased number of neutrophils	Severe aggressive periodontitis
Chédiak-Higashi syndrome	Decreased neutrophil chemotaxis and secretion	Aggressive periodontitis and oral ulceration
	Neutrophil granules fuse to form characteristic giant granules called *megabodies*	Syndrome caused by mutation in the vesicle trafficking regulator gene, *LYST*
Papillon-Lefèvre syndrome	Multiple functional neutrophil defects, including myeloperoxidase deficiency, defective chemotaxis, and phagocytosis	Severe aggressive periodontal destruction at an early age, which may involve primary and permanent dentition Recently associated with mutation in cathepsin C gene
Leukocyte adhesion deficiency type 1 (LAD-1)	Defects in leukocyte function caused by lack of integrin-2 subunit (CD18)	Aggressive periodontitis at an early age and affecting primary and permanent dentition, in individuals who are homozygous for defective gene
	Neutrophil defects include impaired migration and phagocytosis Histologically, almost no extravascular neutrophils are evident in periodontal lesions	
Leukocyte adhesion deficiency type 2 (LAD-2)	Neutrophils fail to express the ligand (CD15) for P- and E-selectins, resulting in impaired transendothelial migration in response to inflammation	Aggressive periodontitis at a young age

From Newman MG, et al: *Carranza's Clinical Periodontology,* ed 12. St. Louis, Saunders, 2015.

resorption; IL-8 is important in attracting inflammatory cells (chemotactic); and tumor necrosis factor (TNF) is important in activating macrophages.

5. *Prostaglandins* are produced from arachidonic acid of cell membranes in response to cyclooxygenases (COX-1 and COX-2). They have widespread proinflammatory effects but can be inhibited by nonsteroidal antiinflammatory drugs (NSAIDs) (e.g., aspirin). However, the negative side effects of these drugs have limited their use as adjuncts in treating periodontal disease.

6. *Pathogenesis of gingivitis*—the development of gingivitis from healthy tissues is characterized in three stages (Box 7-3).

   a. *Stage 1, initial lesion*—2 to 4 days with vascular dilation, infiltration of PMNs, perivascular collagen loss, and increased gingival crevicular fluid flow.

   b. *Stage 2, early lesion*—4 to 7 days with increase in vasculature, lymphocyte infiltration, increased collagen loss, and redness and bleeding on probing.

   c. *Stage 3, established lesion*—14 to 21 days with increased vasculature; mature plasma cells in the tissues; collagen loss; and clinical changes in color, contour, and consistency.

   d. A fourth stage has been described as the *advanced stage,* which is the stage where characteristics of stage 3 move into the PDL and bone to create *periodontitis.*

7. *Pathogenesis of periodontitis*—there are few differences between stage 3 of gingivitis and the destructive lesion of periodontitis except that the inflammatory lesion becomes bigger and moves into the PDL and bone. The severity and extent of periodontal destruction is determined by the magnitude and duration of the inflammatory response. With increased severity of the response, there is an increase in the release of the tissue destructive MMPs and proinflammatory cytokines listed earlier. Risk factors such as smoking, diabetes, and genetic susceptibility to an enhanced or diminished host response may affect the extent and severity of the host response (Figure 7-6).

8. Environmental and systemic factors that may influence the progression of periodontal disease—although bacterial plaque is the primary etiologic factor for periodontal disease, how the host responds to this bacterial challenge is critical in the pathogenic process. The host response varies among individuals and may explain much of the difference in disease severity seen in periodontal disease. Either an insufficient response or an exaggerated host response can lead to more severe forms of disease. Various environmental and systemic influences can have an effect on the periodontium. The magnitude of the inflammatory response can be altered by environmental (smoking/tobacco use), systemic (endocrine disorders and hormonal changes, hematologic disorders,

Table 7-2

Biologic Activities of Selected Matrix Metalloproteinases Relevant to Periodontal Disease

MMP TYPE	ENZYME	BIOLOGIC ACTIVITY
Collagenases	All	Degrade interstitial collagen (type I, II, III) Digest ECM and non-ECM molecules
	MMP-1	Keratinocyte migration and reepithelialization Platelet aggregation
	MMP-13	Osteoclast activation
Gelatinases	All	Degrade denatured collagens and gelatin
	MMP-2	Differentiation of mesenchymal cells with inflammatory phenotype Epithelial cell migration Increased bioavailability of MMP-9
Stromelysins	All	Digest ECM molecules
	MMP-3	Activates pro-MMPs Disrupted cell aggregation Increased cell invasion
Matrilysins	MMP-7	Disrupted cell aggregation Increased cell invasion
Membrane-type MMPs	All	Digest ECM molecules Activate pro-MMP-2 (except MT4-MMP)
	MT1-MMP	Epithelial cell migration Degrade collagen types I, II and III

Adapted from Hannas AR, Pereira JC, Granjeiro JM, et al: The role of matrix metalloproteinases in the oral environment. *Acta Odontol Scand* 65:1, 2007.

ECM, Extracellular matrix; *MMPs,* matrix metalloproteinases; *MT,* membrane type.

immune deficiencies, stress, and psychosomatic disorders), and genetic (polymorphisms in inflammatory genes) influences (see Figure 7-1).

a. *Cigarette smoking is a risk factor for periodontal disease.* Cigarette smokers have more periodontal disease than nonsmokers and exhibit increased attachment and bone loss, an increased number of deep pockets, and an increased amount of calculus formation. There is a dose response with increased risk for disease in individuals who smoke more cigarettes (Tables 7-3 and 7-4).

(1) The number of years of tobacco use, calculated in pack-years, is a significant factor in tooth loss and periodontal disease. The prevalence and severity of periodontal disease in individuals who stop smoking is between that found in current smokers and nonsmokers. Both former smokers and nonsmokers respond better to

Box 7-3

Key Features of Histologic Stages of Gingivitis and Periodontitis

Initial Lesion—Corresponds to Clinically Healthy Gingival Tissues

- Slightly elevated vascular permeability and vasodilation.
- GCF flows out of the sulcus.
- Migration of leukocytes, primarily neutrophils, in relatively small numbers through the gingival connective tissue, across the junctional epithelium, and into the sulcus.

Early Lesion—Corresponds to Early Gingivitis That Is Evident Clinically

- Increased vascular permeability, vasodilation, and GCF flow.
- Large numbers of infiltrating leukocytes (mainly neutrophils and lymphocytes)
- Degeneration of fibroblasts.
- Collagen destruction, resulting in collagen-depleted areas of the connective tissue.
- Proliferation of the junctional and sulcular epithelium into collagen-depleted areas.

Established Lesion—Corresponds to Established, Chronic Gingivitis

- Dense inflammatory cell infiltrate (plasma cells, lymphocytes, neutrophils).
- Accumulation of inflammatory cells in the connective tissues.
- Elevated release of MMPs and lysosomal contents from neutrophils.
- Significant collagen depletion and proliferation of epithelium.
- Formation of pocket epithelium containing large numbers of neutrophils.

Advanced Lesion—Marks Transition from Gingivitis to Periodontitis

- Predominance of neutrophils in the pocket epithelium and in the pocket.
- Dense inflammatory cell infiltrate in the connective tissues (primarily plasma cells).
- Apical migration of junctional epithelium to preserve intact epithelial barrier.
- Continued collagen breakdown resulting in large areas of collagen-depleted connective tissue.
- Osteoclastic resorption of alveolar bone.

Adapted from Page RC, Schroeder HE: Pathogenesis of inflammatory periodontal disease. A summary of current work. *Lab Invest* 34:235-249, 1976.

GCF, Gingival crevicular fluid; *MMPs,* matrix metalloproteinases.

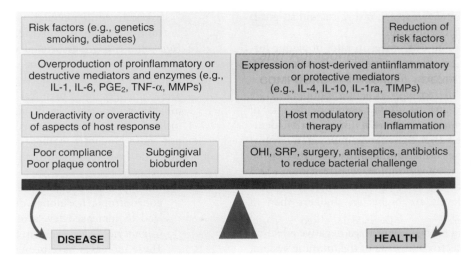

Figure 7-6 The periodontal balance. The balance between periodontal breakdown ("disease") and periodontal stability ("health") is tipped toward disease by risk factors; excessive production of inflammatory cytokines and enzymes (e.g., interleukin-1 and interleukin-6 *[IL-1 and IL-6]*, prostaglandin E$_2$ *[PGE$_2$]*, tumor necrosis factor-α *[TNF-α]*, matrix metalloproteinases *[MMPs]*); and underactivity or overactivity of aspects of the immune-inflammatory host response, poor compliance, and a pathogenic microflora. The balance can be tipped toward health by risk factor modification; upregulation; and restoration of balance between naturally occurring inhibitors of inflammation (e.g., interleukin-4 and interleukin-10 *[IL-4 and IL-10]*, interleukin-1 receptor antagonist *[IL-1ra]*, tissue inhibitors of metalloproteinases *[TIMPs]* and host modulatory therapy *(HMT)* as well as antibacterial treatments such as oral hygiene instructions *(OHI)*, scaling and root planing *(SRP)*, surgery, antiseptics, and antibiotics. *(From Newman MG, et al:* Carranza's Clinical Periodontology, *ed 12, St. Louis, Saunders, 2015.)*

Table 7-3

Effects of Smoking on the Etiology and Pathogenesis of Periodontal Disease

ETIOLOGIC FACTOR	IMPACT OF SMOKING
Microbiology	No effect on rate of plaque accumulation ↑ Colonization of shallow periodontal pockets by periodontal pathogens ↑ Levels of periodontal pathogens in deep periodontal pockets
Immune-inflammatory response	Altered neutrophil chemotaxis, phagocytosis, and oxidative burst ↑ TNF-α and PGE$_2$ in GCF ↑ Neutrophil collagenase and elastase in GCF ↑ Production of PGE$_2$ by monocytes in response to LPS
Physiology	↓ Gingival blood vessels with inflammation ↓ GCF flow and bleeding on probing with inflammation ↓ Subgingival temperature ↑ Time needed to recover from local anesthesia

From Newman MG, et al: *Carranza's Clinical Periodontology,* ed 12. St. Louis, Saunders, 2015.

GCF, Gingival crevicular fluid; *LPS,* lipopolysaccharide; *PGE$_2$,* prostaglandin E$_2$; *TNF-α,* tumor necrosis factor-α; ↓, decreased; ↑, increased.

Table 7-4

Effects of Smoking on Prevalence and Severity of Periodontal Disease

PERIODONTAL DISEASE	IMPACT OF SMOKING
Gingivitis	↓ Gingival inflammation and bleeding on probing
Periodontitis	↑ Prevalence and severity of periodontal destruction ↑ Pocket depth, attachment loss, bone loss ↑ Rate of periodontal destruction ↑ Prevalence of severe periodontitis ↑ Tooth loss ↑ Prevalence with increased number of cigarettes smoked per day ↓ Prevalence and severity with smoking cessation

From Newman MG, et al: *Carranza's Clinical Periodontology,* ed 12. St. Louis, Saunders, 2015.

↓, Decreased; ↑, increased.

periodontal therapy (nonsurgical and surgical) than current smokers.

(2) There are no differences in rates of plaque formation in smokers versus nonsmokers. This finding suggests qualitative rather than quantitative differences in the microflora may be involved in the disease process. Results of checkerboard DNA-DNA hybridization demonstrated that the orange and red microbial complexes were significantly more prevalent in current smokers than in former smokers and nonsmokers. There also is evidence that *T. forsythia* levels are higher in smokers than in nonsmokers.

(3) Smoking exerts a significant negative effect on the protective elements of the immune system. These may include functional alterations in neutrophils (decreased chemotaxis, decreased oxidative burst), reduced levels of IgG2, elevated levels of TNF-α, PGE$_2$, neutrophil elastase, and MMP-8. These findings suggest that smoking not only dampens the response of host defense cells such as neutrophils but also leads to increased release of tissue-destructive enzymes.

(4) There appear to be alterations in the gingival microvasculature in smokers, resulting in decreased blood flow and decreased clinical signs of inflammation.

b. *Smokeless tobacco use* can lead to localized attachment loss and recession at the site of tobacco product placement.

c. *Radiation therapy* to oral tissues can result in increased periodontal attachment loss and tooth loss on the irradiated side. Periodontal health should be established before beginning radiation therapy

d. *Diabetes*—patients with diabetes have a higher prevalence and severity of periodontal disease than individuals without diabetes. Diabetes does not cause periodontal disease, but there is evidence that it alters the response of the periodontal tissues to bacterial plaque.

(1) Patients with poorly controlled diabetes often have enlarged gingival, polyploid gingival proliferations, abscess formation, and loosened teeth. Patients with poorly controlled diabetes often have PMNs that demonstrate impaired chemotaxis, defective phagocytosis, or impaired adherence.

(2) The hyperglycemia that characterizes diabetes leads to nonenzymatic glycosylation of proteins and matrix molecules. These glycated molecules accumulate in various sites and are called *advanced glycosylation end-products* (AGEs). The increase in AGEs as a sequela of

hyperglycemia may play a role in the progression of periodontal disease.

e. *Hormonal changes* associated with puberty, menstruation, pregnancy, use of oral contraceptives, and menopause can affect the periodontium. These changes may manifest as an exaggerated inflammatory response of the gingival tissues to local factors. The hormonal change itself does not cause gingivitis. Rather, it has an impact on how the host responds to the microbial plaque challenge.

(1) *Puberty and related conditions*—increases in gonadotropic hormones during puberty may lead to increased levels of *P. intermedia* and *Capnocytophaga* species in the bacterial plaque. These increases have been associated with the increased gingival bleeding often seen during puberty. Hyperplastic responses of the gingival tissues also have been noted.

(2) *Menstruation*—increased gingival bleeding is often seen during menstruation.

(3) *Pregnancy*—pregnancy gingivitis increases in severity beginning in the second or third month. It is manifest as enlarged, edematous gingival tissues that demonstrate increased ease of bleeding when the patient performs oral hygiene procedures. These changes appear to be associated primarily with increased levels of progesterone, which causes dilation of the gingival microvasculature, circulatory stasis, and increased susceptibility to mechanical irritants. In some cases, the gingival tissues become enlarged to the point that they appear as large masses, which are referred to as *pregnancy tumors* (pyogenic granulomas). These gingival changes seen during pregnancy are usually reversible postpartum, provided that the local etiologic factors have been removed.

(a) Increased levels of *P. intermedia* have been found during pregnancy. This increase appears to be associated with the elevation of systemic levels of estradiol and progesterone, which are proposed to substitute for menadione, a required growth factor for *P. intermedia*.

(b) Immune suppression during pregnancy may contribute to the increased susceptibility to gingival inflammation seen in many women.

(c) Hormonal changes during pregnancy can have an impact on cellular proliferation, differentiation, and keratinization (estrogen effects) and on permeability of the vasculature, the rate and pattern of collagen turnover, and metabolic breakdown of folate (progesterone).

(d) Periodontal treatment during pregnancy should include plaque control through oral hygiene instruction and scaling and root planing. These procedures can be performed any time during the pregnancy, but elective treatment is best performed during the second trimester. Although the safety of performing dental radiographs during pregnancy is well documented, it is recommended that no radiographs be taken during the first trimester. If radiographs are necessary for diagnosis, a protective lead apron must be used.

(e) Medications should be limited during pregnancy. Some local anesthetics (mepivacaine, bupivacaine, procaine) and analgesics (aspirin, ibuprofen, codeine, hydrocodone, oxycodone) commonly used in dental practice must be used with caution. Propoxyphene, commonly used in the past in dentistry, has been withdrawn from the market because of a high risk-to-benefit ratio (see Section 8, Pharmacology). Tetracycline should not be given during pregnancy because this drug can lead to depressed bone growth, enamel hypoplasia, tooth discoloration, and hepatic damage. Ciprofloxacin, metronidazole, gentamicin, vancomycin, and clarithromycin either should be used with caution or should be avoided. Penicillin, erythromycin, and cephalosporins can be used.

(f) *Oral contraceptives*—oral contraceptives may contribute to gingival changes similar to those seen in pregnancy.

(g) *Menopause*—some postmenopausal women present with gingivostomatitis, manifest as dry, shiny oral mucosa that bleeds easily. There also may be thinning of the mucosa. Use of toothbrushes with soft bristles, dentifrices with minimal abrasiveness, and rinses with low alcohol content may be advised. Osteopenia and osteoporosis have been associated with menopause. There is evidence for a probable association between osteoporosis and alveolar bone loss.

(4) *Blood dyscrasias*—patients with leukemia may present with proliferative gingival enlargements that appear bluish red and cyanotic with spongelike consistency. The enlargements are often found in the interdental gingival. As with other gingival alterations, bacterial plaque is the initiating factor. Gingival bleeding, caused by thrombocytopenia, also is often found in leukemic patients. In addition, these patients often have discrete ulcerations in the gingival tissue. Patients with pernicious anemia, iron deficiency anemia, and sickle cell anemia may have a marked pallor to their gingiva. Periodontal manifestations in thrombocytopenia purpura may include swollen, soft, friable gingiva that bleeds easily on probing. Severe periodontal disease may be seen in individuals with neutropenia, agranulocytosis, Chédiak-Higashi syndrome, lazy leukocyte syndrome, leukocyte adhesion deficiency, Down syndrome, and Papillon-Lefèvre syndrome.

(5) *Down syndrome and other syndromes*—increased numbers of *P. intermedia* have been reported in patients with Down syndrome. Hypophosphatasia, congenital heart disease, tetralogy of Fallot, and Eisenmenger's syndrome all are disorders that may be associated with increased severity of periodontal disease.

(6) *Stress*—chronic or long-term stress appears to have effects on the periodontium. People with less stable lifestyles and more negative life events have more periodontal disease than people with more stable lifestyles and fewer negative life events. For example, long-term financial stress in patients with poor coping skills may exacerbate periodontal destruction. Stress not only may induce changes in an individual's behavior, but it also influences the immune system. Stress increases cortisol production, which can subsequently suppress the immune response. In the presence of the microbial challenge that is the primary etiologic factor for periodontal disease, immune suppression may increase the potential for these pathogens to induce disease.

(7) *Nutrition*—the impact of nutrition on periodontal disease is unclear. Although there are no known nutritional deficiencies that alone cause periodontal disease, deficiencies can affect the barrier function of epithelial cells (vitamin A), contribute to osteoporosis of alveolar bone in dogs (vitamin D), contribute to gingivitis (B complex), and increase the severity of gingivitis in the presence of bacterial plaque, leading to severe bleeding, swollen gingival, and loosened teeth (vitamin C). Protein deficiency may lead to altered integrity of the periodontal tissues, resulting in the patient having tissues that are more susceptible to destruction precipitated by bacterial plaque.

(8) *Heavy metals*—ingestion of metals such as bismuth, lead, and mercury can lead to alterations in the periodontium. Bismuth intoxication can lead to discoloration of the gingival margin in areas affected by inflammation; lead intoxication can lead to gingival pigmentation

and ulceration; mercury intoxication also can lead to gingival pigmentation and ulceration.

(9) *Medications*—bisphosphonates inhibit osteoclast activity and are used primarily to treat cancer (intravenous administration) and osteoporosis (usually oral administration). Bisphosphonates are rapidly absorbed in bone, giving them a long half-life. Osteonecrosis of the jaw after dental procedures has been associated with bisphosphonates (bisphosphonate-induced osteonecrosis of the jaw). Dental health care providers should evaluate patients carefully before providing surgical interventions in patients with a history of bisphosphonate use, particularly at higher doses used in treating cancer.

4.0 Treatment Planning

The treatment plan is the outline of therapy designed to establish and maintain oral health. A good treatment plan coordinates therapy across disciplines. Other than managing emergencies, treatment should not be initiated until the treatment plan is established. The primary (short-term) goal of the periodontal treatment plan is elimination of gingival inflammation through the correction of the conditions that cause gingival inflammation. Periodontal treatment also is designed to eliminate pain, arrest soft and hard tissue destruction (loss of attachment), establish occlusal stability and function, reduce tooth loss, and prevent disease recurrence (long-term goals). It is not designed to save all teeth. The periodontal treatment plan takes into consideration the diagnosis, risk factors, and the desires of the patient. Treatment plans should be presented to patients in terms they can understand. They should be informed of the diagnosis, prognosis, and options for treatment. The linkages between periodontal and restorative phases of therapy should be explained to the patient.

A. Phases of periodontal therapy (Box 7-4).
   1. *Preliminary or emergency*—hopeless teeth may be extracted in this phase.
   2. *Nonsurgical (phase I therapy)*—the objective of this phase is to alter or eliminate the microbial etiology and contributing factors to periodontal diseases, leading to reduction in inflammation. This objective is achieved by caries control in patients with rampant caries (including patient education in diet control), removal of local factors (plaque and calculus) through prophylaxis or scaling and root planing, correction of defective restorations, treatment of carious lesions, and institution of oral hygiene practices. It also may include local or systemic antimicrobial therapy,

---

Box 7-4

Phases of Periodontal Therapy

Preliminary Phase

Treatment of Emergencies
- Dental or periapical
- *Periodontal*
- Other—extraction of hopeless teeth and provisional replacement if needed (may be postponed to a more convenient time)

Nonsurgical Phase (Phase I Therapy)

Plaque Control and Patient Education
- Diet control (in patients with rampant caries)
- *Removal of calculus and root planing*
- *Correction of restorative and prosthetic irritational factors*
- Excavation of caries and restoration (temporary or final, depending on whether a definitive prognosis for the tooth has been determined and the location of caries)
- *Antimicrobial therapy (local or systemic)*
- *Occlusal therapy*
- *Minor orthodontic movement*
- *Provisional splinting and prosthesis*

Evaluation of Response to Nonsurgical Phase

Rechecking
- *Pocket depth and gingival inflammation*
- *Plaque and calculus, caries*

Surgical Phase (Phase II Therapy)
- Periodontal therapy, including placement of implants
- Endodontic therapy

Restorative Phase (Phase III Therapy)
- Final restorations
- Fixed and removable prosthodontic appliances
- Evaluation of response to restorative procedures
- Periodontal examination

Maintenance Phase (Phase IV Therapy)

Periodic Rechecking
- *Plaque and calculus*
- *Gingival condition (pockets, inflammation)*
- *Occlusion, tooth mobility*
- Other pathologic changes

From Newman MG, et al: *Carranza's Clinical Periodontology*, ed 12. St. Louis, Saunders, 2015.

minor orthodontic tooth movement, occlusal therapy, and provisional splinting and prostheses. The evaluation phase is designed to determine the effectiveness of treatment provided during phase I therapy through rechecking pocket depths and the presence of inflammation as well as an evaluation for remaining plaque, calculus, and dental caries. It should occur approximately 4 to 8 weeks after the completion of phase I therapy; this permits time for epithelial and connective tissue healing by the formation of a long junctional epithelium.

3. *Surgical (phase II therapy)*—this phase includes all periodontal surgical therapy, including placement of implants and endodontic therapy.

4. *Restorative (phase III therapy)*—this phase includes placement of final restorations and fixed and removable prosthetic appliances, evaluation of the response to these restorations, and periodontal examination.

5. *Maintenance (phase IV therapy)*—periodontal procedures during the maintenance phase include evaluation of oral hygiene status, presence or absence of local factors, condition of the periodontium (pocket depths, attachment levels, mobility, furcation involvements, mucogingival issues and occlusion) and other pathologic changes. This phase should begin after the completion of phase II therapy. This phase may also be called *supportive periodontal therapy*.

B. Risk factors, determinants, indicators, and markers for periodontal disease—risk factors that must be considered when establishing a treatment plan include tobacco smoking, diabetes, and pathogenic bacteria and microbial tooth deposits as well as anatomic factors that favor plaque accumulation (see Section 2.0, Etiology). Other risk determinants, risk indicators, and risk markers that should be considered when developing a periodontal treatment plan include genetic factors, age, gender, socioeconomic status, immune status, osteoporosis, history of previous periodontal disease, and bleeding on probing (Box 7-5). When an at-risk patient is identified, the treatment plan may be modified based on the identified risk factors and the impact they may have on the predicted outcome of treatment.

1. Genetic factors.

a. Studies conducted in twins have shown that genetic factors influence periodontal status. Results from these studies have demonstrated that there is a heritable component to chronic periodontitis.

b. Some studies have shown that polymorphisms in both the interleukin IL-1α and IL-1β genes have been associated with increased IL-1 production and severe chronic periodontitis in nonsmoking subjects. However, other studies have demonstrated limited association of these gene alterations with periodontitis. The presence of these polymorphisms may be only one of several factors related to the risk for periodontal disease.

Box 7-5

Categories of Risk Elements for Periodontal Disease

Risk Factors

Tobacco smoking
Diabetes
Pathogenic bacteria
Microbial tooth deposits

Risk Determinants and Background Characteristics

Genetic factors
Age
Gender
Socioeconomic status
Stress

Risk Indicators

HIV/AIDS
Osteoporosis
Infrequent dental visits

Risk Markers and Predictors

Previous history of periodontal disease
Bleeding on probing

---

c. There is evidence that the risk for aggressive periodontitis may be heritable. Segregation analyses support the role of a major gene in the etiology of these diseases. Genetic and inherited disorders associated with aggressive periodontitis include leukocyte adhesion deficiency types I and II, acatalasia, chronic and cyclic neutropenia, Chédiak-Higashi syndrome, Ehler-Danlos syndrome, Papillon-Lefèvre syndrome, hypophosphatasia, trisomy 21, prepubertal periodontitis, and Kindler syndrome.

d. Alterations in neutrophil and monocyte functions, in the receptor for IgG2, and in IgG2 titers are under genetic regulation. Each of these alterations has been shown to have an impact on periodontal disease.

2. Age.

a. Changes in the periodontium associated with aging include thinning and decreased keratinization of the epithelium, coarser and denser gingival connective tissues, decreases in fibroblasts and organic matrix production in the PDL, increased width of cementum, and more irregular periodontal surface of bone and less regular insertion of collagen fibers.

b. Evidence that age has an impact on the microbial flora is equivocal.

c. The prevalence and severity of periodontal disease increase with age; however, this is most likely due to prolonged exposure to etiologic factors associated with the disease rather than with degenerative changes related to aging. Older adults with periodontal disease generally present with chronic periodontitis. Medical and mental conditions, medications, functional status, lifestyle behaviors, manual dexterity, and disease severity must be considered when developing a treatment plan for these patients. Although some age-related changes occur in the host response, these changes do not appear to be correlated with periodontitis. The risk of dental caries from the exposure of root surfaces through nonsurgical and surgical treatment must be considered as well.

d. Young people with periodontal disease may present with aggressive periodontitis. Although the treatment plan for these patients typically consists of conventional periodontal therapy (patient education, scaling and root planing, frequent maintenance appointments), adjunctive antimicrobial therapy (systemic antibiotics) and host-modifying drugs (systemic sub–antimicrobial dose doxycycline [SDD]) often are necessary to obtain a positive response. In the localized form of disease, several studies support the adjunctive administration of systemic tetracycline or doxycycline. A combination of metronidazole and amoxicillin also has been shown to enhance the response in patients with aggressive periodontitis. Decisions regarding the prognosis for retention of individual teeth and plans for replacing teeth that must be extracted also are important components of the treatment plan for patients with aggressive disease. After stabilization of the periodontium, frequent maintenance visits are important in these patients to allow for early detection and treatment of sites that begin to lose attachment.

3. Gender—males generally have more local factors and more loss of attachment than females. This difference is most likely attributable to preventive habits and practices rather than to physiologic differences.

4. Socioeconomic status—decreased dental awareness and frequency of dental visits and the presence of other risk factors such as smoking are likely contributors to the increased incidence of periodontal disease found in individuals of lower socioeconomic status.

5. Immune status (HIV infection and other systemic factors that influence the immune system)—necrotizing ulcerative periodontitis is often diagnosed in immunocompromised individuals. Dentists should treat a patient presenting with this form of disease in conjunction with the patient's physician to establish potential systemic factors contributing to the disease. Treatment includes local débridement with scaling and root planing, lavage, and oral hygiene instruction. The lesions may be painful, leading to the need for local anesthesia. Antimicrobial agents such as chlorhexidine may be administered. Resolution of any underlying systemic factor may be necessary to treat necrotizing ulcerative periodontitis successfully.

6. Osteoporosis—although there are conflicting studies, the reduced bone mass seen in patients with osteoporosis may have an impact on progression of periodontal disease.

7. Previous history of periodontal disease—patients with the most severe prior loss of attachment are at greatest risk for future loss of attachment.

8. Bleeding on probing—bleeding on probing is the best clinical indicator of gingival inflammation.

9. Stress—emotional stress may interfere with normal immunologic function, and the incidence of necrotizing ulcerative gingivitis increases during periods of stress; both of these suggest a potential relationship between stress and periodontal disease.

5.0 Prognosis

The prognosis is a prediction of the outcome of a disease. It takes into consideration the presence of risk factors for the disease. The prognosis for individual teeth must be considered in the context of the prognosis for the entire dentition. Teeth that will serve as abutments for prosthetic devices must have a periodontal prognosis consistent with their long-term maintenance. Attempts to retain teeth with severe periodontal disease are not advisable if retention jeopardizes adjacent healthy or less affected teeth. The prognosis should be reassessed after the completion of phase I therapy (Box 7-6).

A. *Clinical factors* that affect the prognosis include the patient's age, disease severity, level of plaque control, and patient compliance. Younger patients with evidence of periodontitis generally have a poorer prognosis than older patients with comparable levels of disease. Clinical attachment level is more important than pocket depth in determining prognosis. The amount of bone loss also is important, especially when prosthetic care is part of the treatment plan. The type of bony defect must be considered. Teeth with vertical defects may have a better prognosis than teeth with comparable levels of horizontal bone loss owing to the potential for treating the vertical defect with regenerative therapy. The success of this regenerative procedure is affected by the contour of the vertical defect and the number of remaining walls. Patients with poor plaque control and noncompliant or uncooperative patients also have a poorer prognosis than patients with good oral hygiene practices and demonstrated compliance with recommended treatment.

Overall Clinical Factors

Patient age
Disease severity
Plaque control
Patient compliance

Systemic and Environmental Factors

Smoking
Systemic disease or condition
Genetic factors
Stress

Local Factors

Plaque and calculus
Subgingival restorations

Anatomic Factors

Short, tapered roots
Cervical enamel projections
Enamel pearls
Bifurcation ridges
Root concavities
Developmental grooves
Root proximity
Furcation involvement
Tooth mobility

Prosthetic and Restorative Factors

Abutment selection
Caries
Nonvital teeth
Root resorption

From Newman MG, et al: *Carranza's Clinical Periodontology*, ed 12. St. Louis, Saunders, 2015.

B. *Systemic factors* that affect the prognosis include cigarette smoking, systemic diseases and conditions, genetic factors, and stress. Cigarette smokers not only have a higher prevalence and severity of periodontal disease but also have a decreased healing response to both nonsurgical and surgical therapy. Current cigarette smokers with periodontal disease have a poorer prognosis than patients who have never smoked. However, smokers who successfully complete a cessation program have a better prognosis than current smokers. Patients with poorly controlled diabetes mellitus have a poorer prognosis than patients with well-controlled diabetes mellitus or healthy patients with no history of diabetes mellitus. Diseases that compromise the patient's ability to perform oral hygiene (e.g., Parkinson's disease) or serve as contraindications to recommended surgical periodontal therapy (e.g., uncontrolled diabetes mellitus) are associated with a poorer prognosis. Genetic factors that influence the host response to a microbial challenge also can have an impact on the prognosis. Chronic stress and poor coping mechanisms may also contribute to a poor prognosis.

C. *Local factors* that affect prognosis include plaque or calculus, subgingival restorations, anatomic factors, and tooth mobility. Bacterial plaque is the primary etiologic agent for periodontal disease. Subgingival restorations may contribute to plaque retention, leading to a poorer prognosis. Teeth with short, tapered roots and large crowns have a poor prognosis because of the disproportionate root/crown ratio and reduced root surface available for periodontal support. Cervical enamel projections extending into furcations and enamel pearls serve as plaque retentive areas and interfere with the attachment apparatus. Root concavities, developmental grooves, root proximity, and furcation involvements all create situations that make the tooth difficult to clean and have an impact on the prognosis. In the presence of bacterial plaque, mobile teeth do not respond as well to therapy as nonmobile teeth.

D. *Prognosis*—the prognosis is usually classified as excellent, good, fair, poor, questionable, or hopeless. Characteristics of each classification listed include one or more of the following.

1. *Excellent*—no bone loss, gingival health, good patient cooperation, no secondary systemic or environmental factors.

2. *Good*—adequate alveolar bone support, potential to control etiologic factors and establish maintainable situation, good patient cooperation, no environmental factors, either no systemic factors or well-controlled systemic factors.

3. *Fair*—inadequate alveolar bone, mobility, grade I furcation involvement, potential to establish maintainable situation, adequate patient cooperation, limited environmental or systemic factors.

4. *Poor*—moderate to advanced alveolar bone loss, mobility, grade I and II furcation involvement, questionable patient cooperation, difficult areas to maintain, presence of systemic or environmental factors.

5. *Questionable*—advanced bone loss, grade II and III furcation involvements, mobility, inaccessible areas, presence of environmental or systemic factors.

6. *Hopeless*—advanced bone loss, inability to establish maintainable situation, extraction indicated, uncontrolled environmental or systemic factors.

E. The prognosis varies with the periodontal diagnosis.

1. Patients with a diagnosis of gingivitis associated with dental plaque, which is a completely reversible disease, have a good prognosis if the local initiating factors (usually plaque and calculus) can be reduced or eliminated. The prognosis for patients with

plaque-induced gingival diseases modified by systemic factors and plaque-induced gingival diseases modified by medications is also dependent on elimination of the secondary factors involved. The prognosis for patients with non–plaque-associated gingivitis (e.g., lichen planus, pemphigoid, lupus erythematosus) depends on management of the associated dermatologic disorder.

2. Patients with aggressive periodontitis usually have a poorer prognosis than patients with chronic periodontitis. However, in patients with localized aggressive periodontitis that is diagnosed early, conservative therapy is effective, and the prognosis is good.

3. The prognosis of patients with periodontitis associated with systemic diseases depends on the severity of the systemic disease.

4. The prognosis for patients with necrotizing periodontal diseases is variable, depending on the extent and severity of environmental and systemic factors.

6.0 Therapy

A. Rationale—periodontal therapy is performed to eliminate pain, eliminate gingival bleeding, reduce inflammation, reduce periodontal pockets, arrest destruction of soft tissue and bone, reduce mobility, reduce tooth loss, and prevent the recurrence of disease. The phases of periodontal therapy are outlined in Box 7-4 and Figure 7-7.

1. The removal of bacterial plaque and of factors that favor its accumulation is the primary consideration in local therapy.

2. Systemic administration of antibiotics or host-modifying drugs or both may be used as an adjunct to local therapy.

B. Nonsurgical phase (phase I therapy).

1. Plaque control (see Section 7.0, Prevention and Maintenance).

2. Scaling and root planing.

a. Instrumentation reduces the numbers of subgingival microorganisms and results in a shift in the microflora from disease-associated, gram-negative anaerobes to health-associated, gram-positive, facultative microorganisms.

b. The best evidence for the success of instrumentation is the response of the tissue. Response should be assessed no sooner than 2 weeks after completion of instrumentation.

c. Scaling is the removal of both supragingival and subgingival plaque and calculus. Root planing is the removal of embedded calculus and areas of cementum to produce a clean, hard, smooth surface. The primary objective of scaling and root planing is to restore gingival health by removing these etiologic factors.

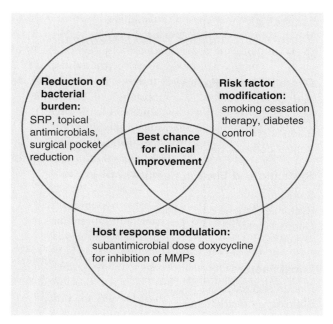

Figure 7-7 Complementary treatment strategies in periodontitis. The best chance for clinical improvement may come from implementing complementary treatment strategies that target different aspects of the periodontal balance. Reduction of the bacterial burden by scaling and root planing *(SRP)* is the cornerstone of treatment and can be augmented by the use of topical antimicrobials and surgical pocket therapy. In addition to this antibacterial treatment approach, the host response can be treated by the use of host modulatory therapy, such as sub–antimicrobial dose doxycycline, for the inhibition of matrix metalloproteinases *(MMPs)*. Risk factor assessment and modification must form a key part of any periodontal treatment strategy, including smoking cessation counseling. These different but complementary treatment strategies can be used as part of a comprehensive management approach. *(From Newman MG, et al: Carranza's Clinical Periodontology, ed 12. St. Louis, Saunders, 2015.)*

d. Sickle scalers are used to remove supragingival calculus. They have two cutting edges and a pointed tip. They have a triangular shape in cross section.

e. Ultrasonic scalers, hoe, chisel, and file scalers are used for removal of tenacious calculus.

f. Curettes are the instrument of choice for subgingival scaling and for root planing. They have a spoon-shaped blade and rounded toe and back and are shaped like a semicircle in cross section.

(1) Universal curettes have two cutting edges and can be used in any area of the mouth. The face of the blade is at a 90-degree angle to the lower shank when seen in cross section from the tip. The blade is curved in one direction.

(2) Area-specific curettes (Gracey curettes) are designed to adapt to specific tooth surfaces. They provide the best access and adaptation to the root surface. The blade is angled 60 to 70

degrees from the lower shank, providing an offset blade. When the lower shank is parallel to the long axis of the tooth, the blade is properly adapted to the root surface. The blade is curved from head to toe and along the side of the cutting edge, providing only one cutting edge that can be accurately adapted to the root surface. When using these instruments, the lower shank must be parallel to the surface being instrumented. Examples of Gracey curettes and the teeth they are designed to adapt to follow.

(a) Gracey 1-2 and 3-4—anterior.

(b) Gracey 5-6—anterior and premolars.

(c) Gracey 7-8 and 9-10—posterior teeth, facial and lingual.

(d) Gracey 11-12—posterior teeth mesial surfaces only.

(e) Gracey 13-14—posterior teeth distal surfaces only.

(3) Gracey curvettes are curettes with shorter, more curved miniblades designed to adapt more closely to the root surface.

(4) Extended-shank curettes have a longer terminal shank, a thinned blade, and a large-diameter terminal shank. They are available in finishing or rigid designs and are used for light scaling or removal of tenacious deposits, respectively.

(5) Mini-bladed curettes have shorter blades than conventional curettes for better adaptation into furcations; developmental grooves; line angles; and tight, deep pockets. They also are available in finishing or rigid designs.

(6) Langer and mini-Langer curettes combine the shank design of Gracey curettes with the universal blade design (90-degree angle of the face and lower shank).

(7) Schwartz periotrievers are magnetized instruments designed to retrieve broken instrument tips from periodontal pockets.

3. *Instrument sharpening*—periodontal instruments must have thin, fine cutting edges to be effective and efficient. The objective of sharpening is to restore this cutting edge after use of the instrument. Instruments can be sharpened using mounted or unmounted stones.

4. Holding and activating hand instruments.

a. Hand instruments are held in the modified pen grasp. A finger rest is established to stabilize the hand and instrument. It provides a firm fulcrum. The fourth finger usually serves as the finger rest. Finger rests may be intraoral or extraoral.

b. Adaptation of the instrument to the tooth surface is important to prevent trauma to soft tissues and the root surface. The lower third of the working end of the instrument (closest to the toe) must be kept in contact with the tooth. This usually means that 1 to 2 mm of the working end of the instrument is adapted to the tooth.

c. When initially inserting an instrument into the pocket, the angulation between the blade and the tooth should be 0 degrees. During scaling and root planing, this angulation is changed to 45 to 90 degrees.

d. The types of strokes used during instrumentation are *exploratory* (a light feeling stroke used with probes and explorers), *scaling* (a short, strong pull stroke used with bladed instruments for the removal of calculus), and *root planing* (a moderate to light pull stroke used for final smoothing and planing of the root surface).

e. Plastic instruments or special metal curettes are available for removing deposits from implant surfaces.

5. Ultrasonic instruments.

a. *Overview*—ultrasonic instruments are used for removing plaque, calculus, and stain from tooth surfaces. The vibrations at the tip of these instruments range from 20,000 to 45,000 cycles/sec. Ultrasonic instrumentation is accomplished by using light, intermittent strokes with the tip parallel to the tooth and in constant motion. A contraindication to the use of ultrasonic instruments includes presence of older cardiac pacemakers. Contraindications to the use of ultrasonic and sonic instruments include patients with communicable diseases that can be spread by aerosol, patients at risk for respiratory disease (patients with immunosuppression or patients with chronic pulmonary diseases), and patients with titanium implants (unless plastic ultrasonic or sonic tips are used).

b. Characteristics.

(1) In *magnetostrictive* ultrasonic instruments, the tip vibrates in an elliptic pattern, meaning that all sides of the tip are active.

(2) In *piezoelectric* ultrasonic instruments, the tip vibrates in a linear (or back-and-forth) pattern, meaning that two sides are more active.

(3) Tips in both units operate in a wet field with a water spray. There are small vacuum bubbles within the spray that collapse, releasing energy in a process termed *cavitation*. This cavitation spray helps flush debris out of the pocket.

6. Sonic instruments—sonic instruments have a handpiece that attaches to a compressed air line. Vibrations range from 2000 to 6000 cycles/sec.

7. Other instruments.

a. A dental endoscope has been designed that consists of a reusable fiberoptic endoscope covered with a disposable sterile sheath. It fits onto specially designed periodontal probes and ultrasonic instruments. It should enable the operator to view subgingival deposits and should aid in their removal.

b. The enhanced visual assessment system uses a series of motor-driven diamond files mounted on a special handpiece to correct overhanging restorations.

c. Rubber cups and bristle brushes are used to remove plaque and stains from the teeth.

d. The prophy-jet delivers a slurry of water and sodium bicarbonate to remove extrinsic stains and soft deposits. It can damage cementum and dentin as well as restorations when used improperly. Its use is contraindicated in patients with respiratory illnesses, hypertension, electrolyte imbalance, and infectious diseases and patients on hemodialysis.

C. Surgery (phase II therapy)—phase II surgical therapy is performed to reduce or eliminate periodontal pockets, correct soft and hard tissue anatomic or morphologic defects, regenerate periodontal tissues, or place implants. The need for surgery is assessed after the completion and evaluation of the success of phase I therapy. Procedures performed at this reevaluation phase include assessment of oral hygiene, clinical attachment levels, and pocket depths. Patients with residual deep pockets, osseous defects, and persistent mucogingival problems who have demonstrated the ability to maintain adequate oral hygiene are candidates for periodontal surgery, provided that there are no medical or psychological contraindications.

1. Flap design and management are important components of periodontal surgery. There are several basic principles of flap design.

a. The base of the flap should be wider than the free margin.

b. The lines of the incision should not be placed over any defect in the bone.

c. Incisions should not be made over a bony eminence.

d. Corners of the flaps should be rounded.

e. Flaps can be classified as either full thickness (mucoperiosteal) or partial thickness (mucosal). In full-thickness flaps, all soft tissue and periosteum are reflected to expose the alveolar bone. In partial-thickness flaps, only the epithelium and the underlying connective tissue are reflected.

f. Depending on how the interdental papilla is managed, flaps can either split the papilla (conventional flap) or preserve it (papilla preservation flap).

g. *Horizontal incisions for full-thickness flaps*—three horizontal incisions are usually associated with a full-thickness flap design.

(1) The first is the *internal bevel incision*— depending on the goal, this incision can be made 0.5 to 1 mm from the free gingival margin (apically displaced flap), 1 to 2 mm from the free gingival margin (modified Widman flap), or just coronal to the base of the pocket (undisplaced flap). It also is known as the *reverse bevel incision*. This incision removes the pocket lining, conserves the outer dimension of the gingiva, and produces a thin sharp flap margin that can be adapted to the bone-tooth junction.

(2) The second is the *crevicular incision*—made from the base of the pocket to the crest of the alveolar bone. The combination of the internal bevel and crevicular incisions creates a collar of tissue around the teeth.

(3) The third is the *interdental incision*—this incision separates the collar of gingiva from the tooth. Reflection of the flap after placement of these three incisions allows for visualization of the alveolar bone.

h. *Vertical incisions for full-thickness flaps*—if the flap is to be positioned apically in a pocket reduction/elimination procedure, vertical releasing incisions that extend beyond the mucogingival junction can be made. These incisions should not be made in the center of the papilla or over the radicular surface of a tooth. Vertical incisions should be avoided on the lingual and in the palate.

i. The *modified Widman flap* uses the three horizontal incisions described previously but is not reflected beyond the mucogingival line. This flap design allows for removal of the pocket lining and exposure of the tooth roots and alveolar bone but does not allow for apical repositioning of the flap.

j. *Periodontal packs*—most surgical sites are covered with a periodontal pack. Packs are placed to protect the surgical wound, minimize patient discomfort, maintain tissue placement, and help prevent postoperative bleeding. Packs usually do not enhance the healing rate of the tissues. Packs usually contain zinc oxide and may be either eugenol-containing or non–eugenol-containing. Antibiotics have been incorporated into some packs. Packs are retained mechanically by interlocking into interdental spaces.

k. *Chlorhexidine*—in the first postoperative week, the patient should rinse with 0.12% chlorhexidine twice daily until normal oral hygiene procedures can be resumed, which is usually during the second postoperative week.

D. Gingival surgery.

1. *Gingivectomy* is an excision of the gingiva. Surgical gingivectomy is performed to eliminate suprabony pockets, gingival enlargements, or suprabony periodontal abscesses. A gingivectomy should not be performed if osseous recontouring is needed, if the

bottom of the pocket is apical to the mucogingival junction, if there is inadequate attached gingiva, or if there is an esthetic concern. The procedure can be performed with scalpels, electrodes, or lasers. A beveled incision is made apical to the pocket depth. The tissue is removed, the area is débrided, and a surgical pack is placed. Healing is by secondary intention with the formation of a protective clot, epithelial migration, and connective tissue repair.

2. *Gingivoplasty* is performed to reshape the tissues where there are deformities, such as gingival clefts or craters, gingival enlargements, and shelflike interdental papillae. It is not performed to reduce or eliminate periodontal pockets. It can be accomplished with a periodontal knife, scalpel, rotary diamond stone, or electrodes.

E. Mucogingival surgery—mucogingival surgical procedures are performed to correct relationships between the gingival and the oral mucous membranes. They include widening of attached gingiva, deepening of shallow vestibules, and resection of aberrant frena.

1. No minimum width of attached gingiva has been established as a standard necessary for gingival health. Persons with excellent oral hygiene may maintain health with almost no attached gingiva. Persons with suboptimal oral hygiene can be helped by the presence of keratinized tissue and vestibular depth.
   a. Widening the attached gingiva can be performed.
      (1) To enhance plaque removal around the gingival margin.
      (2) To improve esthetics by covering denuded root surfaces.
      (3) To reduce inflammation around restored teeth by creating a wider zone of attached gingiva around teeth that serve as abutments for fixed and removable partial dentures and in ridge areas related to dentures.

2. Techniques to increase the width of attached gingiva include free gingival autograft, free connective tissue autograft, and the displaced (apically or laterally) positioned flap.

3. The palate is the most common donor site for the free gingival autograft and the connective tissue autograft. The ideal thickness for the free gingival graft is 1 to 1.5 mm. The success of the graft depends on survival of the connective tissue. In connective tissue autografts, only connective tissue is used from the undersurface of the palatal flap, which is sutured back in primary closure. This results in less discomfort postoperatively.

4. Techniques used for widening the attached gingiva apical to an area of recession can also be used for root coverage. These include the free gingival and connective tissue autograft. Other techniques include the laterally positioned (displaced) flap, the coronally displaced flap, the subepithelial connective tissue graft, and guided tissue regeneration techniques. When planning a laterally positioned (displaced) flap, the donor site should have adequate facial bone and adequate thickness and width of attached gingiva.

5. The Miller classification system for recession is an important consideration when root coverage procedures are planned, when there is severe bone and soft tissue loss interdentally or severe tooth malposition. The prognosis for root coverage for classes I and II is good to excellent; only partial coverage can be expected for class III. Class IV has a very poor prognosis for coverage.
   a. Class I—marginal tissue recession does not extend to the mucogingival junction. There is no loss of bone or soft tissue in the interdental area.
   b. Class II—marginal tissue recession extends to or beyond the mucogingival junction. There is no loss of bone or soft tissue in the interdental area.
   c. Class III—marginal tissue recession extends to or beyond the mucogingival junction. There is bone and soft tissue loss interdentally or malpositioned teeth.
   d. Class IV—marginal tissue recession extends to or beyond the mucogingival junction. There is severe bone and soft tissue loss interdentally or severe tooth malposition.

6. A frenum is a problem if the attachment is too close to the marginal gingiva. Tension from the frenum may pull the gingival margin away from the tooth, creating a situation conducive to plaque retention. A frenectomy is complete removal of the frenum; a frenotomy is incision of the frenum. Both may be used to correct frenum attachment problems, but the frenotomy is usually adequate for relocating the attachment to create a zone of attached gingiva between the gingival margin and the frenum.

7. Deepening the vestibule can be accomplished by the use of free gingival autogenous graft techniques.

8. For all mucogingival procedures, blood supply is the most significant concern. The surgical site also should be free of plaque, calculus, and inflammation. Grafts must be stabilized on the recipient site, and there should be minimal trauma to the surgical site. There must be adequate tissue present at the donor site.

F. Osseous surgery—access to the alveolar bone is accomplished through full-thickness flap reflection. Visualization of the bony architecture allows the clinician to determine the types of bony defects that are present and the extent of those defects.

1. *Osseous crater*—this is an osseous, two-walled concavity in the crest of the interdental bone confined within the facial and lingual walls (Figure 7-8). This defect is best corrected by recontouring the facial and lingual walls to restore normal interdental architecture.

2. *Vertical or angular defects*—the base of the bone defect is located apical to the surrounding bone. These defects can have one, two, or three walls (Figure 7-9) or any combination (Figure 7-10). These defects may be corrected by resective osseous surgery or by periodontal regeneration (for details, see "Resective osseous surgery" and "Periodontal regeneration" further on).

3. *Recontouring*—it is believed that discrepancies in bony contour predispose the patient to recurrence of deep pockets after soft tissue surgery. Resective osseous surgery is the recontouring and removal of alveolar bone to correct these discrepancies— restoring the alveolar bone to the contour that was present before periodontal destruction. It is usually performed in combination with apical repositioning of the gingival flap for pocket reduction or elimination. Because osseous resective surgery is performed at the expense of bony tissue and attachment level, it should be performed only on teeth with moderate bone loss.

4. *Interproximal bone*—in normal alveolar bone morphology, the interproximal bone is more coronal than the facial or lingual/palatal bone (positive architecture). Deviations from this include negative architecture (interproximal bone is apical to the facial or lingual bone) and flat architecture (interproximal bone and radicular bone are at the same height). The embrasure space dictates the interproximal form, and the position of the bony margins follows the contours of the cementoenamel junction.

5. Resective osseous surgery.
   a. Resective osseous surgery can be accomplished through *ostectomy* (removal of tooth supporting bone) or *osteoplasty* (removal of nonsupporting alveolar bone).
   b. After ostectomy, peaks of bone often remain at the line angles. These are called *widow's peaks*. If left, they predispose the patient to recurrence of periodontal pockets in these areas.

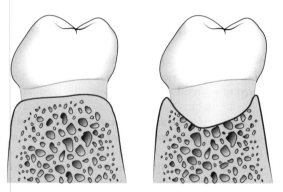

Figure 7-8 Diagrammatic representation of an osseous crater in a faciolingual section between two lower molars. *Left,* Normal bone contour. *Right,* Osseous crater. *(From Newman MG, et al: Carranza's Clinical Periodontology, ed 12. St. Louis, Saunders, 2015.)*

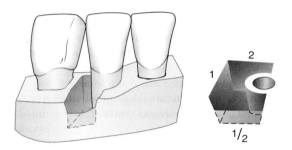

Figure 7-10 Combined type of osseous defect. Because the facial wall is half the height of the distal *(1)* and lingual *(2)* walls, this is an osseous defect with three walls in the apical half and two walls in the occlusal half. *(From Newman MG, et al: Carranza's Clinical Periodontology, ed 12. St. Louis, Saunders, 2015.)*

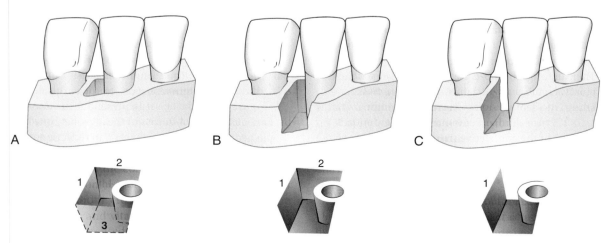

Figure 7-9 One-, two-, and three-walled vertical defects on right lateral incisor. **A,** Three bony walls: distal *(1)*, lingual *(2)*, and facial *(3)*. **B,** Two-wall defect: distal *(1)* and lingual *(2)*. **C,** One-wall defect: distal wall only *(1)*. *(From Newman MG, et al: Carranza's Clinical Periodontology, ed 12. St. Louis, Saunders, 2015.)*

c. Resective osseous surgery is most successful in interproximal bony craters, early furcation involvements, and cases with thick alveolar bone. It should not be performed in areas where there is an esthetic concern.

6. Mechanisms of healing after periodontal treatment.

a. *Regeneration*—growth and differentiation of the same type of tissue (bone, cementum, and PDL) that was damaged through periodontal disease.

b. *Repair*—healing by scar.

c. *New attachment*—embedding of new PDL fibers into new cementum and attachment of gingival epithelium to a previously diseased root surface.

G. Periodontal regeneration—periodontal regeneration (reconstruction) is the formation of new bone, cementum, and PDL. Various techniques have been developed to enhance the likelihood of achieving the goal of regeneration of the periodontium.

1. *Guided tissue regeneration* (GTR) is a method for preventing epithelial migration along the cemental side of a pocket during wound healing after periodontal flap reflection. GTR uses various barrier membranes to cover the bone and PDL before flap replacement in an attempt to exclude the epithelium and connective tissue from the root surface during the healing phase. These barriers also may serve to protect the clot that is formed, allowing for connective tissue attachment during the early phases of wound healing.

2. The root surface can be treated with agents designed to enhance new attachment of gingival tissues after surgical excision. These include citric acid, which is often used in conjunction with free gingival grafts, fibronectin, tetracycline, and various growth factors. Enamel matrix proteins (e.g., Emdogain) have also been used to enhance new attachment.

3. Numerous hard tissue graft materials have been used for restoring periodontal osseous defects, including *autografts* (material to be grafted obtained from the same individual), *allografts* (material to be grafted obtained from a different individual of the same species), and *xenografts* (material to be grafted obtained from a different species). Bone graft materials are evaluated based on their osteogenic potential (ability to induce the formation of new bone by cells contained in the graft), osteoinductive potential (ability of molecules contained in the graft to convert neighboring cells into osteoblasts), and osteoconductive potential (ability of the graft material to serve as a scaffold that favors outside cells to penetrate the graft and form new bone). Three-wall defects are most predictable to respond with bone grafting as opposed to two-wall defects because of better blood supply and cell source proximity. One-wall defects should not be treated with bone grafting.

a. *Autogenous grafts* can be obtained from intraoral sites. Osseous coagulum (a mixture of bone dust and blood obtained from cortical bone), bone blend (bone obtained from a predetermined site that is triturated in an autoclaved plastic capsule and pestle), and cancellous bone marrow transplants (obtained from the maxillary tuberosity, edentulous areas, and healing sockets) are examples of autogenous grafts. Autogenous bone also can be obtained from extraoral sites, such as iliac cancellous marrow bone.

b. *Allograft materials* include undecalcified, freeze-dried bone allograft (osteoconductive material) and decalcified, freeze-dried bone allograft (osteogenic material owing to the presence of bone morphogenetic proteins that are exposed during the demineralization process).

c. Bio-Oss is a *xenograft material* (an anorganic, bovine-derived bone that is an osteoconductive, porous bone mineral matrix).

d. Nonbone graft materials include bioactive glass (PerioGlas, Biogran) and coral-derived materials.

e. Regeneration can be attained without the use of bone grafts in three-walled osseous defects that are meticulously débrided and in periodontal and endodontic abscesses.

f. Regeneration through the placement of bone graft material is most successful in three-walled bony defects. It is least successful in through-and-through (class III) furcation defects.

H. Oral implantology.

1. *Titanium-tissue interaction*—titanium is the material that offers the best biologic attachment to bone and gingival tissue.

a. Titanium implants have a layer of titanium oxide on their surface that is responsible for osseointegration. The oxide content of titanium oxide is essential for the nucleation process that forms calcium phosphate precipitates, which lead to mineralized bone formation.

b. The placement of a titanium implant into a prepared hole in bone leads to bone apposition on the implant surface by mechanisms that are similar to fractured bone healing. The process leading to successful bone apposition on implant surfaces after surgical implant placement is outlined in Figure 7-11. The main goal of implant treatment is to achieve and maintain a stable bone-to-implant connection, also called *osseointegration*. Implants are frequently loaded after 2 to 3 months, when woven bone is still present.

c. The attachment of gingival tissue to a titanium implant is outlined in Figure 7-12, and the blood supply to this area is shown in Figure 7-13. The vascular supply of the periimplant gingival tissue or alveolar mucosa is more limited than the

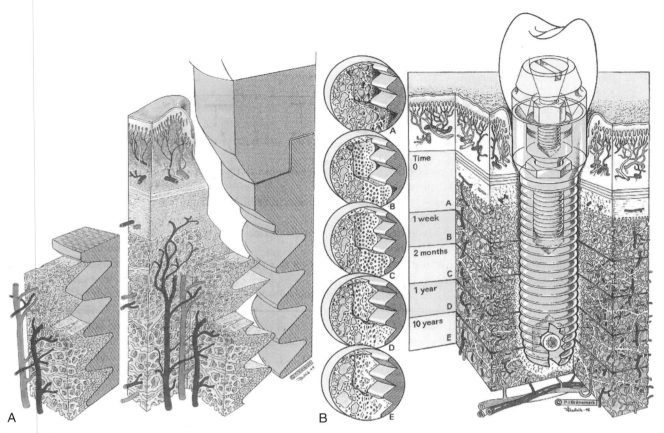

Figure 7-11 A, Three-dimensional diagram of the tissue and titanium interrelationship showing an overall view of the intact interfacial zone around the osseointegrated implant. **B,** Physiologic evolution of the biology of the interface over time. *(From Newman MG, et al: Carranza's Clinical Periodontology, ed 12. St. Louis, Saunders, 2015.)*

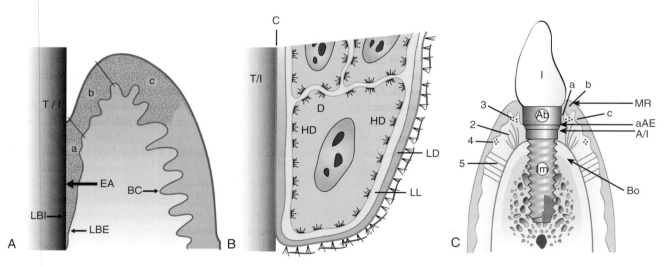

Figure 7-12 A, Histologic scheme of epithelial attachment *(EA)* (identical for tooth and implant). *BC,* Basal complex; *LBE,* lamina basalis externa (only location where cell divisions occur); *LBI,* lamina basalis interna; *T/I,* titanium implant; *a,* long junctional epithelial attachment zone; *b,* sulcular epithelial zone; *c,* oral epithelial zone. **B,** At electron microscopic level, basal complex at epithelial attachment (three most apical cells) and connection with stroma. *C,* Cuticle; *D,* desmosome; *HD,* hemidesmosomes; *LD,* lamina densa; *LL,* lamina lucida. **C,** Implant, abutment *(Ab),* and crown within alveolar bone and soft tissues. *aAE,* Apical (point) of attached epithelium; *A/I,* abutment/implant junction; *Bo,* marginal bone level; *Im,* endosseous part of implant; *MR,* margin of gingiva/alveolar mucosa; *1,* implant crown; *2,* vertical alveolar gingival connective tissue fibers; *3,* circular gingival connective tissue fibers; *4,* circular gingival connective tissue fibers; *5,* periosteal-gingival connective tissue fibers; *a,* junctional epithelium; *b,* sulcular epithelium; *c,* oral epithelium. *(From Newman MG, et al: Carranza's Clinical Periodontology, ed 12. St. Louis, Saunders, 2015.)*

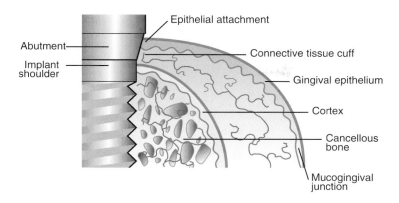

Epithelial attachment

Abutment

Implant shoulder

Connective tissue cuff

Gingival epithelium

Cortex

Cancellous bone

Mucogingival junction

Figure 7-13 Schematic illustration shows the blood supply in the connective tissue cuff surrounding the implant/abutment is scarcer than in the gingival complex around teeth because none originates from a PDL. *(From Newman MG, et al: Carranza's Clinical Periodontology, ed 12. St. Louis, Saunders, 2015.)*

vascular supply around teeth. Because there is no PDL around an implant, the vascular supply may often be missing.

2. Comparison of tissues surrounding natural dentition and osseointegrated implants.
   a. There is no PDL around implants.
   b. There is no supracrestal connective tissue inserting into the implant as in teeth.
   c. When probing around implants, the probe tip may penetrate to the level of bone; on natural teeth, the probe tip stops in the junctional epithelium in health or in the supracrestal connective tissue in disease.
   d. A lack of a PDL means that implants should not be used in growing individuals because implants do not continue to erupt like normal teeth.
3. Clinical applications and evaluation of the patient with implants.
   a. Greater than 90% to 95% success rates can be expected for endosseous titanium implants in healthy patients with good bone and normal healing capacity.
   b. Implants can be placed in edentulous and partially edentulous patients.
   c. Fully edentulous patients seem to benefit the most from implants.
   d. Implant-supported removable or fixed prostheses can be used.
   e. Clinical evaluation requires evaluation of chief complaint; medical history (for risk factors); dental history (for infections, plaque control, previous surgical procedures); intraoral examination (for dental and periodontal health, oral hygiene, jaw relationships, temporomandibular joint [TMJ] conditions); articulated diagnostic study models; hard tissue evaluation (for bone levels); radiographic examination (quantity, quality, and location of bone; can use periapical x-rays, panoramic x-rays, and tomographic imaging); and soft tissue evaluation (extent of keratinized versus nonkeratinized mucosa; quality and quantity of tissue).

4. *Risk factors and contraindications for implants*—risk factors and contraindications for implant therapy are listed in Table 7-5.
5. *Posttreatment evaluation and management of implants*—implant stability is the most important measure of success. It has low sensitivity (cannot accurately determine levels of bone loss) but high specificity (if the implant is mobile, it has probably failed). Intraoral radiographs should be taken at the time of placement, at the time of abutment connection, and regularly thereafter to assess bone levels. Traditional oral hygiene measures should be used, but ultrasonic instruments should be avoided. Plastic instruments or specifically designed curettes should be used for cleaning of implants.
6. Types and prevalence of implant complications.
   a. The most common complication reported for single crowns was abutment or prosthesis screw loosening (2% to 45%).
   b. Loosening rates are higher in posterior than anterior.
   c. Implant fracture is less than 1% of cases.
   d. Technical complications are higher for implants used with overdentures than for implants supporting fixed prostheses.
   e. Implant failures for biologic reasons (periimplantitis, soft tissue lesions)—7% to 8%.
   f. Failure rates in totally edentulous patients are twice that seen in partially edentulous patients.
   g. Failure rates are three times higher in edentulous maxilla compared with edentulous mandible.
   h. No differences for partially edentulous between maxilla and mandible.
7. Biologic complications.
   a. *Periimplantitis*—inflammatory process affecting the tissues around an osseointegrated implant in function, resulting in loss of supporting bone.
   b. *Dehiscence and recession of periimplant soft tissues*—occurs when support for those tissues is lacking or has been lost.

Table 7-5

Risk Factors and Contraindications for Implant Therapy

	RISK FACTOR	CONTRAINDICATION
Medical and Systemic Health-Related Issues		
Diabetes (poorly controlled)	??—Possibly	Relative
Bone metabolic disease (e.g., osteoporosis)	??—Probably	Relative
Radiation therapy (head and neck)	Yes	Relative/absolute
Bisphosphonate therapy (intravenous)	??—Probably	Relative/absolute
Bisphosphonate therapy (oral)	??—Possibly	Relative
Immunosuppressive medication	??—Probably	Relative
Immunocompromising disease (e.g., HIV, AIDS)	??—Possibly	Relative
Psychological and Mental Conditions		
Psychiatric syndromes (e.g., schizophrenia, paranoia)	No	Absolute
Mental instability (e.g., neurotic, hysteric)	No	Absolute
Mentally impaired; uncooperative	No	Absolute
Irrational fears; phobias	No	Absolute
Unrealistic expectations	No	Absolute
Habits and Behavioral Considerations		
Smoking; tobacco use	Yes	Relative
Parafunctional habits	Yes	Relative
Substance abuse (e.g., alcohol, drugs)	??—Possibly	Absolute
Intraoral Examination Findings		
Atrophic maxilla	Yes	Relative
Current infection (e.g., endodontic)	Yes	Relative
Periodontal disease	??—Possibly	Relative

From Newman MG, et al: *Carranza's Clinical Periodontology,* ed 12. St. Louis, Saunders, 2015.

I. Effects of smoking on periodontal therapy—current smokers do not respond as well to periodontal therapy as nonsmokers or former smokers.

J. Pharmacologic therapy.

1. Host modulation—the host immune and inflammatory responses to bacterial plaque are primarily responsible for the destruction of the periodontium. Pharmacologic agents that can modify these responses can be used as adjuncts to conventional mechanical therapy in the prevention and treatment of periodontitis (Figure 7-14).

   a. Systemically administered NSAIDs (e.g., ibuprofen, flurbiprofen, naproxen)—inhibit the formation of prostaglandins (PGE_2).

   b. Bisphosphonates—inhibit bone resorption by osteoclasts; reports of bisphosphonate-related osteonecrosis of the jaw have raised concerns about the use of bisphosphonates to treat periodontitis.

   c. SDD (Periostat)—inhibits MMP destruction of collagen. SDD inhibits MMP-8 and MMP-13. Of the three pharmacologic agents (NSAIDs, bisphosphonates, and SDD), only SDD is approved by the U.S. Food and Drug Administration (FDA) and indicated as an adjunct to scaling and root planing in the treatment of chronic periodontitis. SDD is administered in a 20-mg dose (a typical antimicrobial dose of doxycycline is 100 mg), twice daily for 3 to 9 months. The 20-mg dose inhibits MMPs but has no antibacterial activity. SDD should not be given to patients with a history of allergy or hypersensitivity to tetracyclines, pregnant or lactating women, or children younger than 12 years. Doxycycline concentrates in the skin, and there is an increased risk for sensitivity to sunlight. SDD should be prescribed to coincide with the initiation of scaling and root planing. It should be used only as an adjunct to mechanical therapy. SDD can also be combined with the local delivery of antibiotics to address both the host and the bacterial sides of the disease process. Chemically modified tetracyclines are a newer group of host-modulating

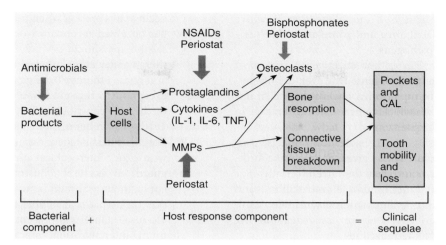

Figure 7-14 Potential adjunctive therapeutic approaches. Possible adjunctive therapies and points of intervention in the treatment of periodontitis are presented related to the pathologic cascade of events. *CAL,* Clinical attachment loss; *IL-1,* interleukin-1; *IL-6,* interleukin-6; *NSAIDs,* nonsteroidal antiinflammatory drugs; *TNF,* tumor necrosis factor. *(From Newman MG, et al: Carranza's Clinical Periodontology, ed 12. St. Louis, Saunders, 2015.)*

drugs in which all antibiotic properties have been removed with retention of the host-modifying, anticollagenolytic properties.

d. Locally administered host-modifying agents include topical NSAIDs and numerous agents used as adjuncts to surgical therapy, including enamel matrix proteins (Emdogain), bone morphogenetic proteins (BMP-2, BMP-7), growth factors (platelet-derived growth factor, insulinlike growth factor), and tetracyclines. Of these agents, only Emdogain and platelet-derived growth factor (GEM 21S) have been approved by the FDA for adjunctive use during surgery.

2. Antiinfective agents act by reducing the number of bacteria present. *Antibiotics* are one type of antiinfective agents. *Antiseptics* are chemical antimicrobial agents that can be applied topically to destroy microorganisms. *Disinfectants* are applied to inanimate objects to destroy microorganisms.

   a. Antibiotics.

   (1) Because the primary initiating agent of periodontal disease is bacterial plaque, systemic antibiotics can be used as adjuncts to mechanical débridement to decrease the number of bacteria in the periodontal pocket. They should not be used as a monotherapy in the absence of mechanical débridement.

   (2) No single antibiotic inhibits all putative periodontal pathogens. A combination of antibiotics may be necessary for significant reduction of the number of bacteria in the periodontal pocket.

   (3) Tetracyclines are often used in the treatment of localized aggressive periodontitis. They can concentrate in the periodontal tissues, inhibit the growth of *A. actinomycetemcomitans,* and exert an anticollagenolytic effect. Tetracyclines are bacteriostatic, are more effective against gram-positive than gram-negative bacteria, and concentrate in the gingival crevicular fluid at levels effective against many periodontal pathogens. Minocycline and doxycycline are commonly used tetracyclines. Both are effective in reducing periodontal pathogens. Advantages include decreased dosing (tetracycline, four times/day; minocycline, two times/day; doxycycline, one time/day), which may improve patient compliance.

   (4) Metronidazole is bactericidal to anaerobic organisms. It disrupts bacterial DNA. It has been used in conjunction with amoxicillin. There can be a disulfiram (Antabuse) effect (severe cramps, nausea, and vomiting) when alcohol is ingested during metronidazole treatment.

   (5) Amoxicillin is a bactericidal, semisynthetic penicillin that is effective against both gram-positive and gram-negative microorganisms. It is susceptible to penicillinase (β-lactamase). Amoxicillin combined with clavulanate potassium (Augmentin) is resistant to many penicillinases.

   (6) Cephalosporins are in the β-lactam family and are similar to penicillins. They are not often used to treat oral infections.

   (7) The spectrum of clindamycin includes anaerobic bacteria, and it can be used when the patient is sensitive to penicillin. It has been associated with pseudomembranous colitis.

(8) Ciprofloxacin is a quinolone that is active against facultative and some anaerobic periodontal pathogens.

(9) Erythromycin is not effective against most periodontal pathogens. However, azithromycin is effective against anaerobes and gram-negative bacilli. It appears to concentrate in gingival tissues.

(10) Bacteriostatic and bactericidal drugs usually should not be given at the same time. However, they may be given serially. For example, metronidazole-amoxicillin and metronidazole-amoxicillin/clavulanate have been used effectively in cases that did not respond to tetracyclines.

(11) Antibiotics also can be delivered locally. Two formulations available in the United States are 10% doxycycline (Atridox) and 2% minocycline (Arestin). These agents are used as adjuncts to mechanical débridement.

(12) Chlorhexidine (2.5 mg) is available in a resorbable delivery system (PerioChip). This agent is used as an adjunct to mechanical débridement.

K. Wound healing, repair, and regeneration.

1. Immediately after suturing to close a periodontal flap, a clot forms that connects the flap to the tooth and alveolar bone. Epithelial cells begin to migrate over the border of the flap 1 to 3 days after surgery. An epithelial attachment is in place 1 week after surgery, consisting of hemidesmosomes and a basal lamina. The clot is replaced by granulation tissue. Collagen fibers appear 2 weeks after surgery. Within 1 month, the gingival crevice is lined with epithelium, and an epithelial attachment is present.

2. Reflection of a full-thickness flap results in bone necrosis at 1 to 3 days and osteoclastic resorption that peaks at 4 to 6 days. Resulting bone loss is approximately 1 mm.

3. Healing of a free gingival graft begins with diffusion of fluids from the recipient bed, adjacent gingiva, and alveolar mucosa. Revascularization starts by the second or third day. Capillaries from the recipient bed proliferate into the graft to form a network of new capillaries. The epithelium undergoes degeneration and sloughing. It is replaced with new epithelium from the borders of the recipient site. The genetic predetermination for the specific character of the epithelium depends on the nature of the connective tissue bed.

L. Splinting and occlusal correction.

1. Overview.

a. Occlusion is a dynamic relationship that involves the teeth, TMJs, and muscles of mastication. A physiologic occlusion is defined as having no signs of dysfunction or disease. In contrast, traumatic occlusion is present when periodontal tissue injury has occurred secondary to occlusal forces. Occlusal therapy should be integrated into periodontal therapy after completion of home care instruction and phase I therapy (scaling and root planing). The exception to this guideline occurs when occlusal forces are contributing to pain or dysfunction. Teeth that remain mobile after phase I therapy should be evaluated for occlusal trauma and treated with either interocclusal appliance therapy (a bite guard) or occlusal adjustment. The purpose of either therapy should be to establish a functional occlusion that is favorable to periodontal health. Occlusal stability is present when there is maximum intercuspation, smooth excursive movements without interferences, and no trauma from occlusion.

b. Each patient should receive a temporomandibular disorder (TMD) screening evaluation that includes examination for maximal interincisal opening, opening and closing pathway, auscultation for TMJ sounds, palpation for TMJ tenderness, and palpation for muscle tenderness. An intraoral examination should include identification of occlusal contacts in maximum intercuspation, guidance in excursive movements, initial contact in centric-relation closure, tooth mobility, and attrition.

2. Signs and symptoms of a *nonphysiologic occlusion* include damaged teeth and restorations, abnormal mobility, fremitus, widened PDL, and possibly pain.

3. *Bruxism* is defined as a parafunctional activity that can include clenching, grinding, gnashing, and bracing of the teeth. Bruxism may contribute to wear and damage to the teeth and restorations, mobility, and muscle pain.

4. Tissue injury occurs when occlusal forces exceed the adaptive capacity of the periodontium. This injury is called *trauma from occlusion* or *occlusal trauma.* The occlusion that causes this damage is termed *traumatic occlusion.* Trauma from occlusion can be caused by alterations in occlusal forces, reduced capacity of the periodontium to withstand occlusal forces, or a combination of both. When trauma from occlusion is the result of occlusal alterations, it is called *primary trauma from occlusion.* An example would be excessive occlusal force, such as a high restoration, on a tooth with a healthy periodontium. When it results from reduced ability of the tissues to resist occlusal forces, it is called *secondary occlusal trauma.* An example would be a normal occlusal force on a tooth with loss of attachment (reduced periodontium).

5. *Occlusal therapy* should be delayed until inflammation is resolved through completion of nonsurgical therapy and implementation of home care. Persistent mobility can be assessed and managed through

occlusal adjustment or treatment with appliance therapy. These appliances are designed to provide a reversible means of redistributing occlusal forces to minimize excessive force on specific teeth.

a. *Occlusal adjustment* or *coronoplasty* is the selective reshaping of occlusal surfaces with the goal of establishing a stable, nontraumatic occlusion. This is an irreversible intervention. It should not be used as a primary means of either preventing or treating TMD. There is evidence that when patients with a defined need for occlusal adjustment receive that treatment, their response to periodontal therapy may be more favorable. However, as with other forms of occlusal therapy, coronoplasty should be deferred until inflammation is resolved. If significant occlusal adjustment is deemed necessary, it should be performed with restorative needs of the patient in mind.

b. *Interocclusal appliance therapy* is used to redistribute occlusal forces and to minimize excessive force on individual teeth.

6. *Splinting*—the most common reason for splinting is to improve patient comfort and function by immobilizing excessively mobile teeth. If splinting is being performed because of mobility, the cause of the mobility should be determined first. If the cause is occlusal trauma, occlusal adjustment should be performed in conjunction with resolution of inflammatory periodontal disease before splinting the teeth.

a. Splinting should be considered in the following situations.

(1) Increasing mobility of teeth.

(2) Mobility that impairs a patient's function.

(3) Migration of teeth.

(4) Prosthetics where multiple abutments are necessary.

b. *Splinting materials*—teeth may be splinted with bonded external materials or appliances, intracoronal appliances, or cast restorations. Regardless of the method used, the splint should be designed such that it does not impinge on the gingival tissues and it allows room for the patient to perform adequate oral hygiene procedures.

M. Special therapeutic problems.

1. *Acute gingival diseases*—acute gingival diseases include acute necrotizing ulcerative gingivitis), acute pericoronitis, and acute herpetic gingivostomatitis.

a. *Treatment of acute necrotizing ulcerative gingivitis* includes evaluation of the medical history, application of topical anesthetic followed by gently swabbing the necrotic lesions to remove the pseudomembrane, and removal of local factors such as calculus (often with ultrasonic instruments unless contraindicated by the medical history). Systemic antibiotics should be prescribed only if there is evidence of lymphadenopathy or fever. The patient should be instructed to avoid alcohol and tobacco, rinse with chlorhexidine, get adequate rest, remove bacterial plaque gently, and take an analgesic as needed for pain. Patients should return in 1 to 2 days for reevaluation and further débridement. Patient should be seen again approximately 5 days later for reevaluation; further counseling regarding diet, rest, and tobacco use; reinforcement of oral hygiene instruction (including chlorhexidine rinses); and periodontal evaluation.

b. *Acute pericoronitis* is treated by gently flushing the area to remove debris and swabbing with antiseptic. Occlusion should be evaluated to ensure the opposing tooth is not in contact with the inflamed tissue. If there is contact, the tissue may need to be excised. Drainage should be obtained if there is evidence that the inflamed tissue is fluctuant; antibiotics should be prescribed if there is evidence of systemic involvement. When the acute condition subsides, the associated tooth should be evaluated for extraction.

c. *Acute herpetic gingivostomatitis* diagnosed early (within 3 days of onset) is treated immediately with antiviral therapy (acyclovir, 15 mg/kg five times daily for 7 days). All patients should receive palliative care, including plaque removal, systemic NSAIDs, and topical anesthetics. Proper nutrition should be maintained. Patients should be made aware of the contagious nature of this disease when vesicles are present.

d. *Aggressive periodontitis.*

(1) Patients with a diagnosis of aggressive periodontitis do not typically respond as predictably to conventional therapy as patients with less aggressive forms of disease, such as chronic periodontitis. An important aspect of managing patients with this form of disease is patient education about the disease in terms of causes and risk factors. Patients should be educated concerning their role in managing the disease.

(2) Resective surgical therapy is often difficult in patients with localized aggressive periodontitis because teeth adjacent to the teeth affected with disease may be completely unaffected. Regenerative surgical therapy may be effective in these cases, especially in patients with localized two-wall or three-wall bony defects.

(3) Various systemic antibiotics have been used as adjuncts to mechanical débridement in the treatment of aggressive periodontitis, including tetracycline; doxycycline; clindamycin; ciprofloxacin; metronidazole; and combinations of amoxicillin-clavulanate, metronidazole-amoxicillin, and metronidazole-ciprofloxacin.

(4) In patients with aggressive periodontitis, severely compromised teeth should be extracted

early. The restorative treatment plan should include plans to accommodate future tooth loss. The use of dental implants should be considered when designing the overall treatment plan for these patients.

(5) Frequent maintenance visits are an important component of treating patients with aggressive periodontitis.

(6) Patients who do not respond to therapy may be classified as *refractory*. These patients may benefit from selective antibiotic therapy in conjunction with the use of host-modifying drugs such as SDD.

e. *Necrotizing ulcerative periodontitis.* Necrotizing ulcerative periodontitis may be associated with immunosuppression. A patient with this diagnosis must be treated in consultation with his or her physician. Resolution or treatment of the systemic condition may be necessary for the periodontal condition to resolve. Treatment of the oral lesions consists of local débridement, lavage, and oral hygiene instruction that may include daily use of antimicrobial agents such as chlorhexidine. These lesions are often painful, leading to the need for local anesthetic during débridement.

f. Abscesses.

(1) *Gingival abscesses* are localized to the gingival tissues, whereas periodontal abscesses involve the deeper supporting structures of the teeth. Gingival abscesses are attributed to plaque, trauma, or foreign body impaction and are treated by débridement and drainage.

(2) *Periodontal abscesses* can be classified as acute or chronic. *Acute abscesses* can be characterized by mild to severe discomfort, localized swelling, presence of a periodontal pocket, mobility, extrusion of tooth in the socket, percussion or biting sensitivity, presence of exudate, elevated temperature, and lymphadenopathy. *Chronic abscesses* usually are not painful, have slight extrusion, have intermittent exudation, are associated with a fistulous tract and deep pocket, and have little systemic involvement.

(a) *Causes*—periodontal abscesses can be attributed to various factors, including untreated moderate to deep periodontal pockets, incomplete calculus removal in periodontal pockets, tooth perforation or fracture, and foreign body impaction.

(b) Periodontal abscesses are treated by first resolving the acute lesion by the establishment of drainage either through the pocket or through an external excision. Patients should be instructed to rinse with warm salt water and to apply chlorhexidine to the area until the signs and symptoms subside

(usually 1 to 2 days). The area is then treated with scaling and root planing and evaluated for possible surgical therapy. Antibiotic therapy is indicated when treating periodontal abscesses if there is evidence of cellulitis, a deep inaccessible pocket, fever, or lymphadenopathy or when treating an immunocompromised patient.

g. Pulpal disease.

(1) Dental caries is the most common cause of pulpal disease. Other causes are direct trauma (e.g., tooth fracture); progressive dental caries; or instrumentation during periodontal, restorative, or prosthetic procedures.

(2) Pulpal infection is polymicrobial, primarily comprising gram-negative anaerobic bacteria. Combined endodontic-periodontal lesions can originate from pulpal necrosis spreading to the periodontium via the apex or accessory canals (primary endodontic lesion/secondary periodontal lesion), or progressive loss of attachment that reaches accessory canals or the apex (retrograde pulpitis; primary periodontal lesion/secondary endodontic lesion). The second mechanism is relatively rare. In true combined lesions (development and extension of an endodontic lesion into an existing periodontal pocket), loss of pulpal vitality should be treated first, followed by periodontal therapy, for resolution to occur.

(3) Both pulpal and periodontal disease can result in abscess formation. Periodontal abscesses are usually not painful; acute endodontic abscesses usually are painful.

h. *Oral malodor*—gingivitis, periodontitis, and tongue coating are the predominant causes of oral malodor. Acute pharyngitis, purulent sinusitis, and postnasal drip also can contribute to the problem. The unpleasant odor originates from volatile sulfur compounds, which include hydrogen sulfide, methylmercaptan, dimethyl sulfide, putrescine, cadaverine, indole, skatole, and butyric or propionic acid. Most of these compounds are formed by oral microorganisms (primarily gram-negative anaerobes) that degrade peptides from various intraoral sources. Treatment strategies include tongue cleaning with either a toothbrush or a tongue scraper, interdental cleaning and toothbrushing, and professional treatment of periodontal disease. Chewing gums, mouth rinses, and toothpastes may be used as adjuncts.

i. *Root sensitivity*—root sensitivity is often a problem after periodontal therapy. Adequate plaque control is essential to reducing or eliminating root sensitivity. Desensitizing agents used by the patient include dentifrices that contain strontium chloride, potassium nitrate, and sodium citrate. These agents act through the precipitation of crystalline salts that block dentinal tubules. Agents that can be professionally applied include cavity varnishes, zinc chloride–potassium ferrocyanide, formalin, calcium hydroxide, dibasic calcium phosphate, sodium fluoride, stannous fluoride, strontium chloride, and potassium oxalate.

j. *Gingival enlargements*—gingival enlargements are usually caused by inflammation (acute and chronic) or are drug-associated. Enlargements associated with acute inflammation are usually treated with scaling and root planing. Chronic enlargements may require surgical removal, either through a gingivectomy procedure or through a flap procedure. Drug-associated gingival enlargement is usually attributable to phenytoin; calcium channel blockers; or cyclosporine, an immunosuppressant. There are both inflammatory and chronic components to these enlargements, so treatment must include removal of plaque and calculus. Surgical therapy may be recommended, but the patient should be aware that the enlargement may recur if he or she continues taking the medication. A discussion with the patient's physician regarding possible discontinuation or substitution of the medication should be part of the treatment plan.

(1) Gingival enlargements associated with blood dyscrasias (e.g., leukemia) should be treated with phase I therapy (scaling and root planing). Adjunctive antibiotic therapy to prevent infection may be indicated.

(2) Gingival enlargements associated with pregnancy should initially be treated by scaling and root planing and oral hygiene instruction. Surgical excision may be indicated if the enlargement creates problems with occluding the teeth.

N. Periodontal restorative considerations—periodontal therapy, including nonsurgical and surgical treatment, should precede extensive restorative care. Periodontal therapy allows for better assessment of margin location; ensures adequate tooth length for retention, optimal tooth stability, and resolution of mucogingival problems; and allow for alveolar ridge reconstruction.

1. Restorative margin placement can be supragingival (least impact on the periodontium), at the marginal gingival crest, or subgingival (greatest impact on the periodontium). Subgingival margins should not impinge on the attachment apparatus. The space for soft tissue above the alveolar bone is termed the *biologic width*. The average human biologic width has been defined as 2 mm; this includes an average width of 0.97 mm for the junctional epithelium and 1.07 mm for the connective tissue attachment. Biologic width violation (i.e., when a restorative margin

is placed ≤2 mm away from the alveolar bone) can lead to inflammation and localized bone loss (Figures 7-15 and 7-16). Because of individual variations in the biologic width, probing to the bone level ("sounding to bone") is recommended to determine the definitive diagnosis of biologic width violation.

2. The location of the interproximal contact can have an impact on the gingival embrasure. Restorations should be designed to allow adequate space for the interproximal papillae. Contacts located too high

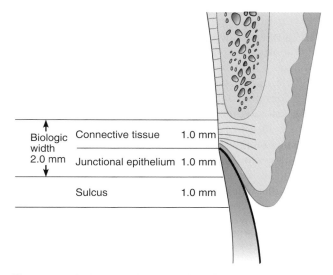

Figure 7-15 Average human biologic width. Connective tissue attachment 1 mm in height; junctional epithelial attachment 1 mm in height; sulcus depth of approximately 1 mm. The combined connective tissue attachment and junctional epithelial attachment, or biologic width, equals 2 mm. *(From Newman MG, et al: Carranza's Clinical Periodontology, ed 12. St. Louis, Saunders, 2015.)*

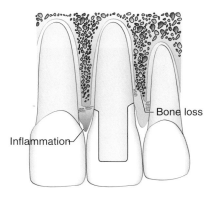

Figure 7-16 Ramifications of a biologic width violation if a restorative margin is placed within the zone of the attachment. On the mesial surface of the left central incisor, bone has not been lost, but gingival inflammation occurs. On the distal surface of the left central incisor, bone loss has occurred, and a normal biologic width has been reestablished. *(From Newman MG, et al: Carranza's Clinical Periodontology, ed 12. St. Louis, Saunders, 2015.)*

coronally can cause an open gingival embrasure. The high coronal contact can be due to diverging root angulation or an excessively tapered tooth. When restoring excessively tapered crowns with an open embrasure space, the margins of interproximal restorations should be placed 1 to 1.5 mm subgingival. This placement successfully moves the contact in an apical direction, closing the embrasure space and allowing for the maintenance of gingival health.

3. Access for oral hygiene procedures is an important aspect of pontic design. The ovate pontic is created by forming a flat or concave receptor site in the alveolar ridge with a diamond bur or electrosurgery. The alveolar bone must be a minimum of 2 mm from the most apical portion of the pontic. This pontic design has a convex undersurface, which makes it easy to clean. The sanitary pontic also has this design but does not contact the soft tissue and is a less esthetic restoration.

4. Teeth with periodontal involvement that are treated by root resection should be restored in a manner that allows for hygiene access. The remaining tooth structure should be reshaped such that, facially and lingually, the contours are a straight line from the margin coronally, whereas the interproximal contours emerge from the margin as either a straight line or slightly convex.

7.0 Prevention and Maintenance

A. Prevention.
1. *Overview*—effective plaque control is key to effective phase I nonsurgical therapy and is an important component of preventive therapy. Good supragingival plaque control can affect the growth and composition of subgingival plaque. Complete plaque removal must be accomplished at least every 48 hours. However, patients with periodontal disease should remove plaque every 24 hours because of enhanced susceptibility to disease.

2. Toothbrushing.
   a. The use of hard bristle toothbrushes, vigorous horizontal brushing, and extremely abrasive toothpastes may lead to cervical abrasions and gingival recession. Soft nylon bristle brushes do not tend to traumatize the gingival tissues. Toothbrushes should be replaced approximately every 3 months.
   b. Powered toothbrushes typically use the mechanical contact of the bristles on the tooth to remove plaque. However, the addition of low-frequency acoustic energy to generate dynamic fluid movement can provide cleaning without direct contact of the bristles. Studies have shown that although powered brushes can remove more plaque, they do not improve measures of gingival inflammation beyond those found with manual brushes. Powered brushes can be beneficial in patients who are poor brushers, patients with dexterity problems, children, and caregivers of individuals who cannot clean their own teeth.
   c. In Bass brushing, the toothbrush bristles are placed at the gingival margin at a 45-degree angle to the tooth. The bristles extend into the gingival sulcus when pressure is applied to the brush in a horizontal direction (Figure 7-17).
   d. Interproximal cleaning—because periodontal disease usually begins in interdental areas, toothbrushing must be augmented with interproximal cleaning.

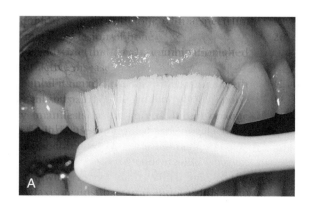
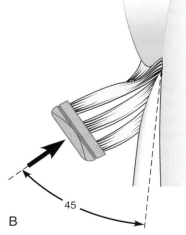

Figure 7-17 **Bass method. A,** Proper position of the brush in the mouth aims the bristle tips toward the gingival margin. **B,** Diagram shows the ideal placement, which permits slight subgingival penetration of the bristle tips. *(From Newman MG, et al:* Carranza's Clinical Periodontology, *ed 12. St. Louis, Saunders, 2015.)*

B. Maintenance.
1. *Overview*—the maintenance phase is initiated after the completion of phase I therapy and reevaluation. It is performed in a continuum with phase II (surgical) therapy and phase III (restorative) therapy. It is essential to long-term preservation of the remaining teeth. The primary rationale for maintenance therapy is continued disruption of bacterial plaque through professional subgingival instrumentation. After completion of phase I therapy, the maintenance interval for the first year should typically be every 3 months. This recommended interval is based on longitudinal clinical studies that evaluated the time required for recolonization of periodontal pockets by proposed pathogens after subgingival débridement. The maintenance interval may be altered after the first year, based on the response of the individual patient to therapy. Factors that can affect the maintenance interval include oral hygiene status, rate of calculus formation, presence and severity of secondary systemic or environmental factors, presence of remaining pockets, complicated prosthetic therapy, recurrent caries, occlusal problems, ongoing orthodontic therapy, and amount of attachment and alveolar bone loss.
2. *Procedures* performed at each maintenance.
   a. Examination—review of medical history; oral pathology examination; evaluation of oral hygiene status; clinical measures to assess for changes in the gingiva, pocket depths, mobility, attachment levels, furcations, and occlusion; caries evaluation; restorative evaluation; and radiographic evaluation when indicated.
   b. Treatment—oral hygiene reinforcement, scaling, polishing, chemical irrigation if indicated.
   c. Establish what is necessary for the next visit—the next maintenance visit, further periodontal treatment, or referral for restorative or prosthetic treatment.

Sample Questions

1. What is dental wear caused by tooth-to-tooth contact called?
   A. Abrasion
   B. Attrition
   C. Erosion
   D. Abfraction
2. Occlusal loading resulting in tooth flexure, mechanical microfractures, and loss of tooth substance in the cervical area is _____.
   A. Abrasion
   B. Attrition
   C. Erosion
   D. Abfraction
3. The distance from the CEJ to the base of the pocket is a measure of _____.
   A. Clinical attachment level
   B. Gingival recession
   C. Probing pocket depth
   D. Alveolar bone loss
4. Your examination reveals a probing pocket depth of 6 mm on the facial of tooth #30. The free gingival margin is 2 mm apical to the CEJ (there is 2-mm recession on the facial). How much attachment loss has occurred on the facial of this tooth?
   A. 6 mm
   B. 2 mm
   C. 8 mm
   D. 4 mm
5. The key feature that differentiates periodontitis from gingivitis is _____.
   A. Loss of clinical attachment
   B. Periodontal pockets greater than 3 mm
   C. Gingival recession
   D. Bleeding on probing
6. In general, what microorganisms are predominant in supragingival tooth-associated attached plaque?
   A. Gram-negative rods and cocci
   B. Gram-negative filaments
   C. Gram-positive filaments
   D. Gram-positive rods and cocci
7. The inorganic component of subgingival plaque is derived from _____.
   A. Bacteria
   B. Saliva
   C. Gingival crevicular fluid
   D. Neutrophils
8. What are the characteristics of the primary (initial) bacterial colonizers of the tooth in dental plaque formation?
   A. Gram-negative facultative
   B. Gram-positive facultative
   C. Gram-negative anaerobic
   D. Gram-positive anaerobic
9. Which of the following is an important constituent of gram-negative microorganisms that contributes to initiation of the host inflammatory response?
   A. Exotoxin
   B. Lipoteichoic acid
   C. Endotoxin
   D. Peptidoglycan
10. Calculus is detrimental to the gingival tissues because it is _____.
    A. A mechanical irritant
    B. Covered with bacterial plaque
    C. Composed of calcium and phosphorus
    D. Locked into surface irregularities
11. Restoration margins are plaque-retentive and produce the *most* inflammation when they are located _____.

A. Supragingival
B. Subgingival
C. At the level of the gingival margin
D. On buccal surfaces of teeth

12. Select from the following list cell types that are part of the innate immune system. (Choose four.)
A. T cells
B. B cells
C. Neutrophils
D. Dendritic cells
E. Plasma cells
F. Monocytes/macrophages
G. Mast cells

13. Which of the following are antigen-presenting cells?
A. Neutrophils
B. T lymphocytes
C. Macrophages
D. Plasma cells

14. Which of the following are the *most* important proteinases involved in destruction of the periodontal tissues?
A. Hyaluronidase
B. Matrix metalloproteinases
C. Glucuronidase
D. Serine proteinases

15. The predominant inflammatory cells in the periodontal pocket are _____.
A. Lymphocytes
B. Plasma cells
C. Neutrophils
D. Macrophages

16. Which of the following are part of preliminary phase therapy?
1. **Treatment of emergencies**
2. **Extraction of hopeless teeth**
3. **Plaque control**
4. **Removal of calculus**
A. 1, 2, and 3
B. 2, 3, and 4
C. 1 and 2 only
D. 2 and 4 only

17. Polymorphisms in which of the following genes have been associated with severe chronic periodontitis?
A. IL-6
B. IL-1
C. TNF
D. PGE$_2$

18. Given the same amount of attachment loss and same pocket depth, a single-rooted tooth and a multirooted tooth have the same prognosis. The closer the base of the pocket is to the apex of the tooth, the worse the prognosis.
A. Both statements are true.
B. Both statements are false.
C. The first statement is true, and the second statement is false.

D. The first statement is false, and the second statement is true.

19. Which of the following is *most* important in determining the prognosis for a tooth?
A. Probing pocket depth
B. Bleeding on probing
C. Clinical attachment level
D. Level of alveolar bone

20. When treating diabetic patients, the most common problems in the dental chair are usually associated with _____.
A. Hyperglycemia
B. Hypoglycemia
C. Insulin deficiency
D. Insulin resistance

21. Offset angulation is a characteristic feature of _____.
A. Sickle scalers
B. Universal curettes
C. Area-specific curettes
D. Chisels

22. Patients with which of the following should *not* be treated with ultrasonic instruments?
A. Deep periodontal pockets
B. Edematous tissue
C. Infectious diseases
D. Controlled diabetes

23. Order the following types of cells by their ability to populate a wound area during the healing process from *fastest* to *slowest*.
1. **PDL cells**
2. **Epithelial cells**
3. **Gingival connective tissue cells**
4. **Bone marrow cells**
A. 1, 2, 4, and 3
B. 2, 3, 1, and 4
C. 3, 2, 1, and 4
D. 1, 3, 4, and 2

24. What is the *most* important procedure to perform during the initial postoperative visits after periodontal surgery?
A. Plaque removal
B. Visual assessment of the soft tissue
C. Periodontal probing
D. Bleeding index

25. When performing a laterally repositioned flap, which of the following must be considered relative to the donor site?
A. Presence of bone on the facial
B. Width of attached gingiva
C. Thickness of attached gingiva
D. All of the above

26. During preparation of implant osteotomy ("drilling" for an implant), the critical temperature that should not be exceeded is _____ at an exposure time of 1 minute.
A. 37°C
B. 47°C

C. 57°C
D. 67°C

27. Which class of bony defect responds best to regenerative therapy?
   A. One-walled
   B. Two-walled
   C. Three-walled
   D. Shallow crater

28. Guided tissue regeneration is a method for preventing
   _____ in a healing surgical site.
   A. Plaque accumulation
   B. Cementum deposition
   C. Epithelial migration
   D. Clot formation

29. The *most* common clinical sign of occlusal trauma is
   _____.
   A. Tooth migration
   B. Tooth abrasion

C. Tooth mobility
D. Tooth attrition

30. For most patients affected with periodontitis, what is the recommended interval for maintenance appointments?
   A. 1 month
   B. 3 months
   C. 6 months
   D. 1 year

31. The minimal mesiodistal space required for the placement of two standard-diameter implants (4.0 mm diameter) between teeth is _____ mm.
   A. 4
   B. 10
   C. 14
   D. 18

Pharmacology

FRANK DOWD

OUTLINE

Pharmacology is a science that bridges basic science and clinical dentistry and medicine. This chapter reviews both aspects. The proper clinical use of drugs requires knowledge and integration of pharmacologic concepts and drugs. This review follows a standard sequence similar to the textbook *Pharmacology and Therapeutics for Dentistry*, ed 6 (St. Louis, Mosby, 2011), by Yagiela et al. Several figures and tables in this review have been taken from that text.

This review is not meant to be a comprehensive treatment of pharmacology but rather a guide to study in preparing for the pharmacology section of Part II of the National Board Dental Examination. Students are referred to other sources, including the above-mentioned text, for more complete discussions in each area of pharmacology. (See also References at the end of this chapter.) This review can help students organize and integrate knowledge of concepts and facts. It can also help students to identify areas requiring more concentrated study.

Cues That Help in Remembering Drugs by Classes

The suffixes of the following generic drug names listed are indicative of the corresponding drug classes:

- "caine" = local anesthetic (e.g., lidocaine)
- "coxib" = cyclooxygenase (COX)-2 inhibitors (e.g., celecoxib)
- "dipine" = dihydropyridine calcium channel blockers (e.g., nifedipine)
- "dronate" = bisphosphonate (e.g., alendronate)
- "fungin" = glucan synthesis inhibitor, antifungal (e.g., caspofungin)
- "gliptin" = dipeptidyl peptidase-4 inhibitor drug for type 2 diabetes (e.g., sitagliptin)
- "glitazone" = peroxisome proliferator activated receptor gamma (PPARγ) activator for type 2 diabetes (e.g., pioglitazone)
- "grel" = P2Y$_{12}$ adenosine diphosphate (ADP) receptor inhibitor in platelets (e.g., clopidogrel)
- "olol" = β-adrenergic receptor blockers (e.g., propranolol)
- "ilol" or "alol" = β-adrenergic receptor blocker that also blocks α_1-adrenergic receptors (e.g., carvedilol)
- "mab" = monoclonal antibodies (e.g., infliximab)
- "onium" or "urium" = quaternary ammonium compounds, usually competitive, peripherally acting skeletal muscle relaxers (e.g., pancuronium)
- "osin" = α_1-adrenergic receptor blockers (e.g., prazosin)
- "oxacin" = fluoroquinolone antibacterial (e.g., moxifloxacin)
- "parin" = heparin or low-molecular-weight heparin (e.g., tinzaparin)
- "prazole" = proton pump inhibitor (e.g., esomeprazole)
- "penem" = carbapenem β-lactam antibacterial (e.g., ertapenem)
- "pril" or "prilat" = angiotensin-converting enzyme (ACE) inhibitors (e.g., captopril)

- "sartan" = angiotensin II receptor blockers (e.g., losartan)
- "statin" = 3-hydroxy-3-methylglutaryl coenzyme A (HMG-CoA) reductase inhibitor antilipid drugs (e.g., lovastatin)
- "teplase" = tissue plasminogen activator drug (e.g., alteplase)
- "triptan" = serotonin 5-HT$_{1B/1D}$ agonist antimigraine drugs (e.g., sumatriptan)

1.0 Principles of Pharmacology

Drugs are the agents studied in pharmacology. These chemicals have their effects through numerous targets in the body. *Targets* refer to the types of sites at which drugs act.

Targets of Drug Action

A. Receptors are proteins on or in cells that mediate the effect of drugs and to which drugs bind with affinity and selectivity. There are five classes of drug receptors.
   1. G protein–linked (seven plasma membrane domain) receptors.
   2. Ion channel receptors.
   3. Transmembrane receptors with cytosolic enzyme domains.
   4. Intracellular nuclear receptors that alter gene expression.
   5. Cell surface adhesion receptors.
B. Enzymes (free or associated with cells) are also subject to inhibition (or stimulation) by certain drugs.
C. Drugs may also act as chemical or physical agents with low selectivity, such as antacids, or high selectivity, such as monoclonal antibodies.

Dose-Response Relationships of Drugs

A fundamental principle in pharmacology is that the effects of drugs are dose-dependent. These effects can be shown on two types of dose-response curves.

A. *Type I*—graded dose-response curves are useful for determining characteristics of agonists and antagonists.
   1. Agonists have intrinsic activity.
   2. Antagonists (pure antagonists) have no intrinsic activity.
   3. If a full agonist has an intrinsic activity of 1 and an antagonist has an intrinsic activity of 0, a partial agonist has an intrinsic activity of more than 0 but less than 1.
   4. D + R ↔ DR → effect, where D = drug concentration, R = receptor concentration, and DR = concentration of drug bound to receptor.
   5. By examining DR, we can investigate the drug binding characteristics to the receptor.
   6. By examining the effect, we investigate the tissue, organ, or organism's response to a drug.

7. *Intrinsic activity* is the maximal effect of a drug (Figure 8-1).
8. *Efficacy* is the effect of a drug as a function of level of binding to its receptor.
9. *Affinity* is a term that refers to the attractiveness of a drug to its receptor. Affinity is usually measured by the dissociation constant (K_d). The lower the K_d, the higher the affinity.
10. *Potency* is the response to a drug over a given range of concentrations (usually measured by the effective concentration of the drug leading to its half maximal effect [EC$_{50}$]) (see Figure 8-1).
11. Graded dose-response curves are also helpful in displaying the effect of antagonists. In Figure 8-2, the tracings in Figure 8-1 have been used to show the effect of antagonists on the response of an agonist. In this case, tracing A slows the effect of an agonist alone compared with the effect of an agonist in the presence of a competitive antagonist (tracing B) and in the presence of a noncompetitive antagonist (tracing C). The pure antagonist has no intrinsic activity.

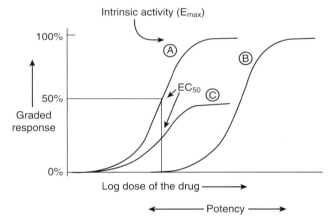

Figure 8-1 Graded dose-response curves of three agonists.

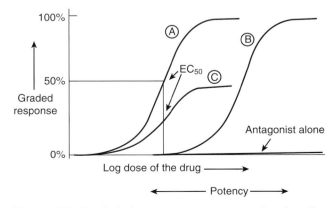

Figure 8-2 Graded dose-response curves showing the effect of antagonists.

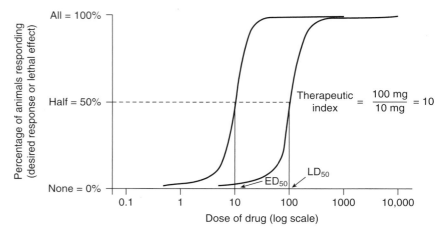

Figure 8-3 Quantal dose-response curves.

B. *Type II Quantal dose-response curves*—quantal dose-response curves look very similar to graded dose-response curves, but the two are quite different. Although both curves determine a response based on dose or concentration of the drug (using a log scale), the y-axis (ordinate) of the quantal dose-response curve indicates the number of subjects responding to a drug. The response is a specific quantitative response (e.g., a 30-mm increase in blood pressure). LD_{50}/ED_{50} = therapeutic index (TI). The TI is an estimate of the margin of safety for the drug (Figure 8-3).

Pharmacokinetics

Pharmacokinetics is the study of what the body does to the drug. It involves absorption, distribution, metabolism, and excretion.

A. Acid-base.

The acid or base properties of a drug and the pH of various body fluids are important considerations for drug distribution (Figure 8-4). Many drugs are either weak acids or weak bases.

1. Weak acids tend to concentrate in compartments of high pH, where they are more charged.
2. Weak bases tend to concentrate in compartments of low pH, where they are more charged.

B. Absorption, distribution, metabolism, and excretion.

1. The kidney is a good example of pH affecting excretion of weak acids and weak bases. Weak acids are excreted more rapidly at higher urinary pH because weak acids are concentrated in the lumen of the kidney tubule.
2. Most drugs are administered by mouth. This involves the portal system of the liver.
3. Some compartments in the body have added barriers against drugs gaining access to the compartment. The best example of such a barrier is the blood-brain barrier.
4. Many cells contain transport systems (mainly P-glycoproteins) that remove drugs from the

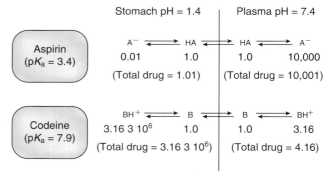

Figure 8-4 Unequal distribution of two drugs across a semipermeable membrane because of the pH of each compartment and the pK_a values of the two drugs. The pH and pK_a of the drug determine the concentration of weak acids and weak bases in various body fluids and are important in determining the rate of absorption and rate of excretion. *(Modified from Yagiela JA, et al: Pharmacology and Therapeutics for Dentistry, ed 6. St. Louis, Mosby, 2011.)*

cytoplasm or that enhance drug excretion (notably anion and cation transporters).

5. Metabolism is important because it usually leads to inactivation of the drug as well as making the drug more water-soluble. If a drug is made active by metabolism, it is called a prodrug.
6. Types of reactions involved in drug metabolism.
   a. Phase I reactions involve reactions such as oxidation, reduction, and hydrolysis.
   b. Phase II reactions involve conjugation, in which a chemical substituent is added to the drug. The most common type of conjugation reaction is glucuronide conjugation.
7. Most metabolism of drugs occurs in the liver.
   a. In the liver, metabolism can be microsomal (includes cytochrome P-450 enzymes).
   b. Alternatively, metabolism in the liver can be nonmicrosomal.

8. Excretion usually occurs in the kidney, especially for more soluble drugs. Processes involved include the following.
   a. Glomerular filtration.
   b. Active tubular secretion.
   c. Passive tubular transfer of the drug either from blood to lumen or from lumen to blood (reabsorption).
9. Most mathematical calculations that involve pharmacokinetics apply to elimination kinetics. The following are among the more important equations. (The following assume first-order kinetics.)
   a. $k_e \times t_{1/2} = 0.693$, where k = first-order rate constant and $t_{1/2}$ = half-time.
   b. $D = Cp_0 \times V_d$, where D is the drug dose (single dose), Cp_0 is the plasma concentration at zero time, and V_d is the apparent volume of distribution.
   c. $Cl = k_e \times V_d$, where k_e is the first-order rate constant of elimination, Cl is the clearance, and V_d is the apparent volume of distribution.
   d. $t_{1/2} = 0.693 \times V_d/Cl$ (this equation is derived from two of the previous equations).
10. In Figure 8-5, plotting plasma concentrations shown (on a log scale) versus time (linear scale) results in a straight line if the drug is eliminated by first-order kinetics. The β phase usually refers to the linear section of the tracing after redistribution and equilibration have occurred. This straight-line plot can be used to determine Cp_0 (plasma concentration at zero time) and $t_{1/2}$. The equations can then be used to determine V_d, k_e, and Cl.
11. Zero-order elimination kinetics refers to the elimination of a constant amount of drug eliminated regardless of dose, as opposed to first-order kinetics, the most common type (see previously), in which a constant percentage of remaining drug is eliminated.
12. Although accumulation of drug in the body can occur with repeated doses, both in first-order and in zero-order elimination, the risk of accumulation is usually greater for zero-order kinetics.

Drug-Drug Interactions

Drugs may interact by acting at the same receptor or signal transduction pathway, or, more commonly, a drug may affect the pharmacokinetics of another drug. The most common form of drug-drug interaction is one drug affecting the metabolism of another drug. Drug-drug interactions based on metabolism involve either induction or inhibition.

A. *Induction of metabolism* is a reaction to certain drugs in which the number of liver cytochrome enzymes increases, resulting in a reduction in the effect of the other drug. Some drugs that induce liver enzyme can also induce P-glycoprotein transporters.
B. *Inhibition of metabolism* is a process by which one drug either competes for metabolism of another or directly inhibits drug-metabolizing enzymes. Some drugs that inhibit liver enzyme can also inhibit P-glycoprotein transporters.
C. Most drug-drug interactions involving metabolism occur in the liver. Induction and inhibition usually involve microsomal enzymes.
D. *Genetics and pharmacology*—enzyme characteristics are important in determining the response to a drug; this is especially true for drug-metabolizing enzymes. The rate of drug metabolism can vary greatly, depending on the cytochrome P-450 isozyme profile of the patient. See also "idiosyncratic reaction," following.
E. Examples of drug-drug interactions in dentistry are presented in Table 8-1.

Adverse Drug Reactions

A. *Toxicity* results when the dose of the drug is excessive for the particular patient. It is due to a similar mechanism of action as the therapeutic effect (extension effect).
B. *Side effect*—an adverse effect that occurs within the therapeutic dose range of the drug.
C. *Drug allergy*—an adverse effect secondary to an immune reaction to a drug.
D. *Idiosyncratic reaction*—an adverse drug reaction that is due to a genetic change usually involving a change in enzyme activity (Table 8-2).

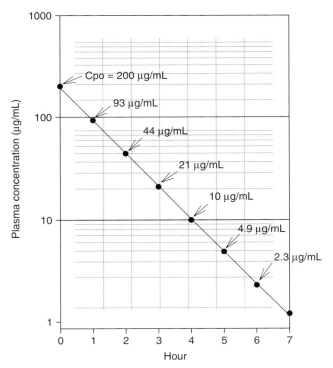

Figure 8-5 Drug plasma concentration on a semilog plot.

Table 8-1

Examples of Drug-Drug Interactions Important in Dentistry

DENTAL DRUG	INTERACTING DRUG	COMMENTS
Diazepam or triazolam	Itraconazole, clarithromycin, or other cytochrome P-450 3A inhibitor	Increased sedation owing to reduced metabolism of benzodiazepine
Tetracyclines	Oral antacids	Reduced absorption of tetracyclines
Aspirin	Anticoagulants	Increased bleeding tendency
Aspirin	Probenecid	Decreased effect of probenecid
Aspirin	Methotrexate	Increased methotrexate toxicity
Acetaminophen	Alcohol	Increased risk of liver toxicity in chronic alcoholics
Local anesthetics	Cholinesterase inhibitors	Antagonism of cholinesterase inhibitor—reduced effectiveness of the cholinesterase inhibitor in the patient with myasthenia gravis

Table 8-2

Idiosyncratic Reactions to Drugs Used in Dentistry

GENETIC ABNORMALITY	DRUGS INVOLVED	IDIOSYNCRATIC RESPONSE
NADH-methemoglobin reductase deficiency	Benzocaine, prilocaine	Methemoglobinemia
Glucose-6-phosphate dehydrogenase deficiency	Aspirin, primaquine, sulfonamides	Hemolytic anemia
Abnormal heme synthesis	Barbiturates, sulfonamides	Porphyria
Low plasma cholinesterase activity	Procaine and other ester local anesthetics	Local anesthetic toxicity
Altered muscle calcium homeostasis	Volatile inhalation anesthetics, succinylcholine	Malignant hyperthermia
Prolonged Q–T interval	Some antipsychotics and antiarrhythmics	Torsades de pointes

Modified from Yagiela JA, et al: *Pharmacology and Therapeutics for Dentistry*, ed 6. St. Louis, Mosby, 2011.

NADH, Reduced nicotinamide adenine dinucleotide.

Miscellaneous Principles

A. Clinical testing of drugs.

After preclinical testing of drugs in animals, clinical testing is conducted in four phases (Table 8-3). After a successful phase III, the drug company submits to the U.S. Food and Drug Administration (FDA) a New Drug Application (NDA) to market the drug.

B. *Drugs and pregnancy*—the relative risks of certain drugs in pregnancy is categorized into risk categories A, B, C, D, and X, with A being considered the safest (adequate and well-controlled studies have failed to demonstrate a risk to the fetus in the first trimester of pregnancy, and there is no evidence of risk in later trimesters). The other extreme is the X category (studies in animals and human beings have demonstrated fetal abnormalities, or there is positive evidence of human fetal risk based on adverse reaction data from investigational or marketing experience, or both, and the potential risk of the drug in pregnant women clearly outweighs the potential benefit).

C. *Drug legislation*—Table 8-4 lists seven drug laws as representative of drug legislation since 1906.

Table 8-3

Drug Testing Phases

PHASE	REMARKS
I	Uses normal volunteers. Safety and pharmacokinetics are assessed.
II	Uses patients who could benefit from the drug. Clinical efficacy, pharmacokinetics, and safety are assessed.
III	Uses larger number of patients, often involving several medical centers. Safety and clinical efficacy are assessed.
IV	Postmarketing surveillance. Safety, patterns of use, and new indications are assessed.

2.0 Autonomic Pharmacology

This section addresses drugs that affect the autonomic nervous system. Because of similarities with the nerves to skeletal muscles (somatic nervous system) and some

Table 8-4

Major Drug Legislative Acts

YEAR	LAW	COMMENTS
1906	Pure Food and Drug Act	Forbade the adulteration and mislabeling of drugs
1914	Harrison Narcotic Act	Regulated opiates and cocaine
1938	Food, Drug, and Cosmetic Act	Mandated the safety of drugs and the role of FDA in enforcing safety
1952	Durham-Humphrey Act	Used restrictions for certain drugs by prescription only
1983	Orphan Drug Amendment	Provided incentives for developing drugs for rare diseases
1997	FDA Modernization Act	Replaced "legend" with label "Rx only"; allowed manufacturer to discuss off-label uses of drugs with practitioners; revised accelerated track approval for drugs that treat life-threatening disorders; made provisions for pediatric drug research; revised interaction of agency with individuals doing clinical trials
2005	Combat Methamphetamine Epidemic Act	Established new regulations for sale of ephedrine, pseudoephedrine, and phenylpropanolamine

Modified from Yagiela JA, et al: *Pharmacology and Therapeutics for Dentistry,* ed 6. St. Louis, Mosby, 2011.

FDA, U.S. Food and Drug Administration.

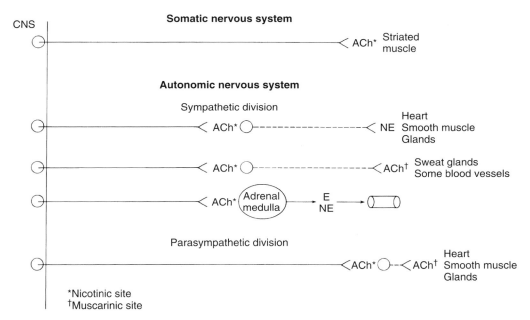

Figure 8-6 Autonomic nerves and somatic nerves to skeletal muscle: synapses and junctions. *(From Yagiela JA, et al: Pharmacology and Therapeutics for Dentistry, ed 6. St. Louis, Mosby, 2011.)*

overlap of drug actions, the nerves to skeletal muscle and the receptors associated with these nerves are also reviewed with the autonomic nervous system.

Organization

A. Organization of the autonomic nervous system.
  1. Most tissues and organs receive innervation from both sympathetic and parasympathetic nervous systems.
  2. All nerve pathways originate from the central nervous system (CNS)—the sympathetics from thoracolumbar outflow and the parasympathetics from cranial-sacral outflow.

Abbreviations, Definitions, and Receptors

ACh: acetylcholine

E: epinephrine

NE: norepinephrine

Cholinergic: pertaining to ACh as in a cholinergic drug, cholinergic nerve, or cholinergic receptor

Adrenergic: pertaining to adrenaline (E) or NE

A. Synapses and junctions.
  1. The synapses (nerve-nerve) and junctions (nerve-effectors) for the autonomic nervous system and somatic nerves to the skeletal muscles are shown in Figure 8-6.

2. The neurotransmitter at each site is identified.
3. It is important to distinguish muscarinic cholinergic sites from nicotinic cholinergic sites.
    a. Muscarinic sites.
        (1) At neuroeffector sites for all postganglionic cholinergic neurons (this is characteristic of all parasympathetic postganglionic nerves).
        (2) At neuroeffector sites of postganglionic sympathetic nerves to the sweat glands and a very few blood vessels (these postganglionic nerves are also cholinergic).
    b. Nicotinic sites.
        (1) At the skeletal neuromuscular junction (involving the somatic nerves).
        (2) At ganglionic sites (note: the same type of nicotinic receptor is present in sympathetic ganglia, parasympathetic ganglia, and the adrenal medulla).
4. The two nicotinic receptors are distinct and different receptor types. There are drugs that can distinguish one from the other.
5. The adrenal medulla secretes the hormones E and NE. There is no ganglion here, but the ACh receptors are ganglionic nicotinic in type.
6. Muscarinic receptors are divided further into M1, M2, M3, M4, and M5 receptors; however, most antimuscarinic drugs are unable to distinguish between the various muscarinic receptors. The roles of the M4 and M5 receptors are unknown.
7. Muscarinic receptors (M1 and M3) are linked to G_q, phospholipase C, and Ca^{2+}, whereas M2 receptors are linked to G_i and a decrease in cyclic adenosine monophosphate (cAMP).
8. Adrenergic receptors are important clinically. Several clinically useful adrenergic drugs are selective for a receptor type (Table 8-5).

Dynamics of Neurotransmission

A. Biosynthetic pathway for ACh.
    Step 1: choline (taken up into nerve via action of permease).
    Step 2: choline acetyltransferase catalyzes the synthesis of ACh from acetyl CoA and choline.
B. Biosynthesis of NE and E.
    Step 1: tyrosine to DOPA (enzyme is tyrosine hydroxylase).
    Step 2: DOPA to dopamine (enzyme is aromatic L-amino acid decarboxylase).
    Step 3: dopamine to NE (enzyme is dopamine beta-hydroxylase).
    Step 4 (mostly in adrenal medulla): NE to E (enzyme is phenylethanolamine N-methyltransferase).
    (Some flow charts show synthesis beginning with phenylalanine.)
C. Tyrosine hydroxylase catalyzes the rate-limiting step in the synthesis. This enzyme is inhibited by metyrosine.

Table 8-5

Adrenergic Receptors, Locations, and Signal Transduction

RECEPTOR TYPE	LOCATION	SIGNALING PATHWAY
α_1*	Blood vessels, radial muscle of eye, sphincter and trigone muscle of bladder, sphincter muscle of GI tract	G_q, PLC, Ca^{2+}
α_2*†	Blood vessels, prejunctional sites that act as autoreceptors†	G_i, ↓cAMP
β_1	Heart, GI tract, salivary glands, adipose tissue (lipolysis), kidney juxtaglomerular cells	G_s, ↑cAMP
β_2‡	Bronchi, blood vessels, heart	G_s, ↑cAMP
β_3	Adipose tissue (lipolysis)	G_s, ↑cAMP

cAMP, Cyclic AMP; *GI*, gastrointestinal; *PLC*, phospholipase C.

*α_1 and α_2 receptors (postjunctional) are associated with vasoconstriction.

†α_2 autoreceptors (prejunctional), when stimulated by agonists, mediate a reduction in release of neurotransmitters.

‡β_2 receptors are associated with vasodilation.

D. The neurotransmitters ACh, NE, and dopamine are stored in vesicles or granules.
E. Termination of transmission by ACh occurs primarily by metabolism by acetylcholinesterase located on postsynaptic or postjunctional membranes.
F. Termination of transmission by NE occurs primarily by reuptake of NE into prejunctional nerves and secondarily into other cells. Monoamine oxidase (MAO) and catechol O-methyltransferase (COMT) play a role in metabolizing NE.

Tissues and Organs

A. Another important part of autonomic pharmacology is linking specific receptors and autonomic pathways to given tissue responses (Table 8-6).
B. Knowing the receptor preference for a drug, the receptors located in a given tissue, and the response to the receptor, one can predict the response to a drug.

Adrenergic Agonists

The receptor preferences for some adrenergic agonists are shown in Table 8-7.

A. Figure 8-7 shows the response to three catecholamines. To determine all of the effects of these drugs, one must remember that, especially for heart rate, the reflex effect mediated by baroreceptors must be taken into account. Notice the role of each receptor and baroreceptor reflex in the various phases of the responses in Figure 8-7.

Table 8-6

Some Important Tissue Receptors and Responses

SYMPATHETIC EFFECTOR	SYMPATHETIC RESPONSE	ADRENERGIC RECEPTOR*	PARASYMPATHETIC RESPONSE
Eye			
Radial muscle of the iris	Contraction (mydriasis)	α_1	—
Sphincter of the iris	—		Contraction (miosis)
Heart			
SA node	Increase in rate	β_1, β_2	Decrease in rate
AV node	Increase in automaticity and conduction velocity	β_1, β_2	Decrease in conduction velocity
Ventricles	Increased contractility, conduction velocity, and automaticity	β_1, β_2	—
Blood vessels	Constriction (α), dilation (β)	$\alpha_1, \alpha_2, \beta_2$	—
Lungs			
Bronchial smooth muscle	Relaxation	β_2	Contraction
GI tract			
Smooth muscle	Decreased motility and tone	$\alpha_1, \alpha_2 \ \beta_1, \beta_2$	Increased motility and tone
Sphincters	Contraction	α_1	Relaxation
Salivary glands	Viscous secretion, amylase secretion	$\alpha_1, \beta_1, \beta_2$	Profuse, watery secretion
Urinary bladder			
Detrusor	Relaxation	β_2	Contraction
Trigone and sphincter	Contraction	α_1	Relaxation

Modified from Yagiela JA, et al: *Pharmacology and Therapeutics for Dentistry,* ed 6. St. Louis, Mosby, 2011.

AV, Atrioventricular; *GI,* gastrointestinal; *SA,* sinoatrial.

*Receptors in bold type have the greatest effect.

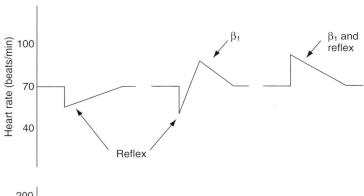

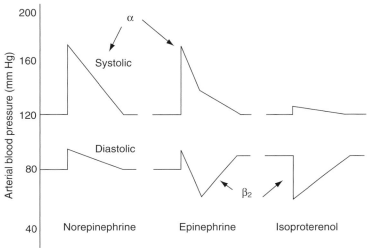

Figure 8-7 Cardiovascular effects of three adrenergic agonists. Some important receptors are linked to responses.

B. Indirectly acting sympathomimetic (sympathetic-type) drugs act by releasing NE. Examples include amphetamines and ephedrine (the latter has both direct and indirect action). These drugs demonstrate tolerance and are orally active, in contrast to E and NE.

Adrenergic Receptor Blockers

A. Table 8-8 shows adrenergic receptor blockers and their adrenergic receptor preferences. Every drug in each column is an antagonist at that receptor. Almost all β blockers end in "olol." Exceptions include carvedilol and labetalol, which block α_1-adrenergic receptors in addition to blocking β_1 and β_2 receptors (not shown in Table 8-8).

B. α-Adrenergic receptor blockers.
   1. Phentolamine and phenoxybenzamine are prototypes of nonselective α-adrenergic receptor blockers (α_1 and α_2) and are rarely used in medicine because of their nonselectivity. However, phentolamine is used in dentistry to reverse soft tissue anesthesia more quickly after procedures involving a local anesthetic with a vasoconstrictor.
   2. Prazosin.
      a. Example of a selective α_1 blocker.
      b. α_1 blockers are used to treat hypertension, heart failure, and benign prostate hypertrophy (α_1 blockers cause vasodilation, reduce afterload and preload of the heart, reduce contraction of smooth muscle in the sphincter and trigone muscles of the bladder, and reduce contraction of the prostate).
      c. *Adverse effects of α_1 blockers*—hypotension (especially first-dose effect), fluid retention, dry mouth, nasal stuffiness.
   3. *Epinephrine reversal*—the vasoconstrictor effect of epinephrine is converted into a vasodilator effect in the presence of an α blocker. The β_2 vasodilator response becomes the major vascular response to epinephrine because α receptors are blocked by the α blocker. This reversal is more complete with nonselective α blockers.

C. β-Adrenergic receptor blockers (β blockers).
   1. Used more often than α blockers.
   2. Some are partial agonists (have intrinsic sympathomimetic activity).
   3. Propranolol is the prototype of nonselective β blockers, but most are selective β_1 receptor blockers.
   4. *β blocker effects*—decrease blood pressure, reduce angina, reduce risk after myocardial infarction, reduce heart rate and force, have antiarrhythmic effect, cause hypoglycemia in diabetics, decrease intraocular pressure.
   5. *Carvedilol*—nonselective β blocker that also blocks α_1 receptors; used for heart failure.

D. Adrenergic neuron blockers.
   1. *Metyrosine*—inhibits tyrosine hydroxylase; used to treat pheochromocytoma.

Table 8-7

Some Adrenergic Agonists, Their Receptor Preferences, and Main Uses

DRUG	USE	RECEPTOR PREFERENCE
Epinephrine	Reverse anaphylaxis, vasoconstriction, bronchodilation	$\alpha_1, \alpha_2, \beta_1, \beta_2, \beta_3$
Norepinephrine	Vasoconstriction	$\alpha_1, \alpha_2, \beta_1$
Isoproterenol	Bronchodilation, reverse heart block	$\beta_1, \beta_2, \beta_3$
Phenylephrine	Nasal vasoconstriction	α_1, α_2
Naphazoline	Nasal vasoconstriction	α_2
Clonidine	Antihypertensive	α_2
Methyldopa	Antihypertensive	α_2
Dexmedetomidine	IV sedation	α_2
Albuterol	Bronchodilation	β_2
Terbutaline	Bronchodilation	β_2
Salmeterol	Bronchodilation	β_2
Dobutamine	Cardiac stimulation	β_1, α_1
Methylphenidate	CNS stimulation	(Indirect action)
Amphetamine	CNS stimulation	(Indirect action)

CNS, Central nervous system; *IV,* intravenous.

Table 8-8

Adrenergic Receptor Blockers

RECEPTOR TYPE BLOCKED	α_1 AND α_2	α_1 SELECTIVE	β_1 AND β_2	β_1 SELECTIVE
Drugs	Phentolamine	Prazosin	Propranolol	Metoprolol
	Phenoxybenzamine	Terazosin	Pindolol	Atenolol
		Doxazosin	Nadolol	Acebutolol
		Tamsulosin	Timolol	Esmolol

Table 8-9			

Cholinergic Receptor Agonists

DRUG	RECEPTOR AFFINITY	STRUCTURALLY SIMILAR TO ACETYLCHOLINE	USE
Acetylcholine	$M \cong N$		Ophthalmic
Bethanechol	$M \gg N$	Yes	To increase GI and urinary tract motility
Methacholine	$M \gg N$	Yes	To test reactivity of airway
Carbachol	$N > M$	Yes	To treat glaucoma
Pilocarpine	$M \gg N$	No, occurs in nature	To treat glaucoma, stimulate salivary flow
Cevimeline	$M \gg N$	No	To stimulate salivary flow
Nicotine*	$N \gg M$	No, occurs in nature	For smoking cessation
Varenicline	$N \gg M$	No	For smoking cessation

GI, Gastrointestinal; *M*, muscarinic; *N*, nicotinic.

*Nicotine acts at both types of nicotinic receptors. It also causes desensitization of nicotinic receptors, leading to receptor blockade in a time-dependent manner.

2. *Reserpine*—depletes granules containing NE in nerve endings, releases NE (rarely used).
3. *Guanethidine and guanadrel*—block adrenergic nerve endings by a series of actions; used rarely for hypertension.
4. *MAO inhibitors*, such as pargyline and tranylcypromine, indirectly reduce granule content of NE but increase it in the cytoplasmic pool of adrenergic neurons. MAO inhibitors should not be used with indirectly acting drugs, such as amphetamines, ephedrine, and tyramine (in many foods and beverages). Newer MAO-A and MAO-B selective inhibitors are available for clinical use.

Dental Implications of α and β Blockers

A. Phentolamine (OraVerse) is used in dentistry to reverse soft tissue anesthesia more quickly after procedures involving a local anesthetic with a vasoconstrictor.
B. The disorders for which these drugs are used often affect dental treatment.
C. β blockers increase the vasoconstrictor response to E but reduce the tachycardia resulting from E.
D. α blockers inhibit the vasoconstrictor response to E and levonordefrin.
E. MAO inhibitors should not be used with indirectly acting sympathetic drugs and with several other drugs such as opioids, especially meperidine.
F. E and levonordefrin have exaggerated effects when given with depleting drugs, such as reserpine, guanethidine, and guanadrel.

Cholinergic Receptor Agonists

A. Most drugs in this group are used for their muscarinic effects. They mimic the effects of postganglionic cholinergic nerves.

B. These drugs are longer lasting than ACh because they are not subject to rapid metabolism similar to ACh (Table 8-9). ACh is metabolized by acetylcholinesterase, located near receptors for ACh. In the plasma and other sites, ACh and many other esters are metabolized by pseudocholinesterase. The other cholinergic agonists used as drugs are metabolized slowly or not at all by these enzymes.
C. ACh given in low doses stimulates mostly muscarinic receptors; in very high doses, more nicotinic effects occur (see Table 8-9).
D. The muscarinic effects of cholinergic agonists include salivation, miosis, bradycardia, bronchoconstriction, increase in gastrointestinal (GI) motility, increased urination, and sweating. (Postganglionic sympathetic nerves to sweat glands release ACh, which stimulates muscarinic receptors.) Vasodilation, another effect of muscarinic receptor agonists, is not as obvious. The vasculature is almost exclusively innervated by the sympathetic system. Why do we get vasodilation from injected muscarinic receptor agonists? Because the blood vessels have muscarinic receptors on their endothelial cells. These receptors are linked to synthesis and release of nitric oxide, which causes vasodilation.
E. Adverse effects of muscarinic receptor agonists are extensions of the effects listed previously.
F. Nicotinic receptor agonists include nicotine itself and varenicline, a partial agonist at the $\alpha_4\beta_2$ type nicotinic receptor. Each is used in smoking cessation.

Anticholinesterases

A. These drugs act as indirect agonists at both muscarinic and nicotinic sites.
B. They inhibit acetylcholinesterase located near both nicotinic and muscarinic receptors.

Table 8-10

Cholinesterase Inhibitors

DRUG	TYPE OF INHIBITION	DURATION OF ACTION	INHIBITORY EFFECT ON PSEUDOCHOLINESTERASE	USES
Edrophonium*	Reversible	Very short	Little	To reverse curare-type drugs, diagnosis
Neostigmine*	Reversible	Extended	Little	To reverse curare-type drugs, to treat myasthenia gravis
Physostigmine	Reversible	Short	Little	For glaucoma, antidote for atropine
Pyridostigmine*	Reversible	Extended	Little	To treat myasthenia gravis
Tacrine	Reversible	Extended	Little	To treat Alzheimer's disease
Donepezil	Reversible	Extended	Little	To treat Alzheimer's disease
Galantamine	Reversible	Extended	Little	To treat Alzheimer's disease
Rivastigmine	Pseudoirreversible	Extended	Little	To treat Alzheimer's disease
Malathion	Irreversible	Long	Substantial	Insecticide
Echothiophate	Irreversible	Long	Substantial	For glaucoma
Sarin	Irreversible	Long	Substantial	Nerve gas
Soman	Irreversible	Long	Substantial	Nerve gas

*Does not enter the central nervous system.

Table 8-11

*Effects of Anticholinesterases**

MUSCARINIC	NICOTINIC
Miosis, salivation, sweating, bradycardia, bronchoconstriction, increased GI motility, urination	Muscle twitching and weakness, tachycardia, increase in blood pressure

GI, Gastrointestinal.

*Central nervous system effects of anticholinesterases include restlessness, ataxia, and respiratory depression.

C. The characteristics of cholinesterase inhibitors vary (Tables 8-10 and 8-11).
D. Drugs that are metabolized by pseudocholinesterase are synergized by pseudocholinesterase inhibitors.
E. Pralidoxime is used to reactivate acetylcholinesterase after irreversible inhibition by an organophosphate (e.g., echothiophate, isoflurophate, sarin, soman).

Autonomics and the Eye

A. Muscarinic receptor agonists stimulate the circular muscle of the eye to contract, decreasing the size of the pupil (miosis). They also cause contraction of the ciliary muscle, leading to focusing for near vision. Contraction of these muscles also leads to enhanced removal of intraocular fluid through the canal of Schlemm and the trabecular network. Uveoscleral drainage through the ciliary muscles also accounts for some removal of intraocular fluid.
B. α_1-Adrenergic receptor agonists stimulate the radial muscle of the eye to contract, increasing the size of the pupil (mydriasis) and in some cases slowing the removal of fluid from the eye.
C. Adrenergic agonists and antagonists and certain prostaglandins reduce formation of intraocular fluid and reduce intraocular pressure.

Antimuscarinic Drugs

A. Block the effect of ACh and all drugs that stimulate muscarinic receptors.
B. Atropine and scopolamine are prototypes.
C. Effects are shown in Table 8-12.
D. Indications are shown in Table 8-13. (A limited number of muscarinic receptor subtype–selective drugs are available.)

Dental Implications of Antimuscarinic Drugs and Cholinergic Drugs

A. Atropine—oral administration is 0.5 mg (adult dose) for reducing salivary flow.
B. Contraindications for using antimuscarinic drugs.
   1. Narrow-angle glaucoma.
   2. Prostate hypertrophy.
   3. Paralytic ileus.
   4. Tachycardia.
C. Reduced salivary flow leads to increased risk of caries.
D. Pilocarpine and cevimeline are used to stimulate salivary flow.

Table 8-12

Effects of Antimuscarinic Drugs

ORGAN	EFFECT
Eye	Mydriasis, cycloplegia (fixation for distant vision)
Salivary glands	Reduced secretion
Lacrimal glands	Reduced secretion
Heart	Tachycardia (moderate and larger doses)
Bronchi	Bronchodilation, reduce secretion
GI tract	Reduced peristalsis, reduced secretion
Bladder	Urinary retention
Sweat glands	Reduced secretion
CNS	
Basal ganglia	Antitremor activity
Vestibular apparatus	Antimotion sickness
Higher centers	Drowsiness or stimulation, depending on drug and dose

CNS, Central nervous system; *GI,* gastrointestinal.

Table 8-13

Antimuscarinic Drugs and Uses

DRUG	USES
Atropine	Prototype, to reduce salivary flow, for antivagal effect during surgery, antidote for physostigmine
Scopolamine	Prototype, for motion sickness
Propantheline	For overactive bladder
Tolterodine	For overactive bladder
Trospium	For overactive bladder
Glycopyrrolate	To reduce stomach acid, to reduce bradycardia during surgery
Homatropine	To cause mydriasis
Cyclopentolate	To cause mydriasis
Tropicamide	To cause mydriasis
Benztropine	To reduce parkinsonian symptoms
Trihexyphenidyl	To reduce parkinsonian symptoms, to treat some dystonias
Oxybutynin	For overactive bladder
Ipratropium	To treat asthma
Pirenzepine (M_1 selective)	To treat peptic ulcers
Darifenacin (M_3 selective)	For overactive bladder
Solifenacin (M_3 selective)	For overactive bladder

Table 8-14

Curare-Type Neuromuscular Junction Blockers

DRUG	HISTAMINE RELEASE	SOME CHARACTERISTICS OTHER THAN MUSCLE RELAXATION
D-tubocurarine	++	Ganglionic blockade
Pancuronium	−	Steroid, has some antimuscarinic effects
Atracurium	+	Metabolized by esterase and Hoffman degradation
Vecuronium	−	Antimuscarinic, steroid
Pipecuronium	−	Steroid
Rocuronium	−	Steroid
Doxacurium	−	Slightly more delayed onset
Mivacurium	+	Metabolized by esterase

Skeletal Neuromuscular Blockers

A. Types.
 1. Depolarizing noncompetitive blockers (succinylcholine).
 2. Nondepolarizing competitive blockers of ACh (curare-type drugs).
B. These drugs are used during surgery for relaxing skeletal muscle, for endotracheal intubation, for treatment of tetanus, and for a few other purposes.
C. They have permanent positive charges and do not enter the CNS, and they are not absorbed after oral administration.
D. The effects of competitive skeletal neuromuscular blockers can be antagonized by cholinesterase inhibitors.
E. The contrasting properties of curarelike drugs are presented in Table 8-14.
F. Dantrolene.
 1. A drug that relaxes skeletal muscle without blocking nicotinic receptors.
 2. Prevents release of Ca^{2+} from the sarcoplasmic reticulum.
 3. Used for prophylaxis against malignant hyperthermia and to overcome muscle contraction and damage secondary to malignant hyperthermia.
 4. Used also for upper motor neuron disorders (e.g., cerebral palsy).
G. Botulinum toxin A (Botox).
 1. Prevents release of ACh from neurons.
 2. Used in ophthalmology to relax extraocular muscles.
 3. Used for muscle dystonias.
 4. Used to remove wrinkles.

3.0 Central Nervous System Pharmacology

Antipsychotic Drugs

A. Indications.
   1. Schizophrenia and other types of psychosis.
   2. Tourette's syndrome.
   3. Huntington's chorea.
   4. Other disorders, such as obsessive-compulsive disorders.
B. Drugs.
   1. Phenothiazines.
      a. Aliphatic derivatives.
         (1) Chlorpromazine.
      b. Piperidine derivatives.
         (1) Thioridazine.
         (2) Mesoridazine.
      c. Piperazine derivatives.
         (1) Fluphenazine.
         (2) Perphenazine.
         (3) Prochlorperazine.
         (4) Trifluoperazine.
   2. Haloperidol resembles piperazine phenothiazines.
   3. Thiothixene resembles piperazine phenothiazines.
   4. Others (e.g., loxapine, pimozide).
   5. Newer and more atypical antipsychotic drugs.
      a. Clozapine.
      b. Olanzapine.
      c. Quetiapine.
      d. Risperidone.
      e. Ziprasidone.
      f. Aripiprazole.
      g. Paliperidone.
C. *Mechanism of action*—treatment of psychosis has been largely based on the dopamine hypothesis. Drugs in the phenothiazine class (as well as haloperidol, thiothixene, and others such as loxapine and pimozide) block dopamine receptors in the mesolimbic and mesocortical pathways. The D_2 receptor is the key antipsychotic receptor. Blocking dopamine receptors is important not only for antipsychotic action but also for other effects, including adverse effects of antipsychotic drugs. Newer and more atypical drugs differ as follows.
   1. They may preferentially inhibit selective dopamine receptors.
   2. They also inhibit serotonin (5-hydroxytryptamine [5-HT]) receptors of the $5-HT_2$ type, accounting for part of their antipsychotic action.
D. Effects of antipsychotic drugs are shown in Table 8-15.
E. Adverse motor effects of antipsychotic drugs.
   1. Acute dystonias.
   2. Akathisia.
   3. Parkinsonism.
   4. Perioral tremor.

Table 8-15

Dopaminergic Cell Groups and Related Effects of Antipsychotics

CELL GROUP	ACTION
Mesolimbic and mesocortical	Antipsychotic effect
Nigrostriatal	Motor side effects
Tuberoinfundibular	Stimulation of prolactin release, galactorrhea
Chemoreceptor trigger zone	Antiemetic effect
Medullary-periventricular	Increased appetite

   5. Malignant syndrome.
   6. Tardive dyskinesia (a more permanent effect that is difficult to reverse).
   7. Many motor-adverse (extrapyramidal) effects can be relieved by antimuscarinic drugs that are able to gain access to the brain because acetylcholine and dopamine oppose each other in the basal ganglia. Blocking muscarinic receptors tends to correct the imbalance of blocking dopamine receptors by antipsychotic drugs.
F. Other adverse effects of antipsychotic drugs.
   1. Antimuscarinic effects.
   2. Orthostatic hypotension.
   3. Convulsions.
   4. Photosensitivity.
   5. Cardiac arrhythmias (long QT syndrome).

Antidepressant Drugs

Drug treatment of depression is based on increasing serotonin (5-HT) or NE (or both) at synapses in selective tracts in the brain; this can be accomplished by different mechanisms. Treatment takes several weeks to reach full clinical efficacy.

A. Drugs.
   1. Tricyclic antidepressants.
      a. Amitriptyline.
      b. Desipramine.
      c. Doxepin.
      d. Imipramine.
      e. Protriptyline.
   2. Selective serotonin reuptake inhibitors (SSRIs).
      a. Fluoxetine.
      b. Paroxetine.
      c. Sertraline.
      d. Fluvoxamine.
      e. Citalopram.
   3. Serotonin norepinephrine reuptake inhibitors (SNRIs).
      a. Venlafaxine.
      b. Duloxetine.

4. MAO inhibitors.
   a. Tranylcypromine.
   b. Phenelzine.
   c. Selegiline (MAO-B selective).
5. Miscellaneous antidepressants.
   a. Bupropion.
   b. Maprotiline.
   c. Mirtazapine.
   d. Trazodone.
   e. St. John's wort.
B. Contrasting mechanisms of action of antidepressants.
   1. Tricyclic antidepressants inhibit reuptake of NE and 5-HT. The inhibition of reuptake leads to a sequence of events that eventually results in an antidepressive effect. Box 8-1 shows this progression.
   2. SSRIs inhibit reuptake only of 5-HT.
   3. SNRIs inhibit reuptake of NE and 5-HT to varying degrees based on concentration.

   4. MAO inhibitors (nonselective) inhibit the metabolism of NE, dopamine, and 5-HT in nerve endings.
   5. Mirtazapine increases the release of NE and 5-HT from nerve endings.
   6. Bupropion increases the release of NE and dopamine. Increasing dopamine in the synapses may contribute to its action, especially in its use in smoking cessation.
   7. Trazodone blocks 5-HT_{2A} and α_1 adrenergic receptors.
   8. St. John's wort reduces the membrane potential of nerves and may indirectly reduce uptake of NE and 5-HT.
C. *Pharmacokinetics*—most of these drugs are lipid-soluble, have long half-lives, and are metabolized.
D. Adverse effects are listed in Table 8-16.
   1. Tricyclic antidepressants are very likely to cause xerostomia. Amitriptyline is especially potent in this regard.
   2. MAO inhibitors should not be used with agents that release catecholamines and serotonin (see Section 2.0, Autonomic Pharmacology). MAO inhibitors should not be used with other antidepressants.

Antimania Drugs

Antimania drugs are used to treat manic-depressive illness.
A. Drugs.
   1. Lithium.
   2. Carbamazepine.
   3. Valproic acid.
   4. Lamotrigine.
B. Mechanisms of action.
   1. Lithium works inside the cell to block conversion of inositol phosphate to inositol.
   2. Carbamazepine blocks sodium channels (see section on antiepileptic drugs).

Box 8-1

Action of Many Antidepressants

Inhibition of reuptake of norepinephrine, serotonin, or both
↓
Increase in synaptic concentrations of neurotransmitter
↓
Desensitization of nerve terminal autoreceptors
↓
Increase of neuronal release of neurotransmitters
↓
Selective changes in postsynaptic receptors

Table 8-16

Comparison of Adverse Effects of Antidepressants

DRUG	SEDATION	SEIZURES	HYPOTENSION	CARDIAC EFFECTS	NAUSEA, VOMITING, DIARRHEA	ANTIMUSCARINIC EFFECTS
Tricyclic antidepressants	+++	+	+++	++	+	++++
Selective serotonin reuptake inhibitors	0	0	0	0	++++	0
Monoamine oxidase inhibitors	0	+	++++	0	+	0
Miscellaneous agents						
Trazodone	++++	+	++	0	+	0
Bupropion	0	++	+	0	0	0
Duloxetine	+	0	+	+	0	0

0, No effect; +, ++, +++, ++++, indicate degree of effect.

3. Valproic acid blocks sodium and calcium channels (see section on antiepileptic drugs).
4. Lamotrigine blocks sodium channels.

C. Lithium toxicity.
   1. Nausea, diarrhea, convulsions, coma, hyperreflexia, cardiac arrhythmias, hypotension.
   2. Thyroid enlargement; increases thyroid-stimulating hormone secretion; may cause hypothyroidism.
   3. Polydipsia, polyuria (lithium inhibits the effect of antidiuretic hormone on the kidney).

D. Clinical applications concerning lithium.
   1. Patients must be warned against sodium-restricted diets because sodium restriction leads to greater retention of lithium by the kidney.
   2. Patients must have regular (e.g., monthly) blood checks because the margin of safety is narrow.

E. Drug-drug interactions of lithium.
   1. Diuretics and newer nonsteroidal antiinflammatory drugs (NSAIDs) reduce lithium excretion and may cause lithium toxicity.

Sedative Hypnotics

Sedative hypnotics work by numerous mechanisms. Most of the drugs enhance chloride channel activity (i.e., increase chloride conductance in the brain). These drugs are used for various purposes depending on the drug, dose, and route of administration.

A. Drugs and their actions.
   1. Benzodiazepines—enhance the effect of γ-aminobutyric acid (GABA) at $GABA_A$ receptors on chloride channels; this increases chloride channel conductance in the brain ($GABA_A$ receptors are ion channel receptors).
   2. Barbiturates—enhance the effect of GABA on the chloride channel but also increase chloride channel conductance independently of GABA, especially at high doses, giving barbiturates greater sedative and hypnotic effects than benzodiazepines. Barbiturates also decrease activation of glutamate α-amino-3-hydroxy-5-methylisoxazole-4-propionic acid (AMPA) receptors.
   3. Zolpidem and zaleplon—work in a similar manner to benzodiazepines but do so only at the benzodiazepine₁ (BZ_1) receptor type. (Both BZ_1 and BZ_2 are located on chloride channels.)
   4. Chloral hydrate—probably similar action to barbiturates.
   5. Buspirone—partial agonist at a specific serotonin receptor ($5\text{-}HT_{1A}$).
   6. Other sedatives (e.g., mephenesin, meprobamate, methocarbamol, carisoprodol, cyclobenzaprine)—mechanisms not well described. Several mechanisms may be involved.
   7. Baclofen—stimulates $GABA_B$ receptors that are linked to the G protein, G_i, resulting in an increase in K^+ conductance and a decrease in Ca^{2+}

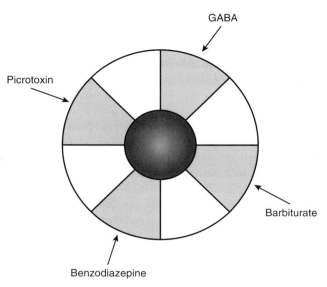

Figure 8-8 Chloride channel with GABA and three drugs. *(Adapted from Sieghart W: GABAA receptors: ligand-gated Cl– ion channels modulated by multiple drug-binding sites,* Trends Pharmacol Sci *13:446-450, 1992. IN Yagiela JA, Dowd FJ, Johnson BS, Mariotti AJ, Neidle EA:* Pharmacology and Therapeutics for Dentistry, *ed 6, St Louis, Mosby, 2011.)*

conductance. (Other aforementioned drugs do not bind to the $GABA_B$ receptor.)
   8. Antihistamines (e.g., diphenhydramine)—block H_1 histamine-1 (H_1) receptors. Doing so in the CNS leads to sedation.
   9. Ethyl alcohol—actions include a likely effect on the chloride channel.
   10. Flumazenil—blocks benzodiazepine receptors (both BZ_1 and BZ_2) and reverses the excessive sedation of sedatives acting at these receptors.

B. Chloride channel.
   Figure 8-8 shows the chloride channel. It is composed of subunits and has several binding domains that include binding domains for GABA, benzodiazepines, and barbiturates. There are two benzodiazepine receptors, BZ_1 (also called omega-1) and BZ_2 (also called omega-2), on the chloride channels, reflecting different subunit structures of the channels.

C. Benzodiazepines.
   1. All benzodiazepines are metabolized, most with active metabolites. Glucuronidation terminates the sedative action. Elimination half-lives vary a great deal from drug to drug.
      a. Triazolam (1 to 2 hours).
      b. Midazolam (2 to 5 hours).
      c. Oxazepam (5 to 15 hours).
      d. Alprazolam (12 to 15 hours).
      e. Lorazepam (10 to 18 hours).
      f. Chlordiazepoxide (5 to 30 hours).
      g. Diazepam (30 to 60 hours).
      h. Flurazepam (50 to 100 hours).

2. α-Hydroxylation is a rapid route of metabolism that is unique to triazolam, midazolam, and alprazolam; this accounts for the very rapid metabolism and short sedative actions of these drugs.
3. Pharmacologic effects of benzodiazepines.
    a. Antianxiety.
    b. Sedation.
    c. Anticonvulsant (including drug-induced convulsions).
    d. Amnesia, especially drugs such as triazolam.
    e. Relax skeletal muscle (act on CNS polysynaptic pathways).
4. Indications.
    a. Intravenous sedation (e.g., midazolam, diazepam, lorazepam).
    b. Antianxiety.
    c. Sleep induction.
    d. Anticonvulsant (e.g., diazepam, clonazepam).
    e. Panic disorders.
    f. Muscle relaxation.
5. Adverse effects.
    a. Ataxia, confusion.
    b. Excessive sedation.
    c. Amnesia (not a desired effect with daytime sedation).
    d. Altered sleep patterns (increase stage 2 and decrease stage 4 sleep).
D. Barbiturates.
    1. *Long-acting*—phenobarbital is used to treat certain types of seizures (see section on antiepileptic drugs).
    2. *Intermediate-acting*—amobarbital, pentobarbital (occasionally used for sleep), secobarbital.
    3. *Short-acting*—hexobarbital, methohexital, thiopental—rarely used as intravenous anesthetics.
    4. Pharmacologic effects of barbiturates.
        a. Similar to benzodiazepines except for the important differences shown in Table 8-17.
        b. Induce an increased synthesis of porphyrins and are contraindicated in certain types of porphyria.
E. Zolpidem and zaleplon.
    1. Short half-lives (zolpidem ≅ 2 hours; zaleplon ≅ 1 hour).

2. Used for insomnia.
3. Selective action at BZ_1 receptor—reduces risk of tolerance and dependence.
4. Do not have anticonvulsant action.
5. Do not greatly affect sleep patterns.
F. Chloral hydrate.
    1. Short-acting sleep inducer—less risk of "hangover" effect the next day.
    2. Little effect on REM sleep.
    3. Metabolized to trichloroethanol, an active metabolite; further metabolism inactivates the drug.
    4. Used for conscious sedation in dentistry. Repetitive doses should not be used.
    5. Can result in serious toxicity if dose is not controlled.
G. Buspirone.
    1. Short half-life (2 to 4 hours).
    2. Relieves anxiety.
    3. Does not act as an anticonvulsant.
    4. Is not a good muscle relaxant.
    5. Minimum abuse potential.
H. Other sedatives—carisoprodol, cyclobenzaprine, and methocarbamol are used for muscle relaxation.
I. Baclofen.
    1. Used in spasticity states to relax skeletal muscle.
    2. Occasionally used in trigeminal neuralgia.
J. Antihistamines (first-generation H_1 receptor blockers).
    1. Used for sedation (e.g., diphenhydramine).
K. Ethyl alcohol—a sedative hypnotic, but not used clinically as a sedative. Its main impact is chronic abuse, which can cause significant damage to the liver, brain, and other organs. Disulfiram inhibits aldehyde dehydrogenase, which when given with ethyl alcohol results in the accumulation of acetaldehyde, leading to adverse effects.

Antiepileptic Drugs

Seizures are caused by inappropriate and excessive activity of motor neurons in the CNS. Seizure activity is either partial or generalized, depending on the extent of hyperactivity. Partial seizures usually involve one side of the brain

---

Table 8-17

Comparison of Benzodiazepines with Barbiturates

CHARACTERISTIC	BENZODIAZEPINES	BARBITURATES
Dose-response profile	Less steep, reaches a plateau at higher doses	Steep, no plateau
Therapeutic index	High	Low
Inducer of liver enzymes	Weak	Strong
Respiratory depression	Lower potential	High potential
Shortens REM sleep resulting in REM rebound	Somewhat	To a significant degree
Potential for abuse	Significant	Higher

Table 8-18

Antiepileptic Mechanisms of Drugs

DRUG	BLOCKS SODIUM CHANNELS	BLOCKS T-TYPE CALCIUM CHANNELS	BINDS TO THE CHLORIDE CHANNEL AND INCREASES ITS CONDUCTANCE	INCREASES GABA
Phenytoin	Yes	—	—	—
Phenobarbital	—	—	Yes	—
Primidone	—	—	Yes	—
Carbamazepine	Yes	—	—	—
Gabapentin*	—	—	—	Yes†
Pregabalin*	—	—	—	Yes†
Tiagabine	—	—	—	Yes‡
Topiramate	Yes	—	Yes	—
Lamotrigine	Yes	—	—	—
Vigabatrin	—	—	—	Yes
Valproic acid	Yes	Yes	—	—
Ethosuximide	—	Yes	—	—
Clonazepam	—	—	Yes	—
Diazepam	—	—	Yes	—
Zonisamide	Yes	Yes	—	—

GABA, γ-aminobutyric acid.

—, No major or known effect.

*Binds to the $\alpha_2\delta$-1 protein subunit of high voltage–activated calcium channels.

†May increase synthesis and release of GABA owing to effect on high voltage–activated calcium channels.

‡Inhibits GABA reuptake.

at the onset, whereas generalized seizures involve both sides at the onset. Although seizure disorders exist in several forms, it is convenient to divide them into partial and generalized, with two subdivisions of the latter, for purposes of determining drug therapy.

A. Types of seizures (brief summary).
   1. Partial seizures.
   2. Generalized seizures.
      a. Tonic-clonic (grand mal).
      b. Absence (petit mal).
B. Mechanisms of action of antiepileptic drugs (Table 8-18)—antiepileptic drugs act through one or more mechanisms.
   1. Inhibition of sodium channels.
   2. Inhibition of T-type calcium channels.
   3. Binding to $\alpha_2\delta$-1 subunits of high voltage–activated calcium channels, which reduces activity of these channels.
   4. Increasing conductance at chloride channels.
   5. Inhibition of AMPA or *N*-methyl-D-aspartate (NMDA) glutamate receptors—as a result of these mechanisms, the seizure focus (foci) or spread of excitation or both are reduced.
C. Phenytoin.
   1. Nonseizure indications—occasionally for trigeminal neuralgia.

2. Pharmacokinetics.
   a. Slow absorption with oral use.
   b. Antacids may decrease absorption.
   c. Highly bound to plasma protein.
   d. Often eliminated by zero-order kinetics.
   e. Metabolized in liver—this can be a basis for drug-drug interactions.
3. Adverse effects.
   a. Gingival hyperplasia, caused by an increase in fibroblast growth and an increase in connective tissue. A similar effect can occur in the face.
   b. CNS—nystagmus, ataxia, vertigo, diplopia.
   c. Hyperglycemia.
   d. Lymphadenopathy.
   e. Osteomalacia secondary to effects on vitamin D and on calcium absorption.
   f. Hirsutism.
   g. Deficiency of folate and megaloblastic anemia.
   h. Congenital defects secondary to in utero effects.
D. Carbamazepine.
   1. Nonseizure indications.
      a. Trigeminal neuralgia.
      b. Manic-depressive illness.
   2. Pharmacokinetics.
      a. Metabolized in the liver.
      b. Inducer of liver enzymes.

3. Adverse effects.
    a. GI upset.
    b. Dizziness, diplopia, blurred vision.
    c. Visual disturbances.
    d. Peripheral neuritis.
    e. Rashes.
    f. Aplastic anemia (rare).
    g. Agranulocytosis (rare).
    h. Jaundice secondary to liver effects.
E. Phenobarbital.
  1. Adverse effects.
    a. Induces liver enzymes (can be an adverse effect).
    b. Sedation.
    c. Neurologic and behavioral effects.
    d. Hepatic toxicity.
    e. Hypersensitivity leading to hematologic side effects.
    f. Osteomalacia.
    g. Respiratory depression.
F. Primidone.
  Acute systemic and CNS toxicity tend to limit use of primidone. Common side effects include sedation, vertigo, nausea, vomiting, ataxia, diplopia, nystagmus, and hepatic and hematologic toxicity.
G. Gabapentin.
  1. Nonseizure indication—neuropathic pain.
  2. Adverse effects.
    a. Sedation.
    b. Ataxia.
H. Valproic acid.
  1. Nonseizure indication—manic depressive illness.
  2. Adverse effects.
    a. Hair loss.
    b. GI upset.
    c. Hyperglycemia.
    d. Hyperuricemia.
    e. Weight gain.
    f. Hepatic toxicity (especially in patients <2 years old and patients receiving other medications).
    g. Thrombocytopenia.
    h. Teratogenic—may cause spina bifida.
I. Ethosuximide.
  1. Adverse effects.
    a. GI irritation.
    b. CNS depression.
    c. Hematologic side effects (uncommon).
    d. Lupus (rare).
J. Rufinamide blocks sodium channels.
K. Seizure indications are shown in Table 8-19.

Anti-Parkinson Drugs

Parkinson's disease involves degeneration of dopaminergic neurons in the nigrostriatal pathway in the basal ganglia. The cause is usually unknown. Sometimes it is associated with hypoxia, toxic chemicals, or cerebral infections.

Table 8-19

Some Indications of Antiepileptic Drugs

DRUG	TONIC-CLONIC	PARTIAL (FOCAL)*	ABSENCE
Phenytoin†	3	3	−1
Phenobarbital	2	2	0
Primidone	1	1	0
Carbamazepine†	3	3	−1
Valproic acid	3	1	3
Ethosuximide	0	0	3
Clonazepam	0	0	2
Lamotrigine	1	2	2
Gabapentin†	1	2	0
Pregabalin†	?	2	?
Tiagabine	1	2	0
Topiramate	2	2	0
Rufinamide	?	3	?

Higher numbers indicate greater effectiveness or desirability. Negative numbers indicate worsening of the condition by the drug. Zero indicates a lack of effect.
*Simple and complex.
†Useful for certain types of neuropathic pain.

A. Strategies for therapy.
  1. Increase dopaminergic receptor stimulation in basal ganglia.
  2. Block muscarinic receptors in the basal ganglia because cholinergic function opposes the action of dopamine in the basal ganglia.
  3. Block NMDA glutamate receptors.
B. Drugs.
  1. Levodopa plus carbidopa (Sinemet).
  2. Bromocriptine, pergolide, pramipexole, ropinirole, apomorphine.
  3. Benztropine, trihexyphenidyl, biperiden, procyclidine.
  4. Diphenhydramine.
  5. Amantadine.
  6. Tolcapone and entacapone.
  7. Selegiline, rasagiline.
C. Mechanisms of action of three drugs affecting DOPA are shown in Figure 8-9.
  1. Levodopa plus carbidopa—levodopa is able to penetrate the blood-brain barrier and is then converted into dopamine. Carbidopa inhibits dopa decarboxylase, which catalyzes the formation of dopamine. Carbidopa does not penetrate the blood-brain barrier; it prevents the conversion of levodopa to dopamine outside the CNS but allows the conversion of levodopa to dopamine inside the CNS.
  2. Bromocriptine, pergolide, pramipexole, ropinirole, and apomorphine are direct dopamine receptor agonists.

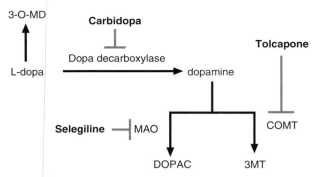

Figure 8-9 Sites of action of carbidopa, MAO inhibitors, and COMT inhibitors. *DOPAC,* Dihydroxyphenylacetic acid; *3-O-MD,* 3-O-methyldopa; *3MT,* 3 methyltyrosine.

3. Benztropine, trihexyphenidyl, biperiden, and procyclidine are antimuscarinic drugs.
4. Diphenhydramine is an antihistamine that has antimuscarinic action.
5. Amantadine releases dopamine and inhibits NMDA receptors.
6. Selegiline is an irreversible inhibitor of MAO-B, which metabolizes dopamine. Selegiline increases the level of dopamine.
7. Tolcapone and entacapone are inhibitors of COMT, another enzyme that metabolizes dopamine.

D. Dopamine and acetylcholine—loss of dopaminergic neurons in parkinsonism leads to unopposed action by cholinergic neurons. Inhibiting muscarinic receptors can help alleviate symptoms of parkinsonism.

E. Adverse effects.
   1. Levodopa.
      a. Therapeutic effects of the drug decrease with time.
      b. Oscillating levels of clinical efficacy of the drug ("on-off" effect).
      c. Mental changes—psychosis.
      d. Tachycardia and orthostatic hypotension.
      e. Nausea.
      f. Abnormal muscle movements (dyskinesias).
   2. Tolcapone, entacapone (similar to levodopa)—hepatotoxicity with tolcapone.
   3. Direct dopamine receptor agonists (similar to levodopa)—apomorphine causes more nausea and vomiting.
   4. Antimuscarinic drugs.
      a. Typical antimuscarinic adverse effects such as dry mouth.
      b. Sedation.
   5. Diphenhydramine (see "antimuscarinic drugs").
   6. Amantadine.
      a. Nausea.
      b. Dizziness.
      c. Edema.
      d. Sweating.

7. Selegiline and rasagiline.
   a. Nausea.
   b. Dry mouth.
   c. Dizziness.
   d. Insomnia and anxiety (mostly selegiline).
   e. Although selegiline and rasagiline are selective for MAO-B, they can still cause excessive toxicity in the presence of tricyclic antidepressants, SSRIs, and meperidine.

F. Indications.
   Parkinson's disease is the obvious major use of the drugs described previously. Parkinson-like symptoms can occur with many antipsychotic drugs. These symptoms are often treated with antimuscarinic drugs or diphenhydramine.

G. Dental implications of anti-Parkinson drugs.
   1. Dyskinesia caused by drugs can present a challenge for dental treatment.
   2. Orthostatic hypotension poses a risk when changing from a reclining to a standing position.
   3. The dentist should schedule appointments at a time of day at which the best control of the disease occurs.
   4. Dry mouth occurs with several of these drugs.

4.0 Anesthetics

Local Anesthetics

The use of local anesthetics dates back at least to the discovery of cocaine, present in the coca plant, followed by the development of benzocaine in the late 19th century. Procaine was developed in 1906, and drugs such as lidocaine were developed later in the 20th century.

A. Drugs.
   1. Esters.
      a. Procaine (Novocain).
      b. Propoxycaine.
      c. Tetracaine (Pontocaine).
      d. Benzocaine (topical only).
      e. Cocaine.
   2. Amides.
      a. Lidocaine (Xylocaine).
      b. Mepivacaine (Carbocaine).
      c. Prilocaine (Citanest).
      d. Bupivacaine (Marcaine).
      e. Etidocaine (Duranest).
      f. Dibucaine.
      g. Articaine (Ultracaine).
      h. Ropivacaine (Naropin).
      i. Levobupivacaine (Chirocaine).
   3. Ketone type—dyclonine (used as a lozenge).
   4. Other chemicals that act like local anesthetics.
      a. H_1 antihistamines such as diphenhydramine.
      b. Saxitoxin.
      c. Tetrodotoxin.

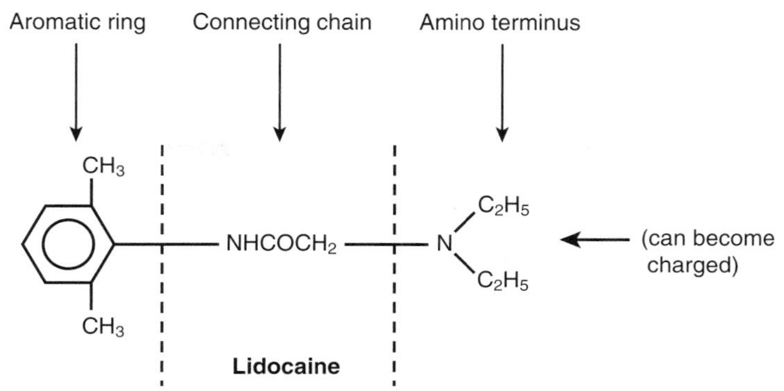

Figure 8-10 Lidocaine.

Table 8-20

Properties of Some Local Anesthetics

DRUG	RELATIVE LIPID SOLUBILITY	RELATIVE ANESTHETIC POTENCY	RELATIVE DURATION OF ANESTHESIA	pK_a	RATE OF ONSET
Procaine	+	+	+	8.9	Slower
Mepivacaine	++	++	++	7.7	Fast
Prilocaine	++	++	++	7.8	Fast
Lidocaine	+++	+++	+++	7.8	Fast
Bupivacaine	++++	++++	++++	8.1	Moderate

Adapted from Yagiela JA, et al: *Pharmacology and Therapeutics for Dentistry,* ed 6. St. Louis, Mosby, 2011.

The greater the number of "+" signs, the greater the relative lipid solubility, potency, and duration of anesthesia.

B. Chemistry.
　　The components of the structure of lidocaine, an example of an amide drug, are shown in Figure 8-10. Note that local anesthetics become more charged as the pH is lowered.
C. Mechanism of action of local anesthetics.
　　1. Block sodium channels in the nerve membrane.
　　2. Prevent depolarization of the nerve.
D. Pharmacokinetics and action of local anesthetics.
　　1. For better solubility, local anesthetics are marketed as the salts of strong acids, such as hydrocloric acid. The pH of the solution in the cartridge is acidic.
　　2. Injection of the drug places the drug in a solution of higher pH because of the buffers in the body. A higher percentage of the drug becomes noncharged and can more readily penetrate through lipid barriers and into nerves. The higher the lipid solubility, the more potent and long-lasting the drug. The lower the pK_a, the faster the onset of action of the drug. At low pH in tissues, anesthesia becomes more difficult to attain because of the presence of a higher percentage of the charged form of the drug (Table 8-20).
E. Vasoconstrictors are used with local anesthetics.
　　1. To increase depth and duration of anesthesia.
　　2. To reduce systemic absorption of local anesthetics.
F. Cardiovascular effects and receptor preferences of two common vasoconstrictors used in dentistry are shown in Table 8-21.

Table 8-21

Some Systemic Effects of Vasoconstrictors

DRUG	ADRENERGIC RECEPTOR PREFERENCE	EFFECT
Epinephrine	$\alpha_1, \alpha_2, \beta_1, \beta_2$	↑ heart rate ↑ blood pressure
Levonordefrin	α_1, α_2	↑ blood pressure

G. *Metabolism*—metabolism of esters occurs primarily in the plasma, whereas amides such as lidocaine are metabolized in the liver by three types of reactions.
　　1. Dealkylation of the amino terminus.
　　2. Hydrolysis of the amide bond.
　　3. Hydroxylation of the aromatic ring.
　　4. The most abundant urinary metabolite of lidocaine is 4-hydroxyxylidine. Metabolism of lidocaine is rapid (terminal half-life ≅ 2 hours).
H. Nerve sensitivity to local anesthetics—nerves that conduct pain sensation (C and Aδ) are smaller and conduct slowly compared with most other nerves. Smaller diameter nerves are more sensitive to local anesthetics (Box 8-2).
I. Effects of local anesthetics at sites other than peripheral nerves leading to adverse effects.

Box 8-2

*Relative Sensitivity of Nerve Fibers
to Local Anesthetics*

(Arranged in decreasing order of sensitivity)
Pain → Temperature → Touch → Pressure → Motor

1. CNS effects.
   a. Lightheadedness.
   b. Dizziness.
   c. Muscle twitching.
   d. Convulsions.
   e. Respiratory arrest.
2. Cardiac effects—some cardiac depression but also specific antiarrhythmic effects.
J. Characteristics of local anesthetics unique to specific drugs or drug classes.
   1. Benzocaine does not have an amino terminus and does not become charged. It is poorly soluble in water, even at low pH.
   2. Esters are metabolized primarily in the plasma; amides are metabolized in the liver.
   3. Esters are more allergenic than amides.
   4. Cocaine is an ester whose metabolism is more complex than other esters.
   5. Cocaine also has sympathetic effects because it inhibits the reuptake of E and NE.
   6. Cocaine also has addictive properties and a euphoric effect most likely secondary to its blockade of reuptake of dopamine in the brain.
   7. All local anesthetics except cocaine are vasodilators at the concentrations used for local anesthesia. However, mepivacaine has less of a vasodilator effect compared with the others and is the drug usually chosen when a vasoconstrictor is not used with the local anesthetic.
   8. Esters show greater apparent toxicity in patients with a hereditary deficiency in plasma esterases.
   9. Prilocaine forms *o*-toluidine on metabolism; this may cause methemoglobinemia.
   10. Allergies are more likely with esters, and they display cross-allergenicity. Amides are much less likely to cause allergies, and cross-allergenicity is apparently less common with the amides. Methylparaben, which was used as a preservative, can also cause allergies. Sulfites, also used as preservatives, can cause intolerance and perhaps should be avoided in steroid-dependent asthmatics.
   11. Bupivacaine is more selective for sensory nerves compared with etidocaine, another long-acting drug.
   12. EMLA is a "eutectic mixture of local anesthetics" such as lidocaine 2.5% plus prilocaine 2.5%. When formulated together, there is an increased solubility of both drugs. Greater penetration is attained by mixing the two drugs, and this is useful for oral topical anesthesia.
   13. Articaine is an amide, but it also has a side chain that is an ester that is required for most of its anesthetic effect. Rapid metabolism of this ester bond gives it a short half-life.
   14. Pregnancy categories—lidocaine, prilocaine (B); mepivacaine, bupivacaine, articaine (C).
K. Drug-drug interactions.
   1. Procaine, which is metabolized to *para*-aminobenzoic acid, may inhibit the antimicrobial effect of sulfonamides.
   2. The systemic effects of esters are increased in the presence of plasma esterase inhibitors.
   3. β-Adrenergic receptor blockers increase the effect of amides owing to lower hepatic blood flow resulting from β blockers.
   4. Basic drugs may compete with lidocaine and other amides at plasma α_1-acid glycoprotein binding sites.
   5. Enzyme inducers decrease the plasma half-life of lidocaine and other amides.
   6. Opioids can increase the systemic toxicity of local anesthetics.
   7. Cimetidine increases plasma levels of lidocaine (reduced metabolism secondary to cimetidine).
   8. Local anesthetics may antagonize the beneficial effect of acetylcholinesterase inhibitors in patients with myasthenia gravis.
L. Calculation of amounts of anesthetic and vasoconstrictor used in one anesthetic cartridge, assuming lidocaine 2% with epinephrine 1 : 100,000 and a cartridge volume of 1.8 mL.
   1. Calculation of the amount of anesthetic used in one cartridge (1.8 mL):

$$\text{Lidocaine } 2\% = 2 \text{ g}/100 \text{ mL}$$

$$\text{Lidocaine } 2\% = 0.02 \text{ g}/\text{mL}$$

$$\text{Lidocaine } 2\% = 0.036 \text{ g}/1.8 \text{ mL}$$

$$\text{Lidocaine } 2\% = 36 \text{ mg}/1.8 \text{ mL}$$

   2. Calculation of the amount of vasoconstrictor used in one cartridge (1.8 mL):

$$\text{Epinephrine } 1 : 100,000$$

$$1 : 1 = 1 \text{ g}/\text{mL}$$

$$1 : 1000 = 1 \text{ mg}/\text{mL}$$

$$1 : 100,000 = 0.01 \text{ mg}/\text{mL}$$

$$1 : 100,000 = 0.018 \text{ mg}/1.8 \text{ mL}$$

$$1 : 100,000 = 18 \text{ μg}/1.8 \text{ mL}$$

General Anesthetics

General anesthetics reduce pain and consciousness. They were developed in the 19th century when nitrous oxide

(N$_2$O) and diethyl ether were developed. Halothane, a prototypical halogenated inhalation anesthetic, was developed in the 1950s, followed by others in that class. Injectable anesthetics have been used for some time, with some important more recent additions to this type of anesthetic.

A. Drugs.
  1. Inhaled anesthetics.
     a. N$_2$O.
     b. Halogen-containing anesthetics.
        (1) Halothane.
        (2) Enflurane.
        (3) Isoflurane.
        (4) Sevoflurane.
        (5) Desflurane.
  2. Injectable anesthetics.
     a. Propofol.
     b. Thiopental.
     c. Ketamine.
     d. Etomidate.
B. Mechanism of action of general anesthetics.
  1. The traditional explanation has been based on the Meyer-Overton hypothesis (i.e., anesthesia occurs when a chemical reaches a certain concentration in the nerve membrane, disrupting its function).
  2. It has been shown more recently that general anesthetics act by various mechanisms. They likely modulate ion channels, such as stimulation of GABA receptors and inhibition of nicotinic cholinergic and NMDA glutamate receptors.
  3. Sites within the CNS most sensitive to the effect of general anesthetics.
     a. Dorsal lamina of spinal cord.
     b. Reticular activating system.
     c. Relay circuits between the thalamus and cortex.
     d. Hippocampus.
C. Stages of general anesthesia based on depth of anesthesia.

1. Stage 1: *analgesia*—amnesia is common. N$_2$O falls in this category when it is used for conscious sedation.
2. Stage 2: *delirium*—excitement phase. This stage begins with unconsciousness.
3. Stage 3: *surgical anesthesia*—progressive loss of reflexes and muscle control.
4. Stage 4: *respiratory paralysis.*

D. Terms applied to the properties of general anesthesia.
  1. *Blood:gas solubility coefficient*—the lower the blood:gas solubility coefficient, the faster the onset and termination of anesthesia. The effect of the blood:gas solubility coefficient on onset of anesthesia is illustrated in Figure 8-11, showing how N$_2$O (which has a very low blood:gas solubility coefficient) approaches plasma steady-state levels fastest.
  2. *Minimum alveolar concentration (MAC)*—the minimum concentration of anesthetic in the alveolus that is sufficient to give no response from a surgical stimulus in 50% of patients.
E. N$_2$O.
  1. Characteristics.
     a. Mechanism includes inhibition of nicotinic cholinergic and NMDA receptors.
     b. Used in conscious sedation (stage 1 anesthesia).
     c. 20% N$_2$O–80% O$_2$ to start. Concentrations of N$_2$O are often increased from there.
     d. Compressed in cylinders at 750 psi (in a liquid state).
     e. Nonflammable and nonexplosive but support combustion.
     f. Inert gas (no chemical changes or combinations in the body are known to occur).
     g. Rapid onset and termination, colorless, tasteless.
     h. Nonirritating, pleasant.
     i. 1.5 times heavier than air.
     j. Blood:gas solubility coefficient = 0.47; induction is fast.

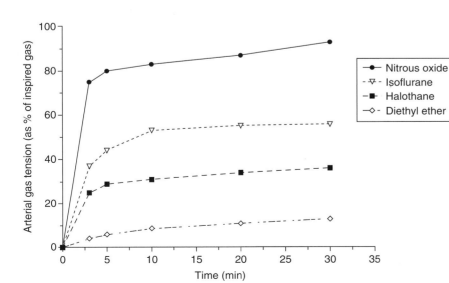

Figure 8-11 Effect of anesthetics on arterial gas tension.

k. Not a respiratory depressant (a weak anesthetic).
l. Minimal depressant effects on myocardial contractibility and cardiovascular system.
m. Low incidence of nausea.
n. No skeletal muscle relaxant properties.
o. Inhibits vitamin B_{12}–dependent methionine synthase by oxidizing the cobalt in cyanocobalamin.
p. Prolonged exposure (e.g., >24 hours) causes bone marrow suppression.
q. Can cause diffusion hypoxia at end of administration if N_2O is not washed out with oxygen.
r. Diffuses into closed air spaces in the body; this is especially noticeable in the bowel.
s. Very useful anesthetic agent because of its analgesic properties.

2. Adverse effects.
a. Decreased mental performance.
b. Decreased audiovisual ability.
c. Decreased manual dexterity.
d. Adverse reproductive effects—reduced fertility with longer and higher exposure.
e. Reports of spontaneous abortion with higher exposure.
f. Reports of neurologic and kidney disease with higher exposure.
g. Bone marrow suppression with longer exposure secondary to vitamin B_{12} effect.

3. Some contraindications to the use of N_2O.
a. Head injury.
b. Chest trauma (pneumothorax).
c. Bowel obstruction, undiagnosed abdominal pain, or marked abdominal distention.
d. Vitreoretinal surgery with intraocular gas (avoid N_2O for at least 3 months).
e. Hypotension—shock.
f. Inability of patient to communicate or follow commands.
g. Chronic obstructive pulmonary disease.

4. Some recommendations to reduce risk of exposure to N_2O.
a. Monitor airborne N_2O (badge) and do leak testing.
b. Maintenance and work practices to reduce exposure.
c. Worker education.
d. Protective gear.
e. Scavenging system.

F. Halogen-containing anesthetics that are inhaled.
1. Characteristics.
a. Mechanism includes ion channel modulation.
b. Widely used clinically.
c. Many advantages over earlier drugs such as diethyl ether (nonexplosive, well tolerated, lower blood:gas solubility coefficient).
d. Dose-dependent decreases in cardiac output and blood pressure.
e. Not analgesic.

Table 8-22

Properties of Anesthetics

ANESTHETIC AGENT	MAC (%)	PARTITION COEFFICIENT AT 37° C BLOOD:GAS
Halothane	0.75	2.3
Isoflurane	1.2	1.4
Enflurane	1.6	1.8
Sevoflurane	2.0	0.65
Desflurane	6.0	0.45
Nitrous oxide	105.0	0.47

Modified from Yagiela JA, et al: *Pharmacology and Therapeutics for Dentistry,* ed 6. St. Louis, Mosby, 2011.

MAC, Minimum alveolar concentration.

2. Table 8-22 compares MAC values and blood:gas solubility coefficients for halogens and N_2O. Notice the range of partition coefficients and MAC values.
3. Unique qualities of certain halogenated anesthetics.
a. Halothane.
(1) Poses a risk with epinephrine.
(2) Associated with hepatitis.
(3) Poor skeletal muscle relaxation.
b. Enflurane.
(1) Good skeletal muscle relaxation.
(2) Less risk with epinephrine.
(3) Not associated with hepatitis.
c. Isoflurane, desflurane, sevoflurane.
(1) Fast-acting.
(2) Similar to enflurane.

G. Injectable anesthetics.
1. Propofol.
a. Agonist at $GABA_A$ receptors.
b. Given intravenously.
c. Rapid onset and termination.
d. Vasodilator.
2. Thiopental.
a. Barbiturate.
b. Fast-acting.
3. Ketamine.
a. Blocks NMDA glutamate receptors.
b. May cause hallucinations on emergence (given with diazepam to avoid this).
c. Increases blood pressure.
4. Midazolam, a benzodiazepine.
5. Neuroleptanesthesia (droperidol plus fentanyl plus nitrous oxide).

H. Antihistamines used for conscious sedation.
1. Promethazine.
2. Hydroxyzine.

I. *Balanced anesthesia*—this term refers to the use of several drugs from the following list to obtain the desired anesthetic effect.

1. Inhaled drugs (N_2O plus a halogen-containing anesthetic).
2. Peripheral skeletal muscle relaxant.
3. Sedative such as a benzodiazepine.
4. Opioid.
5. Others such as scopolamine.

5.0 Analgesics and Antihistamines

Opioids

Opioids are also called narcotic analgesics. However, morphine is also used for pulmonary edema, codeine is also used for cough, and loperamide and diphenoxylate are used exclusively for diarrhea. Opium, from the opium poppy, yields morphine, codeine, and other alkaloids. Newer members of the opioid group of drugs include semisynthetic opium derivatives and synthetic drugs. They act as agonists at one or more of the opioid receptors. A separate group of synthetic drugs has mixed opioid action (i.e., they may antagonize one opioid receptor and stimulate another). In addition, there are endogenous peptides that have opioid-type actions. Naloxone and naltrexone are antagonists at opioid receptors.

A. Mechanism of action of opioids.
   1. Opioids are agonists at opioid receptors, which are in the plasma membranes of neurons, located both presynaptically and postsynaptically.
   2. Stimulation of opioid receptors leads to activation of the G protein, G_i, resulting in a decrease in calcium conductance, which accounts for a decrease in the presynaptic release of neurotransmitters. G_i activation by opioids also increases potassium conductance resulting in an increase in the postsynaptic potential and reduced neuronal conduction.
B. Opioid receptors.
   1. Mu (μ)
   2. Delta (δ)
   3. Kappa (κ)
   4. Each receptor mediates analgesia; however, the μ receptor is also largely responsible for mediating euphoria, reduced GI motility, physical dependence, and respiratory depression. Note the different combinations for drugs and receptors. Morphine and fentanyl are similar in receptor preference to the natural, semisynthetic, and most synthetic opioids.
   5. Opioid receptor preferences of some drugs (Table 8-23).
C. Sites of analgesic action of opioid analgesics.
   1. Descending pathway in the CNS (modulation of pain sensation) including the spinal cord.
   2. Ascending pathway in the CNS (includes pain processing and appreciation, or motivational-affective component of pain).
   3. Peripheral nerve endings.

Table 8-23

Receptor Targets of Opioid Agonists and Antagonists

COMPOUND	MU (μ)	DELTA (δ)	KAPPA (κ)
Morphine	++		+
Fentanyl	+++		
Pentazocine	P		++
Buprenorphine	P		–
Met-enkephalin	++	+++	
β-Endorphin	+++	+++	
Naloxone	–	–	–
Naltrexone	–	–	–

Data from Brunton LL, Chabner BA, Knollman BJ: *Goodman & Gilman's Pharmacological Basis of Therapeutics,* ed 12. New York, McGraw-Hill, 2011.

+, Agonist; –, antagonist; P, partial agonist.

The number of "+" signs indicates relative potency.

D. Effects of morphine and other opioids.
   1. CNS—analgesia, drowsiness, respiratory depression, euphoria, physical dependence, miosis. Head injury is a contraindication.
   2. GI—decreased peristalsis.
   3. Others—histamine release, orthostatic hypotension.
E. Signs and symptoms of acute overdose of morphine and many other opioids.
   1. Coma.
   2. Pinpoint pupil.
   3. Respiratory depression.
F. Pharmacokinetics of morphine.
   1. Significant liver metabolism after oral doses.
   2. The metabolite, morphine-6-glucuronide, is an active metabolite.
   3. $t_{1/2} \sim 3$ hours.
G. Other opioids.
   1. Codeine.
      a. Well-absorbed orally.
      b. $t_{1/2} \sim 3$ hours.
      c. Less potent than morphine.
      d. Converted to morphine by cytochrome P-450 2D6. Patient responses to codeine are variable.
   2. Hydrocodone—similar to codeine.
   3. Dihydrocodeine—similar to codeine.
   4. Meperidine.
      a. Can be used orally.
      b. More potent than codeine but less potent than morphine.
      c. A metabolite, normeperidine, is a CNS stimulant.
      d. Not recommended for long-term pain relief.
      e. Contraindicated with MAO inhibitors.
      f. $t_{1/2} \sim 3$ hours.

5. Methadone.
   a. Used orally.
   b. Used in maintenance for treating opioid addiction as well as for pain.
   c. $t_{1/2}$ ~ 15 to 40 hours.
6. Oxycodone.
   a. Orally useful.
   b. $t_{1/2}$ ~ 3 hours.
   c. More potent than codeine.
   d. OxyContin is controlled-release oxycodone.
7. Heroin.
   a. Diacetylmorphine.
   b. Drug of abuse.
8. Fentanyl—more potent than morphine.
9. Fentanyl congeners (e.g., sufentanil, alfentanil, remifentanil).
10. Propoxyphene has been withdrawn from the market because of high risk/benefit ratio. Risks include cardiac toxicity.
11. Pentazocine.
    a. Mixed-action agonist.
    b. Increases blood pressure.
    c. Orally useful.
    d. Given with naloxone (Talwin NX) to prevent injecting pentazocine.
12. Buprenorphine (see Table 8-23).
13. Opioid antagonists.
    a. Naloxone—short $t_{1/2}$.
    b. Naltrexone—longer $t_{1/2}$.
    c. Alvimopan and methylnaltrexone—do not enter CNS; used in special cases to treat constipation secondary to opioids.
14. Tramadol.
    a. Weak μ receptor agonist.
    b. Also blocks reuptake of norepinephrine and serotonin—leads to analgesia.
15. Diphenoxylate.
    a. Antidiarrheal drug.
    b. Acts directly on opioid receptors in GI tract.
16. Loperamide.
    a. Antidiarrheal drug.
    b. Does not cross blood-brain barrier.
17. Dextromethorphan.
    a. Weak NMDA receptor antagonist.
    b. Used as a cough suppressant but does not act through opioid receptors.
    c. Also has weak analgesic properties.

Nonsteroidal Antiinflammatory Drugs—Nonnarcotic Analgesics

NSAIDs are used to treat pain, fever, inflammation, and some other conditions. NSAIDs are, by definition, antiinflammatory and are analgesics; acetaminophen is an analgesic but has very little antiinflammatory effect and is not an NSAID. Certain NSAIDs (as well as acetaminophen) are also commonly used with opioid analgesics for the treatment of pain. *GI and kidney toxicity are typical adverse effects of NSAIDs, particularly in elderly patients.*

A. Drugs.
   1. NSAIDs.
      a. Aspirin and other salicylates.
      b. Ibuprofen and similar drugs.
      c. Piroxicam.
      d. Other NSAIDs, such as ketorolac, sulindac, and etodolac.
      e. COX-2 inhibitors.
      f. Nabumetone.
      g. Indomethacin.
   2. Acetaminophen.
B. Mechanism of action.
   1. NSAIDs inhibit COX, inhibiting production of prostaglandins and other prostanoids (Figure 8-12).
   2. Most NSAIDs inhibit both forms of COX (COX-1 and COX-2). COX-2 is usually the therapeutic target. NSAIDs have several adverse effects resulting largely from inhibition of COX-1 (Figure 8-13).

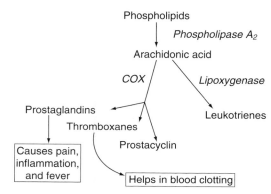

Figure 8-12 Pathway affected by COX and lipoxygenase enzymes.

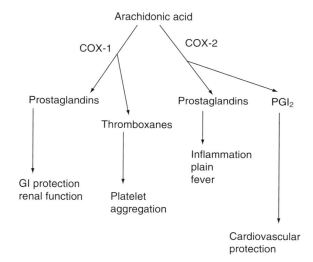

Figure 8-13 Pathways from arachidonic acid.

3. COX-2-selective drugs affect mainly the "right arm" in Figure 8-13 and are generally less irritating to the GI tract.
4. Acetaminophen—the mechanism is still obscure, but it appears to inhibit COX-1 and COX-2 in the CNS and may activate the CB1 cannabinoid receptor as well as the TRPV1 cation channel (vanilloid or capsaicin) receptor.

C. Salicylates.
1. Aspirin is most often used.
2. Indications for aspirin use.
   a. Pain.
   b. Fever.
   c. Inflammation.
   d. Antiplatelet effect.
3. Mechanism of action—irreversible inhibition of COX accomplished by acetylation of the enzyme. This irreversible inhibition is unique to aspirin, even among other salicylates.
   a. Inhibits both COX-1 and COX-2.
   b. Doses vary depending on desired effect (e.g., pain versus inflammation).
   c. The antiplatelet effect lasts beyond the presence of aspirin in the body.
4. Aspirin metabolism—salicylate levels can increase significantly with aspirin overdose. Note the slower rate of metabolism from salicylate to inactive metabolites (Figure 8-14).
5. Acute aspirin toxicity.
   a. Acid-base problems (with increasing doses).
      (1) Initially increases respiration, leading to respiratory alkalosis.
      (2) Medullary suppression can follow, leading to respiratory acidosis.
      (3) Eventually can cause metabolic acidosis.
   b. Carbohydrate metabolism causes release of epinephrine and glucocorticoids (leads to hyperglycemia and depletion of glycogen).
   c. Fever, dehydration, hypokalemia.
6. Chronic aspirin toxicity.
   a. Salicylism.
   b. CNS effects.
   c. Bleeding.
   d. GI disturbances.
   e. Kidney toxicity.

7. Aspirin—contraindications.
   a. Disorders involving excessive bleeding, recent surgery, use of anticoagulants.
   b. Ulcers.
   c. Use of a drug that interacts with aspirin.
   d. Recent viral infection in children and teens (Reye's syndrome may result).
   e. Asthma.
8. Other—NSAIDs that are nonselective COX inhibitors.
   a. Propionic acid derivatives.
      (1) Ibuprofen.
      (2) Naproxen ($t_{1/2} \cong 14$ hours).
      (3) Ketoprofen.
      (4) Oxaprozin ($t_{1/2} \cong 50$ hours).
      (5) These drugs have half-lives of 2 to 4 hours except as noted.
   b. Others (less use in dentistry).
      (1) Etodolac.
      (2) Sulindac.
      (3) Ketorolac (oral use is indicated only as continuation of intravenous or intramuscular administration of ketorolac).
      (4) Piroxicam ($t_{1/2} \cong 50$ hours).
      (5) Nabumetone (more effect on COX-2 than COX-1).
9. Selective COX-2 inhibitor.
   a. Rationale for its use—antiinflammatory effect without as much GI toxicity as occurs with traditional NSAIDs.
   b. Celecoxib (Celebrex).
   c. This drug is associated with added cardiovascular risks in some patients.

D. Acetaminophen and its effects (not an NSAID).
1. Analgesic.
2. Low effect on peripheral COX.
3. Few drug-drug interactions.
4. Not antiinflammatory.
5. Analgesic ceiling is comparable to most NSAIDs.
6. Liver toxicity with higher doses.
7. Acetaminophen metabolism (Figure 8-15).
8. *Acute acetaminophen toxicity*—hepatic necrosis results from toxic metabolites that are produced when, at higher doses, the nontoxic metabolic pathways are saturated (see Figure 8-15). The toxic metabolites deplete glutathione in the liver.

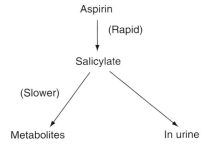

Figure 8-14 Aspirin metabolism.

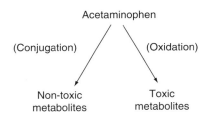

Figure 8-15 Metabolic pathways of acetaminophen.

9. The antidote for liver toxicity secondary to acetaminophen is *N*-acetylcysteine.
10. Acetaminophen is preferred over aspirin when an analgesic or antipyretic drug is indicated and when a condition such as one or more of the following is present.
    a. Patient is asthmatic.
    b. Patient is at added risk of an ulcer.
    c. Patient is experiencing bleeding.
    d. Patient is taking anticoagulants.
    e. Patient is sensitive or allergic to aspirin.
    f. Patient is taking drugs such as probenecid or methotrexate.
    g. Acetaminophen would also be preferable to NSAIDs other than aspirin in most of the above-listed cases as long as an antiinflammatory effect is not the goal.
11. Aspirin, acetaminophen, and ibuprofen (commonly used) are often combined with an opioid such as codeine, hydrocodone, oxycodone, or pentazocine for analgesic use.
12. Other drugs.
    a. Ziconotide inhibits N-type calcium channels and is used intrathecally for severe pain.
    b. Misoprostol, a prostaglandin E_1 analogue, is used to prevent peptic ulcers resulting from NSAIDs (see Figure 8-23).

Drugs for Migraine

Three antimigraine drug classes indicate the importance of serotonin and its receptors in migraine and its alleviation. Vasodilation and inflammation are important functional components of migraine. The dura vessels in the brain and their nerves as well as pain pathways in the brainstem are important targets for these drugs. There are three classes of antimigraine drugs.
A. Triptans.
    1. Example—sumatriptan.
    2. Are agonists at serotonin $5\text{-HT}_{1B/1D}$ receptors.
    3. Used for abortive treatment of migraine.
B. Ergot alkaloids.
    1. Ergotamine and dihydroergotamine.
    2. Act similarly to triptans.
    3. Have considerable vascular toxicity, especially ergotamine.
    4. Used for abortive treatment of migraine.
C. Other drugs used for abortive treatment of migraine.
    1. NSAIDs.
    2. Tramadol.
    3. Isometheptene, a vasoconstrictor.
D. Methysergide.
    1. Blocks 5-HT_2 receptors.
    2. Used for prophylaxis against migraine.
E. Other drugs used for prophylaxis against migraine—β blockers, valproic acid, topiramate, tricyclic antidepressants, calcium channel blockers, ACE inhibitors, angiotensin II receptor blockers.

Antihistamines

Antihistamines are drugs that block histamine receptors. Clinically relevant drugs block either H_1 or histamine-2 (H_2) receptors. Traditionally, the term *antihistamine* is limited to H_1 blockers.
A. Histamine.
    1. Receptors and effects (Table 8-24).
    2. Classification of histamine receptor blockers (Figure 8-16).
    3. H_1 antihistamine drugs.
        a. H_1 receptor blockers (antihistamines) (first-generation).

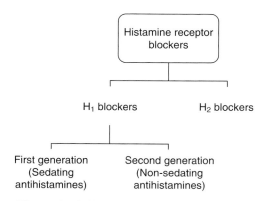

Figure 8-16 Histamine receptor blockers.

Table 8-24			
Histamine Receptor Mechanisms and Effects			
RECEPTOR	**SIGNALING PATHWAY**	**LOCATION**	**EFFECT OF HISTAMINES**
H_1	Inositol 1,4,5-triphosphate and diacylglycerol, leading to ↑ in cell calcium	Bronchi, blood vessels, mucous glands, nerves	Bronchoconstriction, vasodilation, secretion, pain, itch
H_2	Stimulation of adenylyl cyclase leading to ↑ in cAMP	Stomach parietal cells, blood vessels, heart	Acid secretion, vasodilation, increase in force and rate of heart

cAMP, Cyclic adenosine monophosphate.

(1) Diphenhydramine.
(2) Dimenhydrinate (salt of diphenhydramine) (Dramamine).
(3) Pyrilamine.
(4) Hydroxyzine.
(5) Chlorpheniramine.
(6) Promethazine.
b. H$_1$ receptor blockers (nonsedating antihistamines) (second-generation).
(1) Fexofenadine (Allegra).
(2) Loratadine (Claritin).
(3) Desloratadine (Clarinex).
(4) Cetirizine (Zyrtec).
(5) Acrivastine (in Semprex-D).
4. Comparison of first-generation and second-generation histamine receptor blockers.
a. Second-generation drugs do not cross the blood-brain barrier.
b. Second-generation drugs do not cause the drowsiness that occurs with first-generation drugs.
c. Second-generation drugs do not have the antimuscarinic activity that first-generation drugs do.
d. Duration of action—3 to 6 hours for most first-generation drugs; 12 to 24 hours for second-generation drugs.
5. Actions of H$_1$ antihistamines.
a. Block pain and itch from histamine.
b. Block vasodilation from histamine.
c. Block bronchoconstriction from histamine.
d. Useful in mild allergies and colds.
e. Local anesthetic effect (first-generation drugs only).
f. Reduce motion sickness (first-generation drugs only).
g. Promote sleep (first-generation drugs only).
6. Characteristics of H$_1$ nonsedating antihistamines (second-generation drugs).
a. Long half-lives (12 to 24 hours).
b. Do not readily cross blood-brain barrier.
c. Little or no sedation.
d. Higher risk of cardiac arrhythmias (long QT syndrome).
7. H$_2$ receptor blockers.
a. Cimetidine.
b. Ranitidine.
c. Famotidine.
d. Nizatidine.
8. H$_2$ histamine receptor blockers inhibit the action of histamine on the parietal cells of the stomach.
9. Indications for H$_2$ receptor blockers.
a. Dyspepsia.
b. Peptic ulcer.
c. Duodenal ulcer.
d. Gastroesophageal reflux disease (GERD).

10. Adverse effects of H$_2$ receptor blockers.
a. Cimetidine (but not other H$_2$ blockers) has an antiandrogen effect—can lead to impotence, loss of libido, and gynecomastia.
b. Inhibition of liver metabolism occurs with cimetidine and, to a lesser degree, with ranitidine. This inhibition of liver metabolism can lead to an increase in activity of other drugs such as warfarin and carbamazepine.

6.0 Cardiovascular Pharmacology and Diuretics

Antiarrhythmic Drugs

A. Arrhythmias of the heart.
1. Impulse generation.
2. Impulse conduction.
B. Anatomic sites (Figure 8-17).
1. Sinoatrial (SA) node.
2. Atrial myocardium.
3. Atrioventricular (AV) node.
4. His-Purkinje system.
5. Ventricular myocardium.
C. Antiarrhythmic actions—antiarrhythmic drugs do one or more of the following; the electrocardiogram (ECG) changes reflect these effects of drugs.
1. *Reduce automaticity of SA node*—reduce automaticity at phase 4 of the action potential, reducing impulse generation; reduce heart rate and increase the P–P interval on the ECG, reducing abnormal rapid rhythms in the atria.
2. *Reduce conduction velocity in the atria and ventricle*—reduce arrhythmias owing to rapid conduction; effect on the ventricle is widening of QRS complex.
3. *Reduce AV nodal conduction rate*—slow rate of impulses from the atria into the ventricles, resulting in an increase in P–R interval.
4. *Increase refractory period*—in the ventricle this leads to an increase in the Q–T interval.
5. *Reduce His-Purkinje automaticity*—reduce the generation of abnormally rapid and ectopic ventricular arrhythmias.
D. Antiarrhythmic drug classes and how they act.
1. Class I.
a. Block sodium channels.
b. Three divisions (IA, IB, IC) based on how they block sodium channels.
2. Class II—block β-adrenergic receptors.
3. Class III—block potassium channels.
4. Class IV—block calcium channels.
5. Miscellaneous—adenosine stimulates adenosine receptors in the heart; this leads to increased potassium conductance and decreased calcium conductance.
E. Drugs and their principal actions (actions refer to "antiarrhythmic actions" described earlier).

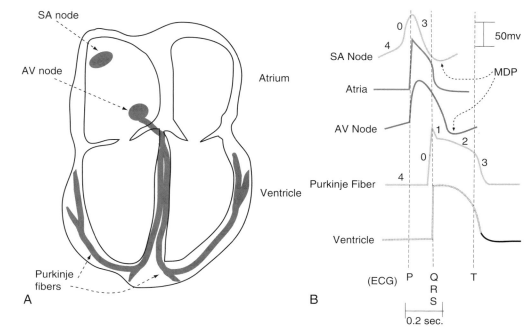

Figure 8-17 Cardiac electrophysiology. **A** and **B,** Drugs affect each site by affecting ion channels. As a result, they affect the action potentials that depend on activity of ion channels. The action potentials are from cells of five regions of the heart. The *dotted vertical lines* indicate the occurrences of the P wave, QRS complex, and T wave on the electrocardiogram compared with the occurrences of the action potentials. *AV,* Atrioventricular; *SA,* sinoatrial; *MDP,* maximum diastolic potential. *(From Yagiela JA, et al: Pharmacology and Therapeutics for Dentistry, ed 6. St. Louis, Mosby, 2011.)*

1. Class IA—quinidine and procainamide.
   a. Reduce automaticity.
   b. Decrease conduction velocity.
   c. Increase refractory period.
2. Class IB—lidocaine; reduces automaticity at abnormal pacemakers in His-Purkinje system and ventricular myocardium.
3. Class IC—flecainide, propafenone.
   a. Reduce automaticity.
   b. Decrease conduction velocity.
4. Class II—propranolol, esmolol.
   a. Reduce automaticity.
   b. Decrease conduction velocity in AV node.
5. Class III—amiodarone, dronedarone, sotalol.
   a. Reduce automaticity.
   b. Increase refractory period.
6. Class IV—verapamil, diltiazem.
   a. Reduce automaticity.
   b. Decrease conduction velocity in AV node.
7. Adenosine.
   a. Reduces automaticity.
   b. Decreases conduction velocity in AV node.
F. General uses of antiarrhythmic drugs (based on sites of action) (Table 8-25).
G. Adverse effects (common, or typical).
   1. Quinidine—cinchonism, hypotension, torsades de pointes.
   2. Procainamide—mental changes, torsades de pointes, lupus.

Table 8-25

Antiarrhythmic Drugs Indicated for Arrhythmias*

CLASS (EXAMPLE)	SUPRAVENTRICULAR	VENTRICULAR
IA (quinidine)	Yes	Yes
IB (lidocaine)	No	Yes
IC (flecainide)	Yes	Yes
II (propranolol)	Yes	Yes
III (amiodarone)	Yes	Yes
IV (verapamil)	Yes	No
Adenosine	Yes	No

*There are many types of arrhythmias in these two general categories.

3. Lidocaine—convulsions.
4. Flecainide—convulsions, cardiac risk with recent myocardial infarction.
5. Propranolol—bronchoconstriction, heart block.
6. Amiodarone—pulmonary fibrosis, thyroid abnormalities, skin discoloration, cornea deposits, peripheral neuropathy. Dronedarone is chemically related to amiodarone but has fewer adverse effects than amiodarone.
7. Calcium channel blockers—flushing, AV node conduction defects, reduced contractility of the heart.

Table 8-26

Elimination Half-Lives of Antiarrhythmic Drugs

DRUG	HALF-TIME
Quinidine	4-10 hr
Lidocaine	1.5-2 hr
Flecainide	12-27 hr
Esmolol	0.2 hr
Amiodarone	25-100 days
Dronedarone	13-19 hr
Adenosine	<10 sec

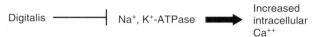

Figure 8-18 Action of digitalis.

8. Adenosine—flushing, asthma, dyspnea, SA nodal arrest, AV nodal block.

H. Half-lives of some antiarrhythmic drugs are compared in Table 8-26.

Drugs Used in Treating Heart Failure

Drugs used for treating heart failure are aimed at reducing vascular resistance, reducing fluid volume, or increasing the force of contraction of the heart.

A. Drugs for chronic heart failure.
   1. Thiazide and loop diuretics.
   2. ACE inhibitors.
   3. Angiotensin II receptor blockers.
   4. Aldosterone antagonists—spironolactone, eplerenone.
   5. β-Adrenergic receptor blockers.
   6. Digitalis.
   7. Vasodilators—nitrates, hydralazine.
B. Mechanisms of action.
   1. Diuretics reduce fluid load.
   2. ACE inhibitors, angiotensin II receptor blockers, and β-adrenergic receptor blockers reduce the vasoconstrictor response and aldosterone-releasing effect of the angiotensin pathway.
   3. Aldosterone antagonists block the effects of aldosterone. Aldosterone has several deleterious effects in heart failure.
   4. β-Adrenergic receptor blockers, in addition to inhibiting renin release, reduce downregulation of β receptors and have an antiarrhythmic effect. Carvedilol is a β blocker used to treat heart failure that also blocks α_1-adrenergic receptors and has an antioxidant effect.
   5. Digitalis—digoxin is the most important drug in this group. It increases the force of contraction of the heart by inhibiting Na^+,K^+-ATPase and indirectly increasing intracellular calcium (Figure 8-18).
      a. Other actions of digitalis.
         (1) Vagal effect on heart.
         (2) Slows AV nodal conduction.
         (3) Increases automaticity in His-Purkinje system.
      b. Adverse effects of digitalis.
         (1) Heart block.
         (2) Ventricular arrhythmias.
         (3) Nausea, vomiting.
         (4) Visual and mental disturbances.
      c. Drug-drug interactions involving digitalis.
         (1) Drugs that lower plasma potassium levels (e.g., thiazide and loop diuretics) increase digitalis toxicity.
         (2) Some antibiotics may reduce metabolism of digoxin in the gut and increase its absorption.
         (3) Quinidine and some other drugs increase the plasma levels of digitalis drugs.
         (4) Epinephrine may increase the risk of ventricular arrhythmias in the presence of digitalis.
C. Drugs used in acute treatment of heart failure.
   1. Dobutamine—catecholamine.
   2. Dopamine—catecholamine.
   3. Inamrinone, milrinone, vesnarinone—inhibit phosphodiesterase III.
   4. Nesiritide—atrial natriuretic peptide.
   5. Tolvaptan—vasopressin receptor antagonist.

Antihypertensive Drugs

A. Drug treatment for hypertension is aimed at one or more of the following.
   1. Reducing cardiac output.
   2. Reducing plasma volume.
   3. Reducing peripheral resistance.
   4. Figure 8-19 shows specific potential targets for antihypertensive drugs. Some, such as ganglionic sites, are rarely used in therapy.
B. Major antihypertensive drugs.
   1. Diuretics.
   2. ACE inhibitors.
   3. Angiotensin II receptor antagonists.
   4. β-Adrenoceptor blockers.
   5. α_1-Adrenoceptor blockers.
   6. Calcium channel blockers.
   7. Direct renin inhibitor (aliskiren).
C. Minor antihypertensive drugs—used only in combination.
   1. Centrally acting antihypertensive drugs.
   2. Hydralazine.
   3. Minoxidil.
   4. Guanethidine.
D. Diuretics.
   1. Include thiazide and loop diuretics (see section on diuretic drugs further on).
   2. Cause enhanced Na^+ and water excretion and reduced fluid volume.

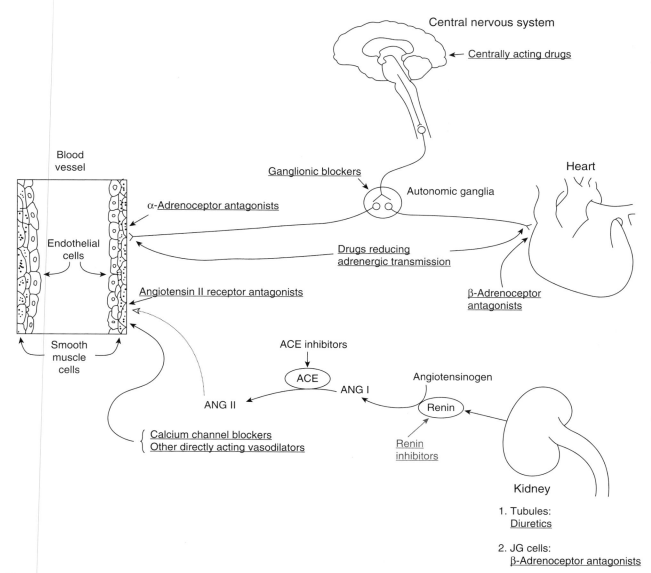

Figure 8-19 Sites of antihypertensive drug action. *ANG,* Angiotensin. *(Modified from Yagiela JA, et al: Pharmacology and Therapeutics for Dentistry, ed 6. St. Louis, Mosby, 2011.)*

3. Mechanism—inhibit Na/Cl cotransport (thiazides); inhibit $Na^+/K^+/2Cl^-$ cotransport (loop diuretics).
4. More effective in volume expanded hypertension.

E. Summary of drugs affecting the renin-angiotensin system (none should be used in pregnancy).
  1. ACE inhibitors.
  2. Angiotensin II receptor antagonists.
  3. β blockers inhibit renin release.
  4. ACE is nonspecific and catalyzes the *breakdown* of bradykinin (Figure 8-20).
  5. Direct renin inhibitors bind to and inhibit the enzyme, renin.

F. ACE inhibitors.
  1. Mechanism of action—inhibition of angiotensin II formation.

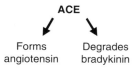

Figure 8-20 Dual function of ACE.

2. Lower angiotensin II leads to less vasoconstriction.
3. Lower angiotensin II leads to less aldosterone secretion and less sodium and water retention.
4. Lower angiotensin leads to less cell proliferation and remodeling. This leads to a long-term benefit for the heart and blood vessels.
5. Drugs (names end in "pril" or "prilat")—examples are captopril, enalapril, lisinopril, fosinopril.

6. ACE inhibitors are especially useful for patients with concomitant congestive heart failure, cardiac arrhythmias, or diabetes mellitus.
7. Adverse effects.
   a. Cough (common).
   b. Hyperkalemia if used with K^+-sparing drugs.
   c. Angioneurotic edema—rare but serious.
   d. Increased bradykinin may play a role in cough and angioneurotic edema.

G. Angiotensin II receptor antagonists.
   1. Drug examples (names end in "sartan").
      a. Losartan
      b. Valsartan
      c. Candesartan
   2. Angiotensin II blockers are used for similar indications as ACE inhibitors; however, fewer adverse effects are associated with angiotensin II blockers because they do not increase bradykinin.
   3. Adverse effects.
      a. Dizziness.
      b. Diarrhea.
      c. Myalgia.

H. β-Adrenergic receptor blockers (names end in "olol," "ilol," or "alol").
   1. Lower blood pressure because of the following.
      a. Reduction of cardiac output.
      b. Reduction of renin release.
      c. CNS—reduction of sympathetic outflow.
   2. Carvedilol, the "ilol" drug, also blocks α_1-adrenoceptors.

I. α-Adrenergic receptor blockers.
   1. Nonselective (α_1 and α_2) phentolamine and phenoxybenzamine—rarely used in medicine; however, phentolamine is used in dentistry to reverse soft tissue anesthesia more quickly after a procedure involving local anesthesia with a vasoconstrictor.
   2. Selective (α_1) (names end in "osin").
      a. Examples—prazosin, terazosin.
   3. Adverse effects.
      a. First-dose effect—hypotension, syncope.
      b. Tachycardia.
      c. Nasal congestion.
      d. Dry mouth.

J. Calcium channel blockers.
   1. Types.
      a. Nifedipine and other dihydropyridines.
      b. Diltiazem.
      c. Verapamil.
   2. The names of the dihydropyridines end in "dipine."
   3. Calcium channel blockers block the L-type calcium channel, reducing vasomotor tone.
   4. Adverse effects.
      a. Flushing.
      b. Headache.
      c. Hypotension.
      d. Gingival hyperplasia.

   e. Pose a risk of adverse cardiac events if the drug is short-acting.
   f. Verapamil and diltiazem are more cardioselective than the dihydropyridines.

K. Other antihypertensive drugs—dilate blood vessels.
   1. Directly acting vascular smooth muscle relaxants.
      a. Hydralazine.
      b. Minoxidil (also used to increase growth of hair).
      c. Diazoxide.
      d. Nitroprusside.
   2. Centrally acting sympatholytics (α_2-adrenoceptor agonists).
      a. α-Methyldopa.
      b. Clonidine.
      c. Guanabenz.
      d. Guanfacine.
   3. Drugs used in hypertensive emergencies.
      a. Nitroglycerin.
      b. Nitroprusside.
      c. Fenoldopam (a D_1-dopamine receptor agonist).
      d. Labetalol.
      e. Diazoxide.
      f. Hydralazine.

L. Drugs for pulmonary hypertension.
   a. Epoprostenol (prostacyclin).
   b. Endothelin receptor antagonists (bosentan, ambrisentan).
   c. Phosphodiesterase type 5 inhibitors (sildenafil, tadalafil).

M. Dental implications of antihypertensive drugs.
   1. Centrally acting drugs cause sedation.
   2. Vasoconstrictors in local anesthetics can be used in these patients, but dose restrictions are recommended.
   3. NSAIDs can inhibit the antihypertensive effect of ACE inhibitors, β blockers, and diuretics.
   4. Orthostatic hypotension can result from centrally acting drugs, α blockers, and direct vasodilators.
   5. Xerostomia is likely from centrally acting drugs and occasionally occurs with other drugs.
   6. ACE inhibitors can alter the sense of taste.
   7. ACE inhibitors can cause angioneurotic edema in a few cases.
   8. ACE inhibitors cause cough in approximately 10% of patients.
   9. Detection of hypertension is important.

Antianginal Drugs

Antianginal drugs work by reducing cardiac rate and force, reducing peripheral vascular resistance, or dilating coronary blood vessels.

A. Drugs.
   1. Nitrates and nitrites (dilate mostly veins).
   2. Calcium channel blockers (dilate peripheral and coronary blood vessels).

3. β-Adrenergic receptor blockers (reduce cardiac rate and force).
4. Antiplatelet drugs (reduce platelet aggregation).
5. Ranolazine improves contractile dysfunction.
6. Lipid-lowering drugs.

B. Nitrates and nitrites (e.g., nitroglycerin, amyl nitrite).
1. Mechanism—donate nitric oxide, which causes vasodilation.
2. Adverse effects.
   a. Headache.
   b. Syncope.
   c. Tachycardia.
   d. Tolerance.
   e. Methemoglobinemia.

C. See previous discussions of β blockers and calcium channel blockers.

D. Other drugs used to reduce the risk of myocardial infarction.
1. Aspirin.
2. Clopidogrel, prasugrel—inhibit the effect of ADP on platelets. They block $P2Y_{12}$ ADP receptors and reduce platelet aggregation.
3. GPIIb-IIIa glycoprotein receptor inhibitors—these bind to GPIIb-IIIa on platelets and reduce aggregation.
   a. Examples—abciximab (a Fab fragment of a monoclonal antibody), eptifibatide, and tirofiban.
4. Ranolazine—inhibits late sodium current and reduces sodium overload in cardiac cells, improving ischemia-induced contractile dysfunction.
5. Lipid-lowering drugs (see "Drugs Used for Blood Lipid Disorders" further on).

E. Dental implications.
1. Stress reduction is important.
2. Gingival hyperplasia may occur with calcium channel blockers.

Diuretic Drugs

Diuretic drugs act on the kidney to cause excretion of sodium and water. These drugs are used in edema states, hypertension, and heart failure. Figure 8-21 indicates where in the kidney they act.

A. Major drugs and their mechanism of action (see Figure 8-21).
1. Thiazides—decrease Na^+ and Cl^- cotransport.
2. Loop diuretics—decrease $Na^+/K^+/2Cl^-$ cotransport.
3. Amiloride, triamterene—decrease Na^+ reabsorption by blocking Na^+ channels.
4. Spironolactone—blocks aldosterone receptor.

B. Thiazides—benzothiadiazines, such as hydrochlorothiazide and related chlorthalidone.
1. Can cause hypokalemia.
2. Reduce Ca^{2+} excretion.
3. Can cause hyponatremia.
4. May increase plasma uric acid.
5. Sometimes used for nephrogenic diabetes insipidus.

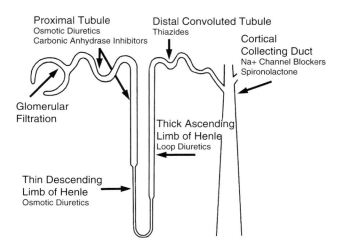

Figure 8-21 Sites of actions of diuretics. *(From Yagiela JA, et al:* Pharmacology and Therapeutics for Dentistry, *ed 6. St. Louis, Mosby, 2011.)*

C. Loop diuretics.
1. Examples—furosemide, bumetanide, torsemide.
2. Have a "high ceiling" or high maximal effect.
3. Can cause hyperuricemia.
4. Can increase excretion of Ca^{2+}.
5. Can cause tinnitus and hearing loss.
6. Can cause hyponatremia and excessive fluid loss.

D. Amiloride and triamterene.
1. K^+-sparing diuretics—reduce the driving force for K^+ movement into the lumen.
2. Used with other diuretics to reduce the risk of hypokalemia.
3. There is a risk of hyperkalemia.

E. Spironolactone and eplerenone.
1. True antagonists of aldosterone.
2. Similar in effects to amiloride and triamterene.

Drugs Used for Blood Lipid Disorders

Drugs are used to reduce abnormally high blood lipid levels. The two major lipoproteins that are targeted are very-low-density lipoproteins (VLDLs) and low-density lipoproteins (LDLs). The primary lipids of VLDLs are the triglycerides, and the primary lipids of LDLs are cholesteryl esters. Higher levels of LDL increase the risk of cardiovascular disease, whereas higher levels of VLDL increase the risk of pancreatitis. Hypercholesterolemia (high LDL) is a very common abnormality.

A. Drugs and their actions.
1. *Fibric acid derivatives*—fenofibrate, gemfibrozil. These agents activate PPARγ nuclear receptor, increase extrahepatic lipoprotein lipase, increase hepatic oxidation of fatty acids, and produce other effects that reduce VLDL and LDL.
2. *HMG-CoA reductase inhibitors (statins)*—atorvastatin, lovastatin, pravastatin, simvastatin. Inhibition of this enzyme leads to reduction in cholesterol

synthesis and an increase in LDL receptors in the liver; this reduces LDL.

3. *Nicotinic acid*—reduces fat cell lipolysis and lowers VLDL.

4. *Bile acid sequestrants*—cholestyramine, colesevelam, colestipol. These agents bind bile acids in the gut, leading to conversion of more cholesterol to bile acids, lowering LDL.

5. *Inhibitors of cholesterol absorption from the intestine*—ezetimibe. These agents prevent cholesterol absorption at the brush border and lower LDL.

B. Adverse effects of drugs used for blood lipid disorders (Table 8-27).

Anticoagulants and Procoagulants

Various drugs are used either to prevent blood coagulation or to dissolve clots. Drugs are sometimes used to enhance clotting in bleeding disorders.

A. Warfarin.

1. Warfarin inhibits the vitamin K–dependent synthesis of factors II (prothrombin), VII (proconvertin), IX (Christmas factor), and X (Stuart-Prower factor) (Figure 8-22).

2. The effect of warfarin takes several days to reach full effect.

3. Antidote—vitamin K (phytonadione).

B. Heparin.

1. Heparin blocks the action of factors Xa (activated) and IIa (thrombin) by stimulating antithrombin III (see Figure 8-22).

2. Heparin acts immediately to reduce blood coagulation.

3. Antidote—protamine.

C. Low-molecular-weight heparins (enoxaparin, dalteparin, tinzaparin) activate antithrombin III, mostly inhibiting factor Xa (not factor IIa). Protamine partially antagonizes these agents.

D. Fondaparinux—inhibits factor Xa by binding to antithrombin III. Protamine is inactive as an antagonist.

E. Direct thrombin inhibitors—lepirudin, bivalirudin, argatroban, dabigatran, rivaroxaban. Protamine is inactive as an antagonist.

F. Antiplatelet drugs—aspirin, dipyridamole (inhibits phosphodiesterase). See also platelet inhibitors under "Antianginal Drugs."

G. Dental implications.

1. The effect of warfarin is measured by the international normalized ratio (INR). Normal INR is 0.8 to 1.2. The typical target INR range for low-intensity anticoagulant therapy is 2.0 to 3.0 and for high intensity therapy is 2.5 to 3.5.

2. Risks from bleeding depend on extent of the surgical procedure and INR; the higher the INR, the greater the risk.

3. Restoration of normal INR after warfarin withdrawal takes several days because of the need to resynthesize clotting factors.

H. Plasminogen activators—used to break down clots by promoting fibrinolysis.

1. Tissue plasminogen activator—alteplase.

2. Tissue plasminogen activator variants—tenecteplase, reteplase.

3. Streptokinase.

4. Urokinase.

I. Plasminogen inhibitor—aminocaproic acid; used to inhibit fibrinolysis.

Table 8-27

Adverse Effects of Antilipid Drugs

DRUG OR DRUG CLASS	ADVERSE EFFECTS
Fibric acid derivatives	Increases the action of warfarin, GI effects, gallstones
HMG-CoA reductase inhibitors	Myalgia, GI effects, impotence
Nicotinic acid	Flushing, itching
Bile acid sequestrants	Hyperchloremic acidosis, GI effects
Probucol	GI effects, cardiac arrhythmias
Ezetimibe	GI effects, back pain

GI, Gastrointestinal; HMG-CoA, 3-hydroxy-3-methylglutaryl coenzyme A.

7.0 Gastrointestinal and Respiratory Pharmacology

Drugs Used to Treat Gastrointestinal Disorders

Drugs are used for various indications related to the GI tract, including to reduce the risk of ulcers and GERD, to alleviate diarrhea, to alleviate constipation, and to promote emesis. Drugs used for increasing or decreasing salivation are discussed in the sections on cholinergic receptor agonists and antimuscarinic drugs.

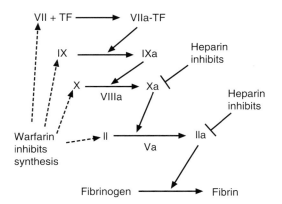

Figure 8-22 Sites of action of heparin and the oral anticoagulants represented by warfarin.

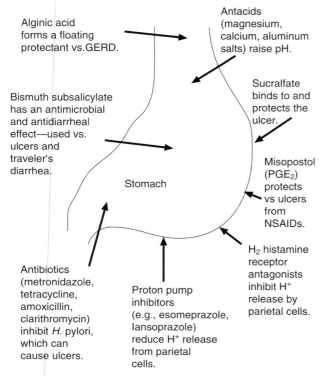

Alginic acid forms a floating protectant vs.GERD.

Antacids (magnesium, calcium, aluminum salts) raise pH.

Sucralfate binds to and protects the ulcer.

Bismuth subsalicylate has an antimicrobial and antidiarrheal effect—used vs. ulcers and traveler's diarrhea.

Misopostol (PGE$_2$) protects vs ulcers from NSAIDs.

Stomach

H$_2$ histamine receptor antagonists inhibit H$^+$ release by parietal cells.

Antibiotics (metronidazole, tetracycline, amoxicillin, clarithromycin) inhibit *H. pylori*, which can cause ulcers.

Proton pump inhibitors (e.g., esomeprazole, lansoprazole) reduce H$^+$ release from parietal cells.

Figure 8-23 Mechanisms of action of antiulcer and anti-GERD drugs.

A. Drugs used to treat ulcers and GERD (Figure 8-23).
B. Emetic—syrup of ipecac stimulates the chemoreceptor trigger zone and the stomach.
C. Antiemetics—usually drugs that control activity in the chemoreceptor trigger zone.
  1. Antihistamines—promethazine, cyclizine.
  2. Droperidol—dopamine receptor antagonist.
  3. Metoclopramide—dopamine and serotonin 5-HT$_3$ receptor antagonist.
  4. Dexamethasone—the mechanism of the antiemetic effect in cancer has not been definitely determined.
  5. Ondansetron—inhibits 5-HT$_3$ receptors.
  6. Dronabinol—a cannabinoid.
  7. Aprepitant—neurokinin (NK1) receptor antagonist.
D. Major laxatives (Figure 8-24).
E. Antidiarrheal drugs.
  1. Magnesium aluminum silicate plus pectin absorbs water and irritants in GI tract.
  2. Diphenoxylate and loperamide stimulate opioid receptors in GI tract.

Drugs Used to Treat Asthma

A. Several different classes of drugs are used to treat asthma (Table 8-28).
B. Other notes.
  1. Epinephrine is used to treat anaphylactic shock. It stimulates α$_1$-adrenergic, α$_2$-adrenergic, β$_1$-adrenergic, and β$_2$-adrenergic receptors. β$_2$ receptor stimulation aids in relieving bronchospasms.

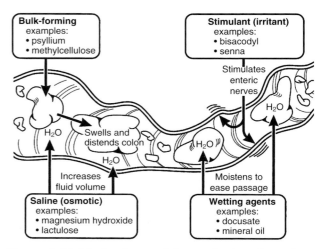

Bulk-forming examples:
• psyllium
• methylcellulose

Stimulant (irritant) examples:
• bisacodyl
• senna

Stimulates enteric nerves

Swells and distends colon

Increases fluid volume

Moistens to ease passage

Saline (osmotic) examples:
• magnesium hydroxide
• lactulose

Wetting agents examples:
• docusate
• mineral oil

Figure 8-24 Mechanisms of the major laxatives. *(From Yagiela JA, et al: Pharmacology and Therapeutics for Dentistry, ed 6. St. Louis, Mosby, 2011.)*

2. Oral glucocorticoids can be given in resistant cases (see Section 8.0, Endocrine Pharmacology). Inhaled corticosteroids, such as beclomethasone and fluticasone, are commonly used.
3. Antimuscarinic anticholinergic drugs—ipratropium, tiotropium. Both of these drugs are quaternary ammonium drugs that are not systemically absorbed after inhalation.
4. Cromolyn, nedocromil—inhibit mast cell degranulation.
5. Leukotriene pathway modifiers—leukotrienes play a key role in asthma treatment.
  a. 5-Lipoxygenase inhibitor—zileuton; blocks the synthesis of cysteinyl leukotrienes.
  b. Cysteinyl leukotriene receptor inhibitors—montelukast, zafirlukast.
6. Omalizumab—a monoclonal antibody; given subcutaneously, binds to IgE and prevents its action at the IgE receptor.
7. Theophylline has a low therapeutic index. Its metabolism is affected by several other drugs, leading to potential problems with theophylline. Theophylline inhibits phosphodiesterase leading to an increase in cAMP. It also stimulates histone deacetylase, reducing inflammatory gene expression. Both mechanisms appear to have benefit in asthma.

8.0 Endocrine Pharmacology

Thyroid Pharmacology

Drugs are used to treat both hypothyroidism and hyperthyroidism.
A. Thyroid hormones.
  1. Bind to intracellular receptors in target cells and activate transcription in the nucleus.

Table 8-28

Antiasthma Drugs

DRUG CLASS	DRUG EXAMPLES	ACTION	COMMENTS
β_2-Adrenergic agonists	Albuterol Metaproterenol Salmeterol	Stimulate β_2 receptors, relax smooth muscle in the lung	Used by inhalation for rapid action (salmeterol is slow-acting); can lead to tachycardia and tremor
Inhaled glucocorticoids	Beclomethasone Budesonide Flunisolide Fluticasone	Increase lipomodulin, which inhibits phospholipase A_2, other mechanisms	Reduce inflammation in airway; can lead to oral candidiasis
Antimuscarinic drug	Ipratropium Tiotropium	Block muscarinic receptors in bronchi, leading to bronchodilation	Used by inhalation; can lead to xerostomia
Methylxanthine	Theophylline	Blocks adenosine receptors, blocks phosphodiesterase leading to an increase in cAMP, causes bronchodilation	Taken orally; watch toxicity (nausea, vomiting, arrhythmias, CNS toxicity)
Leukotriene synthesis inhibitor	Zileuton	Inhibits synthesis of leukotrienes by inhibiting 5-lipoxygenase	Taken orally; reduces inflammation
Leukotriene receptor antagonists	Montelukast Zafirlukast	Block leukotriene (Cys-LT_1) receptors	Taken orally; long-acting
Inhibitors of mast cell degranulation	Cromolyn Nedocromil	Block degranulation of mast cells	Given by inhalation
Anti-IgE monoclonal antibody	Omalizumab	Binds to IgE, preventing its effect at the IgE receptor	Given subcutaneously

cAMP, Cyclic adenosine monophosphate; *CNS,* central nervous system.

2. Used to treat hypothyroidism—T_4 (levothyroxine), T_3 (liothyronine), and T_3 plus T_4 (liotrix) are available for therapy.
3. T_4 has a longer half-life.
4. They are usually used orally.
5. Adverse effects of thyroid hormones.
   a. Nervousness.
   b. Tachycardia, angina, risk with epinephrine.
   c. Nausea, diarrhea.
   d. Tremor, weight loss, heat intolerance.
B. If iodine deficiency causes hypothyroidism, this condition is treated with iodide.
C. *Antithyroid drugs*—used to treat hyperthyroidism (Figure 8-25).
   1. Thioamide drugs—methimazole, propylthiouracil.
      a. Inhibit thyroid peroxidase, inhibiting oxidation of iodide and iodination.
      b. Adverse effects—rash, nausea, agranulocytosis.
   2. Iodides (mostly potassium iodide).
      a. Inhibit release of thyroid hormone and several steps in synthesis.
      b. High doses are used.
      c. Concentrate in thyroid.
      d. Decrease vascularity of thyroid—used before surgery.
      e. Have a short-term effect.
      f. Adverse effects—GI irritation, parotid gland pain, headache, cough.
   3. Radioactive iodide (^{131}I) destroys thyroid cells.

Insulin and Oral Hypoglycemics

Insulin is used to treat both type 1 and type 2 diabetes. It is required for type 1 diabetes because the β cells of the pancreas are devoid of insulin. In type 2 diabetes, drugs other than insulin can often be used because the β cells are able to secrete insulin, albeit in a more sluggish manner.

A. Insulin.
   1. Mechanism of action.
      a. Reduces blood glucose by increasing its uptake and increasing conversion to glycogen and lipid.
      b. Reduces lipolysis.
      c. Increases protein synthesis and cell growth.
      d. Figure 8-26 shows major insulin pathways by which the aforementioned mechanisms are accomplished.
   2. Effects of insulin.
      a. Corrects hyperglycemia of diabetes.
      b. Reduces long-term adverse effects of diabetes.
   3. Drug preparations (Table 8-29).
B. Sulfonylurea oral hypoglycemic drugs—insulin secretagogues.

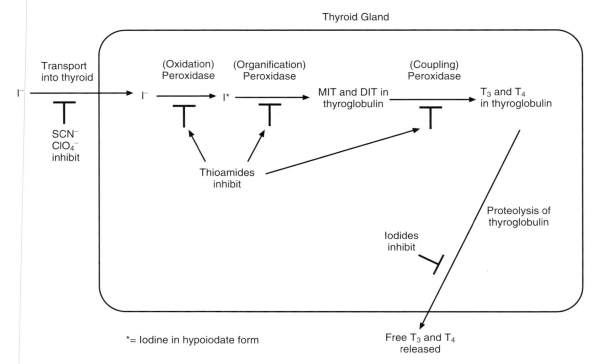

Figure 8-25 Synthesis of thyroid hormones and sites of action of antithyroid drugs. *DIT,* Diiodotyrosine; *MIT,* monoiodotyrosine. *(From Yagiela JA, et al:* Pharmacology and Therapeutics for Dentistry, *ed 6. St. Louis, Mosby, 2011.)*

Table 8-29		
Insulin Preparations		
TYPE	**ONSET***	**DURATION***
Short-Acting		
Regular	30-60 min	4-6 hr
Lispro	15 min	3-5 hr
Aspart	15 min	3-5 hr
Glulisine	15 min	3-5 hr
Long-Acting		
NPH	1-4 hr	12-18 hr
Glargine	1-4 hr	20-24 hr
Detemir	1-4 hr	20-24 hr

Data from Golan DE, et al: *Principles of Pharmacology, The Pathologic Basis of Drug Therapy,* ed 3. Philadelphia, Lippincott Williams & Williams, 2012; and Brunton LL, Chabner BA, Knollman BJ: *Goodman & Gilman's Pharmacological Basis of Therapeutics,* ed 12. New York, McGraw-Hill, 2011.

All of the above-listed preparations incorporate small but important changes in the amino acid sequence of insulin except for regular and NPH insulin.

*After subcutaneous injection.

1. Examples.
   a. Tolbutamide.
   b. Acetohexamide.
   c. Tolazamide.
   d. Chlorpropamide.

e. Glibenclamide.
f. Glipizide.
g. Glimepiride.
2. Mechanism of action.
   a. Close ATP-sensitive potassium channels in cell membranes of β cells.
   b. Stimulate release of insulin from pancreas.
   c. Increase sensitivity of target organs to insulin.
3. Adverse effects.
   a. Hypoglycemia.
   b. GI upset.
   c. Vertigo.
   d. Edema, sodium retention.
4. Indications for sulfonylurea drugs—type 2 diabetes.
C. Other oral hypoglycemic drugs.
   1. Meglitides—repaglinide and nateglinide; insulin secretagogues.
      a. Mechanism—similar to sulfonylureas.
      b. Used orally.
      c. Act like the sulfonylureas.
      d. *Adverse effect*—hypoglycemia.
      e. Used for type 2 diabetes.
   2. Metformin—inhibitor of liver glucose production.
      a. Activates AMP kinase, which regulates energy production.
      b. Used orally.
      c. Reduces gluconeogenesis and lipogenesis in the liver.

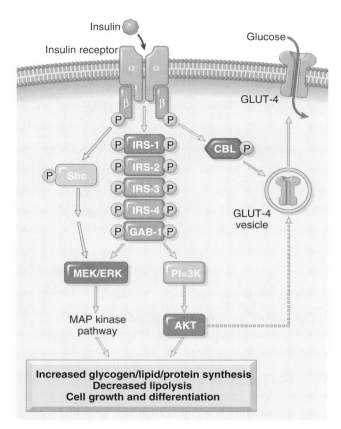

Figure 8-26 Mechanism of action of insulin. Signaling pathways for insulin are shown leading to increases in synthesis, growth, and differentiation. The action of insulin on its receptor leads to phosphorylation (P) of the receptor and key proteins in the signaling pathways. Effects of insulin are realized through numerous mechanisms, including enhancing gene transcription and protein synthesis. The translocation of the glucose transporter (Glut-4) to the plasma membrane, which is stimulated by insulin, is integral to glucose uptake and subsequent glucose use in cells of key target tissues. *AKT,* Protein kinase B; *CBL,* calcineurin B–like protein; *ERK,* extracellular signal–regulated kinases; *IRS,* insulin receptor substrates; *MAP,* mitogen-activated protein; *MEK,* mitogen-activated protein kinase; *PI-3K,* phosphatidylinositol 3′-kinase; *Shc,* Src homology 2 domain-containing. *(Modified from Robbins SL, et al: The endocrine system. In Robbins and Cotran Pathologic Basis of Disease. St. Louis, Saunders, 2010.)*

d. Increases sensitivity to insulin in muscle, liver, and fat cells.
    e. *Adverse effects*—GI problems, lactic acidosis.
    f. Used for type 2 diabetes.
3. Acarbose, miglitol, and voglibose—delayers of carbohydrate digestion.
    a. Inhibit α-glucosidase.
    b. Used orally.
    c. Reduce digestion of carbohydrates in gut.
    d. Decrease glucose absorption.

e. *Adverse effects*—GI problems and malabsorption.
    f. Used for type 2 diabetes.
4. Pioglitazone and rosiglitazone—insulin sensitizers.
    a. Activate transcription factor PPARγ leading to increased insulin sensitivity of muscle, liver, and fat cells.
    b. *Adverse effects*—GI problems, headache, dizziness, liver toxicity.
    c. Used for type 2 diabetes.
    d. Used orally.
5. Pramlintide—amylin analogue.
    a. Amylin analogue that stimulates CNS amylin receptors.
    b. Reduces gastric emptying.
    c. Reduces glucagon release and glucose levels.
    d. Given subcutaneously.
    e. Used in type 1 and type 2 diabetes.
6. Exenatide and liraglutide—is a glucagonlike peptide-1 (GLP-1) analogue.
    a. Analogues of GLP-1 (an incretin).
    b. By stimulating GLP-1, these agents cause insulin secretion, block glucagon release, and reduce food intake.
    c. Given subcutaneously.
7. Sitagliptin and saxagliptin—increase GLP-1 indirectly.
    a. Inhibit dipeptidyl peptidase-4, which inactivates GLP-1.
    b. Actions are due to an increase in GLP-1.
    c. Used orally.
    d. Used in type 2 diabetes.

Adrenal Corticosteroids

Adrenal corticosteroids are composed of mineralocorticoids (e.g., aldosterone) and glucocorticoids (e.g., hydrocortisone). Mineralocorticoids are used as replacement therapy, such as in Addison's disease. Glucocorticoids, although useful in replacement therapy, are most often used as antiinflammatory drugs and antiimmune drugs. Adrenal steroids are used much more often for glucocorticoid effects than for a mineralocorticoid effect.

A. Drugs and their relative potencies as mineralocorticoids and glucocorticoids (as measured by sodium retention and glycogen deposition, respectively) (Table 8-30).
B. Actions of glucocorticoids—all steroid hormones bind to receptors inside the cell, stimulating mRNA synthesis and protein synthesis, resulting in many metabolic effects.
1. Decrease cell uptake of glucose.
2. Stimulate gluconeogenesis.
3. Stimulate lipolysis.
4. Reduce immune and inflammatory responses, partly by inhibiting the nuclear factor, NF-κB.
5. Inhibit action of macrophages.

Table 8-30

Comparison of Steroids

DRUG	POTENCY AS AN ANTIINFLAMMATORY DRUG	SODIUM RETENTION
Aldosterone	0.1	3000
Fludrocortisone	10	3000
Cortisone	0.8	0.8
Hydrocortisone	1	1
Prednisone	4	0.8
Prednisolone	4	0.8
Triamcinolone	5	0
Dexamethasone	25	0
Betamethasone	25	0

Modified from Yagiela JA, et al: *Pharmacology and Therapeutics for Dentistry,* ed 6. St Louis, Mosby, 2011.

Hydrocortisone is assigned an arbitrary number of "1" for comparison purposes. The higher the number, the greater the relative effect of the drug.

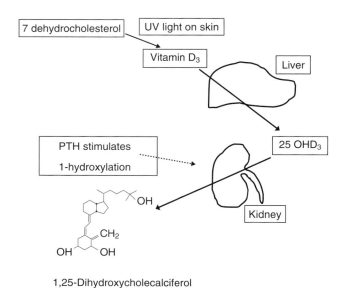

1,25-Dihydroxycholecalciferol
(1,25-dihydroxyvitamin D)

Figure 8-27 Synthesis and activation of vitamin D_3.

6. Inhibit phospholipase A_2 by stimulating the production of lipomodulin.
C. Uses of glucocorticoids.
   1. Asthma.
   2. Inflammatory disease.
   3. Collagen diseases.
   4. Some lymphomas and leukemias.
   5. Cerebral edema.
   6. Rheumatic diseases
   7. Acute attacks of multiple sclerosis.
D. Adverse effects of glucocorticoids.
   1. Insomnia, agitation.
   2. Infections.
   3. Hypertension, atherosclerosis.
   4. Skin and mucosal atrophy.
   5. Negative calcium balance, osteoporosis.
   6. Muscle wasting.
   7. Obesity, glucose intolerance.
   8. Peptic ulcers.
   9. Cataracts.
E. Dental applications.
   1. Glucocorticoids are used to reduce inflammation. Topical application is common. Oral administration is used in more serious cases. Oral glucocorticoids are used in some cases of acute allergies.
   2. Long-term treatment leads to several adverse effects, including risk of infection.

Drugs That Affect Calcium Metabolism

Three major hormones, vitamin D, parathyroid hormone (PTH), and calcitonin, have profound effects on calcium balance, affecting the bones, kidneys, and GI tract. In addition, several other drugs affect calcium metabolism, especially affecting bone.

A. Vitamin D.
   1. Binds to intracellular receptors in target cells and activates transcription in the nucleus.
   2. Derived from dietary sources and from the effect of ultraviolet light on skin.
   3. Increases calcium absorption from the GI tract.
   4. 1,25-Dihydroxyvitamin D_3 is the active form (also known as 1,25-dihydroxycholecalciferol). Ergocalciferol (D_2) is from plant origins.
   5. Synthesis and activation (Figure 8-27).
   6. Action on GI tract.
      a. Acts on intracellular receptor to increase mRNA and protein synthesis.
      b. Increases calcium-binding protein in the gut.
      c. Increases calcium absorption.
      d. In higher doses, vitamin D has additional effects resembling PTH.
   7. Indications.
      a. Vitamin supplementation for optimum health.
      b. Nutritional lack.
      c. Hypoparathyroidism.
      d. Osteoporosis.
      e. Psoriasis.
B. PTH.
   1. Secreted by parathyroid cells when plasma calcium decreases.
   2. Increases cAMP in target cells (bone and kidney).
   3. Simulates osteoclast activity under most conditions.
   4. Stimulates production of active vitamin D in kidney (see Figure 8-27).
   5. Decreases calcium excretion in the kidney.
   6. Increases plasma calcium.
   7. Used in the short molecular form (1-24) (teriparatide) once a day for postmenopausal osteoporosis

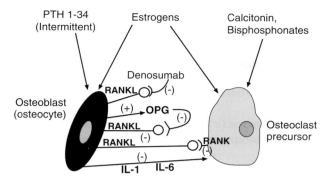

Figure 8-28 Action of several drugs on bone cells. Estrogens act both directly and indirectly to inhibit osteoclast formation and action. Indirect effects include a decrease (−) in the release of cytokines such as interleukin (IL)-1 and IL-6 and receptor activator of nuclear factor kappa-B ligand (RANKL) by osteoblasts. (Stimulation by several cytokines and stimulation of RANK lead to increases in numbers of osteoclasts resulting in bone breakdown.) Estrogens also increase (+) the synthesis and secretion of osteoprotegerin (OPG). OPG binds to RANKL, preventing its binding to receptor activator of nuclear factor kappa-B (RANK) receptors on osteoclast precursors. Denosumab is a monoclonal antibody drug that binds to RANKL and prevents its action at RANK. Many of the effects of intermittent parathyroid hormone 1-34 (PTH 1-34) on osteoblasts are similar to estrogens. Calcitonin and bisphosphonates act directly on osteoclasts and osteoclast precursors to inhibit their activity.

(Figure 8-28). There is a clear difference in the effect on bone between PTH (1-24) given once a day and the hormonal effect of endogenous release of PTH.

C. Calcitonin.
   1. Secreted by parafollicular C cells.
   2. Increases cAMP in osteoclasts, reducing their activity.
   3. Increases calcium excretion in the kidney.
   4. *Indications*—Paget's disease, hypercalcemia, osteoporosis.

D. Other drugs affecting bone (see Figure 8-28).
   1. Bisphosphonates.
      a. Examples—alendronate, pamidronate, tiludronate.
      b. Reduce turnover rate of hydroxyapatite (inhibit osteoclasts by inhibiting prenylation of key proteins).
      c. Used in Paget's disease, osteoporosis, hypercalcemia, and bone metastasis.
      d. *Adverse effects*—GI symptoms; esophageal erosions; osteonecrosis of the jaw, especially in high doses.
   2. Fluoride ion.
      a. Increases osteoblast activity.
      b. Used for dental applications.
   3. A summary of these and other drugs is given in Figure 8-28.
   4. PTH 1-34 (teriparatide) is the shortened form of PTH.

5. Denosumab.
   a. Monoclonal antibody that binds and inhibits receptor activator of nuclear factor kappa-B ligand (RANKL) (see Figure 8-28).
   b. Inhibits formation and activation of osteoclasts.
   c. Used subcutaneously for osteoporosis.
6. Estrogens (see "Sex Hormones," next, and Figure 8-28).

Sex Hormones

Estrogens, progesteronelike compounds (progestins), and androgens are used for various clinical indications. They are steroid hormones with effects on numerous systems of the body. Their action involves binding to intracellular receptors in target cells and activating transcription in the nucleus.

A. Estrogens.
   1. Estradiol is the most potent human estrogenic hormone.
   2. Estrogens have important supportive effects on pregnancy and secondary sex characteristics.
   3. Support bone—stimulate osteoblasts but also reduce RANKL and cytokine gene expression in osteoblasts, ultimately decreasing the number and action of osteoclasts (see Figure 8-28); also inhibit osteoclasts directly.
   4. Reduce LDL and increase high-density lipoprotein.
   5. Indications.
      a. Oral contraception.
      b. Replacement therapy.
      c. Prevention of osteoporosis.
      d. Reduce symptoms of menopause.
   6. Drugs used.
      a. Estradiol.
      b. Ethinyl estradiol.
      c. Mestranol.
      d. Conjugated estrogens.

B. Selective estrogen receptor modulators.
   1. Raloxifene is a major drug.
   2. Estrogen receptor agonist in bone but antagonist in the endometrium and breast.
   3. Used to treat postmenopausal osteoporosis.

C. Progestins.
   1. Progesterone is the natural compound.
   2. Important for sexual development and in pregnancy.
   3. Indications for progestins (progesteronelike compounds).
      a. Oral contraception.
      b. Endometriosis.
      c. Postmenopausal hormone replacement.
      d. Dysfunctional uterine bleeding.
   4. Prevent proliferative effects (and endometrial cancer) from estrogen therapy.
   5. Drugs used.
      a. Norethindrone.
      b. Norethynodrel.

Table 8-31

Composition of Some Oral Contraceptives

	ESTROGEN	PROGESTIN
Desogen, 28-pack	Ethinyl estradiol	Desogestrel
Necon 1/50, 28-pack	Mestranol	Norethindrone
Ortho-Novum 1/35, 28-pack	Ethinyl estradiol	Norethindrone
Yaz	Ethinyl estradiol	Drospirenone
Camila, 28-pack	—	Norethindrone
Seasonale*	Ethinyl estradiol	Levonorgestrel
Plan B†	—	Levonorgestrel
ella†	—	Ulipristal acetate

Combination oral contraceptives are either monophasic or multiphasic, the latter containing varying doses of one or both hormones during the pill cycle.

*Extended (91-day) cycle.

†Emergency contraceptives.

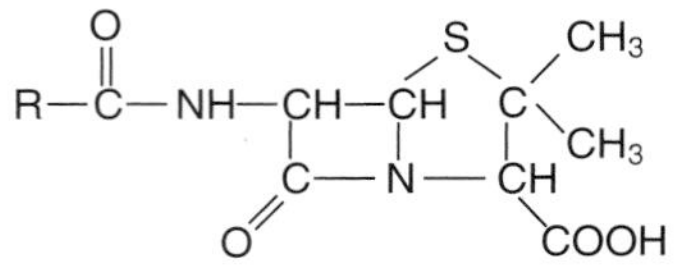

Figure 8-29 Penicillin nucleus.

"cidal" drugs kill bacteria, whereas "static" drugs prevent growth of bacteria. These descriptions are applied to the concentrations of each drug that can reliably be attained in vivo. The spectrum of any antimicrobial drug refers to the extent (broad, extended, or narrow) of the organisms affected by the drug and the specific organisms affected. Extended therapy with a specific drug almost always leads to some resistance of certain organisms to that drug.

Superinfection, defined as a growth of resistant organisms owing to therapy targeting sensitive organisms, is usually more likely to occur with broad-spectrum or extended-spectrum drugs compared with narrow-spectrum drugs. The potency of antibacterial drugs is often estimated using measures such as the minimum inhibitory concentration (MIC).

A. Mechanisms of action of antibacterial drug classes (Table 8-32).
B. Cell wall inhibitors inhibit one of the steps in peptidoglycan synthesis, important in the cell wall.
C. Many antibiotics inhibit ribosomal protein synthesis.
D. Penicillins.
  1. Chemistry—the β-lactam ring gives the name β-lactam to this group of drugs, which includes penicillins (Figure 8-29), cephalosporins, and atypical β-lactams.
  2. Penicillinase is a type of β-lactamase, formed by bacteria, that renders them resistant to many penicillins.
  3. Penicillin G and penicillin V are narrow-spectrum penicillins (Table 8-33).
    a. Penicillin G and V are very similar except that penicillin V is more acid-stable and has a higher bioavailability when given orally.
    b. Penicillin V is often used to treat oral infections caused by a wide variety of sensitive oral bacteria.
    c. Organisms susceptible to penicillin G and V— viridans streptococci, *Streptococcus pyogenes*, *Streptococcus pneumoniae* (gram-positive), *Neisseria gonorrhoeae*, *Neisseria meningitidis*, oral *Bacteroides*, oral *Fusobacterium*, *Leptotrichia buccalis* (gram-negative), *Treponema pallidum*, *Actinomyces israelii*.
    d. Gram-negative cocci are sensitive.
    e. Penicillins, similar to all cell wall inhibitors, are bactericidal against susceptible organisms.
    f. The elimination half-life of penicillins is short. The $t_{1/2}$ for penicillin G and V is about 0.5 hour because of rapid excretion by the kidney, 90% of which is by tubular secretion. Very little drug gets metabolized.

    c. Medroxyprogesterone.
    d. Levonorgestrel.
D. Oral contraceptives.
  1. Types.
    a. Combination estrogen and progestin.
    b. Minipill (progestin only, e.g., Camila).
    c. Emergency (progestin).
  2. Major action of combination and minipill—inhibition of ovulation.
  3. Examples of oral contraceptives (Table 8-31).
  4. Some adverse effects of combination estrogen and progestin.
    a. Hypertension.
    b. Thrombophlebitis.
    c. Gallbladder disease.
    d. Nausea.
E. Fertility drugs.
  1. Antiestrogen—clomiphene.
  2. Human menopausal gonadotropins (menotropins).
  3. Human chorionic gonadotropin (hCG).
  4. Gonadotropin-releasing hormone analogue— gonadorelin (pulsatile use).
  5. Follicle-stimulating hormone (FSH)—follitropin and urofollitropin.
  6. Antiestrogens and gonadorelin stimulate gonadotropin release from the pituitary; menotropins, hCG, and FSH stimulate the ovary directly.

9.0 Antimicrobial Drugs

Antibacterial Drugs

Antibiotics are chemicals produced by microorganisms that inhibit other microorganisms. By this definition, most antibacterial drugs discussed here are antibiotics. Antibacterial drugs are classified as either bactericidal or bacteriostatic;

Table 8-32

Mechanisms of Action and Characteristic Adverse Effects of Antibacterial Drugs

DRUG	MECHANISM OF ACTION, WHAT IS INHIBITED	ADVERSE EFFECTS
Penicillins	Transpeptidase, stage 3 in cell wall synthesis	Allergies, neurotoxicity in high doses
Cephalosporins	Transpeptidase, stage 3 in cell wall synthesis	Allergies, neurotoxicity in high doses, renal toxicity
Macrolides	Translocation step of ribosomal protein synthesis	GI upset, especially with erythromycin, inhibition of drug metabolism, Q–T prolongation*
Clindamycin	Peptide bond formation in ribosomes	Diarrhea, pseudomembranous colitis
Tetracyclines	Binding of aminoacyl-tRNA to ribosome and protein synthesis	Tooth staining, liver toxicity in pregnancy, photosensitivity, Fanconi's syndrome with outdated drug
Sulfonamides	Dihydropteroate synthase step in folic acid synthesis	Crystalluria (some drugs), allergies, psychosis
Streptogramins	Peptide bond formation in ribosomes	Phlebitis, myalgia, arthralgia
Linezolid	tRNA binding to ribosome and initiation of protein synthesis	Myelosuppression, GI effects, peripheral neuropathies
Trimethoprim	Dihydrofolate reductase step in folic acid synthesis	Megaloblastic anemia Leukopenia
Fluoroquinolones	DNA gyrase and topoisomerase IV, transcription	GI upset, CNS toxicity, photosensitivity (some)
Aminoglycosides	Initiation complex of protein synthesis, cause misreading in protein synthesis	Renal toxicity, ototoxicity, neuromuscular blockade
Vancomycin	Transglycosylase in cell wall synthesis	Renal toxicity, ototoxicity, red man syndrome
Metronidazole	Damages DNA after being reduced by nitroreductase	GI effects, metallic taste, oral candidiasis
Chloramphenicol	Peptide bond formation in ribosomes	Bone marrow hypoplasia, aplastic anemia, gray baby syndrome
Bacitracin	Inhibits bactoprenol in cell wall synthesis	Rare adverse effects, used topically

CNS, Central nervous system; *GI,* gastrointestinal.

*Azithromycin given for 5 days has been shown to increase the risk of cardiovascular death in individuals with preexisting cardiovascular risk factors.[1] Azithromycin increases the Q–T interval, which is a likely contributor to the increased risk.

From Ray WA, et al: Azithromycin and the risk of cardiovascular death, *N Eng J Med* 366:1881-90, 2012.

Table 8-33

Comparison of Penicillin Drugs

DRUG CLASS AND/OR DRUGS	SPECTRUM	RESISTANT TO PENICILLINASE?	INDICATIONS	UNIQUE ADVERSE EFFECTS
Penicillin G and V	Narrow	No	Oral infections, many infections caused by sensitive bacteria	—
Methicillin, oxacillin, cloxacillin, dicloxacillin, nafcillin	Narrow	Yes	*Staphylococcus aureus* infections	—
Aminopenicillins (ampicillin, amoxicillin, bacampicillin)	Extended (includes many gram-negative rods)	No	Mixed infections, infections owing to gram-negative rods	Rash in people who have mononucleosis or who take allopurinol
Anti-*Pseudomonas* penicillins (ticarcillin, piperacillin)	Extended	No	Effective against *Pseudomonas, Enterobacter,* and indole-positive *Proteus*	—
Procaine penicillin G (combined with benzathine penicillin)	Narrow	No	IM injection to achieve a more sustained effect of penicillin	—
Benzathine penicillin G	Narrow	No	Long-term, low-level penicillin effect	

IM, Intramuscular.

4. Amoxicillin (see Table 8-33).
  a. Oral extended-spectrum penicillin is used for oral infections and in dental prophylaxis.
  b. Prophylaxis protocol (see Table 8-36).
E. β-Lactamase inhibitors.
  1. Clavulanic acid, sulbactam, and tazobactam.
  2. Used with amoxicillin, ticarcillin, ampicillin, and piperacillin to reduce the effect of plasmid-mediated β-lactamases.
F. Cephalosporins (Table 8-34).
  1. Broad-spectrum drugs.
  2. Characteristics of five generations of cephalosporins (see Table 8-34).
  3. Cephalosporins as options in dental prophylaxis— three cephalosporins are indicated (see Table 8-36).
  4. About 10% cross-allergenicity with penicillins—the risk is greater with patients who have a history of acute or immediate types of allergies.
G. Atypical β-lactams.
  1. Imipenem.
    a. Used with cilastatin, which inhibits imipenem metabolism in the kidney.
    b. Used against *Pseudomonas aeruginosa* and several other gram-negative rods as well as some streptococci.
  2. *Ertapenem, meropenem, doripenem, aztreonam*— similar indications as imipenem.

H. Macrolide antibiotics.
  1. Drugs—erythromycin, clarithromycin, azithromycin, dirithromycin (Table 8-35).
  2. Sensitive organisms.
    a. *Legionella pneumophila.*
    b. *Mycoplasma pneumoniae.*
    c. *Chlamydia pneumoniae.*
    d. Streptococci and some other gram-positive cocci and some gram-negative cocci.
    e. Clarithromycin and azithromycin are more potent than erythromycin and are more effective against *Helicobacter pylori* and *Mycobacterium avium.*
I. Tetracyclines.
  1. Broad spectrum.
    a. Various *Rickettsia* species.
    b. *M. pneumoniae.*
    c. *C. pneumoniae.*
    d. *H. pylori.*
    e. *Borrelia burgdorferi* (Lyme disease).
    f. *Escherichia coli.*
    g. Bacteria associated with refractory and localized aggressive periodontitis.
    h. Bacteria associated with acne.
  2. Representative drugs.
    a. Tetracycline.
    b. Doxycycline.
    c. Minocycline—risk of vestibular toxicity.

Table 8-34

Cephalosporin Generations and Sensitive Organisms

GENERATION	EXAMPLES	SENSITIVE ORGANISMS
1	Cefazolin Cephalexin Cefadroxil	*Escherichia coli, Staphylococcus aureus* (methicillin sensitive), various streptococci
2	a. Cefoxitin b. Cefaclor	a. Oral *Bacteroides* b. *Haemophilus influenzae*
3	a. Cefotaxime, ceftriaxone b. Ceftazidime	a. *Neisseria gonorrhoeae, Neisseria meningitides, E. coli, H. influenzae* b. *Pseudomonas aeruginosa*
4	Cefepime	*P. aeruginosa*
5	Ceftaroline	Multidrug-resistant *S. aureus, Streptococcus pneumoniae, H. influenzae*

Table 8-35

Comparison of Macrolides and Adverse Effects

DRUG	GI UPSET	DRUG-DRUG INTERACTIONS	CHOLESTATIC JAUNDICE	USED IN DENTAL PROPHYLAXIS
Erythromycin	Significant, owing to stimulation of motilin receptor	More	Usually seen only with estolate form	No
Clarithromycin	Less	Less	No	Yes
Azithromycin	Less	Much less	No	Yes
Dirithromycin	Less	Much less	No	No

GI, Gastrointestinal.

J. Clindamycin.
   1. Narrow-spectrum.
   2. Sensitive organisms.
      a. *S. pneumoniae.*
      b. Viridans streptococci.
      c. *S. pyogenes.*
      d. *Staphylococcus aureus* (not methicillin-resistant staphylococci).
      e. Oral *Bacteroides* and some other oral anaerobes.
   3. Uses.
      a. Infections caused by several anaerobic rods and cocci.
      b. Some streptococcal and a few staphylococcal infections.
      c. Oral infections.
      d. Osteomyelitis.
      e. Dental prophylaxis (Table 8-36).
K. Metronidazole.
   1. Antimicrobial spectrum.
      a. Bacteria—limited to anaerobes.
      b. Parasitic infections.
   2. Sensitive organisms and indications.
      a. *Bacteroides.*
      b. *Fusobacterium.*
      c. *Clostridium difficile.*
   3. Contraindications.
      a. Pregnancy.
      b. Alcohol use.
      c. Disulfiram use.
L. Vancomycin.
   1. Narrow-spectrum (gram-positive aerobes and anaerobes).
   2. Sensitive organisms and indications.
      a. *S. aureus*, including methicillin-resistant staphylococci.
      b. Streptococci, enterococci, *C. difficile.*
   3. Administration—given intravenously.
M. Aminoglycosides.
   1. Examples—streptomycin, gentamicin, amikacin, neomycin.
   2. Spectrum limited to aerobes, mostly gram-negative rods.
   3. Sensitive organisms and indications.
      a. *E. coli.*
      b. Enterobacteriaceae.
      c. *Klebsiella pneumoniae.*
      d. *P. aeruginosa.*
   4. Use of streptomycin is largely limited to tuberculosis.
   5. Use of neomycin is topical.
N. Sulfonamides (and trimethoprim).
   1. Examples—sulfamethoxazole, sulfisoxazole, silver sulfadiazine, sulfacetamide (topical).
   2. Spectrum broadened with the addition of trimethoprim—sulfamethoxazole-trimethoprim combination is commonly used.
   3. Organisms sensitive to sulfamethoxazole-trimethoprim combination.
      a. *K. pneumoniae.*
      b. *E. coli.*
      c. *Salmonella* species.
      d. *Shigella* species.
      e. *Pneumocystis jiroveci* (formerly *Pneumocystis carinii*).
      f. *Haemophilus influenzae.*

Table 8-36

*Antibiotic Prophylaxis Guidelines for the Prevention of Bacterial Endocarditis**

	DOSAGE FOR ADULTS	DOSAGE FOR CHILDREN†
Standard regimen (oral)‡		
Amoxicillin	2 g	50 mg/kg
Penicillin allergy (oral)		
Clindamycin *or*	600 mg	20 mg/kg
Cephalexin‡ *or*	2 g	50 mg/kg
Clarithromycin or azithromycin	500 mg	15 mg/kg
Unable to take oral medications		
Ampicillin *or*	2 g IM or IV	50 mg/kg IM or IV
Cefazolin or ceftriaxone	1 g IM or IV	50 mg/kg IM or IV
Penicillin allergy and unable to take oral medications		
Clindamycin	600 mg IM or IV	20 mg/kg IM or IV
Cefazolin‡ or ceftriaxone‡	1g IM or IV	50 mg/kg IM or IV

Wilson W, Taubert KA, Gewitz M, et al: Prevention of infective endocarditis: Guidelines from the American Heart Association. A guideline from the American Heart Association Rheumatic Fever, Endocarditis and Kawasaki Disease Committee, Council on Cardiovascular Disease in the Young, and the Council on Clinical Cardiology, Council on Cardiovascular Surgery and Anesthesia, and the Quality of Care and Outcomes Research Interdisciplinary Working Group. JADA 2008;139(1):3S-23S, American Dental Association, 2007.

IM, Intramuscularly; *IV,* intravenously.

*Single dose 30 to 60 minutes before procedure.

†Total dose for children should not exceed adult dose.

‡Cephalosporins should not be used in patients with a history of immediate allergic reactions (urticaria, angioedema, anaphylaxis) to penicillin.

Table 8-37

Comparison of Antifungal Drugs

CLASS	EXAMPLES	MECHANISM OF ACTION	ADVERSE EFFECTS
Polyenes	a. Amphotericin B b. Nystatin	Combine with ergosterol to form membrane pores	a. Renal toxicity, hemolytic anemia, hypokalemia
Pyrimidine	Flucytosine	Converted to 5-fluorouracil in fungal cell and inhibits thymidylate synthase	Liver toxicity, alopecia, bone marrow suppression
Azoles	a. Ketoconazole	Inhibit ergosterol synthesis (inhibit 14-α-demethylase)	Hormone imbalance (especially ketoconazole), inhibit drug metabolism (especially ketoconazole), liver toxicity
a. Imidazoles b. Triazoles	a. Clotrimazole a. Miconazole b. Fluconazole B. Itraconazole		
Allylamines Benzylamines	Terbinafine Naftifine Butenafine	Inhibit ergosterol synthesis (inhibit squalene monooxygenase) Same as for allylamines	Liver toxicity (only terbinafine is used systemically) Topical only
Echinocandins	Caspofungin Micafungin Anidulafungin	Inhibit glucan synthesis	Release histamine
Other	Griseofulvin	Inhibits mitosis	Photosensitivity, induces liver metabolism, liver toxicity

O. Fluoroquinolones.
   1. Examples—ciprofloxacin, moxifloxacin, norfloxacin, levofloxacin, sparfloxacin.
   2. Spectrum (mostly aerobes) depends to a certain degree on the individual drug.
   3. Sensitive organisms and indications.
      a. *E. coli.*
      b. *H. influenzae.*
      c. *K. pneumoniae.*
      d. *N. gonorrhoeae.*
      e. *M. pneumoniae.*
      f. *L. pneumophila.*
      g. Moxifloxacin is also useful against anaerobes.
P. Bacitracin—topical peptide antibiotic with a spectrum similar to penicillin.
Q. Antituberculosis drugs (first-line)—combination therapy is used for active disease.
   1. Isoniazid—inhibits mycolic acid synthesis.
   2. Rifampin—inhibits DNA-dependent RNA polymerase.
   3. Ethambutol—inhibits synthesis of arabinogalactan.
   4. Pyrazinamide—inhibits mycolic acid synthesis.
   5. Rifabutin—inhibits DNA-dependent RNA polymerase.
R. Dental prophylaxis against bacterial endocarditis from a dental procedure (see Table 8-36).
S. Oral infections.
   1. Among the antibacterial drugs, penicillins are most commonly used for oral infections.
   2. Other antibiotics used for active oral infections.

   a. Macrolides.
   b. Clindamycin.
   c. Tetracyclines (special periodontal applications).
   d. Metronidazole (oral anaerobes).
   e. Others, based on culture and sensitivity tests.

Antifungal Drugs

A. Antifungal drugs (Table 8-37).
B. Comments on specific drugs.
   1. Amphotericin B.
      a. Used systemically.
      b. Very toxic.
      c. Given intravenously (in detergent or lipid medium).
   2. Nystatin.
      a. Used topically.
      b. Often used against oral candidiasis.
C. Indications (Table 8-38).
D. Dental applications—options for treating oral candidiasis.
   1. Clotrimazole oral troches.
   2. Nystatin oral pastilles or rinse.
   3. For more extensive disease.
      a. Fluconazole (oral).
      b. Itraconazole (oral).
      c. Caspofungin (intravenous).

Antiviral Drugs

Antiviral drugs attack the mechanisms used by the viruses to replicate and infect. The mechanism of action of most of

Table 8-38

Indications for Antifungal Drugs

DRUG	INDICATIONS
Amphotericin B	Most systemic fungal infections
Nystatin	Used primarily to treat *Candida albicans*
Clotrimazole, miconazole	Used topically to treat candidiasis
Fluconazole, itraconazole, posaconazole, voriconazole	Used systemically to treat various fungal infections
Flucytosine	Used systemically to treat a limited number of fungal infections (e.g., fungal meningitis)
Caspofungin, micafungin, anidulafungin	Used systemically to treat a limited number of fungal infections, including *Candida* species
Terbinafine	Used orally for dermatophytes
Naftifine	Used topically for dermatophytes
Butenafine	Used topically for dermatophytes

these drugs is to inhibit DNA or RNA synthesis and function. To the extent that this mechanism of action is selective for the virus, human toxicity of the drug is usually lessened. Table 8-39 shows the indications for the antiviral drugs. Table 8-40 shows the mechanism of action of antiviral drugs.

10.0 Antineoplastic Drugs

Antineoplastic drugs are used to inhibit various steps in cancer cell growth. However, these targets are also found in normal cells, and anticancer drugs lead to significant toxicity and have low margins of safety. Combination therapy is often used to enhance the anticancer effect. This approach is more desirable if the drugs have little overlapping toxicity. If possible, it is desirable to target cell components (e.g., enzymes) that are overexpressed in the cancer cell.

A. Mechanisms of antineoplastic drugs. Figure 8-30 shows the sites of action of several anticancer drugs. Figure 8-31 shows the action of anticancer drugs at cell cycle sites. Enzymes that are targets of anticancer drugs are listed in Table 8-41. Adverse effects are an important issue with anticancer drugs. These are presented in Tables 8-42 and 8-43.

B. Dental applications of cancer chemotherapy (Table 8-44).

Table 8-39

Indications for Antiviral Drugs

DRUG	INFLUENZA A	INFLUENZA B	HSV	VZV	CMV	HIV	RSV	HBV, HCV, HPV
Amantadine, rimantadine	+							
Oseltamivir, zanamivir	+	+						
Idoxuridine			+					
Vidarabine, trifluridine			+					
Acyclovir, valacyclovir			+	+				
Famciclovir, penciclovir			+	+				
Foscarnet			+	+	+			
Ganciclovir, valganciclovir					+			
Ribavirin							+	
Reverse transcriptase inhibitors*						+		
Integrase inhibitor (raltegravir)						+		
Protease inhibitors†						+		
Interferon α and α₂b								+

CMV, Cytomegalovirus; *HBV,* hepatitis B virus; *HCV,* hepatitis C virus; *HIV,* human immunodeficiency virus; *HPV,* human papillomavirus; *HSV,* herpes simplex virus; *RSV,* respiratory syncytial virus; *VZV,* varicella-zoster virus.

*Includes both nucleoside (e.g., zidovudine, didanosine, stavudine, zalcitabine, abacavir) and nonnucleoside (e.g., nevirapine, delavirdine) inhibitors.

†Includes saquinavir, indinavir, fosamprenavir, lopinavir, nelfinavir, and ritonavir.

Table 8-40
Mechanism of Action of Antiviral Drugs

DRUG	ANTIVIRAL MECHANISM
Amantadine	Blocks uncoating of virus and blocks replication
Oseltamivir	Inhibits neuraminidase
Vidarabine	Incorporated into DNA/inhibits DNA polymerase
Acyclovir	Inhibits viral DNA polymerase after undergoing phosphorylation
Famciclovir, penciclovir	Inhibit viral DNA polymerase after undergoing phosphorylation
Ganciclovir	Inhibits viral DNA polymerase after undergoing phosphorylation
Foscarnet	Inhibits viral DNA polymerase
Ribavirin	Inhibits several enzymes involved in RNA synthesis
Reverse transcriptase inhibitors	Inhibit viral RNA-dependent DNA polymerase
Protease inhibitors	Inhibit HIV protease and inhibit assembly of infectious virions

Table 8-41
Known Enzyme Targets of Antineoplastic Drugs*

TARGET	DRUG
Dihydrofolate reductase	Methotrexate
DNA polymerase	Cytarabine, fludarabine
Thymidylate synthase	5-Fluorouracil, capecitabine
Topoisomerase	Mitoxantrone, etoposide, teniposide, topotecan, doxorubicin, daunorubicin
Ribonucleoside diphosphate reductase	Hydroxyurea
Caspases	Arsenic trioxide
Tyrosine kinases	Imatinib, gefitinib
Aromatase	Anastrozole, letrozole
Histone deacetylase	Vorinostat

*All listed targets are inhibited by the corresponding drugs except for caspases, which are stimulated by arsenic trioxide.

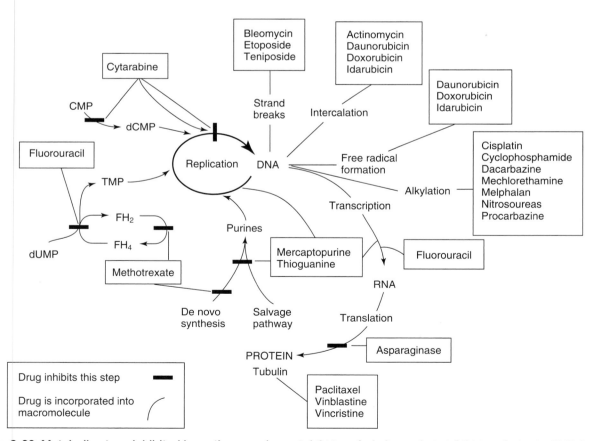

Figure 8-30 Metabolic steps inhibited by anticancer drugs. Inhibition of tubulin results in inhibition of mitosis. *CMP*, Cytidine monophosphate; *FH₂*, dihydrofolate; *FH₄*, tetrahydrofolate; *TMP*, thymidine monophosphate; *UMP*, uridine monophosphate. *(From Yagiela JA, et al: Pharmacology and Therapeutics for Dentistry, ed 6. St. Louis, Mosby, 2011.)*

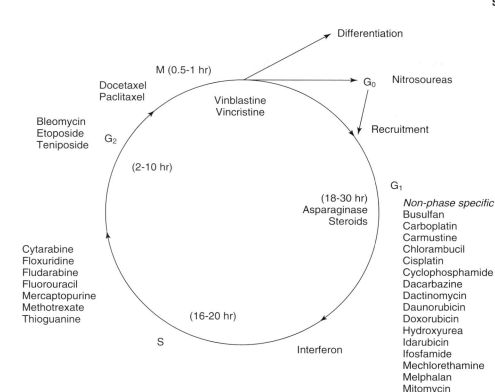

Figure 8-31 Cell cycle sites of anticancer drugs. DNA synthesis occurs during the S phase; M is mitosis and G_0 is the resting phase. *(From Yagiela JA, et al: Pharmacology and Therapeutics for Dentistry, ed 6. St. Louis, Mosby, 2011.)*

Table 8-42

Typical Adverse Effects of Most Antineoplastic Drugs

Myelosuppression	Alopecia
GI toxicity	Dermatotoxicity
Oral mucositis	

GI, Gastrointestinal.

11.0 Toxicology

Heavy metals are often toxic. Other compounds, such as gases and organic chemicals, may be toxic. It is important to know antidotes to the extent they have been identified as well as symptoms of more common toxins.

A. Common toxins and therapy (Table 8-45).

12.0 Prescription Writing

Prescriptions are written for a variety of drugs used in dentistry. The use of abbreviations and Latin terms is generally discouraged. Nevertheless, dentists should know the more common abbreviations used in prescriptions. More importantly, the dentist should know what is required in writing an unambiguous prescription.

A. Prescription

A sample prescription is shown in Figure 8-32, with the terms referring to the various parts of the

Table 8-43

Adverse Effects That Are More Unique to Certain Anticancer Drugs

ADVERSE EFFECT	DRUGS
Cystitis	Cyclophosphamide Ifosfamide
Neurotoxicity	Mechlorethamine Methotrexate Vinblastine Cisplatin Fluorouracil Paclitaxel Docetaxel Teniposide
Pulmonary toxicity, fibrosis	Chlorambucil Melphalan Carmustine Lomustine Bleomycin Mitomycin
Cardiac toxicity	Daunorubicin Doxorubicin Epirubicin Idarubicin Arsenic trioxide
Radiation recall	Daunorubicin Doxorubicin

prescription. Comments are made about various parts of the prescription. In almost every case, the use of generic drug names is preferred. Some states require the dispensing of generic drugs.

A prescription is required for all so-called *legend* drugs (those labeled by the FDA as "Rx only"). Prescriptions can also be used to prescribe over-the-counter drugs.

B. Prescription example (see Figure 8-32).

C. Tables 8-46 and 8-47 provide useful information related to prescriptions.

Table 8-46
Examples of Controlled (Scheduled) Substances

SCHEDULE	EXAMPLES
I	Heroin, 3,4-met hylenedioxymethamphetamine (Ecstasy) (Schedule I drugs may not be prescribed)
II	Morphine, cocaine, oxycodone, fentanyl
III	Codeine* plus acetaminophen tablets
IV	Phenobarbital, diazepam
V	Codeine† cough syrups

*<90 mg codeine per dose unit.

†≤2 mg/mL codeine.

Table 8-44
Adverse Oral Effects of Many Antineoplastic Drugs

EFFECT	TREATMENT
Stomatitis (including mucositis)	Palliative (rinses, protective agents, analgesics)
Salivary gland dysfunction*	Saliva substitutes, pilocarpine, cevimeline
Decreased resistance to infection	More aggressive chemotherapy against bacterial, fungal, and viral infections
Neutropenia, thrombocytopenia	Possible antibiotic prophylaxis for oral procedures, postpone elective surgery, reduce risk of bleeding

*Destruction of salivary gland tissue and resulting xerostomia has been more closely linked to radiotherapy to the head and neck.

Table 8-47
Common Latin Abbreviations and Two Common Weight and Volume Equivalents

b.i.d., t.i.d., q.i.d.	2, 3, 4 times a day
q4h	Every 4 hr
p.r.n.	As needed
Sig	Label
1 grain	= 65 mg
1 ounce	= 30 g or 30 mL

Table 8-45
Some Toxins, Toxic Symptoms, and Therapy

TYPE	TOXIN	SYMPTOMS	THERAPY*
Heavy metal	Mercury a. Elemental b. Inorganic c. Organic	Dyspnea, weakness, GI symptoms, gingivitis, tremor, salivation, kidney dysfunction, neurologic and visual disturbances	a. Chelation (dimercaprol or penicillamine or succimer) b. Chelation (penicillamine, succimer, polythiol resins) c. Chelation (penicillamine, polythiol resin in GI tract, succimer)
Heavy metal	Lead	Metallic taste, hemolysis, renal damage, colic, palsy, mental deterioration, anemia	Chelation (EDTA, dimercaprol, penicillamine, succimer)
Heavy metal	Copper	Anemia, proteinuria, swelling of liver, osteomalacia	Chelation (penicillamine)
Heavy metal	Iron	Abdominal pain, vomiting, acidosis, cardiovascular collapse	Chelation (deferoxamine)
Inorganic anion	Cyanide	Ashen gray appearance, coma, respiratory arrest	Sodium nitrite, sodium thiosulfate
Gas	Carbon monoxide	Mental confusion, tachycardia, coma	Oxygen

EDTA, Ethylenediaminetetraacetic acid; *GI*, gastrointestinal.

*In addition to supportive care.

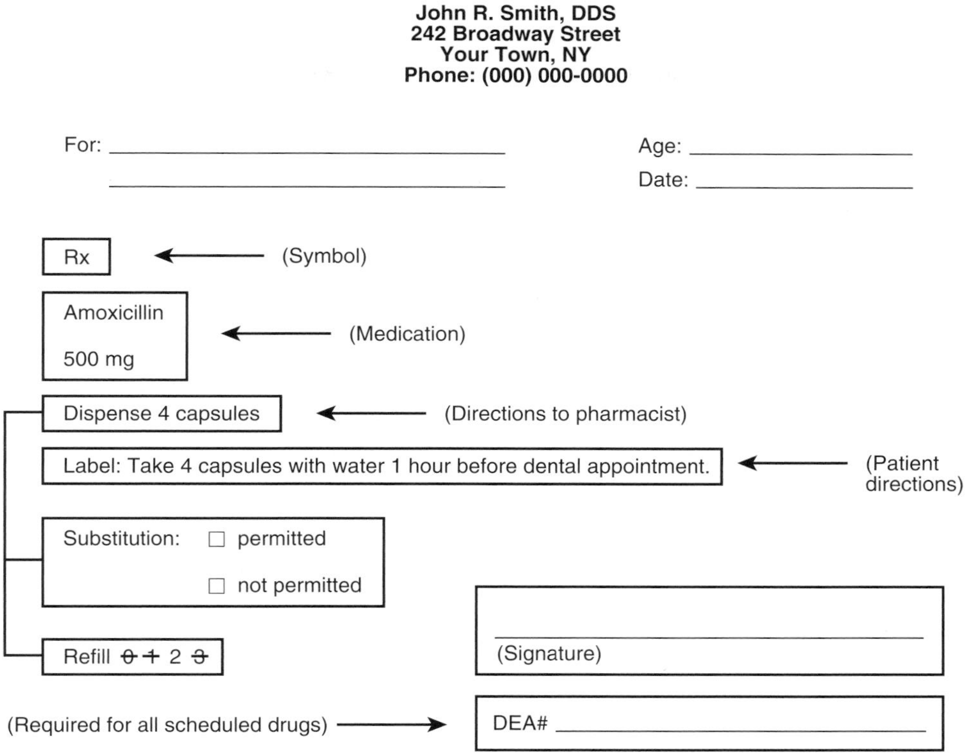

John R. Smith, DDS
242 Broadway Street
Your Town, NY
Phone: (000) 000-0000

For: _____   Age: _____

_____   Date: _____

Rx ← (Symbol)

Amoxicillin
500 mg ← (Medication)

Dispense 4 capsules ← (Directions to pharmacist)

Label: Take 4 capsules with water 1 hour before dental appointment. ← (Patient directions)

Substitution: ☐ permitted
                ☐ not permitted

Refill 0 1 2 3

(Signature)

(Required for all scheduled drugs) → DEA# _____

Figure 8-32 A prescription with various parts identified. In this case, the direction to the pharmacist is in three sections. Notice when the Drug Enforcement Administration (DEA) number is required. Notice the striking out of the unwanted refill numbers.

Bibliography

Ciancio SG, editor: *ADA/PDR Guide to Dental Therapeutics*, ed 5. Chicago, American Dental Association, 2009.

Hersh EV, et al: Reversal of soft tissue anesthesia with phentolamine mesylate in adolescents and adults. *J Am Dent Assoc* 139:1080, 2009.

Malamed SF: *Medical Emergencies in the Dental Office*, ed 6. St. Louis, Mosby, 2007.

Malamed SF: *Handbook of Local Anesthesia*, ed 6. St. Louis, Mosby, 2012.

Tavares M, et al. Reversal of soft tissue anesthesia with phentolamine mesylate in pediatric patients. *J Am Dent Assoc* 139:1095, 2009.

Yagiela JA, et al: *Pharmacology and Therapeutics for Dentistry*, ed 6. St. Louis, Mosby, 2011.

Sample Questions

1. Which drugs tend to concentrate in body compartments with a high pH?
   A. Permanently charged drugs
   B. Drugs that are not charged
   C. Weak organic acids
   D. Weak organic bases
   E. Inorganic ions

2. Drug agonists having the same intrinsic activity also have the same _____.
   A. Maximal effect
   B. Potency
   C. Receptor affinity
   D. Therapeutic index
   E. Aqueous solubility

3. What receptor or signaling pathway is linked *most* directly to α_2-adrenoceptor stimulation?
   A. G_i and a reduction in cAMP
   B. G_s and an increase in cAMP
   C. G_q and calcium
   D. Sodium ion channel
   E. Membrane receptor containing tyrosine kinase

4. What tissue or organ has many muscarinic receptors but lacks innervation to those receptors?
   A. Heart
   B. Parotid gland
   C. Blood vessels
   D. Sweat glands
   E. Urinary bladder

5. Which of the following drugs used in the therapy for parkinsonism does *not* cross the blood-brain barrier?
   A. Amantadine
   B. Carbidopa
   C. Levodopa
   D. Selegiline
   E. Tolcapone

6. After an injection, which of the following drugs would be expected to have the longest duration of action?

(Assume no vasoconstrictor was injected with the local anesthetic.)
   A. Bupivacaine
   B. Lidocaine
   C. Mepivacaine
   D. Prilocaine
   E. Procaine

7. A very low blood:gas solubility coefficient (partition coefficient = 0.47), analgesic effect, and ability to inhibit methionine synthase *best* describes which drug?
   A. Ketamine
   B. Nitrous oxide
   C. Halothane
   D. Isoflurane
   E. Propofol

8. Levonordefrin is added to certain cartridges containing mepivacaine. The desired effect of levonordefrin is due to what pharmacologic effect?
   A. Inhibition of nicotinic cholinergic receptors
   B. Inhibition of muscarinic cholinergic receptors
   C. Stimulation of α-adrenergic receptors
   D. Stimulation of β-adrenergic receptors
   E. Stimulation of dopamine receptors

9. Match each drug with its mechanism of action at the nerve terminal.

   A. Amphetamine _____
   B. Fluoxetine _____
   C. Botulinum toxin _____
   D. Tranylcypromine _____
   E. Physostigmine _____

   1. Blocks the release of a neurotransmitter.
   2. Inhibits an enzyme that metabolizes a neurotransmitter inside the nerve.
   3. Stimulates the release of a neurotransmitter from the cytoplasmic pool.
   4. Inhibits the metabolism of a neurotransmitter at the postjunctional or postsynaptic site.
   5. Prevents the reuptake of a neurotransmitter.

10. Naloxone antagonizes the therapeutic and toxic effects of which drug?
    A. Acetaminophen
    B. Aspirin
    C. Carbamazepine
    D. Fentanyl
    E. Ibuprofen

11. What is the mechanism of the analgesic action of aspirin?
    A. Stimulates μ opioid receptors
    B. Blocks histamine H_2 receptors
    C. Inhibits COX
    D. Inhibits lipoxygenase
    E. Blocks sodium channels in nerves

12. What is the clinical setting for the use of ketorolac by the oral route?
    A. For severe pain
    B. For initial treatment of pain
    C. To continue therapy after an intravenous or intramuscular dose of ketorolac
    D. Only in combination with an opioid
    E. Only in combination with an NSAID

13. At what cell type is the use of H_2 histamine receptor blockers *most* clinically useful?
    A. Beta cells of the pancreas
    B. Basophils
    C. Mast cells
    D. Juxtaglomerular cells
    E. Parietal cells

14. Which class of antihypertensive drug *most* effectively reduces the release of renin from the kidney?
    A. β-Adrenergic receptor blockers
    B. ACE inhibitors
    C. α-Adrenergic receptor blockers
    D. Calcium channel blockers
    E. Angiotensin II receptor blockers

15. The administration of _____ results in "epinephrine reversal" (decrease in blood pressure from epinephrine) if given before administration of epinephrine.
    A. Guanethidine
    B. Propranolol
    C. Phentolamine
    D. Tyramine

16. What is the mechanism of action of enoxaparin?
    A. Inhibition of synthesis of clotting factors II, VII, IX, and X
    B. Activation of antithrombin III with resulting inhibition of clotting factor Xa
    C. Indirect activation of tissue plasminogen activator
    D. Direct inhibition of plasminogen with resulting degradation of fibrin
    E. Dilation of coronary blood vessels

17. Oropharyngeal candidiasis is an adverse effect *most* likely to occur with _____.
    A. Inhaled salmeterol
    B. Inhaled ipratropium
    C. Inhaled nedocromil
    D. Inhaled beclomethasone
    E. Inhaled methacholine

18. Oral antacids are *most* likely to reduce the absorption of which of the following drugs when given orally?
    A. Clarithromycin
    B. Clindamycin
    C. Metronidazole
    D. Penicillin V
    E. Tetracycline

19. A decrease in glycogenolysis in the liver would be expected from which of the following drugs?
    A. Albuterol
    B. Epinephrine

C. Glucagon

D. Insulin

E. PTH

20. What effect does nitroglycerin have on blood vessel smooth muscle?

A. Increase in level of intracellular calcium

B. Increase in level of cyclic guanosine monophosphate (cGMP)

C. Antagonism at α_1-adrenergic receptors

D. Antagonism at β-adrenergic receptors

E. Inhibition of L-type calcium channels

21. Clavulanic acid offers an advantage therapeutically because _____.

A. It inhibits streptococci at a low MIC

B. It inhibits transpeptidase

C. It inhibits penicillinase

D. It inhibits anaerobes at a low MIC

E. It inhibits DNA gyrase

22. Inhibition of which of the following enzymes is *most* responsible for the cell wall synthesis inhibitory effect of penicillin G?

A. β-Lactamase

B. DNA gyrase

C. Nitro reductase

D. Transglycosylase

E. Transpeptidase

23. Which of the following drugs is often combined with sulfamethoxazole for the treatment of respiratory tract and urinary tract infections?

A. Amoxicillin

B. Ciprofloxacin

C. Clindamycin

D. Metronidazole

E. Trimethoprim

24. Which of the following organisms is usually sensitive to clindamycin?

A. *Candida albicans*

B. *Klebsiella pneumoniae*

C. Methicillin-resistant *Staphylococcus aureus*

D. Viridans streptococci

E. *Pseudomonas aeruginosa*

25. Which anticancer drug inhibits the enzyme dihydrofolate reductase?

A. Bleomycin

B. Cisplatin

C. Doxorubicin

D. 5-Fluorouracil

E. Methotrexate

26. A patient has been prescribed glipizide for type 2 diabetes. Arrange the following events, leading to a reduction in plasma glucose, in their order of occurrence as a result of this drug.

_____ A. Insulin release from beta cells

_____ B. Increase in glucose uptake in target cell

_____ C. Closing of ATP-sensitive potassium channels

_____ D. Movement of GLUT-4 to the plasma membrane

_____ E. Stimulation of insulin receptor

27. What events would occur after a submucosal injection of phentolamine in the oral cavity? (Choose three.)

A. Blockade of α-adrenergic receptors

B. Blockade of β-adrenergic receptors

C. Inhibition of sodium channels

D. Blockade of the vasoconstrictor effect of norepinephrine released from neurons

E. Inhibition of protein synthesis in oral bacteria

F. Antagonism of the vasoconstrictor effect of a subsequent injection of epinephrine in the same area of the oral cavity during the same dental appointment

28. Match the proper description with the drug.

_____ A. This is an antimuscarinic drug used to treat overactive bladder.

_____ B. This is an α_2-adrenergic receptor agonist used for intravenous sedation.

_____ C. This drug blocks serotonin 5-HT$_2$ and dopamine D$_2$ receptors and is used for schizophrenia.

_____ D. This sedative selectively inhibits a benzodiazepine receptor subtype.

_____ E. This antiepileptic drug binds to the $\alpha_2\delta$-1 subunit of the high-voltage calcium channel and blocks this channel.

1. Quetiapine
2. Gabapentin
3. Solifenacin
4. Codeine
5. Dexmedetomidine
6. Pilocarpine
7. Zaleplon
8. Carbamazepine

29. Match the enzyme with the drug that inhibits it.

_____ A. Acetylcholinesterase

_____ B. ACE

_____ C. Dipeptidyl peptidase-4

_____ D. DNA-dependent RNA polymerase

_____ E. 14 α-demethylase

_____ F. DOPA decarboxylase

_____ G. MAO B

1. Sitagliptin
2. Terbinafine
3. Aliskiren
4. Fluconazole
5. Neostigmine
6. Ciprofloxacin
7. Lisinopril
8. Lithium
9. Carbidopa
10. Selegiline
11. Rifampin

30. Select the drugs that antagonize the effect of pilocarpine on salivary flow rate. (Choose three.)
    A. Rivastigmine
    B. Benztropine
    C. Metoprolol
    D. Tolterodine
    E. Oxybutynin
    F. Epinephrine

31. Identify which drugs are commonly used in the treatment of herpes simplex viral infections. (Choose two.)
    A. Ganciclovir
    B. Indinavir
    C. Acyclovir
    D. Ribavirin
    E. Penciclovir
    F. Zidovudine

32. Match each adverse effect with the drug it is more typically associated with compared with the other drugs listed.

_____ A. Osteonecrosis of the jaw especially at high doses
_____ B. Cough in 10% of patients taking the drug
_____ C. First dose hypotensive effect
_____ D. Sedation
_____ E. Reye's syndrome in young patients with recent viral infection
_____ F. Methemoglobinemia

1. Terazosin
2. Acetaminophen
3. Pamidronate
4. Prilocaine
5. Lidocaine
6. Diphenhydramine
7. Aspirin
8. Clopidogrel
9. Fosinopril

Prosthodontics

ALEJANDRO PEREGRINA

This review with test questions is intended to serve as a study guide in preparing for the prosthodontic section of Part II of the National Board Dental Examination in the areas of fixed, complete, and removable partial prosthodontics and implant-supported prostheses. This review has been compiled and organized, for the most part, using the following textbooks: Rosenstiel SF, et al: *Contemporary Fixed Prosthodontics*, ed 4 (St. Louis, Mosby, 2006); Carr AB, et al: *McCracken's Removable Partial Prosthodontics*, ed 11 (St. Louis, Mosby, 2005); Zarb GA, et al: *Prosthodontic Treatment for the Edentulous Patient*, ed 12 (St. Louis, Mosby, 2004); Powers JM and Sakaguchi RL: *Craig's Restorative Dental Materials*, ed 12 (St. Louis, Mosby, 2006); Anusavice KJ: *Phillips' Science of Dental Materials*, ed 11 (Philadelphia, Saunders, 2003); and Okeson JP: *Management of Temporomandibular Disorders and Occlusion*, ed 5 (St. Louis, Mosby, 2003). The student is encouraged to consult these or other current textbooks for additional information.

1.0 General Considerations

A. Diagnosis and treatment planning.

Treatment planning in prosthodontics should be based on the individual patient's needs. According to Rosenstiel et al. (2006), treatment should accomplish the following: correct existing disease, arrest decay, prevent future disease, restore function, and improve appearance and oral hygiene.

The sequence, materials, and techniques chosen to treat a patient should take into consideration the expectations and objectives set forth. Partially edentulous patients can be restored with a fixed dental prosthesis (FDP), removable dental prosthesis (RDP), and implant-supported FDP.

1. Considerations when replacing missing teeth.
   a. FDP.
      (1) FDP abutments with half or less of bone support and loss of attachment have a poor prognosis.
      (2) Rigid fixed retainers should be at each end of the pontic except in a cantilever FDP.
      (3) A single retainer cantilever FDP has a poor prognosis.
      (4) Splinting teeth is generally done to distribute occlusal forces; this is recommended where the periodontal surface of the abutment tooth does not provide the needed support for a prosthesis (FDP or RDP).
      (5) Multiple-splinted abutment teeth, nonrigid connectors, or intermediate abutments can compromise the long-term prognosis.
      (6) When replacing the maxillary or mandibular canine, the central and lateral should be splinted to prevent lateral drifting of the FDP.
      (7) Compromised endodontically treated teeth should not be used as retainers.
      (8) Abutment teeth must align to a common path of insertion.
      (9) Occlusal forces that may cause drift or tooth mobility should be avoided.
      (10) Teeth with a short root/crown ratio ($<1:2$) with conical roots should be avoided as abutments.
      (11) Diverging multirooted, curved, and broad labiolingual roots are preferred over fused, single, conical, and round circumferential roots.
      (12) Teeth with a large root surface area (e.g., canines and molars) are better abutments than central incisors and premolars.

(13) The supportive surface area (periodontium) of the abutment teeth should be equal to, but not less than, that of the teeth to be replaced.

(14) Natural teeth exert more force than an RDP or complete denture when opposing an FDP.

b. Indications for RDP.

(1) Where teeth are missing and there are no posterior abutment teeth to support an FDP (distal extension).

(2) Where the span of teeth to be replaced is beyond the load that the existing teeth can bear with an FDP.

(3) Where there is bone loss with a questionable prognosis if restored with an FDP.

(4) Where the cost of an FDP or implants is prohibitive.

c. Complete denture.

(1) Used when all teeth are missing and when an implant-supported prosthesis cannot be used instead. Complete dentures are contraindicated when only the mandibular anterior teeth are present because severe damage to the opposing premaxilla occurs (combination syndrome).

d. Implant-supported prosthesis.

(1) Used for replacing single or multiple teeth instead of conventional FDP, RDP, and complete dentures.

(2) Use is dependent on available bone width and length, type of bone, bone volume, placement away from significant anatomic structures (nerves, adjacent teeth), interocclusal space, and osseointegration.

(3) Used in edentulous patients to support and improve the retention of complete dentures via attachments directly or indirectly retained by the implants.

B. Maxillomandibular relationships, interocclusal records, and anterior guidance—there are two maxillomandibular relationships in which the mandibular teeth can be oriented to the maxillary.

1. *Centric relation (CR)* is considered a terminal hinge position and is defined as "the maxillomandibular relationship in which the condyles articulate with the thinnest avascular portion of their respective discs with the condyle-disc complex in the anterior-superior position against the shapes of the articular eminences" (The glossary of prosthodontic terms, 2005).

2. Maximal intercuspal position, maximum intercuspation (MI), or centric occlusion is defined as "the complete intercuspation of the opposing teeth independent of condylar position" (The glossary of prosthodontic terms, 2005).

a. In 90% of people, CR and MI do not coincide.

b. Casts are often mounted in CR primarily to perform an occlusal analysis to determine whether occlusal corrections are necessary before any definitive prosthodontic treatment or where MI is impossible to maintain (e.g., multiple teeth to restore; complete dentures).

c. Accurate CR interocclusal records require precise manipulation of the mandible by the dentist. The *bimanual manipulation* technique described by Dawson (2007) is recommended.

d. The use of *anterior deprogramming devices* such as a *leaf gauge* or *acrylic resin jig* (known as a Lucia jig) keep the teeth apart and, when left for a determined period of time, can deprogram the existing proprioceptive reflexes and aid to manipulate the mandible into CR.

e. Most common materials used for interocclusal records are wax (Aluwax) and fast-setting elastomeric materials such as polyvinyl siloxane and polyether.

f. Casts mounted with an interocclusal record are mounted more accurately if the material used is selected according to the accuracy of the casts being articulated (casts produced with irreversible hydrocolloid are more accurately mounted with wax records, and casts obtained with elastomeric materials are more accurately mounted with elastomeric registration materials or zinc oxide–eugenol paste).

3. *Anterior guidance* must be preserved, especially when restorative procedures change the surfaces of anterior or posterior teeth that guide the mandible in excursive (lateral, protrusive) movements.

a. The *mechanical anterior guide table* provides limited adjustments that give insufficient information to reproduce the lingual contours of maxillary anterior natural teeth. Their use has been mainly for the fabrication of complete dentures and occlusal appliances.

b. *Custom incisal guide tables* are generally made of acrylic resin and are made to reproduce the surfaces of teeth (usually the lingual concavity and incisal edges of anterior teeth) that have a direct influence in guiding the mandible through all excursive movements.

C. Diagnostic impressions and casts.

1. *Irreversible hydrocolloid* or alginate is the material of choice to produce diagnostic casts. Composition is mainly sodium or potassium salts of alginic acid. The salts react chemically with calcium sulfate to produce insoluble calcium alginate. Diatomaceous earth is added for strength, and trisodium phosphate and other compounds are added to control the setting rate.

2. Most types of trays are suitable to produce acceptable, accurate impressions.

3. Tray adhesive should always be used to prevent distortion at the time of removal.

4. The greater the bulk that irreversible hydrocolloid has, the more favorable the surface area/volume ratio and the lower the susceptibility to water loss or gain and unwanted dimensional change.

5. The tray should be removed 2 to 3 minutes after gelation.

6. The impression should be rinsed and disinfected with glutaraldehyde or iodophor and should be poured within 15 minutes from the time the impression was removed from the mouth.

7. Pouring with American Dental Association type IV or V stone is recommended.

8. Poured impressions should be allowed to set undisturbed for the recommended time, which usually ranges from 30 to 60 minutes depending on the type of stone used.

9. To achieve less distortion of the irreversible hydrocolloid and maximum strength and surface detail of the cast, the poured impression can be stored for 45 minutes in a humidor.

10. Casts should be evaluated for inaccuracies such as voids and nodules that might interfere with proper articulation.

D. Articulators.
   1. *Hand-held casts* provide limited information with respect to the individual arches and tooth alignment.
   2. Nonadjustable articulator.
      a. Does not reproduce the full range of mandibular movement.
      b. The arc of closure is not the same as the patient's arc of closure because the distance between the hinge and the teeth is significantly shorter than in the patient. This difference may affect the construction of restorations, resulting in premature contacts and incorrect ridge and groove direction.
   3. *Semiadjustable articulators*—there are two types of articulators.
      a. *Arcon*, in which the condyles are attached to the lower member of the articulator, and the fossae are attached to the upper member. The mechanical fossae are fixed relative to the occlusal plane of the maxillary cast. This makes them more accurate for fabricating fixed restorations, especially when an interocclusal record is used to mount the mandibular cast.
      b. *Nonarcon*, which has the upper and lower members rigidly attached. The occlusal plane is relatively fixed to the occlusal plane of the mandibular cast. These articulators provide easier control in setting teeth for complete and partial dentures.
         (1) Semiadjustable articulators generally use an *arbitrary facebow* record; this orients the cast in the anterior-posterior and mediolateral position in the articulator to anatomic average values (e.g., the use of the external auditory meatus to stabilize the bow).
         (2) Some semiadjustable articulators allow the use of *kinematic facebows*, allowing more accuracy when mounting casts than with the use of arbitrary facebows. The kinematic facebow is placed on the *hinge axis* (the horizontal axis around which the mandible purely rotates when opening and closing), the location of which has been previously determined. Using the hinge axis is especially necessary when the vertical dimension is altered in the articulator or when an interocclusal record was made at a vertical dimension of occlusion different from the one to be used.
         (3) Most semiadjustable articulators permit some adjustments in the condylar inclination, lateral translation, Bennett angle (side shift), anterior guidance, and intercondylar distance.
   4. *Fully adjustable articulators*—these are capable of duplicating a wide range of mandibular movements but are generally set to follow the patient's border movements. The terminal hinge axis is located, and a pantograph is used to record the mandibular movements. These mandibular movement tracings or recordings are used to set the articulator. The information provided is useful to treat cases in which complex mandibular movements exist that require extensive occlusal mouth rehabilitation. The fully adjustable articulators use a *kinematic facebow* record to orient and articulate the maxillary cast. These articulators can be adjusted to repeat precisely the condylar inclination, Bennett angle (side shift), immediate side shift, rotating condylar movement, and intercondylar distance.

E. Restorative implantology.*

Implants allow patients with single or multiple missing teeth to benefit from implant-supported prostheses with a high degree of success. Implants can be divided in three major groups: *subperiosteal, transosteal,* and *endosteal.* Endosteal implants (root or cylinder, blades form implants) are the most common implants used today. Most implants are made of titanium or titanium alloy with or without hydroxyapatite coating. These materials have the highest biofunctionality. Threaded and nonthreaded designs are available. Many titanium implants today are grit-blasted or acid-etched to roughen the surface to increase the surface area contacting bone.
   1. Treatment planning.
      a. Indications for implants in partially edentulous patients.
         (1) Where there is inability to wear an RDP or complete denture.

---

*Compiled from Rosenstiel et al. (Ch. 13) and McGlumphy (Ch. 2).

(2) Where multiple teeth are missing and a long-span FDP is contraindicated.

(3) Unfavorable number and location of potential natural tooth abutments.

(4) Single tooth replacement that would necessitate preparation of unrestored or minimally restored teeth for an FDP.

b. Contraindications.

(1) Acute illness.

(2) Terminal illness.

(3) Pregnancy.

(4) Uncontrolled metabolic disease.

(5) Unrealistic patient expectation.

(6) Improper patient motivation.

(7) Lack of operator experience.

(8) Inability to restore with prosthesis.

c. Clinical and radiographic evaluation.

(1) Detection of flabby excess tissue.

(2) Bony ridges.

(3) Sharp underlying osseous formations.

(4) Undercuts that would limit implant insertion.

(5) Posterior maxillary and mandibular bone width is visually determined.

(6) Panoramic radiograph is best for initial view to determine approximate bone height and lingual nerve location.

(7) Cephalometric radiographs are used to determine anterior maxillary and mandibular widths.

(8) Computed tomography scans give more accurate information of anatomic landmarks, but higher radiation and expense may limit their use.

d. Preimplantation preparation.

(1) Diagnostic casts to determine the following.

(a) Maxillomandibular relationships.

(b) Interocclusal space.

(c) Existing dentition.

(d) Implant site placement with the aid of diagnostic wax-up.

(e) Construction of surgical templates.

2. Implant placement.

a. Principles for implant placement.

(1) Should be placed entirely in bone.

(2) Must be placed away from significant structures such as inferior alveolar nerve canal, sinus, and incisive foramen.

(3) Ideally, should be placed engaging two cortical plates of bone.

(4) When placing several implants, they should be at least 3 mm apart and 1 mm away from an adjacent tooth (Figure 9-1).

(5) Restorative needs should dictate possible implant selection.

(6) In an elderly edentulous patient, a reduction in the number of implants is recommended: two

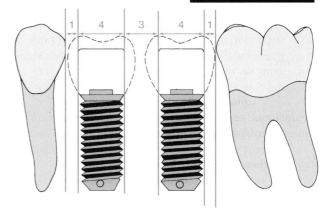

Implants should be placed at least 3 mm apart and 1 mm from adjacent teeth.

Figure 9-1 Recommended minimum distances (in millimeters) between implants and between implants and natural teeth. *(From Rosenstiel SF, Land MF, Fujimoto J: Contemporary Fixed Prosthodontics, ed 4. St. Louis, Mosby, 2006.)*

in the mandible and four in the maxilla (Carr et al. [Ch. 29]).

(7) For additional considerations regarding placement in the maxilla and the mandible, refer to Rosenstiel et al. (Ch. 13).

b. Implant-supported restorations.

(1) Implants support screw-retained or cement-retained restorations.

(2) Implant bodies can be a one-stage restoration, in which the implant bodies project through the soft tissue with a cover screw after surgical placement, or a two-stage restoration, in which, after placement, a cover screw is placed and covered with soft tissue, to be uncovered in a second operation.

(3) Abutment placements are screwed directly into the implant.

(4) Adequate healing time before impression making is 2 weeks in noncritical esthetic areas and 3 to 5 weeks in esthetic areas.

(5) Abutment size and angulation selection depend on the interocclusal space available, the implant long axis position and the orientation of multiple implants to be restored, and type of implant-supported prosthesis to use.

(6) Fixed, detachable prostheses (acrylic resin and metal framework) are indicated where soft tissue and teeth are being replaced with a prosthesis supported by implants (a minimum of five in the mandible and six in the maxilla are recommended) instead of a conventional complete denture (Box 9-1).

Box 9-1

Advantages of Osseointegrated Implants

1. Surgical

a. Documented success rate
b. In-office procedure
c. Adaptable to multiple intraoral locations
d. Precise implant site preparation
e. Reversibility in the event of implant failure

2. Prosthetic

a. Multiple restorative options
b. Versatility of second-stage components
   (1) Angle correction
   (2) Esthetics
   (3) Crown contours
   (4) Screw-retained or cement-retained options
c. Retrievability in the event of prosthodontic failure

From Rosenstiel SF, Land MF, Fujimoto J: *Contemporary Fixed Prosthodontics,* ed 4. St. Louis, Mosby, 2006.

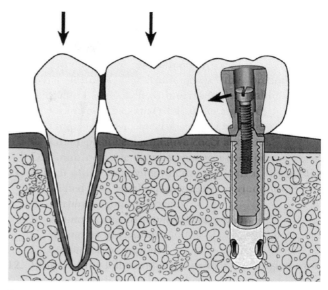

Figure 9-2 When a single implant is attached to a natural tooth, biting forces on the natural tooth and pontic cause stress to be concentrated at the superior portion of the implant. *(From Rosenstiel SF, Land MF, Fujimoto J:* Contemporary Fixed Prosthodontics, *ed 4. St. Louis, Mosby, 2006.)*

c. Guidelines when placing an implant-supported prosthesis.
   (1) Attaching implants to natural teeth is not recommended.
   (2) Two implants can support a three-unit FDP when the crown/implant ratio is favorable.
   (3) If implants are short and crowns are long, one implant to replace each missing tooth is highly recommended.
   (4) When heavier occlusal load is expected, additional implants are recommended to support multiple units or a long edentulous span.
   (5) If retaining the prosthesis by implants and natural teeth, protecting the teeth with telescopic copings (six) is recommended. A single implant attached to a natural tooth causes concentration of stress at the superior portion of the implant (Figure 9-2).
d. Cement-retained implant crown.
   (1) More economical (in some systems).
   (2) Allows minor angle corrections to compensate for discrepancies between the implant inclination and the facial crown contour.
   (3) Easier to use in small teeth than screw-retained implant crown.
   (4) Requires more chair time and has the same propensity to loosen.
e. Screw-retained implant crown.
   (1) Retrievability allows for crown removal, facilitating maintenance (e.g., soft tissue evaluation, calculus removal).
   (2) Future modification capability.
   (3) Access hole is through the occlusal table of posterior teeth or lingual of anterior.
   (4) Main disadvantage is that the screw may loosen during function because of excessive lateral forces, excessive cantilever force, or improperly screwed crowns.
3. *Occlusion*—similar occlusion principles apply to natural teeth and to implants.
   a. Occlusal forces should be directed in the long axis of the implant.
   b. Lateral forces in the posterior part of the mouth are greater and more destructive than lateral forces in the anterior part of the mouth.
   c. When unable to eliminate lateral forces, the occlusion should be balanced so that the stress is distributed over as many teeth as possible (Figure 9-3).

2.0 Complete Dentures

A. Examination.
   1. Clinical examination—one of the purposes of the clinical examination is to detect (recognize) problems in the supporting structures of the denture that might compromise the success of the prosthesis. It includes examination and diagnosis of supporting structures, tongue, floor of mouth, temporomandibular joint, and any existing prosthesis. Critical areas that are frequently missed are tuberosity, retromolar pad, buccal undercuts of tuberosities, and mandibular tori.

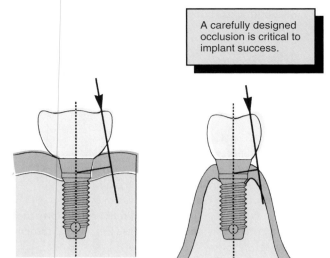

A carefully designed occlusion is critical to implant success.

Figure 9-3 Sharper cusp inclines and wider occlusal tables increase the resultant force on implant components. *(From Rosenstiel SF, Land MF, Fujimoto J:* Contemporary Fixed Prosthodontics, *ed 4. St. Louis, Mosby, 2006.)*

2. Radiographic examination.
  a. Residual root tips.
    (1) *General rule*—root tips with no radiolucency and cortical margin of bone intact may remain; however, the patient should be informed of their presence and risk and of the need to have them removed in the future. They should be removed if the cortical plate is perforated or the periodontal ligament or radiolucent area is enlarging.
  b. Radiolucencies and radiopacities.
    (1) Assess if normal (e.g., salivary gland depression).
B. Conditions that compromise the optimal function of complete dentures.
  1. Preprosthetic treatment.
    a. Soft tissue surgery.
      (1) *Frenectomy*—common for labial, less for buccal, rare for lingual.
        (a) *Labial*—attachment close to ridge crest interferes with good seal and possibly esthetics.
        (b) *Lingual*—high attachment is rare; familial; usually causes speech problem and is noted in children. Historically, lingual frenectomies were performed in children for this condition. Today, speech therapy is generally recommended instead.
        (c) *Surgery*—Z-plasty must include fibrous attachment to bone.
      (2) *Free gingival graft*—necessary for some overdenture teeth.

(3) *Pathologic conditions.*
(4) *Hypermobile ridge*—if inflamed, treat with a tissue conditioner.
  (a) Change one to two times weekly to maintain resiliency of conditioner and healing effect. If effective (2 to 3 weeks), may proceed with impression; in hypermobile tissue, use large relief in the tray or perforate a custom tray.
  (b) If tissue conditioner is ineffective, use electrosurgery or laser surgery to eliminate tissue.
  (c) *Caution:* this procedure might also eliminate the vestibule and risk making it even more difficult to attain a seal. Immediately after surgery, a soft liner must be placed to prevent epulis fissurata from forming.
(5) *Epulis fissurata*—hyperplastic tissue reaction caused by an ill-fitting or overextended flange in a denture.
  (a) *Treatment*—adjust denture border and use tissue conditioner; surgery is indicated if inadequate response.
(6) *Fibrous maxillary tuberosity*—common when large maxillary tuberosities contact mandibular retromolar pads. Radiographs can aid in determining whether soft tissue reduction alone would suffice. Soft relining immediately prevents further problems secondary to an ill-fitting denture.
(7) *Combination syndrome*—believed to be a specific pattern of bone resorption in the anterior portion of edentulous maxillae, caused by wearing a complete denture opposing anterior teeth (partial dentate).
(8) *Benign soft tissue lesions*—excisional biopsy, then reline denture.
(9) *Unknown lesions.*
  (a) Excisional biopsy.
  (b) Incisional biopsy.
  (c) Brush biopsy.
b. Nonsurgical pathologic conditions.
  (1) *Papillary hyperplasia*—found in the palatal vault. Multiple papillary projections of the epithelium caused by local irritation, poor-fitting denture, poor oral hygiene, and leaving dentures in all day and night. Candidiasis is the primary cause.
    (a) *Treatment*—educate patient in oral hygiene; advise patient to leave denture out at night; soak dentures for 30 minutes in a 1% solution of sodium hypochlorite and rinse thoroughly; use tissue conditioner (see *hypermobile ridge* earlier). Patient should brush irritated area lightly with a soft brush.

(2) *Candida albicans—Candida* is characterized by pinpoint hemorrhage or white patches or both. A cytologic smear should be performed to confirm infection.

    (a) *Treatment*—use nystatin or clotrimazole pastilles (note: both contain sugar and should be avoided in diabetic patients) or clotrimazole or nystatin powder in oral suspension. Laser surgery and electrosurgery are difficult and painful on the palatal tissue; because it is easy to go through tissue to bone, it is preferable to try local treatment first.

(3) *Paget's disease of bone*—bone disease characterized by bone resorption followed by attempts at bone repair, leading to bone deformities. The etiology is unknown, and it occasionally involves the maxilla and mandible. A denture or RDP in a patient with this disorder may have to be remade periodically because of bone expansion.

c. *Hard tissue surgery* to eliminate interferences to prosthesis placement.

  (1) *Alveoloplasty*—the improvement of the alveolar bone by surgical reshaping or removal.

  (2) *Pendulous tuberosities* can occur unilaterally or bilaterally and can interfere with denture construction by limiting interarch space. Surgical excision of fibrous tissue, which can be accompanied by bone, is indicated.

  (3) Sharp, spiny, or extremely irregular ridges.

d. Exostoses and tori removal.

  (1) Palatal torus is removed in the following situations.

    (a) It is so large that it fills the vault and prevents the formation of an adequate denture base when it is undercut.

    (b) It extends too far in the posterior direction and interferes with placement of the posterior palatal seal.

    (c) It disturbs the patient psychologically (cancer phobia).

e. Soft tissue surgery (to increase denture base area).

  (1) *Vestibuloplasty*—this technique increases the relative height of the alveolar process by apically repositioning the alveolar mucosa and the buccinator, mentalis, and mylohyoid muscles as they insert into the mandible. After the vestibuloplasty, the periosteum is uncovered. Usually a mucosal graft (from cheek or palate) is placed over the periosteum. If necessary, the use of customized acrylic resin templates or the patient's modified dentures can be used to support the vestibuloplasty in the mandible.

    (a) Lingual vestibuloplasty is more traumatic and is rarely indicated.

  (2) *Reposition neurovascular bundle* (i.e., mental nerve).

f. Augmentation.

  (1) *Bone grafts*—sources include anterior iliac crest of hip and rib. Resorption is unpredictable; often lose greater than 75%.

  (2) *Hydroxyapatite*—biocompatible bone substitute; available as resorbable, nonresorbable, solid, and particulate.

  (3) *Freeze-dried bone.*

  (4) *Connective tissue.*

g. Implants.

C. Occlusion.

1. The *CR record* of an edentulous patient provides the ability to increase or decrease the vertical dimension of occlusion more accurately in the articulator by establishing a radius of the mandible's arc of closure.

2. A *protrusive record* registers the anterior-inferior condyle path at one particular point in the translatory movement of the condyles. Some clinicians use this type of record to determine the amount of space between maxillary and mandibular teeth or occlusal rims to maintain balanced occlusion throughout the mandibular functional range of movement when articulating teeth.

  a. *Christensen's phenomenon* refers to the distal space created between the maxillary and mandibular occlusal surfaces of the occlusion rims of dentures when the mandible is protruded. It is caused by the downward and forward movement of the condyles.

3. *Vertical dimension of rest* or *physiologic rest position of the mandible* is the position when the elevator and depressor muscles are in a state of equilibrium or balance. This position most commonly results in a separation of the maxillary and mandibular teeth of about 3 mm at the first premolar region. This separation is called the *interocclusal space.*

  a. Effects of excessive vertical dimension of occlusion.

    (1) Excessive display of mandibular teeth.

    (2) Complaint of fatigue of muscles of mastication.

    (3) Clicking of the posterior teeth when speaking.

    (4) Strained appearance of the lips.

    (5) Patient unable to wear dentures.

    (6) Discomfort.

    (7) Excessive trauma to the supporting tissues.

    (8) Gagging.

  b. Effects of insufficient vertical dimension.

    (1) Aging appearance of the lower third of the face because of thin lips, wrinkles, chin too near the nose, overlapping corners of the mouth.

    (2) Diminished occlusal force.

    (3) Angular cheilitis (occurs in conjunction with candidiasis).

4. Plane of occlusion—the plane of orientation for complete denture construction is established in the anterior-posterior direction with the maxillary occlusal wax rim parallel to *Camper's line*, which is an imaginary line traced from the ala of the nose to the tragus of the ear, and with the *interpupillary line* in the transverse plane, which is an imaginary line drawn between the pupils of the eyes.

5. Balanced occlusion.
   a. Balanced occlusion requires that the maxillary lingual cusps of the posterior teeth on the non-working side contact the lingual incline of facial cusps of mandibular posterior teeth in conjunction with balanced contact of teeth in the working side.
   b. As the condylar inclination increases, the compensating curve must increase to keep a balanced occlusion.
   c. Anterior guidance in complete denture occlusion should be avoided to prevent dislodgment of the denture bases.

D. Phonetic considerations in the patient with complete dentures.
   1. Speech sounds.
      a. *Fricatives or labiodental sounds f, v, ph* (e.g., "51," "52") are made between the maxillary incisors contacting the wet/dry lip line of the mandibular lip (labiolingual center to the posterior third of the mandibular lip). These sounds help determine the position of the incisal edges of the maxillary anterior teeth.
      b. *Linguoalveolar sounds or sibilants* (sharp sounds: *s, z, sh, ch,* and *j,* with *ch* and *j* being africatives) are made with the tip of the tongue and the most anterior part of the palate or lingual surface of the teeth. These sounds help determine the vertical length and overlap of the anterior teeth. The tongue's anterior dorsum forms a narrow opening near the midline. When there is a small opening, the result is a whistling sound. If the space is large, the *s* sound will be developed as an *sh* sound, like a lisp. A whistling sound with dentures is indicative of having a posterior dental arch form that is too narrow (sounds like "61," "62," "church").
      c. *Linguodental sounds* (tip of the tongue slightly between the maxillary and mandibular teeth, such as "this," "that," "those") help determine the labiolingual position of the anterior teeth. The way *th* sounds are made provides information regarding the labiolingual position of the anterior teeth. If the tip of the tongue is not visible, the teeth most likely are too far anterior (except in class II malocclusion or where there is excessive vertical overlap). The opposite occurs where the tongue extends too far out—the teeth are most likely too far lingual.
         (1) *Vertical dimension*—evaluate during pronunciation of the *s* sound; the interincisal

separation should be 1 to 1.5 mm. This is known as the *closest speaking space.*
      d. The *b, p,* and *m* sounds are made by contact of the lips. Insufficient lip support by the teeth or the labial flange can affect the production of these sounds.

E. Anatomic considerations in complete denture fabrication.
   1. The limiting structures of the maxillary denture.
      a. *In the anterior region*—the labial vestibule, which extends from the right buccal frenum to the left; laterally, from the right and left buccal vestibules extending in the posterior aspect on each side to the right and left hamular notches, respectively.
      b. The *posterior limit* extends to junctions of movable and immovable tissue; this coincides with the line drawn through the hamular notches and approximately 2 mm anterior to the foveae palatina (vibrating line).
      c. *Support for a maxillary complete denture* is provided by the maxillary and palatine bones.
   2. Limiting structures of the mandibular denture.
      a. The *mandibular anterior labial area* extends from the labial frenum to the right and left buccal frenums. The action of the mentalis muscle and the mucolabial fold determines the extension of the denture flange in this area. The mentalis elevates the lower dentures unless this border is established by accurate border molding.
      b. The *mandibular labial frenum* is a band of fibrous connective tissue that helps attach the orbicularis oris muscle. A wide opening stretches and creates a narrow sulcus that limits the extension of the denture border and the thickness of the denture base and affects the position of the mandibular teeth. If the teeth are set too far labial, stability is adversely affected.
      c. The *buccal vestibule* extends posteriorly from the buccal frenum to the lateral posterior corner of the retromolar pad. The buccal vestibule is influenced by the buccinator muscle, which extends from the modiolus anteriorly to the pterygomandibular raphe posteriorly and has its lower fibers attached to the buccal shelf and the external oblique ridge. Proper extension in this area provides the best support for the lower denture. The buccinator muscle fibers run in an oblique fashion and have little displacing action. This area is referred to as the *buccal shelf.* Proper extension is necessary to distribute the load of mastication more widely.
      d. In the *masseter area*, the denture is limited in a lateral direction by the action of this muscle. When the patient occludes with force, a medial force is exerted against this area of the denture base. If this border is overextended, extreme soreness can result.

e. The *retromolar pad* marks the distal termination of edentulous ridge. This structure needs to be covered for support and retention. The integrity of bone in this area is maintained and allows for support.

f. In the *lingual frenum area*, the borders must be established with movements of the tongue. The denture should not be overextended; excessive reduction can result in almost total loss of denture retention. The genioglossus muscle influences the length of this flange during normal movements of the tongue.

g. The *sublingual gland area*—maximum extension desired without overextension. The tongue may rest on this area, helping to retain the denture.

h. The *mylohyoid area*—the flange in this area must accommodate the movement of the muscle in deglutition. In most instances, the flange extends below the mylohyoid ridge. Initially, the extent of this flange is determined by the elevation of the floor of the mouth when the patient wets the lips with the tip of tongue. It is then modified to accommodate this muscle for deglutition.

i. The *retromylohyoid area*—perhaps the most difficult region to manage. This area is limited posteriorly by the action of the palatoglossus muscle and inferiorly by the lingual slip of the superior constrictor muscle. These muscles are activated on swallowing and if impinged on, a sore throat develops.

3. *Maxillary and mandibular lip support* in a patient with complete dentures is provided by the facial surfaces of teeth and the denture base.

F. Retention and stability related to final impression and occlusion.

1. *Denture support* refers to resistance to vertical seating forces.

2. *Denture stability* is necessary to resist dislodgment of a denture in the horizontal direction.

3. *Denture retention* is the ability of the denture to withstand dislodging forces exerted in the vertical plane.

a. Surfaces of a denture that play a part in retention.

(1) *Intimate contact* of the denture base and its basal seat.

(2) *Teeth*—no occlusal prematurities to break retention.

(3) *Design of the labial, buccal, and lingual polished surfaces*—configuration harmonious with forces generated by the tongue and musculature.

b. Factors that influence denture impression surface.

(1) *Adhesion*—saliva to denture and to tissues: primary retentive force.

(a) Proportionate to area covered.

(b) *Close adaptation*—tissue thickness, tissue health, tissue displacement.

(2) *Cohesion* (attraction of molecules for each other) depends on the following.

(a) Area covered.

(b) Type of saliva (thick, ropy—unfavorable; thin, watery—greater retention).

(3) Atmospheric pressure.

(a) Proportionate to area covered.

(b) Depends on peripheral seal.

(c) Effective only when dislodging forces applied.

(4) *Mechanical*—ridge size, shape (undercuts), and interridge distance.

G. Management of abused tissues.

1. Treatment plan for tissue recovery.

a. Removal of dentures.

(1) Abnormal mucoperiosteum beneath the dentures is best treated by complete removal of the dentures until the tissues return to a normal size, shape, color, consistency, and texture. Even the most healthy mouth should receive a 24-hour rest period.

b. Dentures should be kept clean after meals by rinsing them and brushing them (soft brush with no abrasives) at least once a day to remove plaque buildup. They should be soaked for at least 30 minutes in a denture disinfectant solution, which is commercially available.

c. If the patient has dry mouth (*xerostomia*), a saliva substitute or continuous sips of water may be needed.

d. *C. albicans* is normal in the oral cavity, but under trauma or antibiotic usage it may cause generalized inflammation (*candidiasis*). It may involve the corners of the mouth (*angular cheilitis*), which is common in patients with diminished vertical dimension.

e. Therapy.

(1) Nystatin oral rinse four times a day: hold in the mouth for 2 minutes, then expectorate.

(a) Nystatin oral suspension (contains sugar—caution with diabetic patients).

(b) Dispensed: 60 mL of 100,000 units/mL.

(c) Instructions: 4 mL three times daily. After each meal, rinse mouth for 2 minutes.

(2) Nystatin (with triamcinolone acetonide) cream—used for angular cheilitis.

(a) Dispensed: 15-g tube.

(b) Instructions: apply to affected area a small amount four times daily (after meals and bedtime) for 14 days.

(3) See Section 8, Pharmacology, for more options.

f. Resilient liners for dentures—if the tissues are abused, the use of soft acrylic resin liners for several days may be needed for complete recovery. These are placed inside the patient's old dentures to provide an even, cushioned bearing against the mucoperiosteum and aid recovery during periods when the patient must wear dentures.

H. Immediate dentures.
1. Advantages.
   a. The patient avoids the embarrassing period of being without teeth.
   b. Immediate dentures produce the least possible change in the patient's facial appearance because it enables one to place the individual artificial teeth in the exact positions that the natural teeth occupied.
2. Disadvantages.
   a. Wax try-in may not be possible, depending on how many teeth remain before the delivery day. The remaining teeth are extracted at the same time that the denture is scheduled to be delivered.
   b. More time is required for construction and adjustment.
   c. Greater cooperation from the patient is necessary.
   d. Earlier need for rebasing.
3. Technique.
   a. Most procedures are similar to the construction of conventional complete dentures. The main difference is in the impression, which can be challenging because of severe tooth and ridge undercuts. Tray modifications and impression material selection are important to deal with this problem.
   b. The denture teeth are placed by removing the teeth from the cast and placing them in a similar position the natural teeth occupied when the teeth were in an acceptable vertical and horizontal position.
   c. A second problem is that an esthetic tooth try-in generally is not possible because of the presence of

teeth that will be extracted on the day of the denture delivery.
   d. For a detailed description of the technique, review Zarb and Bolender (2004).
I. Overdentures.
1. The advantage is the retention of roots, which decreases bone resorption, while maintaining the proprioceptive fibers within the periodontal ligament.
2. Selection of maxillary teeth as overdenture abutments (Table 9-1).
J. Insertion and postinsertion.
1. Insertion.
   a. Check intaglio surface of denture with finger for nodules or sharp places.
   b. Check contour of polished surface.
   c. Check extension of peripheries with pressure-indicating paste. Reduce lingual flanges in molar area to actual floor of mouth with tongue in opposite cheek.
   d. Check thickness of flanges and any possible interference of the coronoid process against buccal flange of maxillary denture.
   e. Check freedom of frenal and muscle attachments.
   f. Check for pressure areas on impression surface of dentures with pressure-indicating paste. Use digital pressure only, one denture at a time. Special attention is given to hard palate and mylohyoid ridge areas.
   g. Complete final maxillomandibular relation procedures and correction of occlusion. At the time of placement of complete dentures, small occlusal discrepancies are often noted, even though a laboratory remount has been done to correct

Table 9-1

Considerations in Selection of Maxillary Teeth as Overdenture Abutments

MAXILLARY TEETH	ADVANTAGES	DISADVANTAGES
Central incisors	Ideal location; provide protection of the premaxilla	Proximity and alveolar prominence may complicate use
Lateral incisors	Widely separated, facilitating plaque control Tissue undercuts do not pose a problem Path of placement/removal is not compromised Ability to create a flange/peripheral seal	Diminished root surface area
Canines	Longest root of anterior teeth	Diverging facial tissue undercuts Overcontoured flanges Excessive lip support Potentially uncomfortable placement/removal of prosthesis Complicates placement of prosthetic teeth Internal relief to accommodate canines may weaken, create a food trap, compromise peripheral seal

From Zarb GA, Bolender CL: *Prosthodontic Treatment for Edentulous Patients*, ed 12. St. Louis, Mosby, 2004.

laboratory errors. If this is the case, use articulating paper (preferably horseshoe-shaped) to determine premature contacts in CR and in excursions after CR is corrected.

2. Postinsertion.

a. If major occlusal discrepancies are present, a new interocclusal record is made with Aluwax or with an elastic registration material.

b. Occlusal adjustment is checked most accurately in an articulator with accurately remounted dentures with an interocclusal record.

c. *Cheek biting* is due to insufficient horizontal overlap between maxillary and mandibular teeth. It occurs between the facial surface of mandibular teeth and the central aspect of the maxillary teeth. Reducing the facial of mandibular posterior teeth in question can solve the problem.

d. *Overextension* usually causes dislodgment of the denture.

3.0 Removable Partial Prosthodontics

A. Kennedy classification system (Figure 9-4).

1. Class I—bilateral edentulous areas located posterior to the remaining natural teeth.

2. Class II—unilateral edentulous area located posterior to the remaining natural teeth.

3. Class III—unilateral edentulous area with natural teeth remaining both anterior and posterior to it.

4. Class IV—single, but bilateral (crossing the midline), edentulous area located anterior to the remaining teeth.

B. Applegate's rules governing the application of Kennedy classification system.

1. Rule 1—classifications should follow rather than precede any extractions of teeth that might alter the original classification.

2. Rule 2—if a third molar is missing and not to be replaced, it is not considered in the classification.

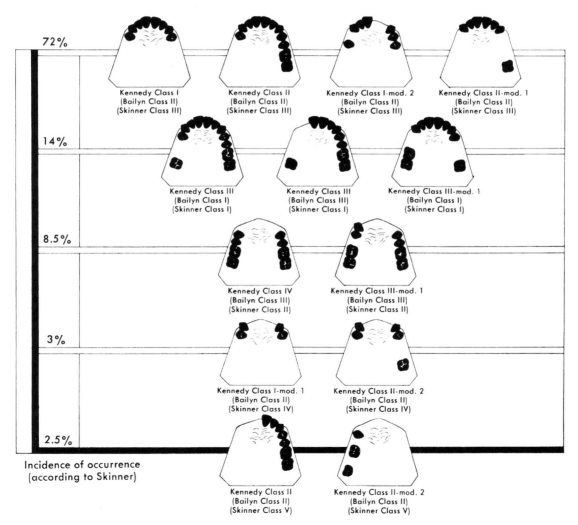

Figure 9-4 Representative examples of partially edentulous arches classified by the Kennedy, Bailyn, and Skinner methods. *(From Carr AB, McGivney GP, Brown, DT: McCracken's Removable Partial Prosthodontics, ed 11. St. Louis, Mosby, 2005.)*

3. Rule 3—if a third molar is present and is to be used as an abutment, it is considered in the classification.
4. Rule 4—if a second molar is missing and is not to be replaced, it is not considered in the classification.
5. Rule 5—the most posterior edentulous area always determines the classification.
6. Rule 6—edentulous areas other than those determining the classification are referred to as modifications and are designated by their number.
7. Rule 7—the extent of the modification is not considered, only the number of additional edentulous areas.
8. Rule 8—there can be no modification areas in class IV arches.

C. Components of an RDP and their use.
  1. Major connectors.
    a. The *function* of the major connector is to connect all the RDP components of one side of the arch with the opposite side to unite them.
    b. Provides *stability* to resist displacement while in function.
    c. Major connector should be *rigid* and not be placed on movable tissue.
    d. Undercut areas and soft and bony prominences (e.g., tori, median palatal suture) should be avoided, removed, or relieved, depending on the severity.
    e. *Relief* should be provided to prevent tissue impingement secondary to distal extension denture rotation.
  2. Types of major connectors.
    a. Maxillary arch.
      (1) *Anterior-posterior palatal strap*—the most rigid major connector for the amount of tissue covered; used in almost any Kennedy class of partial design, especially class II and IV. All major connectors should cross the midline at a right angle rather than on a diagonal.
      (2) *Single palatal strap*—indicated in tooth-borne RDP (Kennedy class III) with bilateral, short-span edentulous areas. The palatal strap should be wide and thin for strength and comfort. The anterior border should be posterior to the rugae.
      (3) *Palatal plate*—can be designed as a wide palatal strap short of the rugae area for distal extension RDP where more than the anterior teeth are present. A complete palatal plate is the most rigid of all major connectors and is indicated when all posterior teeth are missing bilaterally; in a Kennedy class I, modification 1 RDP; and for periodontally compromised teeth, shallow vault, small mouth, or flat or flabby ridges. Various design configurations exist, combined with acrylic resin coverage (see Carr et al., pp. 49-51).
      (4) *U-shaped palatal (horseshoe)*—the least rigid maxillary connector; used only when other, more rigid designs cannot be used. It is commonly used when a large, inoperable palatal torus exists or when anterior teeth need replacement.
      (5) *Single palatal bar*—a palatal bar, by definition, is less than 8 mm in width because the strap width is greater than 8 mm. The bar must be centrally located in the framework and needs bulk to be rigid to provide the needed cross-arch support.
      (6) *Anterior-posterior palatal bars*—similar to the single bar and are configured similarly to the anterior-posterior palatal strap. The main disadvantage is the bar's needed bulk.
    b. Mandibular arch.
      (1) *Lingual bar*—shaped like a half-pear tapered toward the tissue in the superior border and has its greater bulk at the inferior border. For a lingual bar, the depth of the vestibule should exceed 7 to 8 mm. This is the simplest and most commonly used major connector.
      (2) *Lingual plate*—this major connector may be used when the depth of the lingual vestibule is less than 7 mm, when additional loss of teeth is anticipated, when lingual tori are present, and when all posterior teeth are to be replaced bilaterally.
      (3) *Labial bar (swinglock)*—a hinged continuous labial bar located buccal and distal to the remaining dentition. It has a latching mechanism opposite to the hinge. It is indicated when there is a missing canine (e.g., teeth #22, #23, #24, #25, #26), where there are unfavorable tooth or soft tissue contours, and when there are teeth with questionable periodontal prognosis.

  3. A *minor connector* is a rigid component that connects the major connector or base with other components of the partial denture such as rests, indirect retainers, and clasps.
  4. *Beading* is the procedure of scribing a rounded groove (0.05 mm) outlining the anterior and posterior borders of a maxillary major connector. Beading an RDP adds strength to the major connector and maintains tissue contact to prevent food impaction.
  5. *Direct retainer*—the purpose of a clasp is to retain the RDP by means of the abutments. Clasps need adequate encirclement (greater than one half the tooth circumference), retention (retentive arm), stability (minor connector and rest), support (rest), and passivity when seated (engaging the undercut when a dislodging force is applied) (Table 9-2). To prevent horizontal movement of the clasp, this should encircle the tooth more than 180 degrees or one half the circumference of the tooth.
    a. *Retentive clasps* should become active only when dislodging forces are applied to them.

Table 9-2

Function and Position of Clasp Assembly Parts

COMPONENT PART	FUNCTION	LOCATION
Rest	Support	Occlusal, lingual, incisal
Minor connector	Stabilization	Proximal surfaces extending from a prepared marginal ridge to the junction of the middle and gingival one third of abutment crown
Clasp arms	Stabilization (reciprocation)	Middle one third of crown
	Retention	Gingival one third of crown in measured undercut

From Carr AB, McGivney GP, Brown DT: *McCracken's Removable Partial Prosthodontics,* ed 11. St. Louis, Mosby, 2005.

b. There are two types of direct retainers.

(1) *Intracoronal retainer*—composed of a prefabricated machined key and keyway (precision attachment). They are more esthetic than the extracoronal retainer because they eliminate clasps, and the vertical rest directs the forces through the horizontal axes of the abutment teeth.

(2) *Extracoronal retainer*—these are the most common.

(a) *Suprabulge* (originate above the survey line).

(i) Circumferential clasp.

(ii) Ring clasp.

(iii) Combination clasp.

(iv) Embrasure clasp.

(v) Manufactured attachments with interlocking devices (Dalbo attachments) or the use of spring-loaded devices that engage a tooth contour to resist occlusal displacement. These devices have manufactured attachments with flexible clips or rings that engage a rigid cast or attached component to the external surface of an abutment crown.

(b) *Infrabulge* (originate below the survey line).

(i) I bar.

(ii) T bar.

(iii) Bar type.

(iv) Y type.

c. Clasp selection guidelines.

(1) RPI (rest, proximal plate, I bar) and RPC or RPA (rest, proximal plate, and a cast circumferential clasp or an Akers clasp) designs are generally used in Kennedy class I and II arch forms.

(2) Reduction in the torqueing force on abutment teeth is achieved with the use of a wrought wire clasp system; indicated for periodontally weakened teeth or endodontically treated teeth.

(3) A wrought wire direct retainer is indicated if retention is placed on the opposite side of the fulcrum line from the edentulous ridge.

(4) Kennedy class III arch forms use the circumferential design. The occlusal rest seats are located adjacent to the edentulous spaces.

(5) In a distal extension situation, the order of preference of use of clasp assembly is RPI, RPC, and wrought wire.

6. A *reciprocal clasp* or *stabilizing clasp* arm originates from the minor connector and rest. The reciprocal clasp should contact the tooth on or above the height of contour of the tooth, allowing for insertion and removal with passive force. Generally, they are placed on the lingual side.

7. The *indirect retainer* is the component of an RDP located on the opposite side of the fulcrum line to the extension base. It assists the direct retainer to prevent displacement of denture base in an occlusal direction. It consists of one or more rests, their minor connectors, and proximal plates adjacent to the edentulous areas. The indirect retainer should always be placed as far as possible from the distal extension base.

8. *Rests* are critical for the health of the soft tissues underlying the denture resin basis and the minor and major connectors. It should prevent tilting action and should direct forces through the long axis of the abutment tooth.

a. Types of rests.

(1) *Occlusal rest.*

(a) Has a rounded (semicircular) outline form.

(b) One third facial lingual width.

(c) One half width between cusps.

(d) 1.5 mm deep for base metal.

(e) Floor inclines apically toward center.

(f) The angle formed with the vertical minor connector is less than 90 degrees.

(2) *Cingulum rest.*

(a) Inverted "V" or "U" shape.

(b) Mesiodistal length 2.5 to 3 mm.

(c) Labiolingual width 2 mm.

(d) Incisoapical depth 1.5 mm.

(e) Generally contraindicated for mandibular central and lateral incisors.

(3) *Incisal rest.*
(a) Rounded notch at an incisal angle.
(b) 2.5 mm wide; 1.5 mm deep.
(c) Used as an indirect retainer.
(d) Less favorable leverage than lingual rest.
(e) Seldom used because of esthetic compromise.

9. *Proximal plate*—a metal plate that contacts the proximal surface or guide plane of an abutment tooth.

10. *Guide planes*—two or more parallel surfaces in the abutment teeth that provide a path of insertion and removal and can contribute to the retention of an RDP. Guiding planes are parallel to the path of placement of the RDP, preferably to the long axes of the abutment teeth. They should be about one third of the buccolingual width of the tooth and extend 2 to 3 mm vertically from the marginal ridge in the cervical direction.

D. Type of support for RDPs.
1. *Tooth-borne RDPs* should have the rests located next to the edentulous area, providing less opportunity for the framework to flex, and assist in proper placement together with the guide planes.
2. *Distal extension RDPs* rotate when a force is directed on the denture base because of displacement of the soft tissue of the residual ridge and the ligament of the abutment teeth. The altered cast technique records the form of the edentulous segment by means of the metal RDP framework, which holds the custom tray material.

E. Insertion and postinsertion.
Just as in the FDP, the tooth-supported RDP should provide direct resistance to functional forces. Changes in tissue support need to be evaluated with time in the tooth tissue–supported RDP to maintain proper stability.

F. Material science.
1. *Acrylic resins*—the *mechanical properties* of acrylic resin denture bases are affected by several factors.
a. The *molecular weight* of the polymer is indicative of how well the polymethyl methacrylate was cured. The greater the molecular weight, the better the polymerization and the harder the resin.
b. The degree of *cross-linking* within the final polymer is directly proportional to the degree of polymerization.
c. A polymer with a greater molecular weight is formed if more cross-linking occurs.
d. *Shrinkage* of an acrylic resin occurs but is increased when excessive monomer is incorporated to the polymer during the mixture. The volumetric monomer/polymer ratio is 1:3.
e. *Porosity* on an acrylic resin denture base is caused by underpacking with resin at the time of processing or a thick denture base heated too rapidly.
f. *Chemical composition* of denture base resins.

2. *Cobalt-chromium RDPs* fracture when the physical properties of an alloy are altered by the following.
a. *Cold-working*—reduces the percentage elongation. This causes an increase in hardness, which makes the alloy more susceptible to fracture. Chronic flexure of the clasp assembly as an RDP is seated and dislodged as well as during function has the effect of work hardening.
b. These alloys are known to *shrink* approximately 2.3%. This shrinkage is irregular because of irregularities in framework design, and the result is porosity. Sprues used in the thicker sections can reduce shrinkage.
c. A low percent elongation is directly related to greater brittleness. Carbon is present and reacts with other constituents to form carbides. These last during casting and appear in the grain boundaries, which embrittle the alloy.
d. Cobalt-chromium alloys are more rigid compared with gold and palladium alloys.

4.0 Fixed Prosthodontics

A. Tooth preparation for cast fixed prostheses (see Rosenstiel et al.).
1. Conservation of tooth structure by *partial coverage* instead of complete coverage whenever possible is preferred.
2. Minimal *taper* between axial walls conserves tooth structure, prevents undercuts, enhances resistance, and enhances retention (6-degree taper between walls is recommended).
3. Remove tooth structure evenly, considering the morphology of the *pulp.*
4. *Tooth preparation* should allow sufficient space for developing contours and occlusal morphology that is biologically, technically, and esthetically functional (see *buccolingual dimension* later under "Considerations for restoring teeth in a biological, mechanical, and esthetic form"). The labial reduction should be in two planes to avoid overtapering or lack of occlusal clearance or insufficient space for porcelain.
5. Prepare *margins* that are readable and compatible with the materials selected and the design of the final restoration.
6. Margins ideally should be placed *supragingivally* or at the gingival crest whenever possible, for maintenance care, ease of preparation, and impression.
7. Well-executed *finish lines* that are smooth and even facilitate tissue displacement, impression making, die fabrication, waxing, and finishing procedures.
8. Foundation restorations or *cores* should be built to restore missing tooth structure before preparing teeth for crowns.

9. Surgical *crown lengthening* can improve the outcome of a short clinical crown or when the placement of a margin impinges on the normal soft tissue attachment. It is important to maintain the *biologic width* (the combined width of the connective tissue attachment and the junctional epithelium, which averages approximately 2 mm).

10. Factors that affect *retention* are magnitude of the dislodging forces (e.g., sticky food), geometry of the tooth preparation, roughness of the fitting surface of the restoration, the materials being cemented, and the film thickness of the luting agent.

11. *Cements* act by increasing the frictional resistance between tooth and restoration. The cement grains prevent two surfaces from sliding, although they do not prevent one surface from being lifted from another.

12. *Grooves* should be included for additional retention and resistance in short clinical crowns or when retention is compromised.

13. Grooves or *boxes* added to a preparation with good retention do not increase retention significantly, but where a groove limits the path of withdrawal, retention is improved.

14. Teeth with a *large surface area* are more retentive (e.g., long axial walls versus short; molars versus premolars).

15. Root canal–treated teeth restored with *core build-ups* or *post and cores* can serve as abutments. Teeth with short roots or little remaining coronal structure are not recommended because failures can occur.

B. Considerations for restoring teeth in a biologic, mechanical, and esthetic form.
   1. The following are considerations when restoring teeth.
      a. Axial contours should correspond to the *emergence profile* (usually flat or concave) of the tooth to prevent plaque accumulation, gingival inflammation, and bone loss.
      b. The *buccolingual dimension* of a cast restoration is usually determined by the occlusal morphology of the opposing tooth.
      c. *Occlusal point contacts* between opposing teeth are preferred to broad, flat occlusal contacts to prevent wear.
      d. Two *occlusal schemes* are recognized: cusp–marginal ridge and cusp-fossa. Class I occlusion (in general) and unworn teeth have a cusp–marginal ridge scheme. A cusp-fossa arrangement is generally found in class II malocclusion.
      e. Supragingival *margins* are preferred over subgingival (see previously under "Tooth preparation for cast fixed prostheses").
      f. The material used must provide sufficient *strength* to prevent deformation during function. Type I

and II gold alloys are used for intracoronal cast restorations. Type III and IV gold alloys or an alternative to gold alloy are used for crowns and FDPs.
      g. A minimum *metal thickness* of 1.5 mm over centric or occlusal bearing cusps and 1.0 mm over non-bearing or noncentric cusps is needed to withstand occlusal forces when metal alone is used and 2.0 mm when porcelain is used.
      h. Sufficient space for metal (0.5 mm) at the *margin* is required to prevent distortion during function and construction of the restoration (casting, porcelain firing).
      i. Adequate *porcelain thickness* (1.5 mm minimum) is needed to obtain good esthetic results.
      j. The appropriate *retainer* for a tooth with a short clinical crown is a complete crown.
      k. *Partial veneer crowns* include three quarter and seven eighths crowns. Their advantages include conservation of tooth structure, margins being accessible for finishing procedures and inspection, and margins being accessible for hygiene.
   2. A *pontic design* can be classified in two categories: *mucosal* contact and *nonmucosal contact* pontics (Table 9-3).
      a. *Mucosal pontics*—ridge lap, modified ridge lap, ovate, conical, or bullet shape. All of these pontics should be concave and passively contact the ridge.
      b. *Nonmucosal pontics*—sanitary (hygienic) and modified sanitary (hygienic). These are generally used in nonesthetic areas.
      c. A *saddle pontic design* covers the ridge labiolingually, forming a concave area that is not cleansable and for that reason is not used.
   3. Connectors for FDP.
      a. *Rigid connectors.*
         (1) Cast (one-piece casting).
         (2) Soldered (see later under "Dental Materials").
      b. *Nonrigid connector*—indicated when it is impossible to obtain a common path of insertion between FDP abutments.
C. Tissue management for making impressions.
   1. *Fluid control*—saliva can be controlled by the following.
      a. Mechanical means (saliva ejectors, cotton rolls, paper wafers).
      b. Medications such as atropine, propantheline, and hyoscyamine act as antisialogogues (reduce salivary secretions) and should be used with caution.
         (1) Anticholinergic drugs should not be prescribed for patients with glaucoma, especially narrow-angle glaucoma. In the latter case, these drugs can lead to a rapid increase in intraocular pressure and blindness. Anticholinergic drugs should be used with caution in patients with heart disease and patients with urinary retention.

Table 9-3

Pontic Designs

PONTIC DESIGN	APPEARANCE	RECOMMENDED LOCATION	ADVANTAGES	DISADVANTAGES	INDICATIONS	CONTRAINDICATIONS	MATERIALS
Sanitary/ hygienic	2 mm	Posterior mandible	Good access for oral hygiene	Poor esthetics	Nonesthetic zones Impaired oral hygiene	Where esthetics is important Minimal vertical dimension	All-metal
Saddle-ridge-lap		Not recommended	Esthetic	Not amenable to oral hygiene	Not recommended	Not recommended	Not applicable
Conical		Molars without esthetic requirements	Good access for oral hygiene	Poor esthetics	Posterior areas where esthetics is of minimal concern	Poor oral hygiene	All-metal Metal-ceramic All-resin
Modified ridge-lap		High esthetic requirement (e.g., anterior teeth and premolars, some maxillary molars)	Good esthetics	Moderately easy to clean	Most areas with esthetic concern	Where minimal esthetic concern exists	Metal-ceramic All-resin All-ceramic
Ovate		Very high esthetic requirement Maxillary incisors, canines, and premolars	Superior esthetics Negligible food entrapment Ease of cleaning	Requires surgical preparation Not for residual ridge defects	Desire for optimal esthetics High smile line	Unwillingness for surgery Residual ridge defects	Metal-ceramic All-resin All-ceramic

From Rosenstiel SF, Land MF, Fujimoto J: *Contemporary Fixed Prosthodontics*, ed 4. St. Louis, Mosby, 2006.

(2) Glycopyrrolate is an anticholinergic agent used as an adjunct in treatment of peptic ulcer that also reduces secretions.

2. Modes to achieve tissue displacement—tissue displacement is necessary to expose a prepared tooth finish line. This can be achieved by mechanical, a combination of mechanical and chemical, and surgical means.

   a. Mechanical modes.

     (1) *Cords*—stretch the circumferential periodontal fibers by placing them in the gingival sulcus. They can be twisted, braided, or knitted and be preimpregnated or be impregnated with a chemical solution. They are supplied in different size ranges with different diameters, which are selected according to the size of the sulcus to be displaced.

   b. *Mechanical/chemical—impregnated cords* provide better sulcus displacement. Chemicals that contain *aluminum* or *iron* salts cause transient ischemia and shrinkage of the gingival tissue and absorb seepage of gingival fluid. Among these are *aluminum chloride, aluminum sulfate, ferric sulfate,* and *ferric chloride.* Cords preimpregnated with *epinephrine* should be avoided because they can cause tachycardia.

   c. Surgical.

     (1) *Electrosurgery*—when a cord by itself might not achieve the desired tissue displacement, electrosurgery is indicated. To remove minor tissue, the electrosurgery unit is set to a fully rectified electrical current (unmodulated alternating current) and a small electrode.

     (2) Considerations when using electrosurgery.

       (a) It is *contraindicated* in patients using medical devices such as cardiac pacemakers, a transcutaneous electrical nerve stimulation unit, or an insulin pump and in patients with delayed healing.

       (b) Not recommended for thin attached gingiva.

       (c) Use plastic instruments (e.g., mirror, saliva evacuators) instead of metal to prevent burning and tissue destruction of the surface contacted.

       (d) Rapid, single, light stroke made with the electrode.

       (e) When cutting, 5-second intervals should be used.

       (f) The electrode should not contact metallic restorations or tooth structure because this may cause irreversible pulp damage.

D. Impression materials.

Elastic impression materials for final impressions for fixed restorations include reversible hydrocolloid, polysulfide, condensation silicone, polyether, and additional silicone. Advantages, disadvantages, and recommended uses are summarized in Table 9-4. Their composition is as follows:

1. *Reversible hydrocolloids*—These are agar hydrocolloids that, when heated, change from gel to sol between 71° C and 99° C; on cooling, they return to the gel state at 30° C. To heat and temper the material, special equipment is needed. Special trays with internal tubing that connect to a water line are used to cool the material.

2. *Polysulfide polymer*—the base paste main component is a polysulfide polymer, a filler to add strength (titanium dioxide), a plasticizer (dibutyl phthalate), and an accelerator (sulfur). The *reactor* (catalyst) contains lead dioxide and the same filler found in the base, a retarder to control the setting reaction (oleic or steric acid). On polymerizing, *water* is released as a by-product causing dimensional contraction. The cast must be poured within 45 minutes.

3. *Condensation silicone*—the main component in the *base* is polydimethylsiloxane with fillers such as calcium carbonate or silica. The *accelerator* may be stannous octate suspension and alkyl silicate. Similar to polysulfides, the condensation silicones release *alcohol* as a by-product reaction of their polymerization, causing dimensional contraction.

4. *Polyether*—the base paste contains a polyether polymer, colloidal silica as filler, triglycerides, and nonphthalate plasticizer. The *accelerator* paste contains an alkyl-aromatic sulfonate, filler, and a plasticizer. This material has excellent dimensional stability owing to the fact that no volatile by-products are formed. It is very susceptible to change by water absorption. The material is very stable, but it is recommended that the cast be poured promptly for greater accuracy.

5. *Addition silicone (vinyl polysiloxane)*—the addition reaction polymer is terminated with a vinyl group and cross-linked with hydride groups activated by a platinum salt catalyst. No reaction by-products are developed, but hydrogen gas release may occur if a reaction between moisture and residual hydrides of the base polymer occurs. The result is a cast with small voids if the impression is poured soon after removal from the mouth. Platinum or palladium is added by the manufacturer to act as a scavenger for the hydrogen gas. Another option is to wait an hour before pouring to allow the release of gas.

E. Metal-ceramic restorations.

1. Classifications of alloys for metal-ceramic restorations.

   a. *Noble metals* are gold (Au), platinum (Pt), and palladium (Pd). (Silver [Ag] is not considered noble; it is reactive and improves castability but can cause porcelain "greening.")

Table 9-4

Available Elastic Impression Materials

	ADVANTAGES	DISADVANTAGES	RECOMMENDED USES	PRECAUTIONS
Irreversible hydrocolloid	Rapid set Straightforward technique Low cost	Poor accuracy and surface detail	Diagnostic casts Not suitable for definitive casts	Pour immediately
Reversible hydrocolloid	Hydrophilic Long working time Low material cost No custom tray required	Low tear resistance Low stability Equipment needed	Multiple preparations Problems with moisture	Pour immediately Use only with stone
Polysulfide polymer	High tear strength Easier to pour than other elastomers	Messy Unpleasant odor Long setting time Stability only fair	Most impressions	Pour within 1 hr; allow 10 min to set
Condensation silicone	Pleasant to use Short setting time	Hydrophobic Poor wetting Low stability	Most impressions	Pour immediately Take care to avoid bubbles when pouring
Addition silicone	Dimensional stability Pleasant to use Short setting time Automix available	Hydrophobic Poor wetting Some materials release H_2 Hydrophilic formulations imbibe moisture	Most impressions	Delay pouring of some materials Take care to avoid bubbles when pouring
Polyether	Dimensional stability Accuracy Short setting time Automix available	Set material very stiff Imbibition Short working time	Most impressions	Take care not to break teeth when separating cast

From Rosenstiel SF, Land MF, Fujimoto J: *Contemporary Fixed Prosthodontics*, ed 4. St. Louis, Mosby, 2006.

---

b. *High noble alloys* (old term was precious metal) have a noble metal content of 60 wt% or greater and a gold content of 40% or greater.

c. *Noble alloys* (old term was semiprecious metal) have a noble metal content of 25% or greater. (Palladium-copper [Pd-Cu], palladium-silver [Pd-Ag], and palladium-cobalt [Pd-Co] alloys have no stipulation for gold.)

d. *Base metal alloys* (old term was nonprecious metal) contain less than 25% noble metals (nickel-chromuim [Ni-Cr], nickel-chromium-beryllium [Ni-Cr-Be], cobalt-chromium [Co-Cr], titanium [Ti], and Ti alloys).

2. Desirable properties of alloys for metal-ceramic restorations.

 a. Mechanical properties.

 (1) *High yield strength*—minimizes permanent deformation under occlusal force and porcelain fracture secondary to framework deformation.

 (2) *High modulus of elasticity (stiffness)*—minimizes flexure of long-span FDPs and porcelain fracture secondary to framework deformation.

 (3) *Casting accuracy*—base metal alloys are less accurate than gold.

(4) *Biologic compatibility*—can be a problem with Ni and Be in base metal alloys (allergies), and Be dust and vapors are carcinogens.

(5) Corrosion resistance.

(6) The metal coefficient of thermal expansion should be higher than the porcelain to leave the porcelain in compression in a stronger state.

 b. Metal composition.

 (1) *Color*—white, silver, yellow, or gold, depending on its alloy composition (percent of Au, Ag, Pd, and Pt).

 (2) *Density*—base metals are least dense; consider the weight of long-span FDPs.

 (3) *Oxidative elements*—must be present for porcelain to bond to the alloy (tin, indium, and gallium).

3. Bonding of porcelain to metal.

 a. The tooth preparation reduction for metal-ceramic restorations (1.5 to 2.0 mm) must provide space for metal (0.5 mm) and porcelain (1.0 to 1.5 mm).

 b. A metal substructure provides support and increases the strength of the porcelain.

 c. All internal angles where porcelain is veneered should be rounded to prevent stress concentration.

d. The metal-porcelain junction should be at a right angle to avoid porcelain fracture.

e. Occlusal contacts at least 1.5 mm away from porcelain-metal junction.

f. Metal oxide formation is necessary for metal-ceramic bond (*oxidation* of a metal is accomplished by heating the metal structure in a furnace before the application of porcelain).

g. The coefficient of thermal expansion of the porcelain must be slightly lower than that of the metal to place the porcelain in slight compression when cooled.

h. Porcelain is stronger under compressive forces than it is under tensile forces.

4. Metal-ceramic restoration—*porcelain* is composed primarily of feldspar (main constituent), quartz (to strengthen), kaolin (binder), and metallic oxides (give opacity and color). Three layers of porcelain are used to build a ceramic restoration.

a. *Opaque porcelain* must mask the dark oxide color and provide the porcelain-metal bond. Bond strength depends on good wetting of the metal surface. Masking must be accomplished with the minimum thickness of opaque—about 0.1 mm—leaving maximum space to develop a natural appearance with body and incisal porcelains.

b. *Body or dentin porcelain* contains most of the color or shade and is used generally to build most of the crown.

c. *Incisal porcelain* is the most translucent layer of porcelain.

5. Shade selection and color.

a. *Hue* refers to shade or color (red, green, yellow). In the *Vita Lumin Vacuum Shade Guide* (now called Vita Classical Shade Guide; Vita, Bad Sackingen, Germany), A1, A2, A3, A3.5, and A4 are hues similar to the B, C, and D shades. The hue should be selected first.

b. *Chroma* is the saturation or intensity of the color or shade. Once the hue is selected (e.g., A, B, C), the saturation of that hue is selected (e.g., if the B hue was selected, the saturation would be B1, B2). It is always better to choose a shade with a lower chroma, which is easier to alter with surface colorant modifiers.

c. *Value* is the relative lightness or darkness of a color. Shade guides can be arranged in order of increasing lightness to determine whether the value of a tooth is within the range of the shade guide.

d. *Metamerism* is the phenomenon where a color match under a lighting condition appears different under a different lighting condition.

e. *Fluorescence* is the physical property where an object emits visible light when exposed to ultraviolet light (e.g., the dentinal layer of a tooth when exposed to ultraviolet light emits reflected light).

f. *Opalescence* is the light effect of a translucent material (incisal edge of some teeth) appearing blue in reflected light and red-orange in transmitted light.

g. The *Vitapan 3D-Master Shade Guide* (Vita, Bad Sackingen, German) is arranged in five lightness levels and a level for bleached teeth. Each lightness level has sufficient variations in chroma and hue to cover the natural tooth color space.

6. *Characterization*—the art of reproducing natural defects; this can be particularly successful in making a crown blend with the adjacent natural teeth.

a. Chroma and hue adjustment.

(1) The addition of yellow stain increases the chroma of a basically yellow shade. Addition of orange has the same effect on a crown as a yellow-red hue. Too high a chroma is impossible to decrease in hue or increase in value.

(2) *Hue adjustments*—pink-purple moves yellow toward yellow-red, whereas yellow decreases the red content of a yellow-red shade. These are the only two modifications that should be necessary because the hue of a natural tooth always lies in the yellow-red to yellow range.

b. *Value adjustments*—adding a complementary color can reduce value. Violet is used on yellow restorations, which has the added effect of mimicking translucency. Gray is not encouraged because it produces a semitranslucent effect and makes the surface cloudy.

c. *Staining* can cause a loss of fluorescence in the finished restoration and an increase in the metameric effect (a mismatch under some lighting conditions). It usually results in decrease of value.

d. *Glazing*—the degree of gloss or surface luster of a porcelain restoration depends on the autoglazing procedure. Both time and temperature must be carefully controlled. During glazing, the surface layers of porcelain melt slightly, coalescing the particles and filling in surface defects. Glazing must be performed without vacuum.

7. Metal-ceramic failures.

a. Modes of failure in metal-ceramic restorations.

(1) Adhesive failure modes.

(a) Porcelain-metal interface—oxide was not formed.

(b) Oxide-metal interface—contamination of metal.

(c) Porcelain-oxide interface—contamination of oxide surface.

(2) Cohesive failure modes.

(a) Porcelain-porcelain—inclusions or voids; "preferred" type of failure.

(b) Oxide-oxide—oxide layer too thick.

Table 9-5

Comparison of Available All-Ceramic Systems

						BRAND			
	Captek	Ceramco 3	Cerinate	IPS Empress	IPS Empress 2	Empress Cosmo	Finesse	In-Ceram	In-Ceram Spinell
Manufacturer	Precious Chemicals	Dentsply	Den-Mat	Ivoclar	Ivoclar	Ivoclar	Dentsply	Vident	Vident
Crystalline phase	Leucite	Leucite	Leucite	Leucite	Lithium disilicate	Lithium phosphate	Leucite	Alumina	Alumina, spinel
Recommended usage	Crowns	Inlays, onlays, veneers	Inlays, onlays, crowns, veneers	Inlays, onlays, crowns, veneers	Anterior 3-unit FDPs, crowns	Endodontic foundation	Inlays, onlays, crowns, veneers	Crowns, veneers	Crowns, veneers
Fabrication	Sintered on metal foil	Sintered	Sintered	Heat-pressed	Heat-pressed	Heat-pressed	Heat-pressed	Slip-cast and sintered	Slip-cast and sintered
Strength	Low	Low	Medium/low	Medium/low	High	Medium	Medium/low	High	High
Fracture toughness	Medium/low	Medium/low	Medium/low	Medium/low	High	Medium	Medium/low	High	High
Translucency	Opaque	Medium	Medium	Medium	Medium	Medium	Medium	Opaque	Medium
Enamel abrasiveness	Medium	Medium	High	Medium	Low	*	Medium	High	High
Marginal fit	Good	Fair	Fair	Fair	Fair	*	*	Fair	Fair

From Rosenstiel SF, Land MF, Fujimoto J: *Contemporary Fixed Prosthodontics*, ed 4. St. Louis, Mosby, 2006.

CAD/CAM, Computer-aided design/computer-aided manufacturer (or computer-assisted machining); *FDP*, fixed dental prosthesis.

*Not tested.

(c) Metal-metal—not clinically relevant; never happens.

(d) Fracture of a porcelain fused to metal restoration can usually be attributed to inadequate framework design.

   b. Long-span metal-ceramic FDPs may be subjected to bending and may cause cracking or fracture of the porcelain because of its low ductility.

F. All-ceramic restorations.

   All-ceramic restorations are increasingly being used today on anterior and posterior teeth. The main purpose for their use is esthetics. The crystalline phase found on ceramics influences the mechanical and optical properties of the material. For a summary of the properties and use of all-ceramic systems, see Table 9-5.

1. All-ceramic restorations are more prone to fracture if the preparation line angles are not rounded.
2. Ceramic inlays and onlays have better abrasion resistance than composite resins.
3. All-ceramic crowns that are glass infiltrated (feldspathic, leucite, lithium disilicate) are etched with diluted hydrofluoric acid and treated with a silane-coupling agent and bonded to the tooth.
4. All-ceramic crowns with no glass content (zirconia and alumina) are luted to the tooth with conventional or resin cements.
5. Machine grinding of ceramics can induce surface cracks.
6. Repeated loading (chewing) can cause extension of a preexisting defect or crack, reducing the longevity of the restoration.

G. Provisional restorations.

1. *Requirements*—protection, maintain periodontal health, occlusal stability, maintain tooth position, biocompatible, color match.
2. Materials used for provisional restorations (Table 9-6).
   a. Poly ethyl methacrylate.
   b. Polymethyl methacrylate.
   c. Microfilled composite.
   d. Light-cured.
3. Types of materials to produce provisional restorations.
   a. Preformed crowns.
      (1) Cellulose acetate tooth form.
      (2) Polycarbonate crown form.
      (3) Aluminum crown form.

| | **BRAND** | | | | | | | | |
	In-Ceram Zirconia	Mark II	ProCAD	YZ blocs (inVizion)	Cercon Zirconia	Lava	Procera Alumina	Procera Zirconia	Metal-ceramic
Manufacturer	Vident	Vident	Ivoclar	Vident	Dentsply	3M ESPE	Nobel Biocare	Nobel Biocare	Various
Crystalline phase	Zirconia-alumina	Feldspar	Leucite	Zirconia	Zirconia	Zirconia	Alumina	Zirconia	Leucite
Recommended usage	3-unit FDPs	Inlays, onlays, crowns	Inlays, onlays, crowns	Crowns, FDPs	Crowns, FDPs	Crowns, FDPs	Crowns, FDPs	Crowns, FDPs	Crowns, FDPs
Fabrication	Slip-cast and sintered	CAD/CAM	CAD/CAM	CAD/CAM and sintered	CAD/CAM and sintered	CAD/CAM and sintered	CAD/CAM and sintered	CAD/CAM and sintered	Cast framework, sintered porcelain
Strength	Very high	Medium/low	Medium/low	Very high	Very high	Very high	High	Very high	Very high
Fracture toughness	Very high	Medium/low	Medium/low	Very high	Very high	Very high	Very high	Very high	Medium
Translucency	Opaque	Medium	Medium	Opaque	Opaque	Opaque	Opaque	Opaque	Opaque
Enamel abrasiveness	High	Medium	*	*	*	*	*	*	Medium
Marginal fit		Fair	Fair	*	*	*	*	*	Good

Table 9-6

Ranked Characteristics of Representative Provisional Restoration Resins

MATERIAL/CHARACTERISTIC	A	B	C	D	E	F	G	H	I	J	K	L	M	N
Jet (PMMA)	2*	2†	3	1†	1†	3†	1§	2	1	1	2‖	1	3	1
Duralay (PMMA)	1†	—	3	—	—	1	2	1	1	—	1	3	1
Trim (PR′MA)	2†	1†	2	3‡	—	3†	2†	3	1	1	3	1	2	1
Snap (PR′MA)	2†	2†	2	—	—	2†	2	3	1	1	—	1	2	1
Protemp Garant (bis-GMA composition)	1*	1	1	2	2	1	2†	3	2	2	1‖	2	1	2
Unifast LC (light-cured, PR′MA)	2*	2¶	3	—	—	2**	2	1	3	1	—	2	3	2
Triad (light-cured, urethane DMA composition)	2§	3†	1	1	1†	1†	3†	1	3	3	—	3	1	3

From Rosenstiel SF, Land MF, Fujimoto J: *Contemporary Fixed Prosthodontics*, ed 4, St. Louis, Mosby, 2006.

Column heads: *A*, marginal adaptation (indirect); *B*, temperature release during reaction; *C*, toxicity/allergenicity; *D*, strength (fracture toughness); *E*, repair strength (% original); *F*, color stability (ultraviolet light); *G*, ease of trimming and contouring; *H*, working time; *I*, setting time; *J*, flowability for mold filling; *K*, contaminated by free eugenol; *L*, special equipment needed; *M*, odor; *N*, unit volume cost.

Numbers in table: *1*, most desirable; *2*, less desirable; *3*, least desirable.

PMMA, Polymethyl methacrylate; *PR′MA*, poly(R′ methacrylate) (the "R" represents an alkyl group larger than methyl [e.g., ethyl or isobutyl]); *Bis-GMA comp*, microfilled composite; *Ureth. DMA comp.*, urethane dimethacrylate composite.

*Tjan AHL, et al: Marginal fidelity of crowns fabricated from six proprietary provisional materials. *J Prosthet Dent* 77:482, 1997.

†Wang RL, et al: A comparison of resins for fabricating provisional fixed restorations. *Int J Prosthodont* 2:173, 1989.

‡Gegauff AG, Pryor HG: Fracture toughness of provisional resins for fixed prosthodontics. *J Prosthet Dent* 58:23, 1987.

§Koumjian JH, Holmes JB: Marginal accuracy of provisional restorative materials. *J Prosthet Dent* 63:639, 1990.

‖ Gegauff AG, Rosenstiel SF: Effect of provisional luting agents on provisional resin additions. *Quintessence Int* 18:841, 1987.

¶Castelnuovo J, Tjan AH: Temperature rise in pulpal chamber during fabrication of provisional resinous crowns. *J Prosthet Dent* 78:441, 1997.

**Doray PG, et al: Accelerated aging affects color stability of provisional restorative materials. *J Prosthodont* 6:183, 1997.

(4) Tin-silver crown form.

(5) Nickel-chromium crown form.

b. Custom-made.

(1) Impressions are made before preparing teeth with irreversible hydrocolloid or silicones.

(2) Preformed thermoplastic sheets (cellulose acetate or polypropylene) adapted to a cast.

4. Types of provisional restorations.

a. *Direct procedure*—the material used (e.g., acrylic resin) is directly formed intraorally with the aid of a material that has a predetermined tooth form (e.g., a polycarbonate crown).

(1) Disadvantages.

(a) Potential tissue trauma from polymerizing resin.

(b) Poorer marginal fit than indirect method.

b. *Indirect procedure*—an unprepared cast is used to produce a template (e.g., a thermoplastic sheet). The tooth is prepared, and an impression is made of the prepared tooth. The template and the prepared cast are used to produce the provisional restoration with the material of choice (e.g., acrylic resin).

(1) Advantages.

(a) No tissue trauma.

(b) Good marginal adaptation.

H. Delivery of cast restorations.

1. Sequence for crowns and FDPs.

a. Internal surface fit.

b. Adjustments of proximal contacts and pontic-ridge contact relationship.

c. Marginal integrity.

d. FDP stability.

e. Axial contours.

f. Occlusion (centric and eccentric contacts).

2. *Luting agents (cements)*—the thickness of the cement film at the margins should be minimized to reduce dissolution of the luting agent. Through careful technique, a marginal adaptation less than 30 μm can be obtained consistently.

a. Factors that increase the cement space for crowns.

(1) Use of die spacers.

(2) Increased expansion of the investment mold.

b. Comparison, indications, and contraindications for luting agent types (Tables 9-7 and 9-8).

c. Properties and manipulation.

(1) *Zinc phosphate cement* should be mixed by incremental additions every 15 to 20 seconds. Ensuring saturation of the powder with the liquid adds strength to the cement. A frozen slab technique or decreasing the rate of addition of powder to liquid retards the setting cement. The cement film thickness is about 25 μm. Phosphoric acid is very acidic (pH = 3.5).

(2) *Zinc polycarboxylate cement* is more viscous when mixed and has a shorter working time than zinc phosphate cement. It adheres to tooth structure owing to chelation to calcium.

(3) *Glass-ionomer cement* adheres to enamel and dentin and releases fluoride. Its mechanical properties are superior to zinc phosphate and polycarboxylate cements (see Table 9-7).

(4) *Resin-modified glass-ionomer luting agents* have properties similar to glass-ionomer cements but have higher strength and low solubility. They should not be used with all-ceramic restorations because of reports of ceramic fracture, most likely the result of expansion from water absorption.

(5) *Resin luting agents* are unfilled resins that bond to dentin, which is achieved with organophosphonates (2-hydroxyethyl methacrylate or 4-methacryloyloxyethyl trimellitate anhydride). These luting agents are less biocompatible than glass-ionomers if not well polymerized and they provide a greater film thickness than other cements. They are most effective when bonded to tooth structure.

I. Important points about occlusion.

1. *Horizontal forces on teeth* are the most destructive to the periodontium.

2. A *nonworking condyle* moves down, forward, and medially.

3. *Nonworking interferences* generally occur on inner aspects of the facial cusps of mandibular teeth.

4. *In selective grinding* or *occlusal equilibration*, cusp tips should not be reduced; they can be narrowed, or the opposing fossa or marginal ridge can be adjusted.

5. *Terminal hinge position* is when the condyles are in the articular fossae and the mandible is capable of pure rotary opening. In CR, the mandible can rotate around the horizontal axis 20 to 25 mm. It is measured between the maxillary and mandibular incisal edges of the teeth. The horizontal axis around which the *hinge movement* occurs is referred as the *hinge axis*.

6. *Translation* is the motion of a body in which all of its points move in the same direction at the same time. When the condyle is said to translate, the condyle and the disc translate together during jaw opening beyond the point where motion is purely rotational. Translation occurs within the superior cavity of the joint between the disc-condyle complex and the articulator fossa. The lateral pterygoid is responsible for condylar translation.

7. *Canine protected occlusion* is a form of mutually protected occlusion in which the canine teeth disocclude or aid in separating the posterior teeth in excursive

Table 9-7

Comparison of Available Luting Agents

PROPERTY	IDEAL MATERIAL	ZINC PHOSPHATE	POLY-CARBOXYLATE	GLASS-IONOMER	RESIN IONOMER	COMPOSITE RESIN	ADHESIVE RESIN
Film thickness (μm)*	Low	$\leq$25	<25	<25	>25	>25	>25
Working time (min)	Long	1.5-5	1.75-2.5	2.3-5	2-4	3-10	0.5-5
Setting time (min)	Short	5-14	6-9	6-9	2	3-7	1-15
Compressive strength (MPa)	High	62-101	67-91	122-162	40-141	194-200	179-255
Elastic modules (GPa)†	Dentin = 13.7 Enamel = 84-130‡	13.2	Not tested	11.2	Not tested	17	4.5-9.8
Pulp irritation	Low	Moderate	Low	High	High	High	High
Solubility	Very low	High	High	Low	Very low	High to very high	Very low to low
Microleakage	Very low	High	High to very high	Low to very low	Very low	High to very high	Very low to low
Removal of excess	Easy	Easy	Medium	Medium	Medium	Medium	Difficult
Retention	High	Moderate	Low/moderate	Moderate to high	High§	Moderate	High

From Rosenstiel SF, Land MF, Fujimoto J: *Contemporary Fixed Prosthodontics,* ed 4, St. Louis, Mosby, 2006.

*White SN, Yu Z: Film thickness of new adhesive luting agents. *J Prosthet Dent* 67:782, 1992; see also Figure 31-2 in Rosenstiel et al (2006).

†Rosenstiel SF, et al: Strength of dental ceramics with adhesive cement coatings. *J Dent Res* 71:320, 1992.

‡O'Brien WJ: *Dental Materials and Their Selection,* ed 2. Chicago, Quintessence Publishing, 1997, p 351.

§Cheylan JM, et al: In vitro push-out strength of seven luting agents to dentin. *Int J Prosthodont* 15:365, 2002.

movements of the mandible. When preparing maxillary or mandibular anterior teeth, a mechanical or custom anterior guide table is used to preserve a record of the degree of disocclusion given by the linguoincisal concavity on maxillary teeth and the buccoincisal contour of the mandibular teeth.

8. *Group function occlusion* is seen when the maxillary and mandibular teeth of multiple posterior teeth contact in lateral excursive movements on the working side. This type of occlusion is seen in some natural dentitions and is used in restoring some dentitions with the idea of distributing the occlusal forces.

9. A *facebow transfer* positions the maxillary cast in three dimensions.
   a. Relating the maxillary cast to the condylar elements anteroposteriorly.
   b. Relating the maxillary cast vertically with some third point of reference.
      (1) Relating the maxillary cast with a tentative occlusal plane, which is parallel to the alatragus line, orbitale, or incisal pin notch. This precise positioning does the following.
      (a) Allows the teeth to be within a close radius of the correct arc of closure when the articulator is used in hinge movement.
      (b) Allows the teeth to reproduce more accurately the lateral arc during excursions.
      (c) Minimizes occlusal discrepancies caused by changes in vertical dimension (e.g., mounting cast with interocclusal records).
         (i) In complete denture construction, the facebow transfer record can be preserved by means of a plaster index of the occlusal surfaces of the maxillary denture before removing the denture from the articulator and cast after processing and occlusal adjustment is completed.

J. Dental materials.
   1. Common materials used in prosthodontics and their application (Table 9-9).

Table 9-8

Indications and Contraindications for Luting Agent Types

RESTORATION	INDICATION	CONTRAINDICATION
Cast crown, metal-ceramic crown, partial FDP	1, 2, 3, 4, 5, 6, 7	—
Crown or partial FDP with poor retention	1	2, 3, 4, 5, 6, 7
MCC with porcelain margin	1, 2, 3, 4, 5, 6, 7	—
Casting on patient with history of posttreatment sensitivity	Consider 4 or 7	2
Pressed, high-leucite, ceramic crown	1, 2	3, 4, 5, 6, 7
Slip-cast alumina crown	1, 2, 3, 4, 6, 7	5
Ceramic inlay	1, 2	3, 4, 5, 6, 7
Ceramic veneer	1, 2	3, 4, 5, 6, 7
Resin-retained partial FDP	1, 2	3, 4, 5, 6, 7
Cast post-and-core	1, 2, 3, 5, 6	4, 7

KEY:			
LUTING AGENT TYPE	CHIEF ADVANTAGES	CHIEF CONCERNS	PRECAUTIONS
1. Adhesive resin	Adhesive, low solubility	Film thickness, history of use	Moisture control
2. Composite resin	Low solubility	Film thickness, irritation	Use bonding resin, moisture control
3. Glass-ionomer	Translucency	Solubility, leakage	Avoid early moisture exposure
4. Reinforced ZOE	Biocompatible	Low strength	Only for very retentive restorations
5. Resin ionomer	Low solubility, low microleakage	Water sorption, history of use	Avoid with ceramic restorations
6. Zinc phosphate	History of use	Solubility, leakage	Use for "traditional" cast restorations
7. Zinc polycarboxylate	Biocompatible	Low strength, solubility	Do not reduce powder/liquid ratio

From Rosenstiel SF, Land MF, Fujimoto J: *Contemporary Fixed Prosthodontics*, ed 4. St. Louis, Mosby, 2006.

FDP, Fixed dental prosthesis; *MCC,* metal-ceramic crown; *ZOE,* zinc oxide–eugenol.

2. Gypsum.
   a. The *setting expansion* of any gypsum product is a function of calcium sulfate dihydrate crystal growth. Some is the result of thermal expansion.
   b. Dental gypsum classification.
      (1) Type I—plaster, impression plaster.
      (2) Type II—model plaster.
      (3) Type III—dental stone.
      (4) Type IV—dental stone, high strength (die stone).
      (5) Type V—high strength.
   c. The *particle size* shape of dental gypsum products differs, requiring different *water/powder ratios.* Type I and II plasters require a higher water/powder ratio than type III and IV stones.
   d. A thinner mix of a gypsum base product decreases the degree of *exothermia,* decreasing setting expansion.
   e. Increasing the water/powder ratio increases the setting time and decreases strength. The increase in water/powder ratio decreases the number of nuclei of crystallization per unit volume and increases the amount of space between crystallizing nuclei, increasing porosity when drying. This causes a decrease in the interaction of dihydrate crystals and diminishes any outward thrust of the mass. Consequently, setting expansion is decreased.
   f. Potassium sulfate and sodium chloride *accelerate* setting of gypsum, whereas sodium citrate and borax *retard* setting.
   g. *Manipulation*—when *hand spatulating,* powder is added and allowed to settle into the water for about 30 seconds. This minimizes the amount of air incorporated into the mix during initial spatulation. Spatulation to wet and mix the powder uniformly with the water requires about 1 minute at 2 revolutions per second. A *power-driven mechanical spatulator* requires that the powder initially be wet by the water, as with hand mixing. The mix is spatulated for 20 seconds on the low-speed drive of the mixer. Vacuuming during mixing reduces the air entrapped in the mix.

Table 9-9	
Common Materials Used in Prosthodontics and Their Application	
Amalgam	Commonly used for conservative restorations where esthetics is not a concern. It is underused as a core buildup material for crowns. Mechanical properties are inferior to cast metal and ceramic restorations.
Composite	Commonly used for conservative restorations where esthetics are desired. Also used as a core buildup material with some inferior physical properties (moisture and thermal expansion) compared with amalgam.
Cast metal	*Extracoronal restorations or crowns* are used to replace tooth structure damaged secondary to caries or trauma, as retainers for FDP, and as retainers for RDP. Strengthens and protects a tooth.
	Intracoronal restorations or inlay (gold) are used for conservative restorations with better physical properties than amalgam. They require removal of more tooth structure than amalgam.
Metal-ceramic	Similar to cast metal restorations but used where esthetics are a consideration because porcelain is bonded to the metal.
Complete ceramic	Crowns, inlays, and laminate veneers made with dental porcelain are used instead of the above materials where good esthetics are desired.
	Drawbacks include fracture potential and in some ceramic materials marginal fit.

FDP, Fixed partial prosthesis; *RDP,* removable dental prosthesis.

h. The poured cast should be allowed to set for 45 to 60 minutes before separating it from the impression.
i. Casts can be disinfected by immersion in a 1:10 dilution of sodium hypochlorite for 30 minutes or with iodophor spray.
3. Investments and casting.
   a. Investments *expand* during *setting*, when heated (*thermal*). When additional expansion is desired, use a *hydroscopic* technique by placing the invested ring in water while setting. Investment expansion provides a larger mold for the metal being cast, which compensates for the contraction that the metal experiences when it solidifies. Investments commonly used in dentistry are as follows.
      (1) *Gypsum-bonded investments* are used for casting alloys containing 65% to 75% gold at temperatures near 1100° C. They have a gypsum binder.
      (2) *Phosphate-bonded investments* are used for casting metal-ceramic alloys because of their capability to withstand high temperatures (1100° C). They have a metallic oxide and phosphate binder. Gas and oxygen torches are used for melting metal-ceramic alloys.
      (3) *Silica-bonded investments* are used for casting base metal alloys for frameworks for dental prostheses. They have a silica gel binder.
   b. *Quenching* is the procedure performed on a metal when it is brought to an elevated temperature and is cooled rapidly. It is usually performed when a complete gold crown is cast and immediately quenched in water. This softens the alloy owing to

change in the phase structure of the alloy, making it more malleable for finishing procedures.
   c. *Sprues* should always be larger in diameter than the cross-section area of the pattern where they are attached.
   d. *Crucibles* should always be used with only one type of alloy to prevent contamination, regardless of the type of casting being performed.
4. *Soldering*—procedure to join metal components by heating a piece of metal (solder) that melts at a temperature slightly lower than the metals to be joined together.
   a. The recommended *gap* or *distance* between the parts to be joined should be 0.25 mm (the thickness of a typical business card) for accuracy.
   b. *Soldering flux* dissolves surface oxides and allows the melted solder to wet and flow onto the adjoining alloy surfaces. Flux is composed of borax, potassium fluoride (some fluxes), and boric acid.
   c. *Antiflux* restricts the flow of solder away from undesired surfaces and is applied on areas such as occlusal grooves and margins. Graphite and iron oxide (rouge) are antifluxes.

Bibliography

The glossary of prosthodontic terms. *J Prosthet Dent* 94: 10, 2005.

Anusavice KJ: *Phillips' Science of Dental Materials*, ed 11. Philadelphia, Saunders, 2003.

Beuer F, Schweiger J, Edelhoff D: Digital dentistry: an overview of recent developments for CAD/CAM generated restorations. *Br Dent J* 204:505, 2008.

Carr AB, McGivney GP, Brown T: *McCracken's Removable Partial Prosthodontics*, ed 11. St. Louis, Mosby, 2005.

Dawson PE: *Evaluation, Diagnosis, and Treatment of Occlusal Problems*, ed 2, St. Louis, Mosby, 1989.

Okeson JP: *Management of Temporomandibular Disorders and Occlusion*, ed 5. St. Louis, Mosby, 2003.

Powers JM, Sakaguchi RL: *Craig's Restorative Dental Materials*, ed 12. St. Louis, Mosby, 2006.

Rosenstiel SF, Land MF, Fujimoto J: *Contemporary Fixed Prosthodontics*, ed 4. St. Louis, Mosby, 2006.

Zarb GA, et al: *Prosthodontic Treatment for the Edentulous Patient*, ed 12. St. Louis, Mosby, 2004.

Sample Questions

1. The impression material that is mainly composed of sodium or potassium salts of alginic acid is ____.
   A. Polyether
   B. Irreversible hydrocolloid
   C. Polyvinyl siloxane
   D. Polysulfide

2. A patient with complete dentures presents with angular cheilitis. A review of recent medical history revealed that vitamin deficiency is not a factor. A possible predisposing factor is ____.
   A. Excessive vertical dimension of occlusion
   B. A closed or insufficient vertical dimension of occlusion
   C. Improper balance of the occlusion
   D. Poor contour of the denture base

3. All of the following are a feature of papillary hyperplasia *except* one. Which one is the *exception*?
   A. It is a proliferative bone disease
   B. It can be caused by wearing dentures at night
   C. It can be caused by poor oral hygiene
   D. It can be caused by an ill-fitting denture

4. For optimal esthetics when setting maxillary denture teeth, the incisal edges of the maxillary incisors should follow the ____.
   A. Lower lips during smiling
   B. Upper lips during smiling
   C. Lower lips when relaxed
   D. Upper lips when relaxed

5. Excessive monomer added to acrylic resin results in ____.
   A. Increased expansion
   B. Increased heat generation
   C. Increased shrinkage
   D. Increased strength

6. What is the purpose of adjusting the occlusion in dentures?
   A. To obtain balanced occlusion
   B. To stabilize dentures
   C. To obtain even occlusal contacts
   D. All of the above

7. Which of the following may be a consequence of occlusal trauma on implants?
   A. Widening of the periodontal ligament
   B. Soft tissue sore area around the tooth
   C. Bone loss
   D. All of the above

8. Which of the following is *true* of an occlusal rest for an RDP?
   1. **One third facial lingual width of the tooth**
   2. **1.5 mm deep for base metal**
   3. **2.0 mm labiolingual width of the tooth**
   4. **Floor inclines apically toward the center of the tooth**
   A. All of the above
   B. 1, 3, and 4
   C. 1, 2, and 4
   D. 3 and 4

9. A patient is unhappy with the esthetics of an anterior metal-ceramic crown, complaining that it looks too opaque in the incisal third. The reason for this is most likely ____.
   A. Using the incorrect opaque porcelain shade
   B. Inadequate vacuum during porcelain firing
   C. Not masking the metal well enough with the opaque
   D. The tooth was prepared in a single facial plane

10. An endodontically treated tooth was restored with a cast post-and-core and a metal-ceramic crown. The patient complains of pain, especially on biting, 3 months later. Radiographic findings and tooth mobility tests are normal. The *most* probable cause of pain is ____.
    A. A loose crown
    B. Psychosomatic
    C. A vertical root fracture
    D. A premature eccentric contact

11. For an occlusal appliance used for muscle relaxation to be effective, the condyles must be located in their most stable position from a musculoskeletal perspective. This is ____.
    A. Centric occlusion
    B. At the vertical dimension of rest
    C. Centric relation
    D. Maximum intercuspal position

12. A diagnostic wax-up is indicated when ____.
    A. Reestablishing anterior guidance
    B. A provisional fixed prosthesis is to be fabricated
    C. Uncertainty exists regarding esthetics
    D. All of the above

13. Which of the following is the *most* important predictor of clinical success of a cast post and core?
    A. Amount of remaining coronal tooth structure
    B. Post length
    C. Post diameter
    D. Positive horizontal stop

14. Factors associated with bone loss include ____.
    A. Initial implant instability
    B. Excessive occlusal force

C. Inadequate hygiene

D. Inadequate prosthesis fit

E. All of the above

15. Which of the following statements is true concerning the evaluation of the occlusion on a cast restoration?

A. The restoration is in proper occlusion if it holds shim stock.

B. The restoration is in proper occlusion if the adjacent teeth hold shim stock.

C. The restoration is in proper occlusion when articulating paper marks multiple points of contact on the restoration.

D. A, B, and C.

E. None of the above.

16. In a Kennedy class I arch in which all molars and the first premolar are missing and the rest of the teeth have good periodontal support, the preferred choice of treatment is _____.

A. RDP replacing all missing teeth

B. FDP replacing the missing premolar and RDP replacing the molars

C. Implant-supported crowns replacing the first premolars and RDP replacing the molars

D. A and B are preferred over C

E. B and C are preferred over A

17. The surveyor is used to _____.

A. Aid in the placement of an intracoronal retainer

B. Block out a master cast

C. Measure a specific depth of an undercut

D. All of the above

E. A and B

18. A dentist is preparing all maxillary anterior teeth for metal-ceramic crowns. Which of the following procedures is necessary to preserve and restore anterior guidance?

A. Protrusive record

B. Template for provisional restorations

C. Custom incisal guide table

D. Interocclusal record in centric relation

19. A radiolucency near the apex of tooth #28 is seen radiographically. The tooth is asymptomatic and does not have caries or periodontal problems. What is the *most* likely cause of the radiolucency?

A. Submandibular fossa

B. Periapical granuloma

C. Complex compound odontoma

D. Mental foramen

20. The minor connector for a mandibular distal extension base should extend posteriorly about _____.

A. Two thirds the length of the edentulous ridge

B. Half the length of the edentulous ridge

C. One third the length of the edentulous ridge

D. As long as possible

21. The characteristics of a major connector that contribute to health and well-being include which of the following?

A. It is rigid and provides unification of the arch stability

B. It does not substantially alter the natural contour of the lingual surface of the mandibular alveolar ridge or the palatal vault

C. It contributes to the support of the prosthesis

D. All of the above

E. Only A and B

22. When does an FDP that was cast in one piece need to be sectioned?

A. When a cantilever pontic is used

B. When the fit cannot be achieved or verified with a one-piece cast

C. When single crowns are adjacent to the FDP

D. Always to achieve a good fit

23. When soldering an FDP, what is the effect of flux when heated on the area to be soldered?

A. To remove oxides from the metal surface

B. To displace metal ions from the area

C. To change the composition of the alloy

D. To reduce the surface tension of the metal

24. Which component of an RDP is spoon-shaped and slightly inclined apically from the marginal ridge of a tooth?

A. Indirect retainer

B. Minor connector

C. Rest

D. Lingual bar

25. Metamerism invariably involves _____.

A. A color difference between two objects under one or more illuminants

B. One object having a lower chroma than another

C. One object having a lower lightness than another

D. A significant color change of one object as it moves from one illuminant to another

26. A patient has generalized severe alveolar bone loss with resulting teeth mobility for the maxillary and mandibular anterior and posterior teeth. All remaining teeth need to be extracted. The patient has opted to have immediate maxillary and mandibular complete dentures. The patient does not want to wait for healing after all the teeth are extracted before dentures can be constructed mainly because of esthetic concerns. What is the *best* esthetic option for the patient that would minimize drastic changes in the supporting tissue the day of the delivery of the immediate denture?

A. Extract all the anterior teeth, leave the posterior teeth to maintain the vertical dimension, construct an immediate denture, and extract the posterior teeth the day of delivery of the immediate denture

B. Extract the posterior teeth, leave the anterior teeth, wait a month for healing, construct the dentures, and extract the anterior teeth the day of delivery of the immediate dentures

C. Extract all the teeth because it is very difficult to predict the esthetic outcome of immediate dentures when most of the posterior and anterior teeth are present

D. Extract only the worst posterior and anterior teeth, and construct the immediate complete dentures; extract the remaining teeth the day of the delivery of the dentures

27. In the scenario for question 26, if constructing an immediate denture, which of the following constitutes the *most* difficult procedure?
    A. Border molding before the final impression with existing teeth
    B. Sequencing the treatment plan
    C. Delivery of the complete dentures
    D. All are equally difficult

28. A 55-year-old patient presents with a DO amalgam in tooth #14 and a cervical abfraction on the buccal surface. The patient complains of pain when chewing and sensitivity to cold liquids but only while drinking the cold liquids. The clinical examination and radiographs reveal no apparent abnormalities except for mild discoloration of the lingual distal cusp. An ice test is positive immediately, and there is pain when occluding with a tooth sleuth. What is the *most* likely cause of the pain, and what treatment does the tooth require?
    A. The tooth has an occlusal prematurity and needs an occlusal adjustment
    B. The abfraction causes the sensitivity, and a cervical restoration is needed

C. The tooth has a crack and requires a crown
D. None of the above

29. The preparation of a tooth for a Zirconia crown can be the same as for _____.
    A. Metal-ceramic crown
    B. Full metal crown
    C. All-ceramic crown
    D. All of the above

30. You are evaluating an FDP replacing tooth #4 because the margins are open secondary to probable distortion during the manufacture of the prosthesis. Which (if any) of the following should you do first *before* deciding to section between one of the retainers and the pontic to see if the fit improves and to obtain a solder relationship for the prosthesis?
    1. **Assessment and adjustment of occlusal relationships**
    2. **Assessment and adjustment of proximal contacts**
    3. **Assessment and adjustment of axial contours**
    4. **Assessment of marginal integrity**
    A. All are correct
    B. 1, 2 and 3 are correct
    C. 2, 3 and 4 are correct
    D. 2 and 4 are correct
    E. 1 and 4 are correct

Sample Examination

Endodontics

1. A patient complains of recent severe pain to percussion of a tooth. The *most* likely cause is _____.
   A. Acute periradicular periodontitis
   B. Chronic periradicular periodontitis
   C. Reversible pulpitis
   D. Irreversible pulpitis

2. Which of the following statements regarding post preparation is *not* correct?
   A. The primary purpose of the post is to retain a core in a tooth with extensive loss of coronal structure.
   B. The need for a post is dictated by the amount of remaining coronal tooth structure.
   C. Posts reinforce the tooth and help to prevent vertical fractures.
   D. At least 4 to 5 mm of remaining gutta-percha after post space preparation is recommended.

3. Prolonged, unstimulated night pain suggests which of the following conditions of the pulp?
   A. Pulpal necrosis
   B. Mild hyperemia
   C. Reversible pulpitis
   D. Periodontal abscess

4. A nasopalatine duct cyst is located between _____.
   A. Two maxillary central incisors
   B. Maxillary central and lateral incisors
   C. Maxillary lateral and canine
   D. Maxillary canine and first premolar

5. The severity of the course of a periradicular infection depends on the _____.
   A. Resistance of the host
   B. Virulence of the organisms
   C. Number of organisms present
   D. Both A and B only
   E. All of the above

6. Informed consent requires that the patient be advised of all of the following *except* one. Which one is the *exception*?
   A. Benefits of endodontic treatment
   B. Cost of endodontic treatment
   C. Risks of endodontic treatment

7. Which of the following statements *best* describes pulpal A-delta fibers compared with C fibers?
   A. Larger unmyelinated nerve fibers with slower conduction velocities
   B. Larger myelinated nerve fibers with faster conduction velocities
   C. Smaller myelinated nerve fibers with slower conduction velocities
   D. Smaller unmyelinated nerve fibers with faster conduction velocities

8. When compared with the bisecting-angle technique, the advantages of the paralleling technique in endodontic radiology include all of the following *except* one. Which one is the *exception*?
   A. Significant decrease in patient radiation
   B. More accurate image of the tooth's dimensions
   C. Easier to reproduce radiographs at similar angles to assess healing after treatment
   D. Most accurate image of all dimensions of the tooth and its relationship to surrounding anatomic structures

9. The primary reason for designing a surgical flap with a wide flap base is to _____.
   A. Avoid incising over a bony protuberance
   B. Obtain maximum access to the surgical site
   C. Maintain an adequate blood supply to the reflected tissue
   D. Aid in complete reflection

10. The apical portion of the maxillary lateral incisor usually curves to the _____.
   A. Facial
   B. Palatal
   C. Mesial
   D. Distal

11. Aqueous ethylenediamine tetraacetic acid (EDTA) is primarily used to _____.
   A. Dissolve organic matter
   B. Dissolve inorganic matter
   C. Kill bacteria
   D. Prevent sealer from extruding out of the canal space

12. A noncarious tooth with deep periodontal pockets that do not involve the apical third of the root has developed an acute pulpitis. There is no history of trauma other than a mild prematurity in lateral excursion. What is the *most* likely explanation for the pulpitis?
   A. Normal mastication and toothbrushing have driven microorganisms deep into tissues with subsequent pulp involvement at the apex.
   B. During a general bacteremia, bacteria settled in this aggravated pulp and produced an acute pulpitis.
   C. Repeated thermal shock from air and fluids getting into the deep pockets caused the pulpitis.

D. An accessory pulp canal in the gingival or the middle third of the root was in contact with the pockets.

13. On a radiograph, the facial root of a maxillary first premolar would appear distal to the lingual root if the ____.
    A. Vertical angle of the cone was increased
    B. Vertical angle of the cone was decreased
    C. X-ray head was angled from a distal position relative to the premolar
    D. X-ray head was angled from a mesial position relative to the premolar

14. If a canal is ledged during instrumentation, the *best* way to handle the problem is to ____.
    A. Continue instrumenting at the ledge; although it may take some time, you will eventually bore your way to patency in the periodontal ligament space
    B. Stop immediately and fill to where the ledge begins
    C. Bind your irrigating needle in the canal and use short bursts of irrigant to loosen any debris blocking the canal; this will reopen the natural canal
    D. Prebend the tip of a small file, lubricate, and try to negotiate around the ledge
    E. Place citric acid or ethylenediamine tetraacetic acid in the canal to soften the dentin; a small Gates Glidden or other rotary can be used to bypass the ledge

15. Which of the following factors affects long-term prognosis of teeth after perforation repair?
    A. Size of the defect
    B. Location of the defect
    C. Time elapsed between the perforation and its repair
    D. All of the above

16. Which of the following statements *best* describes treatment options for a separated instrument (e.g., finger spreader) at the filling stage of treatment?
    A. Immediately attempt to remove the instrument.
    B. Do not attempt removal, and proceed to obturation.
    C. Attempt to bypass the obstructed instrument.
    D. Both A and C are options.

17. Endodontically treated posterior teeth are more susceptible to fracture than untreated posterior teeth. The *best* explanation for this is ____.
    A. Moisture loss
    B. Loss of root vitality
    C. Plastic deformation of dentin
    D. Destruction of the coronal architecture

18. There is a horizontal root fracture in the middle third of the root of tooth #10 in an 11-year-old patient. The tooth is mobile and vital. How should this be treated?
    A. Extract
    B. Immediate pulpectomy and splint
    C. Splint and observe
    D. Do nothing and follow-up in 10 to 14 days

19. Which of the following is the *best* radiographic technique to identify a suspected horizontal root fracture in a maxillary anterior central incisor?
    A. Multiple Waters' projections
    B. Multiple angulated periapical radiographs in addition to a normal, parallel-angulated, periapical radiograph
    C. Panoramic radiograph
    D. Reverse Towne's projection

20. An 8-year-old boy sustained a traumatic injury to a maxillary central incisor. Electrical and thermal vitality tests performed 1 day later failed to elicit a response from the tooth. This finding dictates ____.
    A. Pulpectomy
    B. Apexification
    C. Calcium hydroxide pulpotomy
    D. Delay for the purpose of reevaluation

21. Twisting a triangular wire best describes the manufacturing process of a ____.
    A. Reamer
    B. Barbed broach
    C. Hedström file
    D. K-Flex file

22. Direct pulp cap is recommended for teeth with ____.
    A. Carious exposures
    B. Mechanical exposures
    C. Calcification in the pulp chambers
    D. Closed apices more than teeth with open apices

23. Which of the following is the treatment of choice for a 7-year-old child with a nonvital tooth #30 with buccal sinus tract?
    A. Gutta-percha filling
    B. Gutta-percha filling followed by root-end surgery
    C. Extraction
    D. Apexogenesis
    E. Apexification

24. Which of the following is the main side effect of bleaching an endodontically treated tooth?
    A. External cervical resorption
    B. Demineralization of tooth structure
    C. Gingival inflammation

25. What is the safest recommended intracoronal bleaching chemical?
    A. Hydrogen peroxide
    B. Sodium perborate
    C. Sodium hypochlorite
    D. Carbamide peroxide

26. Pulp capping and pulpotomy can be more successful in newly erupted teeth than in adult teeth because ____.
    A. A greater number of odontoblasts are present
    B. Of incomplete development of nerve endings
    C. An open apex allows for greater circulation
    D. The root is shorter

27. Zinc oxide eugenol is a good temporary restoration because ____.

A. It is less irritating

B. It has increased strength over other restorations

C. It provides a good seal

D. It is inexpensive

28. During a routine 6-month endodontic treatment recall evaluation, you note a marked decrease in the radiographic size of the periradicular radiolucency. Which of the following is the *most* appropriate treatment plan?

A. Extraction

B. Nonsurgical endodontic retreatment

C. Recall the patient in another 6 months

D. Surgical endodontic retreatment

29. What is the radiographic sign of successful pulpotomy in a permanent tooth?

A. Open apex

B. Apex has formed

C. Loss of periradicular lucency

D. No internal resorption

30. Which of the following statements is *false* regarding internal root resorption?

A. It happens rarely in permanent teeth.

B. It appears as an asymmetrical "moth-eaten" lesion in radiographs.

C. Chronic pulpal inflammation is the primary cause.

D. Prompt endodontic therapy stops the process.

31. An emergency patient is diagnosed with symptomatic irreversible pulpitis and symptomatic apical periodontitis of tooth #12. Which of the following is the *best* treatment protocol for this patient?

A. Anesthesia followed by incision and drainage

B. Anesthesia followed by extraction

C. Anesthesia followed by pulpectomy

D. Prescribe antibiotic for 1 week and follow with nonsurgical endodontic treatment

32. In which of the following conditions is elective root canal therapy contraindicated?

A. AIDS

B. Recent myocardial infarction (MI)

C. Leukemia

D. Radiotherapy

E. Second trimester of pregnancy

33. What is the *best* timing for performing incision and drainage at an area of infection?

A. When the swelling is hard and diffuse

B. When the area is the most painful

C. When the area is large

D. When the swelling is localized and fluctuant

34. Endodontic infection usually is polymicrobial. What is the predominate type of microorganism found in a tooth that requires endodontic therapy?

A. Aerobic bacteria

B. Facultative bacteria

C. Obligate anaerobic bacteria

D. Yeast microorganisms

35. The "danger zone" of mandibular molars for perforations during canal instrumentation is _____.

A. The periphery at the level of the dentinocemental junction

B. Within 2 mm of the apex

C. The furcation area

D. The periphery of the access at the level of the cementoenamel junction

36. What is the treatment of choice for an 8-year-old patient who has a 1-mm intrusion injury of tooth #8?

A. Extract the tooth

B. Perform pulpotomy immediately

C. Immediately splint the tooth for 10 to 14 days

D. Allow the tooth to reerupt

37. On routine radiographic survey of a new patient, you notice a circle-shaped radiolucency at the midroot and over the pulpal outline of tooth #6. You take a second mesially angulated radiograph and confirm the radiolucency is part of the pulp canal outline. After a vital response to cold testing, your diagnosis and subsequent treatment plan are _____.

A. Internal resorption and completion of nonsurgical endodontic treatment

B. Internal resorption and surgical repair of the defect

C. External root resorption and forced orthodontic eruption to expose the defect

D. External root resorption and extraction

38. During a nonvital bleaching procedure, if a barrier material is not placed between the root canal filling and bleaching material, the tooth can be subjected to _____.

A. External cervical resorption

B. Demineralization of tooth structure

C. Gingival inflammation

D. Poor color improvement

39. A healthy 32-year-old man presents with localized fluctuant swelling associated with a necrotic pulp and an apical diagnosis of acute apical abscess for tooth #5. The principal modality or modalities for treating a localized fluctuant swelling include which of the following?

A. Administration of antibiotics

B. Achievement of drainage

C. Removal of the source of infection

D. Both A and C

E. Both B and C

40. Which of the following statements *most* accurately describes the manufacturing process for a K-type hand instrument?

A. Grinding a stainless steel wire to a tapered square or triangular cross section

B. Twisting a square or rhomboid (cross section) nontapered silver metal blank

C. Grinding a silver metal blank to a nontapered square or rhomboid cross section

D. Both B and C

E. All of the above

Operative Dentistry

1. A good preventive and treatment strategy for dental caries includes ____.
   A. Limiting cariogenic substrate
   B. Controlling cariogenic flora
   C. Elevating host resistance
   D. All of the above

2. Which of the following statements regarding caries risk assessment is correct?
   A. The presence of restorations is a good indicator of current caries activity.
   B. The presence of restorations is a good indicator of past caries activity.
   C. The presence of dental plaque is a good indicator of current caries activity.
   D. The presence of pit-and-fissure sealants is a good indicator of current caries activity.

3. Which of the following is considered a reversible carious lesion?
   A. The lesion surface is cavitated.
   B. The lesion has advanced to the dentin radiographically.
   C. A white spot is detected on drying.
   D. The lesion surface is rough or chalky.

4. Which of the following statements about indirect pulp caps is *false*?
   A. Some leathery caries may be left in the preparation.
   B. A liner is generally recommended in the excavation.
   C. The operator should wait at least 6 to 8 weeks before reentry (if then).
   D. The prognosis of indirect pulp cap treatment is poorer than the prognosis of direct pulp caps.

5. Smooth surface caries refers to ____.
   A. Facial and lingual surfaces
   B. Occlusal pits and grooves
   C. Mesial and distal surfaces
   D. Both A and C

6. How many blades does a finishing bur have compared with a cutting bur?
   A. Fewer blades
   B. Same number of blades
   C. More blades
   D. Number of blades is unrelated to the bur type

7. The use of the rubber dam is best indicated for ____.
   A. Adhesive procedures
   B. Quadrant dentistry
   C. Teeth with challenging preparations
   D. Difficult patients
   E. All of the above

8. A rubber dam is inverted to ____.
   A. Prevent the dam from tearing
   B. Prevent the underlying gingiva from accidental trauma

   C. Provide a complete seal around the teeth
   D. All of the above

9. For a dental hand instrument with a formula of 10-8.5-8, the number 10 refers to ____.
   A. The width of the blade, in tenths of a millimeter
   B. The primary cutting-edge angle, in centigrades
   C. The blade length, in millimeters
   D. The blade angle, in centigrades

10. The tooth preparation technique for a class I amalgam on a mandibular first molar does *not* include which of the following?
    A. Maintaining a narrow isthmus width
    B. Initial punch cut placed in the most carious pit
    C. Establishment of pulpal depth of 1.5 to 2 mm
    D. Orientation of bur parallel to the long axis of the tooth

11. When placement of proximal retention locks in class II amalgam preparations is necessary, which of the following is *not* correct?
    A. One should not undermine the proximal enamel.
    B. One should not prepare locks entirely in the axial wall.
    C. Even if deeper than ideal, one should use the axial wall as a guide for proximal lock placement.
    D. One should place locks 0.2 mm inside the dentinoenamel junction (DEJ) to ensure that the proximal enamel is not undermined.

12. When the gingival margin is gingival to the cementoenamel junction (CEJ) in a class II amalgam preparation, the axial depth of the axiogingival line angle should be ____.
    A. 0.2 mm into sound dentin
    B. Twice the diameter of a No. 245 carbide bur
    C. 0.75 to 0.80 mm
    D. The width of the cutting edge of a gingival marginal trimmer

13. Which of the following statements about class V amalgam restorations is *not* correct?
    A. The outline form is usually kidney-shaped or crescent-shaped.
    B. Because the mesial, distal, gingival, and incisal walls of the tooth preparation are perpendicular to the external tooth surface, they usually diverge facially.
    C. Using four corner coves instead of two full-length grooves conserves dentin near the pulp and may reduce the possibility of a mechanical pulp exposure.
    D. If the outline form approaches an existing proximal restoration, it is better to leave a thin section of tooth structure between the two restorations (<1 mm) than to join the restorations.

14. When preparing a class III or IV composite tooth preparation, which of the following statements regarding placement of retention form is *false*?
    A. Placement of retention form often involves gingival and incisal retention.

B. Placement of retention form is placed at the axio-gingival line angle regardless of the depth of the axial wall.

C. Placement of retention form may be needed in large preparations.

D. Placement of retention form is usually prepared with a No. ¼ round bur.

15. In the conventional class I composite preparation, retention is achieved by which of the following features?
   1. **Occlusal convergence**
   2. **Occlusal bevel**
   3. **Bonding**
   4. **Retention grooves**
   A. 2 and 4
   B. 1 and 3
   C. 1 and 4
   D. 2 and 3

16. The success of an amalgam restoration depends on all of the following features of tooth and cavity preparation *except* one. Which one is the *exception*?
   A. Butt-joint cavosurface margin that results in a 90-degree margin for the amalgam
   B. Adequate tooth removal for appropriate strength of the amalgam
   C. Divergent (externally) preparation walls
   D. Adequate retention form features to lock the amalgam mechanically in the preparation

17. Many factors affect tooth/cavity preparation. Which of the following would be the least important factor?
   A. Extent of the defect
   B. Size of the tooth
   C. Fracture lines
   D. Extent of the old material

18. Which of the following statements about an amalgam tooth/cavity preparation is *true*?
   A. The enamel cavosurface margin angle must be 90 degrees.
   B. The cavosurface margin should provide for a 90-degree amalgam margin.
   C. All prepared walls should converge externally.
   D. Retention form for class V amalgam preparations can be placed at the dentinoenamel junction (DEJ).

19. A "skirt" feature for a gold onlay preparation ____.
   A. Has a shoulder gingival margin design
   B. Is prepared by a diamond held perpendicular to the long axis of the crown
   C. Is used only for esthetic areas of a tooth
   D. Increases both retention and resistance forms

20. Causes of postoperative sensitivity with amalgam restorations include all of the following *except* one. Which one is the *exception*?
   A. Lack of adequate condensation, especially lateral condensation in the proximal boxes
   B. Voids

C. Extension onto the root surface
D. Lack of dentinal sealing

21. Factors that affect the success of dentin bonding include all of the following *except* one. Which one is the *exception*?
   A. Dentin factors such as sclerosis, tubule morphology, and smear layer
   B. Tooth factors such as attrition, abrasion, and abfraction
   C. Material factors such as compressive and tensile strengths
   D. C-factor considerations

22. Which of the following statements regarding carving a class I amalgam restoration is *false*?
   A. Carving may be made easier by waiting 1 or 2 minutes after condensation before it is started.
   B. The blade of the discoid carver should move parallel to the margins resting on the partially set amalgam.
   C. Deep occlusal anatomy should not be carved.
   D. The carved amalgam outline should coincide with the cavosurface margins.

23. The generally accepted maximum thickness of a composite increment that allows for proper cure is ____.
   A. 1 to 2 mm
   B. 2 to 4 mm
   C. 4 to 6 mm
   D. There is no maximum thickness restriction.

24. The setting reaction of dental amalgam proceeds primarily by ____.
   A. Dissolution of the entire alloy particle into mercury
   B. Dissolution of the copper from the particles into mercury
   C. Precipitation of tin-mercury crystals
   D. Mercury reaction with silver on or in the alloy particle

25. What is the half-life of mercury in the human body?
   A. 5 days
   B. 25 days
   C. 55 days
   D. 85 days
   E. 128 days

26. Restoration of an appropriate proximal contact results in all of the following *except* one. Which one is the *exception*?
   A. Reduces or eliminates food impaction at the interdental papilla
   B. Provides appropriate space for the interdental papilla
   C. Provides increased retention form for the restoration
   D. Maintains the proper occlusal relationship

27. The best way to carve amalgam back to occlusal cavosurface margin is to ____.
   A. Use visual magnification
   B. Use a discoid-cleoid instrument guided by the adjacent unprepared enamel

C. Make deep pits and grooves

D. Use a round finishing bur after the amalgam has set

28. Major differences between total-etch and self-etching primer dentin bonding systems include all of the following *except* one. Which one is the *exception*?
    A. The time necessary to apply the material
    B. The amount of smear layer removed
    C. The bond strengths to enamel
    D. The need for wet bonding

29. Which of the following statements is *not* true regarding bonding systems?
    A. Although dentin bonding occurs slowly, it results in a stronger bond than to enamel.
    B. Enamel bonding occurs quickly, is strong, and is long-lasting.
    C. One-bottle dentin bonding systems may be simpler but are not always better.
    D. Dentin bonding is still variable because of factors such as sclerosis, tubule size, and tubule location.

30. A casting may fail to seat on the prepared tooth because of all of the following factors *except* one. Which one is the *exception*?
    A. Temporary cement still on the prepared tooth after the temporary restoration has been removed
    B. Proximal contacts of casting are too heavy or too tight
    C. Undercuts present in prepared tooth
    D. The occlusal of the prepared tooth was underreduced

31. For a gold casting alloy, which of the following is added primarily to act as a scavenger for oxygen during the casting process?
    A. Copper
    B. Palladium
    C. Silver
    D. Zinc

32. All of the following are likely to indicate the need for restoration of a cervical notch *except* one. Which one is the *exception*?
    A. Patient age
    B. Esthetic concern
    C. Tooth is symptomatic
    D. Tooth is deeply notched axially

33. When comparing pin retention with slot retention for a complex amalgam restoration, which of the following statements is *false*?
    A. Slots are used where vertical walls allow opposing retention locks.
    B. Slots provide stronger retention than pins.
    C. Slots and grooves can be used interchangeably.
    D. Pin retention is used primarily where there are few or no vertical walls.

34. All of the following statements about slot-retained complex amalgams are true *except* one. Which one is the *exception*?

A. Slots should be 1.5 mm in depth.

B. Slots should be 1 mm or more in length.

C. Slots may be segmented or continuous.

D. Slots should be placed at least 0.5 mm inside the dentinoenamel junction (DEJ).

35. Bonding of resins to dentin is *best* described as involving ____.
    A. Mechanical interlocking
    B. Ionic bonding
    C. Covalent bonding
    D. van der Waals forces

36. Which one of the following acids is generally recommended for etching tooth structure?
    A. Maleic acid
    B. Polyacrylic acid
    C. Phosphoric acid
    D. Tartaric acid
    E. Ethylenediamine tetraacetic acid

37. The principal goals of bonding are ____.
    A. Sealing and thermal insulation
    B. Strengthening teeth and esthetics
    C. Esthetics and reduction of postoperative sensitivity
    D. Sealing and retention
    E. Retention and reduction of tooth flexure

38. Triturating a dental amalgam ____.
    A. Reduces the size of the alloy particles
    B. Coats the alloy particles with mercury
    C. Reduces the crystal sizes as they form
    D. Dissolves the alloy particles in mercury

39. Which of the following is a primary contraindication for the use of a composite restoration?
    A. Occlusal factors
    B. Inability to isolate the operating area
    C. Nonesthetic areas
    D. Extension onto the root surface

40. Which of the following materials has the highest linear coefficient of expansion?
    A. Amalgam
    B. Direct gold
    C. Tooth structure
    D. Composite resin

41. Which of the following is the *most* common pin used in restorative procedures?
    A. Friction-locked pin
    B. Cemented pin
    C. Amalgam pin
    D. Self-threaded pin

42. A cervical lesion should be restored if it is ____.
    A. Carious
    B. Very sensitive
    C. Causing gingival inflammation
    D. All of the above

43. With regard to the mercury controversy related to the use of amalgam restorations, which of the following statements is *not* correct?

A. Scientific evidence is lacking that amalgam poses health risks to humans except for rare allergic reactions.

B. Alternative amalgamlike materials with low or no mercury content have promise.

C. True allergies to amalgam rarely have been reported.

D. Efforts are under way to reduce the environmental mercury to which people are exposed to lessen their total mercury exposure.

44. Compared with amalgam restorations, composite restorations are _____.
    A. Stronger
    B. More technique-sensitive
    C. More resistant to occlusal forces
    D. Not indicated for class II restorations

45. Which of the following statements regarding the choice between doing a composite or amalgam restoration is *true*?
    A. Establishing restored proximal contacts is easier with composite.
    B. The amalgam is more difficult and technique-sensitive.
    C. The composite generally uses a more conservative tooth/cavity preparation.
    D. Only amalgam should be used for class II restorations.

46. Eburnated dentin has which of the following characteristics? (Choose all that apply.)
    A. Is sclerotic dentin
    B. Indicates recent poor hygiene
    C. Usually appears as a white patch
    D. Is firm to the touch of an explorer
    E. Is usually seen in older patients

47. Rounding internal cavity preparation angles is part of what form in cavity preparation?
    A. Resistance form
    B. Retention form
    C. Convenience form
    D. Outline form

48. Which of the following terms refers to tooth structure loss in the cervical area secondary to biomechanical loading?
    A. Abfraction
    B. Abrasion
    C. Attrition
    D. Erosion

49. For a mechanical pulp exposure that is noncarious and the exposure is less than 1.0 mm, what is usually the *most* appropriate treatment?
    A. No pulp treatment
    B. Direct pulp cap
    C. Indirect pulp cap
    D. Endodontic therapy

50. A beveled shoulder design around a capped cusp of a gold onlay preparation is termed a _____.

A. Skirt
B. Stubbed margin
C. Secondary flare
D. Groove extension bevel
E. Collar

51. After completing the tooth preparation for the application of an etch-and-rinse (total-etch) three-step dental adhesive, what is the next step?
    A. Apply adhesive
    B. Rinse etchant and leave surface wet
    C. Apply two to three layers of primer
    D. Etch enamel and dentin with phosphoric acid for 10 to 15 seconds
    E. Light-cure

Oral and Maxillofacial Surgery and Pain Control

1. You have placed a dental implant for replacement of tooth #9. Preoperatively, you obtained a panoramic and a periapical film. During the surgery, you used a crestal incision, series of drills, and paralleling pins as necessary. On restoration of the crown, obtaining ideal esthetics is difficult because the implant is placed too close to the labial cortex, causing the restoration to appear overcontoured. Which of the following techniques could *most* adequately have prevented this problem?
    A. Using an anterior surgical template
    B. Obtaining preoperative tomograms of the alveolus
    C. Using a tissue punch technique
    D. Using a smaller size of implant

2. The third molar impaction *most* difficult to remove is the _____.
    A. Vertical
    B. Mesioangular
    C. Distoangular
    D. Horizontal

3. On a panoramic radiograph of a 13-year-old patient, there is evidence of crown formation of the third molars but no root formation yet. These teeth fall into the category of impacted teeth.
    A. True
    B. False

4. Which of the following is *not* appropriate treatment for an odontogenic abscess?
    A. Placing the patient on antibiotics and having him or her return when the swelling resolves
    B. Surgical removal of the source of the infection as early as possible
    C. Drainage of the abscess with placement of surgical drains
    D. Close observance of the patient during resolution of the infection

E. Medical management of the patient to correct any compromised states that might exist

5. Before the exploration of any intrabony pathologic lesion, which type of biopsy must *always* be done?
    A. Cytologic smear
    B. Incisional biopsy
    C. Excisional biopsy
    D. Aspiration biopsy

6. You are performing a 5-year follow-up examination on a 43-year-old patient with an implant. When comparing radiographs, you estimate that there has been almost 0.1 mm of lost bone height around the implant since it was placed. Which of the following is indicated?
    A. Removal of the implant and replacement with a larger size implant
    B. Removal of the implant to allow healing before another one can be placed 4 months later
    C. Remaking the prosthetic crown because of tangential forces on the implant
    D. The implant is doing well; this amount of bone loss is considered acceptable

7. The major mechanisms for the destruction of osseointegration of implants are _____.
    A. Related to surgical technique
    B. Similar to those of natural teeth
    C. Related to implant material
    D. Related to nutrition

8. After completing your postoperative instructions for dental implant placement for replacement of tooth #14, your patient asks you how long it will be before she can get her new tooth. Which of the following is *most* correct to allow complete osseointegration?
    A. 3 weeks
    B. 6 weeks
    C. 3 months
    D. 6 months

9. The imaging evaluation of the temporomandibular joint (TMJ) is most likely to include any of the following *except* one. Which one is the *exception*?
    A. Panoramic radiographs
    B. TMJ tomograms
    C. Xeroradiography
    D. Magnetic resonance imaging

10. When is distraction osteogenesis preferred over a traditional osteotomy?
    A. When a large advancement is needed
    B. When a small advancement is needed
    C. When exacted interdigitation of the occlusion is needed
    D. When the treatment needs to be done in a very short period of time
    E. Distraction osteogenesis is always preferred over a traditional osteotomy

11. The most common mandibular surgical osteotomy to advance the mandible is _____.

A. Le Fort I osteotomy
B. Segmental maxillary osteotomy
C. Bilateral sagittal split osteotomy
D. Intraoral vertical ramus osteotomy

12. Obstructive sleep apnea syndrome (OSAS) often results in all of the following *except* one. Which one is the *exception*?
    A. Excessive daytime sleepiness
    B. Aggressive behavior
    C. Personality changes
    D. Depression

13. Which of the following procedures would be considered the *least* invasive surgical treatment for temporomandibular joint complaints?
    A. Splint therapy
    B. Arthrocentesis
    C. Arthroscopy
    D. Disc removal
    E. Total joint replacement

14. A 23-year-old college student is suspected to have sustained a mandible fracture during an altercation. Which of the following statements is *false*?
    A. At least two x-rays should be obtained.
    B. The most common x-ray obtained is a panoramic radiograph.
    C. The most likely area for this patient's mandible to be fractured is the mandibular dental alveolus.
    D. Point tenderness, changes in occlusion, step deformities, and gingival lacerations all should be noted on physical examination.

15. Which of the following is *not* a classification of mandible fractures?
    A. Anatomic location
    B. Description of the condition of the bone fragments at the fracture site
    C. Angulation of the fracture and muscle pull
    D. Le Fort level

16. Although the state-of-the-art treatment for facial fractures is internal rigid fixation using bone plates and screws, a proper occlusal relationship must be established before fixation of the bony segments if the reduction is to be satisfactory.
    A. True
    B. False

17. Which of the following statements regarding possible complications resulting from dental extractions is *true*?
    A. Patients with numbness lasting more than 4 weeks should be referred for microneurosurgical evaluation.
    B. Infections are common, even in healthy patients.
    C. Dry socket occurs in 10% of patients with third molar extractions.
    D. Teeth lost into the oropharynx are usually swallowed and do not require further intervention.

18. Which of the following statements regarding the possibilities for reconstruction of an atrophic edentulous ridge before denture construction is true?
    A. Dental implants are used only as a last resort after bone grafting attempts have failed.
    B. Distraction osteogenesis is too new a technique to be applied to ridge augmentation.
    C. Potential bone graft harvest sites for ridge reconstruction include rib, hip, and chin.
    D. The need for ridge augmentation is more common in the maxilla than in the mandible.

19. You are evaluating a patient 5 days after extraction of tooth #17. The patient complains of a severe throbbing pain that started yesterday, 4 days after extraction. The patient *most* likely has which of the following conditions?
    A. Dry socket
    B. Subperiosteal abscess
    C. Periapical periodontitis in tooth #18
    D. Neuropathic pain

20. Which of the following patients would *not* be expected to experience delayed healing of an extraction site?
    A. A patient older than 60 years of age
    B. A patient younger than 10 years of age
    C. A patient with diabetes
    D. A patient with a heavy smoking habit

21. All of the following are desirable properties of an ideal local anesthetic *except* one. Which one is the *exception*?
    A. It should have sufficient potency to give complete anesthesia even if harmful results occur at therapeutic doses
    B. It should be relatively free from producing allergic reactions
    C. It should be stable in solution and readily undergo biotransformation in the body
    D. It should be either sterile or capable of being sterilized by heat without deterioration

22. What is the direct effect of local anesthetics on blood vessels in the area of injection?
    A. Constriction
    B. Dilation
    C. Sclerosis
    D. Thrombosis

23. All of the following describe lidocaine as packaged in dental cartridges *except* one. What one is the *exception*?
    A. Provided in a 2% solution
    B. Provided with or without epinephrine
    C. Has a $pK_a = 8.1$
    D. Has a rapid onset

24. All of the following are reasons that 25-gauge needles are preferred to smaller diameter needles *except* one. Which one is the *exception*?
    A. Greater accuracy in needle insertion for 25-gauge needles

B. Increased rate of needle breakage for 25-gauge needles
    C. Aspiration of blood is easier and more reliable through a larger lumen
    D. There is no difference in pain of insertion

25. A 1.0-mL volume of a 2% solution contains ____.
    A. 18 mg
    B. 20 mg
    C. 36 mg
    D. 54 mg

26. During local anesthetic administration, the patient should be placed in a ____ position.
    A. Trendelenburg
    B. Supine
    C. Reclined
    D. Semisupine

27. According to Malamed, slow injection is defined as the deposition of 1 mL of local anesthetic solution in not less than ____.
    A. 15 seconds
    B. 30 seconds
    C. 60 seconds
    D. 2 minutes

28. The ____ nerve block is recommended for management of several maxillary molar teeth in one quadrant.
    A. Posterior superior alveolar
    B. Inferior alveolar
    C. Long buccal
    D. Nasopalatine

29. In an adult of normal size, penetration to a depth of ____ mm places the needle tip in the immediate vicinity of the foramina, through which the posterior superior alveolar nerves enter the posterior surface of the maxilla.
    A. 10
    B. 16
    C. 20
    D. 30

30. The ____ nerve block is useful for dental procedures involving the palatal soft tissues distal to the canine.
    A. Nasopalatine
    B. Greater palatine
    C. Long buccal
    D. Inferior alveolar

31. At about what threshold does elevation of cardiovascular signs occur with epinephrine that is injected in a local anesthetic solution in a patient with cardiovascular compromise?
    A. 40 μg
    B. 100 μg
    C. 200 μg
    D. 1000 μg

32. According to Malamed, the maximum local anesthetic dose of lidocaine (with or without vasoconstrictor) is ____.

A. 1.5 mg/kg
B. 2.0 mg/kg
C. 4.4 mg/kg
D. 7.0 mg/kg

33. Which of the following injections, when properly performed, does *not* lead to pulpal anesthesia?
   A. Inferior alveolar
   B. Lingual
   C. Posterior superior alveolar
   D. Infraorbital (true anterior superior alveolar nerve block)

34. The optimal volume of local anesthetic solution delivered for a true anterior superior alveolar nerve block is usually about _____.
   A. 0.5 mL
   B. 1.0 mL
   C. 1.5 mL
   D. 1.8 mL

35. The local anesthetic agent that is *most* appropriate for use in *most* children is _____.
   A. 3% mepivacaine
   B. 2% mepivacaine with 1:20,000 levonordefrin
   C. 2% lidocaine with 1:100,000 epinephrine
   D. 0.5% bupivacaine with 1:200,000 epinephrine

36. Which of the following local anesthetics causes the *least* amount of vasodilation?
   A. Lidocaine
   B. Mepivacaine
   C. Bupivacaine
   D. Articaine

37. According to Malamed, how many cartridges of 2% lidocaine can be safely administered to a child weighing 40 lb?
   A. Three cartridges
   B. One cartridge
   C. Nine cartridges
   D. Two cartridges

38. If a local anesthetic has a low pK_a, it usually has a _____.
   A. Greater potency
   B. Higher degree of protein binding
   C. Faster onset of action
   D. Greater vasodilating potential

39. What areas are anesthetized with correct administration of the (long) buccal injection?
   A. Soft tissues and periosteum buccal to the mandibular molar teeth
   B. Soft tissues and periosteum lingual to the mandibular molar teeth
   C. Soft tissues and periosteum lingual to the mandibular premolar teeth
   D. Soft tissues and periosteum buccal to the mandibular premolar teeth

40. Which local anesthetic is *most* hydrophobic and has the highest degree of protein binding?
   A. Mepivacaine
   B. Lidocaine
   C. Bupivacaine
   D. Procaine

41. A portion of which cranial nerve is anesthetized when performing an infraorbital nerve block?
   A. VII
   B. V
   C. III
   D. II

42. Which of the following local anesthetics has the shortest half-life?
   A. Lidocaine
   B. Prilocaine
   C. Bupivacaine
   D. Articaine

43. In odontogenic infections such as abscesses, which groups of organisms should be the usual targets of empiric therapy with antibiotics?
   A. Fungi and enveloped viruses
   B. Methicillin-resistant *Staphylococcus aureus*
   C. Methicillin-sensitive *S. aureus* and aerobes
   D. Streptococcal species and anaerobes

44. Which of the following are reasons for removing an impacted tooth? (Choose all that apply.)
   A. Prevention of pericoronitis
   B. Asymptomatic full bony impaction in a 65-year-old patient
   C. Prevention of periodontal disease in a tooth adjacent to the impacted tooth
   D. Prevention of odontogenic cysts and tumors

45. Which biopsy procedure should be used initially for a soft tissue lesion deep to the oral mucosa?
   A. Incisional
   B. Excisional
   C. Aspiration
   D. Hard tissue
   E. Mucoperiosteal flap

46. The pK_a of a local anesthetic is most likely to determine which of its characteristics?
   A. Potency
   B. Duration of action
   C. Risk of allergy
   D. Compatibility with a vasoconstrictor
   E. Rate of onset of anesthesia

47. Which nerve block results in anesthesia of palatal soft tissue from canine to canine?
   A. Nasopalatine
   B. Greater palatine
   C. Mental
   D. Anterior superior alveolar
   E. Posterior superior alveolar

Oral Diagnosis

1. Which of the following is a potential sequela of an acute periapical abscess?

A. Central giant cell granuloma
B. Peripheral giant cell granuloma
C. Osteosarcoma
D. Periapical granuloma
E. Periapical cemento-osseous dysplasia

2. Which of the following odontogenic cysts occurs as a result of stimulation and proliferation of the reduced enamel epithelium?
A. Dentigerous cyst
B. Lateral root cyst
C. Radicular cyst
D. Odontogenic keratocyst
E. Gingival cyst

3. Two cystic radiolucencies in the mandible of a 16-year-old boy were lined by thin, parakeratinized epithelium showing palisading of basal cells. All teeth were vital, and the patient had no symptoms. This patient most likely has which of the following?
A. Odontogenic keratocysts
B. Periapical granulomas
C. Periapical cysts
D. Traumatic bone cysts
E. Ossifying fibromas

4. When a diagnosis of odontogenic keratocyst is made, the patient should be advised regarding the _____.
A. Need for full-mouth extractions
B. Association with colonic polyps
C. Associated recurrence rate
D. Likelihood of malignant transformation
E. Need for additional laboratory studies

5. A painless, well-circumscribed 1 cm × 3 cm radiolucent lesion with radiopaque focus was found in the posterior mandible of an 11-year-old boy. Which of the following should be included in a differential diagnosis?
A. Ameloblastic fibro-odontoma
B. Paget's disease
C. Dentigerous cyst
D. Ameloblastoma
E. Langerhans' cell disease

6. Herpes simplex virus is the cause of which of the following?
A. Minor aphthous ulcers
B. Herpetiform aphthae
C. Herpetic whitlow
D. Herpangina
E. Herpes zoster

7. A 12-year-old patient presents with premature loss of primary teeth. On radiographic examination, a sharply marginated lucency is seen in the area of tooth loss. A biopsy specimen shows a round cell infiltrate with numerous eosinophils. Which of the following diagnoses is suggested?
A. Cherubism
B. Gardner's syndrome
C. Paget's disease

D. Fibrous dysplasia
E. Langerhans' cell disease

8. A 15-year-old patient has a numb lower lip and pain in her right posterior mandible. A radiograph shows uniform thickening of the periodontal membrane space of tooth #30. The tooth shows abnormally increased mobility. Which one of the following diagnoses should be seriously considered?
A. Periapical cyst
B. Periapical granuloma
C. Traumatic bone cyst
D. Ameloblastoma
E. Malignancy

9. Which of the following signs or symptoms suggests a chronic benign process?
A. Paresthesia
B. Pain
C. Vertical tooth mobility
D. Uniformly widened periodontal membrane space
E. Sclerotic bony margins

10. Which of the following features are shared by central and peripheral giant cell granulomas?
A. Microscopic appearance
B. Clinical behavior
C. Recurrence rate
D. Similar forms of treatment
E. Radiographic appearance

11. Diffuse soft swelling of the lips and neck after the ingestion of drugs, shellfish, or nuts is known as _____.
A. Fixed drug reaction
B. Anaphylaxis
C. Urticaria
D. Acquired angioedema
E. Contact allergy

12. A 7-year-old patient presents with a quadrant of teeth showing abnormal formation of both enamel and dentin. All of his other teeth appear clinically normal. Radiographically, the affected teeth can be described as "ghost teeth." The patient has _____.
A. Regional odontodysplasia
B. Dens evaginatus
C. Dentin dysplasia
D. Ectodermal dysplasia
E. Cleidocranial dysplasia

13. An adult patient presents with a 0.5 cm × 0.5 cm submucosal mass in the posterior lateral tongue. A biopsy specimen shows a neoplasm composed of glandlike elements and connective tissue elements. It is covered by normal-appearing epithelium. This could be which of the following?
A. Oral wart
B. Pleomorphic adenoma (mixed tumor)
C. Granular cell tumor
D. Idiopathic leukoplakia
E. Peripheral giant cell granuloma

14. Oral squamous cell carcinomas manifest typically in which of the following ways?
    A. Vesicular eruption
    B. Pigmented patch
    C. Inflamed pustule
    D. Submucosal swelling
    E. Indurated nonhealing ulcer

15. A clinical differential diagnosis of an asymptomatic submucosal lump or nodule in the tongue would include all of the following *except* one. Which one is the *exception*?
    A. Traumatic fibroma
    B. Neurofibroma
    C. Granular cell tumor
    D. Salivary gland tumor
    E. Dermoid cyst

16. Ectopic lymphoid tissue would *most* likely be found in which of the following sites?
    A. Hard gingiva
    B. Soft gingiva
    C. Floor of mouth
    D. Dorsum of tongue
    E. Vermilion of the lip

17. Schwann's cell is the cell of origin for which of the following tumors?
    A. Odontogenic myxoma
    B. Rhabdomyoma
    C. Neurofibroma
    D. Mixed tumor
    E. Leiomyoma

18. A 43-year-old man presents with an asymptomatic anterior palatal swelling. A radiograph shows a 1 cm × 1 cm lucency and divergence of tooth roots #8 and #9. All teeth in the area are vital. What lesion does this *most* likely represent?
    A. Periapical granuloma
    B. Aneurysmal bone cyst
    C. Nasopalatine duct cyst
    D. Globulomaxillary lesion
    E. Dermoid cyst

19. The globulomaxillary lesion of bone _____.
    A. Is associated with the crown of an unerupted tooth
    B. Occurs between maxillary lateral and canine teeth
    C. Typically causes pain
    D. Typically manifests as a mixed lucent-opaque lesion with ill-defined margins
    E. Is always associated with a nonvital tooth

20. A generalized red, atrophic tongue would suggest all of the following *except* one. Which one is the *exception*?
    A. Vitamin B deficiency
    B. Pernicious anemia
    C. Chronic candidiasis
    D. Iron deficiency anemia
    E. Peripheral giant cell granuloma

21. Nevoid basal cell carcinoma syndrome includes multiple basal cell carcinomas, bone abnormalities, and _____.
    A. Osteomas
    B. Café au lait macules
    C. Odontogenic keratocysts
    D. Hypoplastic teeth
    E. Lymphoma

22. All of the following lesions characteristically manifest in individuals younger than age 20 years *except* one. Which one is the *exception*?
    A. Traumatic bone cyst
    B. Adenomatoid odontogenic tumor
    C. Ameloblastic fibroma
    D. Compound odontoma
    E. Ameloblastoma

23. Oral and genital lesions are seen in patients with _____.
    A. Behçet's syndrome
    B. Peutz-Jeghers syndrome
    C. Herpangina
    D. Wegener's granulomatosis
    E. Hairy leukoplakia

24. A 32-year-old man presented with a 1 cm × 2 cm macular red-blue lesion in the hard palate. The lesion was asymptomatic and had been present for an unknown duration. He had no dental abnormalities and no significant periodontal disease. This lesion could be all of the following *except* one. Which one is the *exception*?
    A. Vascular malformation
    B. Nicotine stomatitis
    C. Ecchymosis
    D. Kaposi's sarcoma
    E. Erythroplasia

25. Bremsstrahlung radiation results from _____.
    A. X-rays interacting with electrons
    B. Electrons interacting with electrons
    C. Electrons interacting with nuclei
    D. L shell electrons falling into the K shell
    E. Photons interacting with nuclei
    F. Photons converting into electrons

26. X-rays are produced in most conventional dental x-ray machines _____.
    A. Continuously during operation
    B. When there is a large space charge
    C. Half the time during operation
    D. When the anode carries a negative charge
    E. Only when the beam is collimated
    F. Only during the first half of each second

27. Deterministic effects _____.
    A. Show a severity of response proportional to dose
    B. Are seen only in the oral cavity
    C. Are found after exposure to low levels of radiation
    D. Result from particulate radiation such as alpha and beta particles but not x-rays
    E. None of the above

28. In the radiolysis of water, ____.
    A. Free radicals are formed, which are nonreactive
    B. The presence of dissolved oxygen reduces the number of free radicals
    C. The formation of free radicals is the "direct effect"
    D. The resultant free radicals may alter biologic molecules
    E. Two of the above
    F. None of the above

29. The radiosensitivity of cells depends on ____.
    A. Mitotic future
    B. Mitotic activity
    C. Degree of differentiation
    D. All of the above
    E. None of the above

30. Rectangular collimation is recommended because it ____.
    A. Deflects scatter radiation
    B. Decreases patient dose
    C. Increases film density
    D. Increases film contrast

31. It is acceptable for the operator to hold the film in a patient's mouth ____.
    A. If the patient is a child
    B. If the patient or parent grants permission
    C. If the patient has a handicap
    D. If no film holder is available
    E. Never

32. Comparing screen film/intensifying screen combinations with direct-exposure films reveals that screen film/intensifying screen combinations ____.
    A. Render less resolution
    B. Require more exposure
    C. Require special processing chemistry
    D. Are preferred for intraoral radiography

33. It is important that the film base be ____.
    A. Opaque
    B. Very rigid
    C. Flexible
    D. Completely clear
    E. Sensitive to x-rays

34. Excessive vertical angulation causes ____.
    A. Overlapping
    B. Foreshortening
    C. Elongation
    D. Cone-cutting

35. Which of the following statements about obtaining the most geometrically accurate image is *false*?
    A. The film should be parallel to the object.
    B. The central ray should be parallel to the object.
    C. The central ray should be perpendicular to the film.
    D. The object-to-film distance should be short.
    E. The object-to-anode distance should be long.

36. The size of the x-ray tube focal spot influences radiographic ____.
    A. Density
    B. Contrast
    C. Resolution
    D. Magnification
    E. Both C and D

37. The primary function of developer is to ____.
    A. Reduce crystals of silver halide to solid silver grains
    B. Reduce solid silver grains to specks of silver halide
    C. Remove unexposed silver halide crystals
    D. Remove exposed silver halide crystals

38. If an exposed radiograph is too dark after proper development, you should ____.
    A. Place it back in the fixer
    B. Place it back in the developer
    C. Decrease development time
    D. Increase milliamperage
    E. Decrease exposure time
    F. Decrease development temperature

39. The radiolucent portions of the images on a processed dental x-ray film are made up of ____.
    A. Microscopic grains of silver halide
    B. Microscopic grains of metallic silver
    C. A gelatin on a cellulose acetate base
    D. Unexposed silver bromide

40. The purpose of the "penny test" is to check ____.
    A. Developer action
    B. Fixer action
    C. For proper development temperature
    D. For proper safelighting conditions

41. Proper radiographic infection control includes all of the following *except* one. Which one is the *exception*?
    A. Wearing gloves while making radiographs
    B. Disinfecting x-ray machine surface
    C. Covering working surfaces with barriers
    D. Sterilizing nondisposable instruments
    E. Sterilizing film packets

42. Occlusal radiographs are useful for all of the following *except* one. Which one is the *exception*?
    A. For views of the temporomandibular joint (TMJ)
    B. For displaying large segments of the mandibular arch
    C. When the patient has limited opening
    D. When there are sialoliths in the floor of the mouth
    E. When there is buccal-lingual expansion of the mandible

43. From the following list, select the systemic diseases that involve a defect in the immune system. (Choose all that apply.)
    A. Celiac sprue
    B. Sarcoidosis
    C. Amyloidosis
    D. Behçet's syndrome
    E. Crohn's disease
    F. Neurofibromatosis

44. Sjögren's syndrome is characterized by which of the following conditions? (Choose all that apply.)

A. Xerostomia
B. Aphthous ulcers
C. Hairy leukoplakia
D. Keratoconjunctivitis sicca
E. Lymphocyte infiltration in minor salivary glands

45. Which of the following apply to filtration of an x-ray beam in a modern x-ray unit? (Choose all that apply.)
    A. Decreases the mean energy of the x-ray beam
    B. Reduces patient exposure by removing lower energy photons
    C. Provided by an aluminum filter
    D. Required to be 1.5 mm thick for 70 kVp

46. On a radiograph, you observe a radiolucency extending from the distal aspect of the maxillary canine to the posterior wall of the maxilla above the tuberosity. The *most* likely cause of this radiolucency is ____.
    A. Dentigerous cyst
    B. Ameloblastoma
    C. Zygomatic process of the maxilla
    D. Maxillary sinus

47. Discoid lupus erythematosus has all of the following characteristics *except* one. Which one is the *exception*?
    A. Produces oral lesions that resemble erosive lichen planus
    B. Predominately affects middle-aged women
    C. Involves damage to the heart and kidney
    D. Affects the skin of the face and scalp

Orthodontics and Pediatric Dentistry

1. Which of the following types of malocclusions is *most* common?
   A. Class I malocclusion
   B. Class II malocclusion
   C. Class III malocclusion
   D. Open bite malocclusion

2. According to Scammon's growth curves, which of the following tissues has a growth increase that can be used to help predict timing of the adolescent growth spurt?
   A. Neural tissues
   B. Lymphoid tissues
   C. Reproductive tissues

3. Which of the following is the *least* reliable way to predict the timing of the peak of the adolescent growth spurt for an individual?
   A. Plotting changes in height over time on a growth curve
   B. Following eruption timing of the dentition
   C. Taking a hand-wrist radiograph to assess skeletal development
   D. Observing changes in secondary sex characteristics

4. In a patient with incomplete cleft palate, which of the following aspects is *most* likely to remain open?

A. Anterior aspect
B. Middle aspect
C. Posterior aspect
D. Right aspect

5. Children in the primary dentition *most* often present with ____.
   A. An increased overbite
   B. A decreased overbite
   C. An ideal overbite
   D. A significant open bite

6. During the mixed dentition, a 1-mm diastema develops between the maxillary incisors. Which of the following is *most* likely to happen?
   A. The diastema will need orthodontic intervention to be closed
   B. The diastema will resolve once the canines erupt
   C. The diastema will resolve only when all of the permanent teeth erupt
   D. The diastema will continue to widen as permanent teeth erupt

7. A patient with the maxillary first permanent molar mesiobuccal cusp sitting distal to the buccal groove of the mandibular first molar has which type of malocclusion?
   A. Class I
   B. Class II, division 1
   C. Class II, division 2
   D. Class III

8. An adult patient with a class II molar relationship and a cephalometric ANB angle of 2 degrees has which type of malocclusion?
   A. Class II dental malocclusion
   B. Class II skeletal malocclusion
   C. Class I dental malocclusion
   D. Class II skeletal malocclusion

9. Which of the following would be the preferred method of overbite correction in a patient who displays excessive maxillary incisor at rest, has an excessive lower face height, and has a deep overbite?
   A. Eruption of posterior teeth to rotate the mandible open
   B. Intrusion of maxillary incisors
   C. Intrusion of mandibular incisors
   D. Flaring of maxillary and mandibular incisors

10. In tooth movement, the formation of a hyalinized zone on the pressure side is due to ____.
    A. Application of light, continuous forces
    B. Application of heavy forces
    C. Normal forces of mastication
    D. Abnormal swallowing patterns

11. Which of the following reactions is *least* likely to be observed during orthodontic treatment?
    A. Root resorption
    B. Devitalization of teeth that are moved
    C. Mobility of teeth that are moved
    D. Development of occlusal interferences

12. Root resorption is correlated to the pattern of stress distribution in the periodontal ligament (PDL) and type of tooth movement.
    A. True
    B. False
13. Putting a force through which of the following points would cause pure translation of a tooth without rotation, tipping, or torque?
    A. Center of rotation
    B. Center of resistance
    C. Center of the bracket
    D. Apex of the root
14. Doubling the force applied at the bracket of a tooth would have what effect on the moment affecting tooth movement?
    A. Moment would decrease by 50%
    B. Moment would not change
    C. Moment would double
    D. Moment would increase fourfold
15. Two equal and opposite forces that are not collinear applied to a tooth are called _____.
    A. The center of resistance
    B. The center of rotation
    C. Root movement
    D. A couple
16. A wire extending from the molars to the incisors is activated to intrude the incisors. What is the side effect on the molars?
    A. Molars tip forward and intrude
    B. Molars rotate mesiobuccally
    C. Molars tip distally and extrude
    D. Molars rotate distobuccally
17. Class II elastics are used by stretching an elastic between which of the two following points?
    A. From the posterior to the anterior within the maxillary arch
    B. From the posterior to the anterior within the mandibular arch
    C. From the posterior of the maxillary arch to the anterior of the mandibular arch
    D. From the posterior of the mandibular arch to the anterior of the maxillary arch
18. What makes it possible for nickel-titanium archwires to exhibit superelastic behavior?
    A. This behavior is based on a reversible transformation within the austenitic phase.
    B. This behavior is based on a reversible transformation between the austenitic and martensitic phases.
    C. This behavior is based on a reversible transformation within the martensitic phase.
    D. This behavior is based on an irreversible transformation within the martensitic phase.
19. What is a second-order bend?
    A. Bend to position a tooth buccolingually
    B. Bend to provide angulation of a tooth in mesiodistal direction (tip)

C. Bend to provide correct angulation of a tooth in labiolingual direction (torque)
    D. Bend to rotate a tooth
20. When class III elastics are used, the maxillary first molars _____.
    A. Move distally and intrude
    B. Move mesially and extrude
    C. Move mesially and intrude
    D. Move only mesially; there is no movement in the vertical direction
21. An adolescent patient presents to your office with a skeletal and dental class II malocclusion and a deep bite. Which of the following would be a proper treatment plan for this patient?
    A. Reverse-pull headgear, extrusion arch, and full fixed appliances
    B. Reverse-pull headgear, intrusion arch, and full fixed appliances
    C. Extraction of maxillary first premolars, extrusion arch, and full fixed appliances
    D. Extraction of maxillary first premolars, intrusion arch, and full fixed appliances
22. When using a cervical-pull headgear, the forces generated on the maxillary first molar cause this tooth to move in which of the following ways?
    A. Mesially and to extrude
    B. Distally and to extrude
    C. Mesially and to intrude
    D. Distally and to intrude
23. Which of the following depicts the usual order of extraction of teeth if serial extraction is chosen as the treatment to alleviate severe crowding?
    A. Primary second molars, primary first molars, permanent first premolars, primary canines
    B. Primary canines, primary first molars, permanent first premolars
    C. Primary first molars, primary second molars, primary canines
    D. Primary canines, permanent canines, primary first molars, permanent first premolars
24. Closure of a 2-mm maxillary midline diastema should be accomplished orthodontically in an 8-year-old child in which of the following circumstances?
    A. If the lateral incisors are missing
    B. If the space creates an esthetic concern and the child is being teased about it
    C. If there is also deep overbite present
    D. If mild crowding is also present
25. In a patient with missing permanent maxillary lateral incisors, the decision of whether to substitute canines in the lateral spaces depends on all of the following *except* one. Which one is the *exception*?
    A. Amount of crowding in the maxillary arch
    B. Interarch relationship between the maxillary and mandibular dentition
    C. Esthetic appearance of the permanent canines

D. Type of orthodontic appliance used to align the teeth

26. All of the following may be indications to consider extraction of permanent teeth in an orthodontic patient *except* one. Which one is the *exception*?
   A. Excessive crowding
   B. Class II interarch relationship
   C. Flat lip profile
   D. Anterior open bite

27. Which of the following is an advantage of fixed wire retention compared with a removable Hawley-type retainer?
   A. Does not require the patient to remember to wear it
   B. Is easier to clean
   C. Design can be altered to achieve minor tooth movements
   D. Can incorporate an acrylic bite plate to avoid relapse of overbite correction

28. The preferred surgical procedure to correct a class II malocclusion owing to a deficient mandible is ____.
   A. Maxillary impaction
   B. Maxillary setback
   C. Mandibular setback
   D. Mandibular advancement

29. Which of the following is considered to be the *least* stable orthognathic surgical movement?
   A. Advancement of the mandible
   B. Advancement of the maxilla
   C. Superior movement (impaction) of the maxilla
   D. Inferior movement of the maxilla

30. Your patient exhibits enamel hypoplasia near the incisal edges of all permanent incisors and cuspids except for the maxillary lateral incisors, which appear normal. At what age would you suspect some kind of systemic problem?
   A. Before birth
   B. From birth to 1 year of age
   C. From 1 to 2 years of age
   D. From 2 to 3 years of age

31. Fluorosis is the result of excessive systemic fluoride during which stage of tooth development?
   A. Initiation
   B. Morphodifferentiation
   C. Apposition
   D. Calcification

32. Why are implants not generally performed on a 12-year-old patient with congenitally missing lateral incisors?
   A. The patient likely would be unable to tolerate the surgical procedure.
   B. Waiting for the crowns is too much of an esthetic issue with most children that age.
   C. The gingival tissue will recede as the child gets older.

D. The implants will appear to submerge as the child gets older.

33. On the health history form, the mother of a 6-year-old new patient notes that the child is moderately mentally challenged. The dentist should ____.
   A. Refer to a pediatric dentist
   B. Use a Tell-Show-Do technique of behavior management
   C. Use conscious sedation
   D. Use restraints after obtaining informed consent

34. The functional inquiry questionnaire reveals that a mother has had negative dental experiences and remains very nervous regarding her dental care. How would this most likely influence her 3-year-old child's reaction to dentistry?
   A. Increase the likelihood of a negative behavior
   B. Increase the likelihood of a positive response to dentistry
   C. Cause an initial positive reaction, which changes to a negative reaction with the slightest stress.
   D. Maternal anxiety has little effect on a child's behavior in a dental setting.

35. Which of the following local anesthetic techniques is recommended for anesthetizing a primary mandibular second molar that is to be extracted?
   A. Buccal and lingual infiltration adjacent to the second primary molar
   B. Inferior alveolar nerve block
   C. Inferior alveolar nerve block and lingual nerve block
   D. Inferior alveolar, lingual, and buccal nerve block

36. In the primary dentition, the mandibular foramen is located where in relation to the plane of occlusion?
   A. Higher than the plane of occlusion
   B. Much higher than the plane of occlusion
   C. Lower than the plane of occlusion
   D. The same level as the plane of occlusion

37. What is the minimum alveolar concentration of nitrous oxide (vol %)?
   A. 50
   B. 75
   C. 95
   D. 105

38. After administration of a local anesthetic, most patients can be maintained in conscious sedation at ____.
   A. 20% to 40% nitrous oxide
   B. 20% to 40% oxygen
   C. 50% nitrous oxide
   D. 10% nitrous oxide

39. In a 9-year-old patient, the mandibular left first primary molar has a large, carious lesion on the distal and on the occlusal, and the tooth has greater mobility than what you would normally expect. You should ____.
   A. Take a radiograph of the area
   B. Perform a pulpotomy

C. Perform a pulpectomy

D. Extract the tooth and consider space maintenance

40. Why are rounded internal line angles desirable in the preparation of amalgam restorations in primary teeth?

A. They increase retention

B. They conserve tooth structure

C. They increase resistance

D. They decrease internal stresses in the restorative material

41. A 7-year-old patient has a very large, carious lesion on tooth T. What radiologic factors should be used to determine the best treatment of choice between pulpotomy and primary endodontics?

A. Furcation involvement

B. External root resorption

C. Internal root resorption

D. Two of the above

E. All of the above

42. Which pulpotomy medicament demonstrates better success rates than formocresol?

A. Mineral trioxide aggregate

B. Calcium hydroxide

C. Resin-modified glass ionomer cement

D. Fifth-generation bonding agents

43. The pulp tissue of primary teeth _____.

1. **In general is smaller proportionately than permanent pulps in relation to tooth crown size**

2. **Is closer to the outer surface of the tooth than the permanent teeth**

3. **Follows the general surface contour of the crown**

4. **Has the mesial pulp horn closer to the surface than the distal pulp horn**

A. 1, 2, and 4 are correct

B. 2, 3, and 4 are correct

C. 1, 3, and 4 are correct

D. 1, 2, 3, and 4 are correct.

44. The following teeth are erupted in an 8-year-old patient. What is the space maintenance of choice?

3	A	B	C	7	8	9	10	H	I		14
30	T	S	R	26	25	24	23	M	L	K	19

A. Band-loop space maintainer

B. Lower lingual holding arch

C. Nance holding arch

D. Distal shoe space maintainer

45. The following teeth are erupted in a 4-year-old patient. What is the space maintenance of choice?

A	B	C	D	E	F	G	H	I	J
S	R	Q	P	O	N	M	L	K	

A. Band-loop space maintainer

B. Lower lingual holding arch

C. Nance holding arch

D. Distal shoe space maintainer

46. If the fluoride level in the drinking water is greater than 0.6 ppm at any age, no supplemental systemic fluoride is indicated. If the patient is younger than 12 months old, no supplemental systemic fluoride is indicated, whatever the water fluoride level.

A. The first statement is *true*, and the second statement is *true*.

B. The first statement is *true*, and the second statement is *false*.

C. The first statement is *false*, and the second statement is *true*.

D. The first statement is *false*, and the second statement is *false*.

47. A 1-year-old patient has his first dental examination. The dentist reviews with the parent when to expect the next teeth to erupt, teething, and oral hygiene tips for toddlers and discusses fluoride issues with bottled water and toothpaste. The term that describes this proactive approach to dental care is _____.

A. Risk assessment

B. Probability counseling

C. Anticipatory guidance

D. Preventive support counseling

48. Most natal and neonatal teeth are primary teeth. They should be extracted.

A. The first statement is *true*, and the second statement is *true*.

B. The first statement is *true*, and the second statement is *false*.

C. The first statement is *false*, and the second statement is *true*.

D. The first statement is *false*, and the second statement is *false*.

49. The "willful failure of parent or guardian to seek and follow-through with treatment necessary to ensure a level of oral health essential for adequate function and freedom from pain and infection" is a definition of _____.

A. Munchausen syndrome by proxy

B. Emotional abuse

C. Parental corruption

D. Neglect

50. Where do lesions commonly occur in the primary form of acute herpetic gingivostomatitis?

A. Buccal mucosa

B. Tonsils and hard and soft palate

C. Tongue

D. Gingiva

E. All of the above

51. Localized aggressive periodontitis in the primary dentition is seen most commonly in the primary molar area. It is most common in Asian children.

A. The first statement is *true*, and the second statement is *true*.

B. The first statement is *true*, and the second statement is *false*.

C. The first statement is *false*, and the second statement is *true*.

D. The first statement is *false*, and the second statement is *false*.

52. In an 8-year-old patient, tooth #8 was avulsed and was replanted within 30 minutes. What is the *best* splint to use?
    A. Rigid fixation for 7 days
    B. Rigid fixation for 2 months
    C. Nonrigid fixation for 7 days
    D. Nonrigid fixation for 2 months

53. In an 8-year-old patient, teeth #8 and #9 have approximately 50% of their crowns erupted. The patient fell from a skateboard 1 month ago and hit teeth #8 and #9 on the sidewalk. The radiograph today shows open apices of these teeth, normal periodontal ligament, and no apparent periapical radiolucency. The patient has no reaction to electrical pulp tests. What is your treatment of choice?
    A. Calcium hydroxide pulpotomy
    B. Formocresol apexification technique
    C. Calcium hydroxide apexification technique
    D. Repeat examination and radiographs in 6 weeks

54. A permanent incisor with a closed apex is traumatically intruded. What is the treatment of choice?
    A. Gradual orthodontic repositioning and calcium hydroxide pulpectomy
    B. Surgical repositioning and calcium hydroxide pulpectomy
    C. Gradual orthodontic repositioning and conventional endodontic therapy
    D. Surgical repositioning and conventional endodontic therapy

55. Which of the following is the *most* likely cause of pulpal necrosis after trauma to a tooth?
    A. Ankylosis
    B. Calcific metamorphosis
    C. Pulpal hyperemia
    D. Dilaceration

56. What is the sequence of treatment when orthodontic therapy is involved as part of an interdisciplinary plan?
    A. Orthodontic alignment
    B. Caries control
    C. Periodontal surgery including bone recontouring
    D. Placement of full coverage crown

57. From the following, select the bones that grow primarily by endochondral bone formation. (Choose three.)
    A. Maxilla
    B. Mandible
    C. Ethmoid
    D. Frontal
    E. Occipital
    F. Sphenoid

58. According to Scammon's growth curves, which of the following tissues has a growth increase that can be used to help predict timing of the adolescent growth spurt?
    A. Neural tissues
    B. Lymphoid tissues
    C. Reproductive tissues

59. Which of the following features characterize the primary dentition? (Choose two.)
    A. Spacing between the teeth
    B. Crowding of the teeth
    C. Increased overbite
    D. Decreased overbite
    E. Ideal overbite
    F. Anterior crossbite

60. An adult patient with a class II molar relationship and a cephalometric ANB angle of 2 degrees has which type of malocclusion?
    A. Class II dental malocclusion
    B. Class II skeletal malocclusion
    C. Class I dental malocclusion
    D. Class II skeletal malocclusion

61. Which of the following reactions is *least* likely to be observed during orthodontic treatment?
    A. Root resorption
    B. Devitalization of teeth that are moved
    C. Mobility of teeth that are moved
    D. Development of occlusal interferences

62. Doubling the force applied at the bracket of a tooth would have what effect on the rotational tendency during tooth movement?
    A. The moment would decrease by 50%.
    B. The moment would not change.
    C. The moment would double.
    D. The moment would increase fourfold.

63. Which of the following statements describe accurately the "ugly duckling" stage of occlusal development? (Choose three.)
    A. This is considered to be a normal stage of occlusal development.
    B. It requires treatment whenever it is observed.
    C. It occurs in the primary dentition.
    D. It occurs in the mixed dentition.
    E. The crowding that occurs in the maxillary incisors is likely to continue to worsen over time as the permanent canines erupt.
    F. The small diastema created between the maxillary central incisors is likely to close as the permanent canines erupt.

64. When class III elastics are used, the maxillary first molars _____.
    A. Move distally and intrude
    B. Move mesially and extrude
    C. Move mesially and intrude
    D. Move only mesially; there is no movement in the vertical direction

65. Order the sequence of steps when performing serial extraction treatment.

A. A decision is made that the patient definitely needs extraction of permanent teeth to provide room for alignment in the future
B. Extraction of the permanent first premolars
C. Extraction of the primary canines
D. Extraction of the primary first molars

66. A 7-year-old patient has a 4-mm maxillary midline diastema. Which of the following should be done?
A. Brackets should be placed to close it.
B. A radiograph should be taken to rule out the presence of a supernumerary tooth.
C. Nothing should be done. It will close on its own.
D. Nothing should be done. Treatment should be deferred until the rest of the permanent dentition erupts.

67. Reduction of overbite can be accomplished most readily by which of the following treatment strategies?
A. Intruding maxillary incisors
B. Uprighting maxillary and mandibular incisors
C. Using a high-pull headgear to the maxillary molars
D. Using a lip bumper

68. Match the stage of tooth development with the anomaly.

A. Initiation _____
B. Histodifferentiation _____
C. Morphodifferentiation _____
D. Calcification _____

1. Excessive systemic fluoride ingestion
2. Peg permanent lateral incisor
3. Dentinogenesis imperfecta
4. Congenitally missing tooth

69. Which of the following are consistent with dentinogenesis imperfecta? (Choose three.)
A. Internal root resorption
B. Primary and permanent teeth affected
C. Pitted enamel
D. Enamel chips easily
E. Small or absent pulp chambers or canals
F. Normal tooth color

70. Order the process of tooth formation. Match each letter with its proper sequence number.

1. _____   A. Apposition
2. _____   B. Histodifferentiation
3. _____   C. Calcification
4. _____   D. Initiation
5. _____   E. Proliferation

Patient Management

1. A patient is sitting in the chair immediately after an extraction. She says, "Thank you. That wasn't as bad as I expected, but my sister told me that the first night after having a tooth pulled is very painful. What if the medication you're giving me isn't strong enough?" Choose the *most* appropriate response.
A. "Did she make you feel worried about that?"
B. "It sounds like you're worried that you might not have enough pain relief when you're home."
C. "I understand your concern."
D. "Don't worry. I'll give you plenty of pain medicine."
E. "It sounds like your sister had a unusually bad experience. Don't believe what others tell you, and certainly don't let that worry you. You'll be fine."

2. During admission, a patient interrupts you on numerous occasions with stories about past dental experiences while you are attempting to take a complete medical history. Your *best* response would be _____.
A. Say nothing, listen to the patient, and finish your intake as best you can.
B. Say, "I'd like to focus on your present experience and right now I need to know your medical history."
C. Say, "It seems like you've had some important experiences and I would like to hear more about them, but first, let's discuss this health questionnaire before we address them, okay?"
D. Say, "I don't need to know the details of your dental history. Please inform me of the experiences asked about in the questionnaire."
E. Say, "We have about 30 minutes to complete this questionnaire and get started in your examination, so let's focus on that."

3. A 7-year-old child has a history of recurrent pain and discomfort in a second molar, which has a necrotic pulp. You present the treatment options to the parents. "There are several ways in which we can treat this problem. We could do a pulpectomy in which we .... We could do something called a pulpotomy, which involves .... We could apply a pulp cap, which is .... We could remove the tooth. Or we could leave the tooth untreated for now and see how things go." You have phrased the options so that they are in what you believe to be the order of descending desirability, and you have indicated that to the patient. Which option is most likely to be chosen by the parents?
A. Pulpectomy
B. Pulpotomy
C. Pulp cap
D. Extraction
E. No treatment

4. Which of the following statements regarding motivation is *false*?
A. Motivation is strengthened when a person succeeds and is weakened when a person fails to achieve his or her goals.
B. Motivation is increased when the person focuses on long-term goals.
C. Motivating a person can be achieved by generating interest, showing your concern, and providing information.

D. Encourage a sense of personal acceptance in the face of the inevitable difficulties involved in breaking old habits and establishing new ones.

E. Help a patient cope with relapses by emphasizing the knowledge gained.

5. Which of the following statements about behavioral contracts is *false*?

A. It is a legal and binding agreement between health care professional and patient.

B. It helps solidify an agreement with a patient.

C. It should always be open to modification.

D. It helps clarify agreements.

E. The clinician should give a copy to the patient and keep one for himself or herself.

6. A 6-year-old patient likes to tell you stories about school. Each time he begins a story, you stop working to listen. After three long sessions, you realize that the child is attempting to avoid or delay the dental work by telling stories. You decide that from this point on you are going to continue working while engaged in conversation with the patient. At first, the child tells you more stories about school and tries other strategies to get your attention and stop your work. He eventually settles down and allows you to work, whether or not you are engaged in conversation. This is an example of _____.

A. Shaping

B. Extinction

C. Modeling

D. Stimulus control

E. Power

7. Which of the following is *not* a factor in the appraisal of stress?

A. Familiarity—how familiar the situation is; the less familiar, the more stressful it may seem

B. Predictability—how predictable the situation is; the less predictable, the more stressful it may seem

C. Controllability—how controllable the situation seems to be; the less controllable, the more stressful it may seem

D. Imminence—the more imminent the situation is, the more stressful it may seem

E. Positive or negative valence—whether the situation is positive or negative; positive situations (e.g., a wedding) are typically experienced as less stressful than negative situations (e.g., a divorce)

8. The substitution of a relaxation response for an anxiety response (using a relaxation strategy such as diaphragmatic breathing) when one is exposed to a hierarchy of feared stimuli is called _____.

A. Progressive muscle relaxation

B. Habituation

C. Flooding

D. Systematic desensitization

E. Biofeedback

9. Which of the following statements regarding the relationship between pain and fear is *false*?

A. Fear initially inhibits pain owing to a release of endorphins from the pituitary, resulting in an analgesic effect.

B. Although muscle tension contributes to the experience of anxiety, it does not contribute to the perception of pain.

C. Any autonomic activation causes one to have a lower pain threshold.

D. Catastrophic thinking and a perceived lack of control are common factors that influence pain perceptions.

E. Misattribution occurs when patients identify an event as painful because they can identify a fearful stimulus.

10. Which of the following is an example of a cognitive strategy that may be useful in pain management?

A. Address expectations by providing information and addressing any questions or concerns

B. Suggest to patients that they learn to identify, evaluate, and eliminate maladaptive thinking

C. Encourage patient efforts to address their anxiety and pain management

D. Suggest to patients that they learn to generate, evaluate, and apply more realistic thinking

E. All of the above

11. Which of the following scenarios is an example of classical conditioning?

A. You teach an anxious patient diaphragmatic breathing (unconditional stimulus [US]), which naturally induces the physiologic relaxation response (unconditional response [UR]). You seat the anxious patient in the dental chair for an examination (conditional stimulus [CS]) and ask the patient to use diaphragmatic breathing during the examination (US). While using the breathing skills, the patient feels more relaxed (conditional response [CR]).

B. You teach an anxious patient diaphragmatic breathing (US), which naturally induces the physiologic relaxation response (UR). You ask the patient to practice that technique at home (CS) and use it during procedures to reduce the subjective experience of anxiety (CR).

C. You teach an anxious patient diaphragmatic breathing (US), which naturally induces the physiologic relaxation response (UR). You seat the anxious patient in the dental chair for an examination (CS) and ask the patient to use diaphragmatic breathing during the examination (US). The focus on breathing serves as a distraction (US) from what the patient feels is threatening and fearful (CR), and the patient reports less anxiety (CR).

D. You teach an anxious patient diaphragmatic breathing (US), which naturally induces the physiologic relaxation response (UR). You seat the anxious patient in the dental chair for an examination (CS) and ask the patient to use diaphragmatic breathing during the examination (US). After a number of these experiences, the patient feels relaxed during the examination while using the breathing technique (UR) and without using it at all (CR).

E. None of the above

12. The best strategy for addressing dental fear that is based on distrust of the dentist is to _____.

A. Use distraction techniques
B. Use cognitive coping strategies
C. Enhance informational and behavioral control
D. Teach diaphragmatic breathing
E. Reassure the patient that he or she can trust you

13. What behavior can you typically expect from an anxious patient in the dental chair?

A. He or she is more likely to sit still, hands clasped together.
B. He or she is more likely to sit casually, legs crossed, reading a magazine.
C. He or she is more likely to keep to himself or herself and not speak unless spoken to.
D. He or she is more likely to fidget in the chair, moving his or her hands and feet.
E. Both A and C.

14. With no other intervention or instruction, which of the following is *most* likely to trigger a physiologic relaxation response?

A. Observing one's own physiologic responses (e.g., heart rate, blood pressure)
B. Muscle tensing
C. Reassurance
D. Thought stopping
E. Diaphragmatic breathing

15. A 32-year-old man is fearful of receiving injections. You decide to use a cognitive-behavioral strategy with him to help him through an injection. You have already instructed him in diaphragmatic breathing and ask him to practice this skill throughout the procedure. First, you show him the syringe. You talk about the characteristics of the needle. Next, you place the needle in his mouth with the cap on. You simulate the procedure with the cap on. You then simulate the procedure with the cap off. Eventually, you proceed with the injection. What does this procedure exemplify?

A. Habituation
B. Cognitive control
C. Flooding
D. Systematic desensitization
E. Behavior modification

16. Principles of operant conditioning teach us that _____.

A. If you praise your 5-year-old patient and reward him for keeping his legs still while you are drilling, this will make the child happy and more likely to like you and less likely to resist your requests.

B. If you praise your 5-year-old patient and reward him for keeping his legs still while you are drilling, this will increase the likelihood that he will remain still in similar situations in the future.
C. If you make the dental environment a child-friendly place, your young patient will be more comfortable.
D. If you pair the dental chair with having a parent present, the child will be less likely to be anxious.
E. None of the above.

17. According to research on anxiety disorders, it has been suggested that _____ is the *most* important component of systematic desensitization.

A. Cognitive restructuring
B. Progressive muscle relaxation
C. Diaphragmatic breathing
D. Exposure
E. Psychoeducation

18. Sarah S. is a young child who consistently presents as anxious, hypervigilant, and upset during dental visits. Sarah is often accompanied by her parent, who appears to be very concerned about the child and wants to be involved at all times in her evaluation and treatment. During this visit, Sarah's treatment requires an injection and a rubber dam application, which you anticipate may lead to increased anxiety. Which strategy would be the *least* effective in completing the rubber dam application?

A. Tell-Show-Do
B. Distraction
C. Ask the child to be a helper
D. Structure time
E. Rehearsals

19. Which of the following factors are involved in the cognitive appraisal of a threat?

A. Interference, adaptability, longevity, and reactance
B. Adaptability, preventability, inevitability, and constancy
C. Controllability, familiarity, predictability, and imminence
D. Validity, reliability, adaptability, and predictability
E. Accountability, reliability, validity, and familiarity

20. A patient has difficulty inhibiting the gag reflex during x-ray procedures. You suggest that the patient take several x-ray packets home and practice holding the packets in his or her mouth for increasingly longer periods of time. Which of the following techniques does this best exemplify?

A. Reinforcement
B. Graded exposure
C. Modeling
D. Behavioral control
E. Systematic desensitization

21. When faced with a frightened child patient, which would be the *most* appropriate or effective response?

A. Ask the child about his or her fears
B. Reschedule the appointment for a later date
C. Reassure the child
D. Tell the child that dentistry should not be frightening
E. Chastise the child

22. Research suggests that life events and perceived stress or distress _____ predictors of self-reported health concerns.
A. Are
B. Are not
C. Are sometimes
D. Have little to do with
E. None of the above

23. Patients experiencing stress and anxiety typically require _____ interpersonal distance for comfortable interaction.
A. Greater
B. Less
C. The same as patients who are not experiencing stress and anxiety
D. Individualized
E. Behaviorally controlled

24. Which of the following statements about the use of silence as an interviewing technique is *true*?
A. It permits and encourages patient participation.
B. It is a nonverbal technique for showing interest in the patient.
C. It is a nonverbal technique for encouraging the patient to speak.
D. It is done by silently attending to the patient, while maintaining eye contact.
E. All of the above

25. How do people typically respond to stress?
A. Physiologically (fight-or-flight response, i.e., autonomic arousal)
B. Cognitively (beliefs of self-efficacy, stress appraisal)
C. Behaviorally (e.g., disturbed sleep or appetite, impaired attention, acting out)
D. Emotionally (e.g., anxiety, anger, fear)
E. All of the above

26. Which of the following indices is *not* reversible?
A. DMFT
B. GI
C. PI
D. OHI-S
E. None of the above

27. The recommended level of fluoride for community water supply systems in the United States ranges from _____.
A. 0.2 to 0.5 ppm
B. 0.7 to 1.2 mL
C. 1.2 to 1.5 ppm
D. 0.2 to 0.5 mL
E. 0.7 to 1.2 ppm

28. The supplemental fluoride daily dosage schedule for a 5-year-old child who lives in a community where the concentration of fluoride in the drinking water is less than 0.3 ppm is _____.
A. 0 mg
B. 0.10 mg
C. 0.25 mg
D. 0.50 mg
E. 1 mg

29. What type of epidemiology is primarily used in intervention studies?
A. Descriptive
B. Analytical
C. Observational
D. Experimental
E. None of the above

30. A researcher follows a group of individuals in a population over 10 years to determine who develops cancer and then evaluates the factors that affected the group. What type of study is this?
A. Cross-sectional
B. Case-control
C. Randomized
D. Prospective cohort
E. Retrospective cohort

31. A group of researchers undertook a study to assess the relationship between squamous cell carcinoma and chewing tobacco. The researchers determined past exposure records among subjects who had been diagnosed with the disease. This type of study was a _____.
A. Clinical trial
B. Community trial
C. Retrospective cohort study
D. Case-control study
E. Randomized clinical trial

32. Which part of a scientific article summarizes the background and focus of the study; the population sampled; and the experimental design, findings, and conclusion?
A. Introduction
B. Background
C. Literature review
D. Methods
E. Abstract

33. In what section of a scientific article does the researcher interpret and explain the results obtained?
A. Summary and conclusion
B. Results
C. Discussion
D. Abstract
E. None of the above

34. The following were the scores for six dental students in their Restorative Dentistry examination: 56, 64, 68, 46, 82, 86. The median is _____.
A. 68
B. 64

C. 67

D. 40

E. 66

35. A correlation analysis shows that as the income of the population increases, the number of decayed teeth decreases. An expected value for this correlation coefficient (r) would be _____.

A. 0

B. 1

C. −1

D. 2

E. −2

36. A test result that erroneously excludes an individual from a specific diagnostic or reference group is called _____.

A. Erroneous

B. False positive

C. False negative

D. Mistaken

E. None of the above

37. Which of the following statements about transmissible diseases is *false*?

A. The risk of transmission after percutaneous injury is higher for hepatitis B virus (HBV) than for HIV.

B. Hepatitis C virus (HCV) and HIV are both caused by an RNA virus.

C. A vaccine to immunize against HBV is available.

D. The average risk of infection for HBV after a needle-stick injury falls between that for HCV and HIV.

E. All of the above

38. In HIV diagnosis, the Western blot assay is used to confirm the results of a positive enzyme-linked immunosorbent assay test. We can say that the Western blot test would confirm a _____.

A. True-positive result

B. True-negative result

C. False-positive result

D. False-negative result

E. None of the above

39. Which of the following statements about the hepatitis B virus (HBV) vaccination is *true*?

A. The HBV vaccine must be offered to all potentially exposed dental workers.

B. The HBV vaccine must be free to all potentially exposed dental workers.

C. At the time of employment, each person should be asked to provide documentation of previous immunizations.

D. Three doses of HBV vaccine are given to confer immunity.

E. All of the above

40. Which of the following terms refers specifically to the process where an antimicrobial agent destroys (germicide) or avoids the growth (microbiostatic) of pathogenic microorganisms on inanimate surfaces?

A. Antisepsis

B. Microbacterial control

C. Sterilization

D. Disinfection

E. Asepsis

41. Which of the following is the *most* common method of sterilization?

A. Dry heat

B. Ethylene oxide

C. Glutaraldehyde at 2%

D. Autoclave

E. Chemiclave

42. A set of precautions designed to prevent transmission of HIV, hepatitis B virus (HBV), and other bloodborne pathogens when providing first aid or health care is known as _____.

A. Asepsis

B. Infection control

C. Sterilization

D. Disinfection

E. Standard infection control procedures

43. Which of the following chemical agents is *not* a disinfectant?

A. Iodophors

B. Sodium hypochlorite

C. Synthetic phenol

D. Isopropyl alcohol

E. Glutaraldehyde

44. Which of the following recommendations must be followed when handling mercury?

A. Train personnel involved in the handling of mercury

B. Work in properly ventilated areas

C. Use high-volume evacuation systems when finishing or removing amalgams

D. Avoid direct skin contact with the metal

E. All of the above

45. According to the U.S. Centers for Disease Control and Prevention (CDC), the acceptable water quality in a dental office should be _____.

A. Less than 125 CFU/mL

B. Less than 250 CFU/mL

C. Less than 500 CFU/mL

D. Less than 750 CFU/mL

E. Less than 1000 CFU/mL

46. Which of the following American Dental Association Principles of Ethics states that a dentist has a duty to respect the patient's right to self-determination and confidentiality?

A. Patient autonomy

B. Nonmaleficence

C. Beneficence

D. Justice

E. Veracity

47. Which of the following are characteristics of proper documentation in a dental record?

A. Specific
B. Objective
C. Complete
D. Timely
E. All of the above

48. Which of the following is an arrangement between a plan and a group of dentists whereby the providers agree to accept certain payments (usually less than their usual fees) in anticipation of a higher volume of patients?
    A. PPO
    B. Capitation
    C. HMO
    D. IPA
    E. None of the above

49. Which of the following agencies monitors and prevents disease outbreaks, implements disease prevention strategies, and maintains national health statistics?
    A. CDC
    B. FDA
    C. DEA
    D. IHS
    E. None of the above

50. Which of the following federal agencies is the principal agency of the U.S. government for protecting the health of all Americans and providing essential human services?
    A. DHHS
    B. NIH
    C. HRSA
    D. AHRQ
    E. None of the above

51. Which of the following statements pertain to a case-control study? (Choose all that apply.)
    A. Patients with a specific condition or disorder are compared with controls.
    B. A general population is followed through time to see who develops a disease.
    C. Investigators seek an association with or cause for (e.g., lifestyle or dietary habits) a condition.
    D. Investigators seek to establish a temporal relationship between a cause and a condition.

52. Which of the following are common subsections of the methods section of a scientific article? (Choose all that apply.)
    A. Sampling strategy
    B. Measurement strategies and measurement instruments
    C. Experimental design
    D. Commentary on the results
    E. Statistical analytical procedures

53. In a measurement of a set of data, the median is defined as the _____.
    A. Average of the set of data
    B. Most frequent measurement in a set of data

C. Mean of a set of data
D. Middle measurement in a set of data

54. Which statistical test is used to analyze whether or not the means of several groups are equal and generalizes a t test to more than two groups?
    A. Analysis of variance (ANOVA)
    B. χ^2 test
    C. Correlation coefficient
    D. Multiple regression

55. Which characteristic does *not* apply to community water fluoridation?
    A. Prevents tooth decay in all age groups
    B. Water fluoridation usually requires supplemental systemic fluoride treatment in children younger than 12 years of age
    C. Approximately 75% of the U.S. population have proper water fluoridation
    D. The optimal fluoride level in the water supply is 0.7 to 1.2 ppm

56. For which of the following infectious diseases is there an effective immunization?
    A. Hepatitis A virus (HAV)
    B. Hepatitis B virus (HBV)
    C. HIV/AIDS
    D. Tuberculosis
    E. Hepatitis C virus (HCV)

57. The National Fire Protection Association color and number method is used to identify easily information about various hazardous chemicals on the material safety data sheets and product labels. Which color identifies the reactivity or stability of a chemical?
    A. Blue
    B. Red
    C. Yellow
    D. White

58. Which of the following are required informational elements for informed consent? (Choose all that apply.)
    A. Explanation of the procedure in understandable terms
    B. Reasons for the procedure and the benefits and risks of the procedure and anticipated outcome
    C. Any alternatives and their risks and benefits, including no treatment at all
    D. The costs of the procedure and the alternatives

Periodontics

1. Loss of tooth substance by mechanical wear is _____.
   A. Abrasion
   B. Attrition
   C. Erosion
   D. Abfraction

2. The width of keratinized gingiva is measured as the distance from the _____.

A. Free gingival margin to the mucogingival junction
B. Cementoenamel junction to the mucogingival junction
C. Free gingival groove to the mucogingival junction
D. Free gingival margin to the base of the pocket

3. Which of the following *best* distinguishes periodontitis from gingivitis?
A. Probing pocket depth
B. Bleeding on probing
C. Clinical attachment loss
D. Presence of suppuration

4. A 22-year-old college student presents with oral pain, erythematous gingival tissues with blunt papillae covered with a pseudomembrane, spontaneous gingival bleeding, and halitosis. There is no evidence of clinical attachment loss. What form of periodontal disease does this patient *most* likely have?
A. Gingivitis associated with dental plaque
B. Localized aggressive periodontitis
C. Generalized chronic periodontitis
D. Necrotizing ulcerative gingivitis

5. Which of the following methods of radiographic assessment are *best* for identifying small volumetric changes in alveolar bone density?
A. Bitewing
B. Periapical
C. Subtraction
D. Panoramic

6. What tooth surfaces should be evaluated for furcation involvement on maxillary molars?
A. Palatal, facial, and distal
B. Mesial, distal, and palatal
C. Facial, palatal, and mesial
D. Facial, mesial, and distal

7. What bacterial species are found in increased numbers in the apical portion of tooth-associated attached plaque?
A. Gram-negative rods
B. Gram-positive rods
C. Gram-positive cocci
D. Gram-negative cocci

8. What are the major organic constituents of bacterial plaque?
1. **Calcium and phosphorus**
2. **Sodium and potassium**
3. **Polysaccharides and proteins**
4. **Glycoproteins and lipids**
A. 1 and 2
B. 2 and 3
C. 3 and 4
D. 2 and 4

9. Although many plaque bacteria coaggregate, which of the following bacteria is believed to be an important bridge between "early colonizers" and "late colonizers" as plaque matures and becomes more microbiologically complex?

A. *Porphyromonas gingivalis*
B. *Streptococcus gordonii*
C. *Haemophilus parainfluenzae*
D. *Fusobacterium nucleatum*

10. What features *best* characterize the predominant microflora associated with periodontal health?
A. Gram-positive, anaerobic cocci and rods
B. Gram-negative, anaerobic cocci and rods
C. Gram-positive, facultative cocci and rods
D. Gram-negative, facultative cocci and rods

11. Which of the following microorganisms is frequently associated with localized aggressive periodontitis?
A. *Porphyromonas gingivalis*
B. *Actinobacillus actinomycetemcomitans*
C. *Actinomyces viscosus*
D. *Streptococcus mutans*

12. Which of the following is the primary etiologic factor associated with periodontal disease?
A. Age
B. Gender
C. Nutrition
D. Bacterial plaque

13. Inadequate margins of restorations should be corrected primarily because they _____.
A. Cause occlusal disharmony
B. Interfere with plaque removal
C. Create mechanical irritation
D. Release toxic substances

14. Light smokers are likely to have less severe periodontitis than heavy smokers. Former smokers are likely to have more severe periodontitis than current smokers.
A. Both statements are *true*.
B. Both statements are *false*.
C. The first statement is *true*, and the second statement is *false*.
D. The first statement is *false*, and the second statement is *true*.

15. Well-controlled diabetics have more periodontal disease than nondiabetics. Well-controlled diabetics generally can be treated successfully with conventional periodontal therapy.
A. Both statements are *true*.
B. Both statements are *false*.
C. The first statement is *true*, and the second statement is *false*.
D. The first statement is *false*, and the second statement is *true*.

16. Oral contraceptives can cause gingivitis. Oral contraceptives can accentuate the gingival response to bacterial plaque.
A. Both statements are *true*.
B. Both statements are *false*.
C. The first statement is *true*, and the second statement is *false*.
D. The first statement is *false*, and the second statement is *true*.

17. Which of the following cells produce antibodies?
    A. Neutrophils
    B. T lymphocytes
    C. Macrophages
    D. Plasma cells

18. Defects in which inflammatory cell have most frequently been associated with periodontal disease?
    A. T lymphocyte
    B. Mast cell
    C. Plasma cell
    D. Neutrophil

19. What is the major clinical difference between the established lesion of gingivitis and the advanced lesion of periodontitis?
    A. Gingival color, contour, and consistency
    B. Bleeding on probing
    C. Loss of crestal lamina dura
    D. Attachment and bone loss
    E. Suppuration

20. Which interleukin (IL) is important in the activation of osteoclasts and the stimulation of bone loss seen in periodontal disease?
    A. IL-1
    B. IL-2
    C. IL-8
    D. IL-10

21. Scaling and root planing are used in which phases of periodontal therapy?
    1. **Initial (hygienic)**
    2. **Surgical (corrective)**
    3. **Supportive (maintenance)**
    A. 1 only
    B. 1 and 2 only
    C. 2 and 3 only
    D. 1 and 3 only
    E. 1, 2, and 3

22. What is the *most* objective clinical indicator of inflammation?
    A. Gingival color
    B. Gingival consistency
    C. Gingival bleeding
    D. Gingival stippling

23. A 25-year-old patient presenting with generalized marginal gingivitis without any systemic problems or medications should be classified with which periodontal prognosis?
    A. Good
    B. Fair
    C. Poor
    D. Questionable

24. Instrumentation of the teeth to remove plaque, calculus, and stains is defined as ____.
    A. Coronal polishing
    B. Scaling
    C. Gingival curettage
    D. Root planing

25. Scalers are used to remove supragingival deposits. Curettes are used to remove either supragingival or subgingival deposits.
    A. Both statements are *true*.
    B. Both statements are *false*.
    C. The first statement is *true*, and the second statement is *false*.
    D. The first statement is *false*, and the second statement is *true*.

26. Which of the following is *not* a characteristic of sickle scalers?
    A. Two cutting edges
    B. Rounded back
    C. Cutting edges meet in a point
    D. Triangular in cross section
    E. Used for removal of supragingival deposits

27. The modified Widman flap uses three separate incisions. It is reflected beyond the mucogingival junction.
    A. Both statements are *true*.
    B. Both statements are *false*.
    C. The first statement is *true*, and the second statement is *false*.
    D. The first statement is *false*, and the second statement is *true*.

28. The free gingival graft technique can be used to increase the width of attached gingival tissue. Apically displaced full-thickness or partial-thickness flaps can also be used to increase the width of attached gingiva.
    A. Both statements are *true*.
    B. Both statements are *false*.
    C. The first statement is *true*, and the second statement is *false*.
    D. The first statement is *false*, and the second statement is *true*.

29. Miller class I recession defects can be distinguished from class II defects by assessing the ____.
    A. Location of interproximal alveolar bone
    B. Width of keratinized gingiva
    C. Involvement of the mucogingival junction
    D. Involvement of the free gingival margin

30. The reshaping or recontouring of nonsupportive alveolar bone is called ____.
    A. Ostectomy
    B. Osteoplasty
    C. Osteography
    D. All of the above

31. How many walls does an interdental crater have?
    A. One
    B. Two
    C. Three
    D. Four

32. During the healing of a surgically treated intrabony (infrabony) pocket, regeneration of a new periodontal ligament, cementum, and alveolar bone occurs only

when cells repopulate the wound from which of the following sources?
A. Gingival epithelium
B. Connective tissue
C. Alveolar bone
D. Periodontal ligament

33. Which of the following is *least* likely to be successfully treated with a bone graft procedure?
A. One-walled defect
B. Two-walled defect
C. Three-walled defect
D. Class III furcation defect

34. When osseointegration occurs, which of the following *best* describes the implant-bone interface at the level of light microscopy after osseointegration?
A. Epithelial attachment
B. Direct contact
C. Connective tissue insertion
D. Cellular attachment

35. The *most* effective topical antimicrobial agent currently available is ____.
A. Chlorhexidine
B. Stannous fluoride
C. Phenolic compounds
D. Sanguinarine

36. What is the active ingredient in PerioChip?
A. Doxycycline
B. Tetracycline
C. Metronidazole
D. Chlorhexidine

37. How many days does it usually take for surface epithelialization to be complete after a gingivectomy?
A. 3 to 7
B. 5 to 14
C. 14 to 18
D. 20 to 27

38. The most obvious clinical sign of trauma from occlusion is increased tooth mobility. The most obvious radiographic sign of trauma from occlusion is an increase in the width of the periodontal ligament space.
A. Both statements are *true*.
B. Both statements are *false*.
C. The first statement is *true*, and the second statement is *false*.
D. The first statement is *false*, and the second statement is *true*.

39. Trauma from occlusion refers to the ____.
A. Occlusal force
B. Damage to the tooth
C. Injury to the tissues of the periodontium
D. Widened periodontal ligament

40. Which of the following is the primary reason for splinting teeth?
A. For esthetics
B. To improve hygiene
C. For patient comfort
D. As a preventive measure

41. In the treatment of an acute periodontal abscess, the *most* important first step is to ____.
A. Prescribe systemic antibiotics
B. Reflect a periodontal flap surgery
C. Obtain drainage
D. Prescribe hot salt mouth washes

42. Which of the following medications often result in overgrowth of gingival tissues?
A. Penicillin, calcium channel blockers, phenytoin
B. Calcium channel blockers, phenytoin, and cyclosporine
C. Cyclosporine, penicillin, and cephalosporins
D. Ampicillin, tetracycline, and erythromycin

43. Which of the following is the *most* important preventive and therapeutic procedure in periodontal therapy?
A. Professional instrumentation
B. Subgingival irrigation with chlorhexidine
C. Patient-administered plaque control
D. Surgical intervention

44. How many hours after brushing does it usually take for a mature dental plaque to reform?
A. 1 to 2
B. 5 to 10
C. 12 to 24
D. 24 to 48

45. Placing the toothbrush bristles at a 45-degree angle on the tooth and pointing apically so that the bristles enter the gingival sulcus describes which brushing technique?
A. Charter
B. Stillman
C. Bass
D. Roll

46. Systemically administered subantimicrobial doses of doxycycline are sometimes used to treat chronic periodontitis because the doxycycline inhibits which enzyme?
A. Amylase
B. β-Lactamases
C. Metalloproteinases
D. Cyclooxygenases
E. 5-Lipoxygenase

47. Place in their order of sequence (earliest first), the events that normally take place after suturing is done to close a periodontal flap.
A. Collagen fibers appear
B. Epithelial cells begin to migrate
C. Clot formation
D. An epithelial attachment is in place

48. For which conditions (occurring either alone or together) are systemic antibiotics indicated for treatment of acute necrotizing ulcerative gingivitis? (Choose two.)

A. Foul oral smell

B. Pain

C. Lymphadenopathy

D. Fever

E. Presence of a pseudomembrane

49. Regarding furcation involvement of a periodontal pocket, what grade of involvement would include cul-de-sac formation with a definite horizontal component but without complete bone loss in the furcation?

A. I

B. II

C. III

D. IV

50. In plaque formation, which two organisms are the earliest colonizers?

A. *Prevotella* species and *Capnocytophaga* species

B. *Porphyromonas gingivalis* and *Aggregatibacter actinomycetemcomitans*

C. *Streptococcus* species and *Actinomyces* species

D. *Campylobacter* species and *Fusobacterium nucleatum.*

Pharmacology

1. Tight capillary cell junctions resulting in an added barrier to the entry of drugs is *most* characteristic of which organ or tissue?

A. Adrenal gland

B. Brain

C. Heart

D. Liver

E. Lung

2. A prescription for which of the following drugs requires a valid Drug Enforcement Administration (DEA) number on the prescription?

A. Amoxicillin

B. Carbamazepine

C. Dexamethasone

D. Diphenhydramine

E. Oxycodone

3. What would be the effect of prior administration of a competitive drug antagonist on the concentration-response profile of a drug agonist on a graded concentration-response curve? (Assume that both drugs act at the same receptor.)

A. The agonist curve would shift to the left.

B. The agonist curve would shift to the right.

C. The agonist curve would not change.

D. The agonist curve would not shift but would reach a lower maximal effect than the curve with agonist alone.

E. The agonist curve would both shift to the left and have a lower maximal effect.

4. How many human drug testing phases are carried out before a drug is marketed?

A. One

B. Two

C. Three

D. Four

5. In what situation is the postganglionic nerve of the sympathetic system a cholinergic nerve?

A. The nerves to the eye

B. The nerves to the heart

C. Most nerves to blood vessels

D. Most nerves to sweat glands

E. Most nerves to salivary glands

6. Which of the following is a nicotinic receptor?

A. Receptor for the neurotransmitter at the skeletal-neuromuscular junction

B. Receptor for the neurotransmitter at the junction between the postganglionic sympathetic nerve and sweat glands

C. Receptor for the neurotransmitter at the junction between the postganglionic parasympathetic nerve and the parotid gland

D. Receptor for the neurotransmitter at the junction between the postganglionic sympathetic nerve and blood vessels

E. Receptor for the neurotransmitter at the junction between the postganglionic parasympathetic nerve and the heart

7. Which of the following effects is a typical effect of an antimuscarinic drug?

A. Bronchoconstriction

B. Lacrimation

C. Miosis

D. Sweating

E. Urinary retention

8. The administration of which compound would provide "epinephrine reversal" (decrease in blood pressure from epinephrine) if given before administration of epinephrine?

A. Atropine

B. Guanethidine

C. Propranolol

D. Phenoxybenzamine

E. Tyramine

9. Motor adverse effects from phenothiazine antipsychotic drugs are due to drug effects in what region of the brain?

A. Chemoreceptor trigger zone

B. Cerebrum

C. Cerebellum

D. Nigrostriatal pathway

E. Mesolimbic pathway

10. A patient is administered haloperidol. Along with the haloperidol, the patient also receives benztropine. What is the *most* likely reason for administering the benztropine?

A. To reduce the effects of histamine release

B. To aid in the therapeutic response to haloperidol

   C. To reduce the motor adverse effects of haloperidol

   D. To overcome a decrease in salivary flow resulting from haloperidol

   E. To reduce the rate of kidney excretion of haloperidol

11. The benzodiazepine receptors BZ_1 and BZ_2 are located on which ion channel?
   A. Calcium
   B. Chloride
   C. Magnesium
   D. Potassium
   E. Sodium

12. Methemoglobinemia is an adverse effect associated with which local anesthetic as a result of its metabolism to *o*-toluidine?
   A. Lidocaine
   B. Mepivacaine
   C. Prilocaine
   D. Bupivacaine
   E. Benzocaine

13. Which of the following drugs poses the greatest risk of a cardiac arrhythmia when administered at the same time as epinephrine?
   A. Desflurane
   B. Halothane
   C. Isoflurane
   D. Propofol
   E. Sevoflurane

14. Local anesthetics act on what type of receptor?
   A. Ion channel receptor
   B. Nuclear receptor
   C. Seven-membrane domain receptor linked to G_s
   D. Seven-membrane domain receptor linked to G_q
   E. Membrane receptor with tyrosine kinase activity

15. Which of the following drugs lacks the amine terminus that other anesthetics have and is used only topically?
   A. Procaine
   B. Mepivacaine
   C. Lidocaine
   D. Benzocaine
   E. Prilocaine

16. Injecting a local anesthetic into an area of inflammation would _____.
   A. Increase the rate of onset of anesthesia
   B. Decrease the rate of metabolism of the anesthetic
   C. Reduce the net anesthetic effect of the drug
   D. Reduce the vasodilator effect of the local anesthetic
   E. Reduce the need for a vasoconstrictor with the local anesthetic

17. Which two drugs have mechanisms of analgesic action that are most similar?
   A. Fentanyl, ibuprofen
   B. Aspirin, codeine
   C. Oxycodone, acetaminophen
   D. Ibuprofen, naproxen
   E. Aspirin, ibuprofen

18. Your patient takes a small daily dose of aspirin (82 mg) prescribed by the patient's physician. The object of this therapy is *most* likely what mechanism?
   A. To mimic the effect of endogenous endorphins
   B. To inhibit the production of prostaglandin E_1
   C. To inhibit the production of thromboxane A_2
   D. To inhibit the production of arachidonic acid
   E. To inhibit the production of leukotrienes

19. Your patient indicates that he is taking medication for atrial fibrillation. He reports that a blood test has indicated that he has an international normalized ratio (INR) value of 4.0. An emergency dental extraction is now required. Which postoperative medication would pose the greatest risk for an adverse effect in this patient?
   A. Acetaminophen
   B. Amoxicillin
   C. Aspirin
   D. Codeine
   E. Ibuprofen

20. Which drug blocks H_1 histamine receptors but is *least* likely to cause sedation?
   A. Diphenhydramine
   B. Hydroxyzine
   C. Fexofenadine
   D. Albuterol
   E. Famotidine

21. The use of selective cyclooxygenase-2 inhibitors has been restricted or discontinued more recently because of what type of adverse effects?
   A. Carcinogenesis
   B. Cardiovascular disorders
   C. Convulsive disorders
   D. Striated muscle disorders
   E. Skeletal disorders

22. Sodium reabsorption in the thick ascending limb of the loop of Henle is inhibited by which drug?
   A. Bumetanide
   B. Chlorthalidone
   C. Hydrochlorothiazide
   D. Spironolactone
   E. Triamterene

23. Torsades de pointes, or polymorphic ventricular tachycardia, is linked *most* closely to what characteristic of the electrocardiogram (ECG)?
   A. Inverted T wave
   B. Shorter P–R interval
   C. Shorter P–P interval
   D. Longer Q–T interval
   E. Normal ECG

24. Which antihypertensive drug also increases bradykinin levels?
   A. Candesartan
   B. Furosemide

C. Lisinopril
D. Metoprolol
E. Nifedipine

25. Which one of the following drugs enters the target cell and acts on a nuclear receptor?
    A. Diazepam
    B. Epinephrine
    C. Insulin
    D. Prednisone
    E. Heparin

26. Inhibiting α-glucosidase and reducing glucose absorption from the gastrointestinal tract is the mechanism of action of _____.
    A. Acarbose
    B. Acetohexamide
    C. Glyburide
    D. Metformin
    E. Pioglitazone

27. Which of the following drugs blocks the aldosterone receptor?
    A. Amiloride
    B. Triamterene
    C. Losartan
    D. Spironolactone
    E. Furosemide

28. Which of the following drugs is *most* selective as a glucocorticosteroid?
    A. Aldosterone
    B. Dexamethasone
    C. Fludrocortisone
    D. Hydrocortisone

29. Stimulation of gluconeogenesis and lipolysis are most characteristic of which hormone?
    A. Calcitonin
    B. Cortisol
    C. Insulin
    D. Parathyroid hormone
    E. Progesterone

30. Fanconi's syndrome resulting from outdated tetracyclines affects predominantly which organ?
    A. Brain
    B. Heart
    C. Kidney
    D. Pancreas
    E. Stomach

31. Methicillin-resistant staphylococci are *most* likely to be inhibited by which drug?
    A. Amoxicillin
    B. Clarithromycin
    C. Clindamycin
    D. Vancomycin
    E. Penicillin V

32. Which of the following organisms is usually clinically sensitive to clarithromycin but not to penicillin V?
    A. Viridans streptococcus
    B. *Leptotrichia buccalis*

C. *Mycoplasma pneumoniae*
D. *Streptococcus pneumoniae*
E. *Streptococcus pyogenes*

33. What is the approximate elimination half-time for penicillin V?
    A. 0.5 hour
    B. 2 hours
    C. 4 hours
    D. 8 hours
    E. 12 hours

34. _____ has an antibacterial spectrum that is limited to anaerobes.
    A. Amoxicillin
    B. Clarithromycin
    C. Clindamycin
    D. Gentamicin
    E. Metronidazole

35. Which drugs are very susceptible to metabolism by serum cholinesterases? (Choose two.)
    A. Carbachol
    B. Articaine
    C. Bethanechol
    D. Acetylcholine
    E. Pilocarpine

36. Match the antidiabetic drug with its mechanism of action.

    A. Glibenclamide _____
    B. Metformin _____
    C. Rosiglitazone _____
    D. Sitagliptin _____
    E. Miglitol _____

    1. Inhibits α-glucosidase and delays carbohydrate digestion in the gut
    2. Activates transcription factor PPARγ, leading to increased insulin sensitivity in tissues
    3. Inhibits dipeptidyl peptidase-4, increasing the level of glucagonlike peptide
    4. Increases the release of insulin
    5. Activates adenosine monophosphate (AMP) kinase, reducing liver glucose production, gluconeogenesis, and lipogenesis

37. Which antiepileptic drugs bind to the $\alpha2/\delta$-1 protein subunit of high-voltage–activated calcium channels and inhibit these channels? (Choose two.)
    A. Gabapentin
    B. Phenobarbital
    C. Carbamazepine
    D. Ethosuximide
    E. Pregabalin

38. Which of the following benzodiazepines have the shortest half-lives? (Choose two.)

A. Chlordiazepoxide
B. Diazepam
C. Lorazepam
D. Midazolam
E. Triazolam

39. Which of the following reactions are *not* involved in the metabolism of lidocaine? (Choose two.)
A. Hydroxylation of the aromatic ring
B. Cleavage of the aromatic ring
C. Dealkylation of the amino terminus
D. Hydrolysis of the amide bond
E. Hydrolysis of an ester bond

40. Flumazenil blocks the receptors stimulated by which of the following drugs? (Choose all that apply.)
A. Baclofen
B. Buspirone
C. Diazepam
D. Zolpidem
E. Zaleplon

Prosthodontics

1. The incisive papilla provides a guide for the anterior-posterior placement of maxillary anterior denture teeth. The labial surfaces of natural teeth are generally 8 to 10 mm anterior to this structure.
A. Both statements are *true*.
B. The first statement is *true*, and the second statement is *false*.
C. The first statement is *false*, and the second statement is *true*.
D. Both statements are *false*.

2. Which of the following statements is *true* concerning vertical dimension of rest (VDR)?
A. VDR is a physiologic rest position.
B. VDR is a position of the mandible when opening and closing muscles are at rest.
C. VDR is a postural relationship of the mandible to maxilla.
D. VDR is the amount of jaw separation controlled by jaw muscles when they are in a relaxed state.
E. All of the above

3. All of the following are characteristics of a postpalatal seal of complete dentures *except* one. Which one is the *exception*?
A. Compensates for shrinkage of the acrylic resin caused by its processing
B. May reduce the gag reflex
C. Improves the stability of the maxillary denture
D. It is most shallow in the midpalatal suture area

4. Which of the following is the *most* likely cause of an occlusal rest fracture?
A. Inadequate rest-seat preparation
B. Improper rest location

C. Structural metal defects
D. Occluding against the antagonist tooth

5. The primary purpose of a maxillary denture occlusal index is to ____.
A. Maintain the patient's vertical dimension
B. Maintain both correct centric and vertical relation records
C. Maintain the patient's centric relation
D. Preserve the face-bow record

6. An edentulous patient with a diminished vertical dimension of occlusion is predisposed to have which of the following conditions?
A. Epulis fissurata
B. Pemphigus vulgaris
C. Papillary hyperplasia
D. Angular cheilosis

7. When performing a diagnostic occlusal adjustment on diagnostic casts, the mandibular cast should be mounted to the maxillary cast in an articulator using which of the following?
A. Centric relation interocclusal record
B. Hinge articulator
C. Maximum intercuspation wax record
D. Face-bow transfer

8. When border molding a mandibular complete denture, the extension of the lingual right and left flanges are *best* molded by having the patient ____.
A. Purse the lips
B. Wet the lips with the tongue
C. Open wide
D. Swallow
E. Count from 50 to 55

9. The main function of the direct retainer of a removable partial denture is ____.
A. Stabilization
B. Retention
C. Support
D. Add strength to the major connector

10. Lack of reciprocation of a removable partial denture (RPD) clasp is likely to cause ____.
A. Tissue recession because of displacement of the RPD
B. Insufficient resistance to displacement
C. Fracture of the retentive clasp
D. Abutment tooth displacement during removal and insertion

11. Centric relation is the maxillomandibular relationship in which the condyles are in their most ____.
A. Posterior position with the disc interposed at its thickest avascular location
B. Posterior position with the disc interposed at its thinnest locale
C. Superior position with the disc in its most anterior position
D. Superior-anterior position with the disc interposed at its thinnest location

12. The denture base of a mandibular distal extension removable partial denture (RPD) should cover ____.
    A. The retromolar pads
    B. All undercut areas and engage them for retention
    C. The hamular notch
    D. The pterygomandibular raphe

13. A good landmark for anterior-posterior positioning of the anterior maxillary teeth in a complete denture is the ____.
    A. Residual ridge
    B. Incisive papilla
    C. Incisal foramen
    D. Mandibular wax rim

14. Which one of the following is a purpose or characteristic of the postpalatal seal?
    A. Provides a seal against air being forced under the denture
    B. Usually should extend posterior to the foveae palatinae
    C. Improves the stability of the maxillary denture
    D. Is carved deeper in the midpalatal suture area

15. The ____ is used as a guide to verify the occlusal plane.
    A. Ala-tragus line
    B. Interpupillary line
    C. Camper's line or plane
    D. All of the above

16. Balanced occlusion is less important during chewing than during nonchewing events. This difference occurs because the time teeth are in contact during nonchewing events is much greater than the time teeth are in contact during chewing.
    A. Both statements are *true*.
    B. The first statement is *true*, and the second statement is *false*.
    C. The second statement is *true*, and the first statement is *false*.
    D. Both statements are *false*.

17. Which of the following conditions can be caused in an edentulous patient by an ill-fitting denture flange?
    A. Papillary hyperplasia
    B. Epulis fissurata
    C. Candidiasis
    D. Fibrous tuberosity

18. Inadequate rest-seat preparation for a removable partial prosthesis can cause ____.
    A. Tooth mobility
    B. Ligament widening
    C. Occlusal rest fracture
    D. Occlusal rest distortion

19. Which of the following is the main disadvantage of resin-modified glass ionomer compared with conventional glass ionomer?
    A. Reduced fluoride release
    B. Increased expansion
    C. Reduced adhesion
    D. Cost

20. You are planning to replace a maxillary central incisor with a fixed prosthetic device. The edentulous space is slightly wider than the contralateral tooth. To achieve acceptable esthetics, you should ensure that ____.
    A. The line angles of the pontic are placed in the same relationship as the contralateral tooth
    B. The pontic is made smoother than the contralateral tooth
    C. The pontic has a higher value than the contralateral tooth
    D. The line angles are shaped to converge incisally on the pontic

21. Polycarboxylate cement achieves a chemical bond to tooth structure. The mechanism for this bond is ____.
    A. Ionic bond to phosphate
    B. Covalent bond to the collagen
    C. Chelation to calcium
    D. These cements do not form a chemical bond

22. Which of the following properties of a gold alloy exceeds a base metal alloy in numerical value?
    A. Hardness
    B. Specific gravity
    C. Casting shrinkage
    D. Fusion temperature

23. Which of the following impression materials has the highest tear strength?
    A. Polyether
    B. Polysulfide
    C. Addition silicone
    D. Condensation silicone

24. Chroma is the aspect of color that indicates ____.
    A. The degree of translucency
    B. The degree of saturation of the hue
    C. Combined effect of hue and value
    D. How dark or light a shade is

25. For an alloy to be considered noble metal, it should ____.
    A. Contain at least 25% silver
    B. Contain at least 25% platinum or palladium
    C. Contain 40% gold
    D. Contain at least 80% gold

26. The purpose of fabricating a provisional restoration with correct contours and marginal integrity is ____.
    A. For protection
    B. To supervise the patient's dental hygiene and give the patient feedback during this stage
    C. To preserve periodontal health
    D. All of the above

27. A compomer cement ____.
    1. **Is indicated for cementation of metal-ceramic crowns**
    2. **Is indicated for cementation of all-ceramic restorations**
    3. **Is indicated for some all-ceramic crowns, inlays, and veneers with some contraindications**

4. **Has low solubility and sustained release of fluoride**
   A. All are correct.
   B. 1, 2, and 3 are correct.
   C. 1, 3, and 4 are correct.
   D. 2, 3, and 4 are correct.

28. Heating the metal structure in a furnace before opaque application in a metal-ceramic crown is necessary to ____.
    1. **Harden the metal**
    2. **Oxidize trace elements in the metal**
    3. **Eliminate oxidation**
    A. 1 only
    B. 1 and 2
    C. 1 and 3
    D. 2 only
    E. 3 only

29. Which of the following are probably not clinically significant in terms of influencing the retention of a cemented restoration?
    1. **Tooth preparation**
    2. **Surface texture**
    3. **Casting alloy**
    4. **Tooth taper**
    5. **Luting agent**
    A. 1, 3, and 4
    B. 1, 2, 3
    C. 1, 2, 3, 5
    D. 3 and 5

30. Which articulator is capable of duplicating the border mandibular movements of a patient?
    A. Nonadjustable
    B. Arcon
    C. Non-arcon
    D. Fully adjustable

31. Tooth #30 is endodontically treated after a conservative access cavity was made through a typical MO amalgam restoration. The restoration of choice is a ____.
    A. Chamber-retained amalgam foundation
    B. Custom cast post and core
    C. Wire post and core
    D. Parallel-sided prefabricated post with cast core

32. Potential problems in connecting implants to natural teeth include all of the following *except* one. Which one is the *exception*?
    A. Stress is concentrated at the superior portion of the implant
    B. Breakdown of osseointegration
    C. Cement failure on the natural abutment
    D. Screw or abutment loosening
    E. Fracture in the connector area of the prosthesis

33. A minor connector of a removable partial denture ____.
    A. Should be thin so as not to interfere with the tongue
    B. Should be located on a convex embrasure surface
    C. Should conform to the interdental embrasure
    D. All of the above
    E. A and C only

34. The design of a restored occlusal surface depends on the ____.
    1. **Contour of the articular eminence**
    2. **Position of the tooth in the arch**
    3. **Amount of lateral shift in the rotating condyle**
    4. **Amount of vertical overlap of anterior teeth**
    A. 1 and 3
    B. 2, 3, and 4
    C. 2 and 4 only
    D. 3 and 4 only
    E. All of the above

35. Which of the following is a main function of a guide plane surface contacted by a minor connector of a removable partial denture (RPD)?
    A. Provides a positive path of placement and removal for the RPD
    B. Can provide additional retention
    C. Aids in preventing cervical movement
    D. All of the above
    E. Only A and B

36. Which of the following components of a removable partial denture (RPD) must be rigid?
    A. Major connector, minor connector, and retentive clasp
    B. Wrought wire clasp, rests, and minor connector
    C. Minor connector, rest, and major connector

37. Which type of clasp is generally used on a tooth-supported removable denture?
    A. Circumferential cast clasp
    B. Combination clasp
    C. Wrought wire clasp

38. Which of the following disinfectants can be used with alginate impressions?
    A. Alcohol
    B. Iodophor
    C. Glutaraldehyde
    D. All of the above
    E. B and C only

39. A dentist replaces an amalgam on tooth #5 and notices a small pulpal exposure. The dentist elects to perform a direct pulp cap procedure. Which of the following *best* predicts success of the procedure?
    A. Size of the lesion
    B. Isolation of the lesion
    C. Use of calcium hydroxide
    D. Age of the patient

40. In a tooth-supported removable partial denture (RPD) with a circumferential cast clasp assembly, there is ____.
    A. More than 180 degrees of encirclement in the greatest circumference of the tooth
    B. A distal rest on the tooth anterior to the edentulous area

C. A mesial rest on the tooth posterior to the edentulous area

D. Only B and C

E. All of the above

41. What is a nonrigid connector?

A. An appliance composed of a key and keyway that is used to connect one piece of a prosthesis to another

B. An appliance that is used to connect two crowns rigidly fixed

C. A bar appliance that is used to maintain a space for a tooth that has not erupted

D. None of the above

42. The distance between the major connector on a maxillary removable partial denture framework and the gingival margins should be at least _____.

A. 3 mm

B. 2 mm

C. 6 mm

D. 15 mm

43. The _____ is the component that is responsible for connecting the major connector with the rest and clamp assembly.

A. Bar

B. Minor connector

C. Proximal plate

D. Guide plane

44. The three dimensions of the Munsell Color Order System, the basis for shade guides such as Vita Lumin, are _____.

A. Absorption, scattering, and translucency

B. Color, translucency, and gloss

C. Size, shape, and interactions with light

D. Hue, value, and chroma

45. The purpose of applying a layer of opaque porcelain in a metal-ceramic restoration is to _____.

A. Create a bond between the metal and porcelain

B. Mask the metal oxide layer and provide a porcelain-metal bond

C. Create the main color for the restoration

D. A and B are correct

E. A, B, and C are correct

46. The light effect of a translucent material (e.g., incisal edge of some teeth) appearing blue in reflected light and red-orange in transmitted light is called _____.

A. Metamerism

B. Opalescence

C. Value

D. Chroma

E. Fluorescence

47. Which of the following are considered noble elements? (Choose all that apply.)

A. Silver

B. Gold

C. Platinum

D. Palladium

E. Chromium

48. Reversible hydrocolloid is composed of _____.

A. Polysulfide polymer

B. Agar

C. Polyether polymer

D. Polydimethylsiloxane

49. Electrosurgery is contraindicated under what conditions? (Choose all that apply.)

A. Patient with a transcutaneous electrical nerve stimulation (TENS) unit

B. Patients with a cardiac pacemaker

C. Patients with an insulin pump

D. Patients with delayed healing

50. Regarding extracoronal retainers in a removal dental prosthesis, which ones originate above the survey line? (Choose all that apply.)

A. Circumferential clasp

B. I bar

C. T bar

D. Ring clasp

Answer Key for Section 1

1. **C.** Until apical closure occurs, teeth do not respond normally to electrical pulp testing. In addition, a traumatic injury may temporarily alter the conduction capability of nerve endings or sensory receptors, or both, in the pulp. A patient with a vital pulp may not experience any sensation right after trauma.

2. **D.** The perception of pain in one part of the body that is distant from the actual source of the pain is known as "referred pain." Teeth may refer pain to other areas of the head and neck. Referred pain is usually provoked by stimulation of pulpal C-fibers, the slow conducting nerves that when stimulated cause an intense, dull, slow pain. The pain always radiates to the ipsilateral side. Posterior teeth may refer pain to the opposite arch or periauricular area. Mandibular posterior teeth tend to transmit referred pain to the periauricular area more often than maxillary posterior teeth.

3. **D.** External root resorption is a process that is initiated in the periodontium, in contrast to internal root resorption, which begins within the root canal system. There are three main types: inflammatory root resorption, replacement resorption, and cervical resorption. Although some types are located only along the apical and lateral end, replacement resorption can be located anywhere along the root. However, external root resorption is characterized radiographically by margins that are less well defined, ragged, and irregular.

4. **A.** Cracks extend deep into the dentin and are usually propagated mesiodistally in posterior teeth, often in the region of the marginal ridge. Dyes and transillumination are very helpful in the visualization of cracks. However, it is often impossible to determine how extensive a crack is until the tooth is extracted.

5. **E.** In chronic apical abscess, a continuously or intermittently draining sinus tract usually drains into the oral mucosa. The exudate can also drain through the gingival sulcus of the involved tooth, mimicking a periodontal lesion with a "pocket." However, this is not a true periodontal pocket because there is not a complete detachment of connective tissue from the root surface. Treatment is with conventional root canal therapy. Antibiotics are not needed because the infection is localized and draining. If the tract does not heal within a few weeks, root end surgery may be required to treat accessory canals that are inaccessible. However, if left untreated, it may become covered with an epithelial lining and become a true periodontal pocket.

6. **B.** Confirmation of clinical diagnosis should be made before treatment is rendered. Access is the first and arguably most important phase of nonsurgical root canal therapy. The objectives are (1) to achieve straight-line access to the apical foramen or curvature of the canal, (2) to locate all root canal orifices, and (3) to conserve sound tooth structure.

7. **A.** NaOCl is the most widely used irrigant and has effectively aided canal preparation for years. NaOCl is a good tissue solvent as well as having an antimicrobial effect. It acts as a lubricant for root canal instrumentation. It is toxic to vital tissue, so a rubber dam should always be used. The antibacterial action of NaOCl is based on its effects on the bacterial cell wall. When the cell wall is disrupted, the vital contents of the bacteria are released. The bacterial membrane and intracellular associated functions cease. NaOCl is an effective necrotic tissue solvent. Because it fulfills all these requirements, NaOCl remains the main irrigating solution of choice in endodontic treatment.

8. **A.** Ledges can sometimes be bypassed; the canal coronal to the ledge must be sufficiently straightened to allow a file to operate effectively. This straightening may be achieved by anticurvature filing (file away from the curve). Precurve the file severely at the tip and use it to probe gently past the ledge. Otherwise, clean to the ledge and fill it, but you must warn the patient of poorer prognosis.

9. **B.** Apical perforations occur through the apical foramen or the body of the root (a perforated new canal). Generally, the more subcrestally located the lesion, the better the prognosis. However, all perforations have an inherently worsened prognosis.

10. **C.** Often the radiographic interpretation of a vertical root fracture is the pattern of bone loss occurring in a "teardrop" shape.

11. **A.** Periodontal abscess occurs with preexisting periodontitis and is characterized by localized purulent inflammation of the periodontal tissues. It is also known as *lateral periodontal abscess* or *parietal abscess*. This acute infection occurs in the walls of periodontal pockets as a result of the invasion of bacteria into the periodontal tissues. Although

abscesses usually occur spontaneously in patients with untreated periodontitis, they are more common in patients with periodontitis and a systemic disease such as diabetes, in which there is a reduced ability to combat infections. In some cases, an abscess can occur a few days after dental cleaning as a result of mechanical disruption of junctional epithelium, allowing the bacteria to gain entrance into the tissues. This is not the same as acute apical abscess because the involved tooth usually is vital. Abscesses tend to worsen as time goes on. Symptoms include tenderness or pain and the site of the abscess being warm to the touch. Symptoms of discomfort or pain depend mainly on the site of the abscess, although larger ones—because they are a source of infection within the body—can cause fever, chills, sweating, and malaise.

12. **A.** Lingering spontaneous pain is evidence of C-fiber stimulation. Even in degenerating pulps, C fibers may respond to stimulation. The excitability of C fibers is less affected by disruption of blood flow compared with A-delta fibers. C fibers are often able to function in hypoxic conditions (e.g., at the early stage of pulpal necrosis.)

13. **D.** Symptomatic apical periodontitis is characterized by *pain*, commonly triggered by chewing or percussion. It is usually caused by localized inflammation of the periodontal ligament in the periradicular region. Symptomatic apical periodontitis alone is *not* indicative of irreversible pulpitis. Tenderness to percussion is a pathognomonic symptom of symptomatic apical periodontitis.

14. **A.** In a periodontal abscess, the pulp vitality test would be within normal limits.

15. **E.** Patients with cracked teeth may experience pain in the tooth on biting or chewing. However, the discomfort is not constant, as with a decay-induced toothache or abscess. Often the pain is mimicked only when a patient bites a certain way. The tooth may be more sensitive to cold temperatures. If the crack worsens, the tooth may become loose. Many people with cracked tooth syndrome have symptoms for months, but it is often difficult for them to explain what is wrong because the symptoms are not consistent. Some patients present with asymptomatic cracks that are only clinically evident.

16. **B.** True-combined lesions are treated initially as primary endodontic lesions with secondary periodontal involvement. Periodontal surgical procedures are almost always indicated. The prognosis of a true-combined periodontal-endodontic lesion is often poor or even hopeless, especially when periodontal lesions are chronic with extensive loss of attachment.

17. **B.** The patient is displaying characteristic signs of irreversible pulpitis. The treatment of choice is to remove the source of pulpitic infection by initiating endodontic therapy. The scenario in the question is considered an endodontic emergency, and treatment should be rendered to relieve the patient's pain.

18. **C.** The best treatment of symptomatic irreversible pulpitis with a corresponding bony lesion is removal of the source of infection via pulpectomy.

19. **B.** The current recommendation for patients with a recent MI is to postpone dental or surgical treatment for at least 6 months. Risk for a second MI in patients with recent MI if given a general anesthetic is as follows: 0 to 3 months after MI, 31% risk of reinfarction; 3 to 6 months after MI, 15% risk of reinfarction; more than 6 months after MI, 5% risk of reinfarction. It is recommended to defer elective care for at least 6 months after MI.

20. **D.** Incision and drainage techniques work best for fluctuant abscesses, so as to release purulent exudate. Local anesthesia should be obtained first. An incision should be placed at the most dependent part of the swelling. The incision should be wide enough to facilitate drainage and allow blunt dissection. After irrigation, a drain may be placed to maintain patency of the wound.

21. **C.** Many studies have shown definitively the predominant role of gram-negative obligate anaerobic bacteria in endodontic periapical infections. Earlier studies generally implicated facultative organisms, but improved culturing techniques established the predominance of obligate anaerobes.

22. **C.** "Danger zone" refers to the distal area in the mesial root in mandibular molars. Usually a straight layer of dentin, it becomes a preferable site for strip perforation during instrumentation. "Safety zone" is described as the mesial area of the root, with a thicker layer of dentin, slightly touched by the endodontic instruments.

23. **D.** In an intrusive dental injury, the patient may complain of pain. The patient's tooth is misaligned, or there is no sense of tooth mobility. This type of displacement has the worst prognosis. For intruded primary teeth, allow teeth to reerupt before possible repositioning. For intruded adult teeth, allow reeruption and then stabilize.

24. **A.** Internal resorption begins on the internal dentin surface and spreads laterally. It may or may not reach the external tooth structure. The process is often asymptomatic and becomes identifiable only after it has progressed enough to be detectable radiographically. The etiology is unknown. Trauma is often, but not always, implicated. Resorption that occurs in inflamed pulps is characterized histologically by dentinoclasts, which are specialized,

multinucleated giant cells similar to osteoclasts. Treatment is prompt endodontic therapy. However, when external perforation has caused a periodontal defect, the tooth is often lost.

25. **A.** Internal bleaching alone causes 3.9% of external cervical root resorption (also referred to as *peripheral inflammatory root resorption*). The presence of a barrier (base material) between the root filling material and the internal bleaching material should be approximately 4 mm to prevent this resorption.

26. **E.** Emergency treatment of localized swelling associated with an endodontic infection is to achieve drainage either through the root canal or by incision and drainage and to remove the source of infection. Administration of antibiotics is considered with the concomitant presentation of fever and malaise and for diffuse swelling (cellulitis).

27. **A.** The manufacturing process of a K-type instrument (K-file or K-reamer) is grinding a stainless steel wire to a tapered square or triangular cross-section.

28. **D.** Irrigation of the root canal system is a critical component in nonsurgical endodontic treatment. Benefits of irrigation include dissolution of organic debris, disinfection of complex anatomy that is not accessible by instrumentation, destruction of endodontic pathogens, and removal of the smear layer. Additionally, irrigation acts as an intracanal wetting medium.

29. **B.** In a primary infection gram-negative bacteria are the most common pathogens. In post-treatment disease most (but not all) gram-negative bacteria are eliminated. Bacteria persisting after chemomechanical debridement are typically gram-positive facultative anaerobes exhibiting the ability to adapt to antimicrobial treatment. Samples typically include Pseudoamibacter micra, Actinomyces species, Propionibacterium species, *Parvimonas alactolyticus, lactobacilli, and Enterococcus faecalis*.

30. **C.** The maxillary first premolar has a pronounced mesial crown concavity making this tooth vulnerable to mesial perforation after access opening particularly when the tooth is restored with a full crown.

31. **B.** Irrigation with saline and not hydrogen peroxide is advocated for treating a NaOCl accident. Additional treatment includes cold compresses within the first 24 hours and warm compresses after to control swelling, analgesics for pain control and antibiotics for patients at increased risk for secondary infection.

32. **A.** EDTA is a decalcifying chelating agent used in buffered solution in concentrations between 15 and 17%. Ethylenediaminetetraacitic acid acts as a chelator and typically targets calcium ions and removes the smear layer from root canal walls.

33. **D.** In comparing accuracy among the three pulp diagnostic tests, a cold test or heat test exhibits the highest sensitivity or the ability to identity teeth with pulpal disease and highest specificity or the ability to identify teeth without pulpal disease.

34. **B.** Composition of gutta-percha for clinical endodontic use is: gutta-percha (19%-22%), zinc oxide (59%-79%), heavy metal salts (1%-17%), waxes or resins (1%-4%).

35. **C.** Avulsion. To have pulp space infection, the pulp must first become necrotic. This will occur in a fairly serious injury in which displacement of the tooth results in severing of the apical blood vessels.

36. **E.** All of the choices are true. *Suppurative apical periodontitis:* continuously or intermittently draining sinus tract, usually drains into the oral mucosa. The exudate can also drain through the gingival sulcus of the involved tooth, mimicking a periodontal lesion with a "pocket." However, this is not a true periodontal pocket because there is not a complete detachment of connective tissue from the root surface. It should be treated with conventional root canal therapy. Antibiotics are not needed, since the infection is localized and draining. If the tract does not heal within a few weeks, root-end surgery may be required. If left untreated, however, it may become covered with an epithelial lining and become a true periodontal pocket.

37. **B.** A history of recent restoration of the tooth in question. *Focal sclerosing osteomyelitis* (FSO) consists of a localized, usually uniform zone of increased radiopacity adjacent to the apex of a tooth that exhibits a thickened periodontal ligament space or an apical inflammatory lesion. The size of the lesions usually measure less than 1 cm in diameter. There is no radiolucent halo surrounding this type of lesion. The osteitis microscopically appears as a mass of dense sclerotic bone.

FSO is most often found in patients younger than 20 years of age, around the apices of mandibular teeth (most commonly molars) with large carious lesions and chronically inflamed pulps or with recent restorations. Most sources agree that the associated tooth may or may not be vital.

Gender is not a predisposing factor. FSO can be asymptomatic or the patient can experience mild pain, depending on the cause. FSO is usually discovered upon radiographic analysis. It represents a chronic, low-grade inflammation.

38. **B.** They are eliminated by the natural defenses of the body. Obturation prevents coronal leakage and bacterial contamination and seals the remaining irritants in the canal. After root canal obturation, the remaining bacteria should have lost their source of nutrition, becoming susceptible to the body's immune system.

Answer Key for Section 2

1. **B.** A restored or sealed tooth indicates potential past carious activity but not current activity. The presence of plaque biofilm does not indicate caries presence. Sealants are used for preventive purposes, not caries treatment.

2. **D.** When doing an indirect pulp cap, some caries may be left; a liner (usually calcium hydroxide) is usually placed over the excavated area, and the area may be assessed 6 to 8 weeks later. Regardless, the prognosis for an indirect pulp cap is better than the prognosis for a direct pulp cap.

3. **D.** Smooth-surface caries occurs on any of the axial (facial, lingual, mesial, and distal) tooth surfaces but not the occlusal.

4. **E.** The advantages and benefits of rubber dam usage are reflected in all of the items listed. The rubber dam isolation increases access and visibility.

5. **A.** The first number is the width of the blade or primary cutting edge in tenths of a millimeter (0.1 mm). The second number of a four-number code indicates the primary cutting edge angle, measured from a line parallel to the long axis of the instrument handle in clockwise centigrades. The angle is expressed as a percent of 360 degrees. The instrument is positioned so that this number always exceeds 50. If the edge is locally perpendicular to the blade, this number is normally omitted, resulting in a three-number code. The third number (second number of a three-number code) indicates the blade length in millimeters. The fourth number (third number of a three-number code) indicates the blade angle, relative to the long axis of the handle in clockwise centigrades.

6. **C.** Retention locks, when needed in class II amalgam preparations, should be placed entirely in dentin, not undermining the adjacent enamel. They are placed 0.2 mm internal to the DEJ, are deeper gingivally (0.4 mm) than occlusally (i.e., they fade out as they extend occlusally and translate parallel to the DEJ). If the axial wall is deeper than normal, the retention lock is not placed at the axiofacial or axiolingual line angles but rather is positioned 0.2 mm internal to the DEJ. If placed at the deeper location, it may result in pulp exposure, depending on the location of the axial wall depth.

7. **D.** Because of the typical shape of a carious lesion in the cervical area, the resulting restoration is kidney-shaped or crescent-shaped, and the extensions are to the line angles, resulting in the mesial and distal walls diverging externally. The convexity of the tooth in the gingival one third results in the occlusal and gingival walls diverging externally. Several retention groove designs are appropriate, including four corner coves, occlusal and gingival line angle grooves, or circumferential grooves. However, as with any restoration, if there is only a small amount of tooth structure (<1 mm) between the new and existing restoration, it is best to join the two restorations together and prevent the possibility of fracture of the small amount of remaining tooth structure.

8. **B.** Typically, the class I composite preparation has occlusally converging walls that provide primary retention form. The actual bonding also provides retention form. However, an occlusal bevel is not indicated on class I preparations, and retention grooves are not used.

9. **B.** A tooth preparation is dictated by the extent of the carious lesion or old restorative material, the creation of appropriate convenience form for access and vision, and the anticipated extensions necessary to provide an appropriate proximal contact relationship. Fracture lines present should normally be included in the restoration. However, it is rare that the size of the tooth affects the design of the tooth preparation.

10. **B.** Although the amalgam margin must be 90 degrees, the enamel margin may not be 90 degrees, especially on the occlusal surface. Most walls converge occlusally, but many class V amalgam preparations have walls that diverge externally. No retention form should be placed at the DEJ; otherwise, the adjacent enamel would be undermined and subject to fracture.

11. **C.** The primary causes of postoperative sensitivity for amalgam restorations are voids (especially at the margins), poor condensation (that may result in a void), or inadequate dentinal sealing. Extension onto the root surface does not result in increased sensitivity.

12. **B.** Amalgam carving should result in coincidence with the cavosurface margin and should not result in deep occlusal anatomy because such form may create acute amalgam angles that are subject to

fracture. Depending on the condensation rate of the amalgam used, waiting a couple of minutes before initiating carving may allow the amalgam to harden enough that the carving is easier and over-carving is minimized. When carving the occlusal cavosurface margin, the discoid carver should rest on the adjacent unprepared enamel, which will serve as a guide for proper removal of amalgam back to the margin.

13. **D.** The trituration process mixes the amalgam components, and the reaction results in the alloy particle being coated by mercury and a product being formed.

14. **C.** Proper proximal contacts reduce the potential for food impaction, preserving the health of the underlying soft tissue. A missing proximal contact may result in tooth movement that has an adverse effect on the occlusal relationship of the tooth. Having a correct contact does not enhance the retentive properties of the restorative material.

15. **A.** Self-etch adhesive systems differ from etch-and-rinse (total-etch) adhesive systems by removing less of the smear layer (they use a less potent acid), creating a weaker bond to enamel (especially non-prepared enamel), and not requiring wet bonding that may be necessary for most etch-and-rinse systems. Although fewer actual materials may be needed with some self-etch systems, they need to be applied in multiple coats, and the time necessary to apply the materials is similar for both systems.

16. **D.** Occlusal reduction would not affect the ability to seat a casting. However, temporary cement, heavy proximal contacts, or tooth undercuts could keep the casting from seating completely.

17. **A.** If a patient has a notched cervical area that is very sensitive or esthetically objectionable, restoration is usually indicated. If the notched area is very deep, adverse pulpal or gingival responses may occur. Although more notched areas are encountered in older patients, a patient's age is not a factor in the need for restoration.

18. **A.** The longer a slot, the better. They should be inside the DEJ and prepared with an inverted cone bur to a depth of 1 mm.

19. **C.** Although some self-etch bonding systems use milder acid, the primary acid system used for etching tooth structure is phosphoric acid.

20. **B.** Triturating (mixing) the amalgam particle with the mercury is intended to result in coating the particles with a surface of mercury and creating the desirable phases in the set amalgam. All of the alloy particle is not dissolved in the mercury, and the size is not significantly reduced.

21. **D.** Composite materials exhibit more dimensional change (2.5 times greater than tooth structure) when subjected to extreme changes in temperature than the other choices. Direct gold is slightly higher than tooth structure, and amalgam is about twice as high as tooth structure.

22. **D.** All of these factors indicate that a cervical lesion should be restored. In addition, if the lesion is large and the pulpal or gingival tissues are in jeopardy, it should be considered for restoration.

23. **B.** Composite restorations are more technique-sensitive than amalgam restorations because the bonding process is very specific (requiring exact, correct usage of the various materials and an isolated, noncontaminated field), and the insertion and contouring of composites are more demanding and time-consuming. Composites are not stronger than amalgam and have similar wear resistance compared with amalgams. Composites are indicated for class II restorations.

24. **B.** The constant contraindication for using a composite restoration is the inability to isolate the operating area properly. Occlusal wear of composite is similar to that of amalgam. Extension onto the root surface may result in gap formation with composite but also results in initial leakage with amalgam, indicating that there is no ideal material for root-surface extended restorations. A high C-factor (class I) can be largely overcome by using (1) a liner under the composite, (2) a filled adhesive, and (3) incremental insertion of the composite.

25. **C.** The restoration of a proximal contact is easier with amalgam than composite. Amalgam is easier to use and is less technique-sensitive. Either material can be used for class II restorations. Because an amalgam restoration requires a tooth preparation that has (1) a specified depth (for strength of the amalgam), (2) cavosurface marginal configurations that result in 90-degree amalgam margins, and (3) undercut form to its walls or secondary retention form features, they require more tooth structure removal than composite tooth preparations. Composite tooth preparations require (1) removal of the fault, defect, or old material; (2) removal of friable tooth structure; and (3) no specific depths—they are more conservative.

26. A—4; B—2; C—3; D—1.

27. **A, C, E, G.** Abraded or eroded noncarious lesions are restored when the area is cariously involved (**A**), when there is intolerable sensitivity unresponsive to conservative desensitizing measures (**C**), when the area is to be involved in the design of a removable partial denture (**E**), and the patient desires an esthetic improvement (**G**). The restoration of these lesions has no impact on phonetics, restoration is not needed when the defect is shallow and it does not compromise the structural integrity of the tooth, and restoration is unnecessary because the tooth is treated endodontically.

28. **A, B, D, G.** Light marginal staining not compromising esthetics, recurrent caries that can be adequately treated by a repair restoration, and shallow ditching around an amalgam restoration are not reasons to replace an existing restoration.

29. A—3; B—2; C—1; D—4.

30. A—5; B—3; C—1; D—4; E—2; F—6.

31. A—6; B—2; C—5; D—3; E—1; F—4.

32. **A, C.** Skirts increase retention and resistance forms. They do not provide bracing (collars do), enhance esthetics, provide pulp protection, or improve draw.

Answer Key for Section 3

1. **D.** The superficial temporal, pterygomandibular, masseteric, and submental spaces are potentially involved in odontogenic infection. There is no rhinosoteric space.

2. **B.** Depending on the ramus relationship, mesioangular and vertical impactions may not require removal of bone or sectioning of the tooth. Horizontal impaction always requires removal of bone and sectioning.

3. **E.** A patient with severe infection and systemic involvement, unless immunocompromised, is expected to present in a febrile state, or a temperature of greater than 100° F. All the other items refer to symptoms that indicate potential airway emergency.

4. **D.** Criteria for implant success include mean vertical bone loss of less than 0.02 mm annually after the first year of service. In this question, no further treatment is necessary at this time.

5. **C.** Implants should be placed a minimum of 2 mm from the inferior alveolar canal.

6. **A.** In myofascial pain dysfunction, the source of the pain and dysfunction is muscular. Dysfunction is associated with decreased opening or inability to chew.

7. **D.** Periodontal management is the first step in the management of this patient. If the patient is unwilling, or unable, to maintain adequate hygiene before placement of orthodontic appliances, their subsequent placement would make the periodontal situation more difficult. For the same reasons, dental decay should be treated before beginning orthodontic treatment. The final prosthetic management should not be completed before the underlying skeletal anomaly is addressed because the occlusion would be constructed to the best—and final—anatomic location.

8. **C.** Systemic sequelae of obstructive sleep apnea syndrome include hypertension, cor pulmonale, and cardiac arrhythmia.

9. **C.** Tissue symmetry, tenderness, joint noises, dental health, and occlusion and range of motion all are critical components of the physical examination in the patient with TMJ complaints. Although the length of the soft palate is important in the evaluation of patients with sleep apnea, patients with snoring, patients being sedated, or patients needing complete denture construction, it does not contribute directly to TMJ dysfunction.

10. **C.** Maxillary fractures may be classified as Le Fort I, II, or III. Le Fort III is the highest and most severe classification.

11. **C.** Chronic sinusitis is not a relative contraindication to most elective oral surgical procedures. Unstable chest pain should be evaluated by an internist or cardiologist before any dental treatment. Radiation to the jaws and a history of clotting disorders both would require further investigation of the health history and likely alter the patient's treatment plan to lessen the likelihood of osteoradionecrosis or of bleeding complications.

12. **B.** Disc displacement without reduction can result in decreased range of motion because the condyle becomes restricted by the anteriorly displaced disc, limiting translation.

13. **B, D, F.** Choice **A** is incorrect because antibiotics used to treat odontogenic infections should be effective against streptococci and oral anaerobes. *S. aureus* is commonly seen on respiratory tract and skin, not on oral mucosa. Choice **C** is incorrect because high-grade fever resulting from infection suggests systemic involvement, and antibiotic therapy should be initiated. Choice **E** is incorrect because narrow-spectrum antibiotics are preferred over broad-spectrum antibiotics because of less likelihood in altering the normal flora and less impact on the development of resistant strains.

14. **A, C, E.** Mesioangular impacted third molars are the least difficult to remove because the withdrawal path does not run into the mandibular ramus as distoangular impacted third molars do. It is easier to remove a tooth with roots that are one half to one third formed because such length prevents the tooth from "spinning in place" compared with teeth with less formed roots. Finally, teeth with fused conical roots are less difficult to extract because there are no undercuts compared with diverged or dilacerated roots.

15. **A—1, B—4, C—2, D—3.** Incisional biopsy is often used in lesions larger than 1 cm in size, as opposed to excisional biopsy, which is often used in lesions less than 1 cm. Osteomyelitis is an infection and

inflammation of the bone. A hard tissue bone biopsy is required to reach a definitive diagnosis of osteomyelitis. Aspiration or fine-needle biopsy on a soft tissue lesion deep to mucosa should be done first to confirm if the entity is truly cystic, vascular, or solid. Otherwise, an attempt to obtain a biopsy specimen of a soft tissue lesion that is vascular in origin, such as an arteriovenous malformation, can result in hemorrhagic complications.

16. **B, C.** Bupivacaine is not approved by the Food and Drug Administration for use in children younger than 12 years. In children, the most significant safety issue with respect to local anesthetics is related to overdose. Overdose is most often directly related the volume of the drug injected. Lidocaine allows the greatest volume to be injected safely.

17. **B.** Most local anesthetics packaged in dental cartridges are tertiary amines. At the present time, the only local anesthetic packaged in dental cartridges that has an ester bond is articaine, but the bond in the connecting chain in the drug molecule is an amide.

18. **D.** Bupivacaine is packaged in dental cartridges only as a 0.5% solution. Likewise, lidocaine is always a 2% solution (in the United States), and articaine is always a 4% solution. Mepivacaine is packaged in both 2% and 3% solutions in the United States.

19. **A.** The larger the lumen of the needle, the easier it is to determine whether the needle is actually in a vessel. The needle length is irrelevant, as is the patient. The injection performed is relevant in regard to the frequency of obtaining a positive aspiration but not the reliability of the aspiration per se.

20. **D.** The palatal tissue from canine to canine bilaterally is the premaxilla. The nasopalatine injection anesthetizes this area.

21. **C.** The pK_a for lidocaine or prilocaine is 7.8, for mepivacaine is 7.7, and for bupivacaine is 8.1.

22. **D.** By definition, a 2% solution of any drug contains 20 mg/mL. A dental cartridge of local anesthesia has a fluid volume of 1.8 mL. 20 mg × 1.8 = 36 mg of lidocaine per cartridge. Three cartridges of 2% lidocaine with 1 : 100,000 epinephrine contain 108 mg.

23. **D.** All mandibular molars are anesthetized by the inferior alveolar nerve block. The other three answer choices are maxillary injections.

24. **D.** The degree of hydrophobicity and protein binding are the most important factors in determining duration of action of a local anesthetic. Bupivacaine is highly hydrophobic (lipophilic) and is 95% bound to protein. The other listed agents are less hydrophobic and are 55% to 75% bound to protein.

25. **A.** All amide local anesthetics are biotransformed in the liver. One available local anesthetic also has an ester side chain, which means it has some degree of extrahepatic biotransformation (outside the liver). This drug is articaine and is the most appropriate drug for patients with liver disease.

26. **D.** The inferior alveolar nerve block has a stated success rate of 85%, the lowest of any intraoral injection. Lingual and nasopalatine injections are close to 100% successful, and the posterior superior alveolar nerve block is also much more than 85% effective.

27. **A, B, C.** Vasocontrictors prolong the duration of action of local anesthetic preparations by keeping the drug at the site of action longer. Agents with greater protein binding have a greater attraction for receptor sites and remain within sodium channels for a longer time, which prolongs the duration of action of the drug. Although lipid solubility is primarily related to potency, it is secondarily related to duration of action because lipid solubility is directly related to protein binding. The pK_a determines the onset of the local anesthetic, not the duration. The pH and concentration of the local anesthetic have no relationship to the duration of action.

28. **A, B, D, E, F.** See chemical structure of articaine, demonstrating both an amide and an ester linkage. Articaine is packaged as a 4% drug, in the highest concentration of all local anesthetics in dentistry. The amide component of articaine is biotransformed in the liver where the ester component of articaine is biotransformed in the plasma (an extrahepatic site).

Answer Key for Section 4

1. **C.** In pemphigus vulgaris, autoantibodies attach to antigens (desmoglein) found in desmosomes that keep keratinocytes linked to each other. Cells eventually separate from each other (acantholysis), resulting in short-lived intraepithelial vesicles or bullae.

2. **D.** Condyloma latum is one of the lesions that may be seen in secondary syphilis, which is caused by *Treponema pallidum.* All the other lesions listed may be associated with HPV.

3. **D.** Hairy leukoplakia is viral in origin and shows intranuclear inclusions in infected epithelial cells. Hairy leukoplakia is caused by EBV, a herpesvirus. Intranuclear epithelial inclusions are also seen other herpesvirus infections (e.g., HSV infections).

4. **E.** Odontogenic myxomas are connective tissue neoplasms that contain little collagen; this gives them an embryonic look microscopically.

5. **D.** This triad of signs defines primary Sjögren's syndrome. The patient has secondary Sjögren's syndrome if rheumatoid arthritis or other autoimmune disease is present.

6. **C.** Recurrent intraoral herpes infections occur only in the hard palate and hard gingiva except in patients with AIDS. A history of blister (vesicle) formation and recurrence are also supportive of this diagnosis.

7. **A.** Nodular fasciitis is a rapidly developing reactive lesion that typically does not recur after excision. Fibromatosis is an aggressive nonencapsulated lesion that is associated with a significant potential for recurrence. The other lesions listed are malignancies and require more than simple excision to prevent recurrence.

8. **E.** Traumatic bone cysts characteristically occur in the body of the mandible of teenagers. They are pseudocysts because they have no epithelial lining. They are empty cavities.

9. **C.** Cherubism is a fibro-osseous lesion that occurs in teenagers. Characteristically, it manifests with ill-defined margins and a "ground-glass" appearance radiographically. The other features described also support this diagnosis.

10. **B.** The maculopapular rash of rubeola (measles) is preceded by the herald sign of Koplic's spots (punctate ulcers of the buccal mucosa).

11. **D.** Destructive inflammation in the three sites noted is characteristic of Wegener's granulomatosis.

12. **A, C, E, G.** Central giant cell granulomas, jaw lesions in patients with hyperparathyroidism (so-called brown tumors), and jaw lesions in cherubism all microscopically demonstrate significant numbers of osteoclastlike, multinucleated giant cells distributed within a fibrovascular matrix. Aneurysmal bone cysts contain similar types of tissues and cells, including multinucleated giant cells, but also demonstrate a prominent pseudocystic architecture.

13. **A—4, B—6, C—2, D—1, E—3, F—5.** For choice **A,** minor aphthous stomatitis is the most common form of this disorder and is usually characterized by the development of a single, superficial ulcer of nonkeratinized mucosal areas such as buccal mucosa. For choice **B,** the reticular form of lichen planus often manifests with asymptomatic, interlacing white lines in a bilateral distribution. Buccal mucosa is a common site for these lesions, although tongue and gingiva are also affected often. For choice **C,** infiltration of gingival tissues by leukemic cells may occur in some patients, most commonly patients with chronic monocytic leukemia. The gingival appears enlarged because of malignant cell infiltration, and the tissue is often red, boggy, and hemorrhagic. For choice **D,** the tongue is the most common site in the body for the development of a granular tumor. This is a benign proliferation or aggregation of cells with features similar to Schwann's cells that results in a firm, often yellow nodule in the substance of the tongue. For choice **E,** amalgam tattoo is the most common pigmented lesion in the oral cavity. For choice **F,** mucous extravasation phenomenon is a pool of extraductal mucin that collects after traumatic severance of the minor salivary gland duct. The lower lip is the most common location for this reactive lesion.

14. **A, D, E.** Aphthous or aphthouslike ulcers may develop in patients with celiac sprue, Behçet's syndrome, or Crohn's disease, all examples of diseases in which immune system dysfunction is an important factor in the pathogenesis. Although oral manifestations may be variable, lesions in patients with sarcoidosis, amyloidosis, and neurofibromatosis typically manifest as submucosal nodules and masses.

15. **C, D.** X-ray beam B was produced with a higher mA and higher exposure time (s). Both these factors increase the total number of photons produced.

However, the peak or mean energies of the x-ray beam do not change.

16. **A, D.** The mean energy of an x-ray beam is influenced by the kilovoltage setting on the machine. As the kilovoltage setting is increased, the mean energy of the beam increases. The amount of built-in filtration that preferentially absorbs low-energy photons also results in an increase in the mean energy of the beam.

17. **D.** When heated, the filament releases electrons (thermionic emission).

18. **B.** Basal epithelial cells are the most mitotically active of the cells on the list and are the most radiosensitive.

19. **A—1, 4; B—2, 3, 5.** Thyroid cancer and heritable effects are stochastic effects. Xerostomia, cataract formation, and oral mucositis are deterministic effects.

20. **A.** The probability of photoelectric interactions is directly proportional to the cube of the atomic number. Enamel has the highest effective atomic number.

21. **A.** Silver halide in an x-ray film is sensitive to x-rays and visible light. Sodium thiosulfate is a component of the fixer. Gelatin is used to suspend the silver halide crystals, but is not radiosensitive. Rare earth elements are used in intensifying screens.

22. **A.** The effective dose considers the dose absorbed by each tissue and weighs the dose depending on the type of tissue exposed. The numerical effective doses from different examinations can be directly compared. The higher the effective dose, the higher the estimated risk.

23. **B.** Use the rule of "SLOB": *Same Lingual, Opposite Buccal*.

24. **D.** Cone-cutting results from misalignment of the x-ray tube. Use a film-holding device with an external guide.

25. **B.** If proper processing procedures are followed, the developer will become depleted with age and need changing.

26. **D.** Visible light exposes all the silver bromide crystals, and the film is black after processing.

27. **A.** Daily check of the processing solution temperature, whether using automatic processing or manual tanks, and comparison with the manufacturer's recommended values improves image quality. The other procedures are useful but can be performed less frequently.

28. **D.** Prudence suggests that radiographic examinations of a pregnant patient should be kept to a minimum consistent with the patient's dental needs.

29. **D, E.** Radiographs demonstrate calcified structures such as bone and teeth. Radiographic examination does not permit evaluation of the depth of the soft tissue pocket. Additionally, intraoral radiographs are two-dimensional images; they are unable to characterize loss of specific bony walls of a periodontal defect and do not depict three-dimensional anatomy.

Answer Key for Section 5

1. **C.** According to available data, approximately 15% of adolescents have severe crowding that would require major expansions or numerous extractions to resolve. The other statements are false. Crowding in the primary dentition is very rare and would indicate crowding will occur in the permanent dentition; spacing in the primary dentition is normal; and African-Americans generally have less crowding than whites.

2. **B.** The cranial base includes, from anterior to posterior, the ethmoid, sphenoid, and occipital bones.

3. **C.** Reproductive tissues grow at the same time as the adolescent growth spurt, and the appearance of secondary sexual characteristics can be used to help predict the timing of growth.

4. **B.** Young children often present with minimal overbite or anterior edge-to-edge relationship. Habits such as thumb sucking increase the likelihood that less overbite will be present.

5. **A.** The molars are class II, but the skeletal relationship described by a normal ANB measurement is normal, so the malocclusion is dental in origin.

6. **B.** Root resorption is common during orthodontic treatment, although lesions often resolve on the root surface. Mobility of teeth is also common as the PDL reorganizes and widens during tooth movement. It is uncommon for teeth to become devitalized as a result of orthodontic movement, unless they have also been substantially compromised by injury or infection.

7. **C.** Because M = Fd, doubling the force would double the moment, or tendency to rotate, tip, or torque.

8. **D.** Class II elastics work in the direction that would be used to correct a class II malocclusion, to pull the mandibular teeth forward and the maxillary teeth distally.

9. **B.** Class III elastics are worn from the maxillary first molars to the mandibular canines. The force system created by class III elastics produces mesial movement and extrusion of the maxillary first molars.

10. **B.** Primary canines are extracted to encourage alignment of the crowded incisors. However, the incisors align and upright, borrowing space otherwise needed for eruption of the permanent canine. Primary first molars are extracted to encourage eruption of the first premolar so that it may be extracted to make room for the permanent canine to erupt.

11. **B.** When a large diastema greater than 2 mm is present, it likely will not close on its own. Diagnostic tests, such as a radiograph, should be performed to rule out the presence of a supernumerary tooth, usually a mesiodens.

12. **A.** Intruding incisors would decrease overbite while uprighting teeth, and using a high-pull headgear could make overbite correction more difficult. A lip bumper would likely have little effect on overbite.

13. **A.** Initiation and proliferation are the only possibilities for congenitally absent teeth, the bud and cap stages, respectively. In the histodifferentiation stage, the teeth are present; failure in this stage results in structural abnormalities of the enamel and dentin. Failure in the morphodifferentiation stage results in size and shape abnormalities.

14. **A.** For any child patient, it is imperative to discuss any kind of physical restraint with the parent to obtain an informed consent. An informed consent includes recommended treatment, reasonable alternatives to that treatment, and the risk of no treatment. If the dentist wants to use a firm voice control, it is recommended that a discussion take place beforehand as well.

15. **A.** Conscious sedation is defined as a minimally depressed level of consciousness as opposed to deep sedation or general anesthesia. There are four stages of anesthesia (analgesia → delirium → surgical anesthesia → respiratory paralysis), and the patient is conscious only in the first stage (analgesia). The patient should be able to maintain an airway and respond to stimulation and command.

16. **A.** Both of these statements are true. As a result of these differences, there are modifications in preparation design for class II amalgams. Beveling the gingival seat of class II amalgams is not recommended. There is a greater convergence from cervical to occlusal of the buccal and lingual walls of class II amalgam preparations because of the broad and flat contact areas.

17. **B.** There have been concerns regarding the bloodborne spread of formocresol at least since 1983, when a study was published describing the tissue changes induced by the absorption of formocresol from pulpotomy sites in dogs. Ferric sulfate and mineral trioxide aggregate have been demonstrated to be reasonable alternatives to formocresol.

18. A. A band-loop space maintainer would work well in this case because the maxillary first bicuspid normally erupts before the loss of either the second primary molar or the primary cuspid.

19. D. The patient's overbite and overjet improved from the previous examination, and so it is likely that the patient's thumb-sucking habit had decreased significantly. The mother stated that the patient sucks his thumb only while falling asleep. When thumb sucking occurs for a limited time per day, not only is tooth movement normally associated with thumb sucking unlikely, but also it is possible for teeth to return to a more normalized position. The risk of malocclusion as related to habitual activity is a function of amount of time per day the habit is practiced, the duration of the habit in terms of weeks and months, and the intensity of the habit. Because the occlusion seems to be improving and because the habit has significantly decreased, the best treatment is to counsel the parent regarding thumb sucking and recall the patient in 3 months.

20. A. Orthodontic closure of a midline diastema is accomplished before the periodontal surgery. If a frenectomy is performed before orthodontic treatment, it is possible that scar tissue could form in the area, which may impede orthodontic tooth movement.

21. D. Unless it can be determined that the primary tooth is impinging on the permanent successor, intruded primary teeth are left alone in the hopes that they will spontaneously reerupt. Intruded permanent teeth have a poorer prognosis. If there is an open apex, an intruded permanent tooth should be closely monitored for spontaneous eruption. An intruded permanent tooth with a closed apex should be repositioned orthodontically, and a calcium hydroxide pulpectomy should be performed 2 weeks after the injury.

22. D. Replanting primary teeth has a poor prognosis but could be considered if performed within 30 minutes. A primary tooth that is replanted is likely to require splinting. The patient should be placed on antibiotics, be restricted to a soft diet, and undergo a primary endodontic procedure accomplished.

23. B. Because the exposure site is likely significantly contaminated from the injury that occurred 24 hours previously, direct pulp capping with calcium hydroxide is contraindicated. A calcium hydroxide pulpectomy should not be the automatic procedure performed because continued root elongation and closure of the pulp canal will likely not occur. A calcium hydroxide pulpotomy is preferable for a traumatized tooth with an open apex with either a large exposure or a small exposure of several hours or days postinjury. Clinically, the tooth should be anesthetized, and, under sterile conditions, the clinician should open the pulp chamber to search for healthy pulp tissue. It is likely that vital tissue will be present within 24 hours of the injury.

24. B. An extruded permanent incisor with an open apex should be repositioned, splinted, and monitored closely for loss of vitality. Because of the open apex, the tooth may remain vital and continue to develop; immediate pulp treatment is contraindicated.

25. C. The other three answer choices may occur as the result of trauma but do not cause loss of vitality. Pulpal hyperemia causes increased intrapulpal pressure and swelling, which may result in an interruption of the pulp's blood supply. Without an adequate blood supply, the pulp becomes necrotic. This process can take time, and symptoms (either radiographic or clinical) may not manifest for weeks or months. Typically, follow-up examination and radiographs are indicated at 1-, 2-, and 6-month intervals after a traumatic incident.

26. A—1, B—3, C—2, D—4. When heavy forces are applied during orthodontic treatment, the tooth is moved in the direction in which the force is pushing, compressing the PDL on the side toward which the tooth is moving. The area of the compressed PDL becomes necrotic or hyalinized. Cell migration occurs from surrounding bone marrow spaces, and undermining resorption occurs. As the force dissipates over time and repair occurs, frontal resorption can begin to occur.

27. C. Beta titanium is a titanium and molybdenum alloy that does not contain nickel. Stainless steel used in orthodontic wires is generally 8% nickel and 18% chromium. Cobalt chromium has a small amount of nickel in its composition. Nickel titanium is the wrong answer because it has "nickel" in its name.

28. B. Acid etching of the enamel performed during the orthodontic bonding procedure causes microporosities in enamel, which are filled with bonding primer and resin to achieve a mechanical interlocking between the tooth and composite resin material. The composite itself can be chemically cured or light-cured. However, the bond between the tooth and resin is mechanical, not chemical.

29. C. The width of the permanent incisors is greater than the deciduous or primary incisors, so it is normal and desirable for there to be spacing between primary incisors so that the permanent successors have adequate space to erupt. However, this extra space is not the leeway space. The term *leeway space* refers to the extra width of the primary canine, primary first molar, and primary second molar (combined) compared with their permanent successors (permanent canine and first and second premolars). This extra leeway space becomes available when these posterior teeth exfoliate, and the permanent teeth, which are typically smaller, erupt.

30. **A.** *Low/load deflection* means that a low amount of force is required to create a particular amount of deflection of a wire. That means that the wire is very flexible compared with a high load/deflection wire (a stiffer wire), which would require a greater amount of force to deflect it the same amount. If the amount of force change per unit of deflection is small, the amount of force delivered does not change much as the wire is activated more and more. Increasing the length of a wire (by adding loops or helices to its design) makes it more springy (less stiff), reducing its load/deflection.

31. **D.** When the permanent dentition is fully erupted, there is little or no likelihood that crowding will resolve on its own without intervention. Widening of the dental arches during occlusal development continues to occur naturally to a small degree during growth until the permanent canines are erupted. There is some increase in space available for the dentition as the permanent premolars erupt to replace the primary molars owing to the leeway space. However, there is no increase in the length of the mandible that occurs within the dental arches during growth. The mandible grows by addition of bone at the condyle and deposition of bone at the posterior ramus. Resorption of bone at the anterior border of the ramus provides room for the posterior teeth (first molar, second molar and, perhaps later, third molar) to erupt but does not provide room for anterior dental crowding to resolve.

32. **A—3, B—2, C—4, D—1.** It is important to observe the behavior of the child to better treat the patient.

33. **A—3, B—1, C—4, D—2.** It is important to know these stages in order to effectively manage the expectations of the patient and to prevent deeper stages that may lead to nausea, vomiting, and other adverse outcomes.

34. **B, C, D.** The enamel is thinner and the pulp chambers are relatively larger; therefore, restorative preparations must be shallower than typical permanent teeth. The greater constriction at the cement-enamel junction allows for a retentive area for stainless steel crowns; however, this feature also may cause a problem in attaining a gingival seat when a class II preparation is prepared too cervically. Interproximal contacts are broader and flatter in primary teeth and therefore, preparations for primary teeth are altered by preparing relatively wider gingival seats with increased convergence to the occlusal, thereby removing more lateral interproximal decay while maintaining a conservative occlusal outline form.

35. **A, C, D.** Choice **A**: Pulp therapy is generally contraindicated in children who have serious illnesses. Extremely serious complications secondary to acute infection can arise should the pulp therapy fail. Choice **B**: A patient's chronologic age has little to do with decisions regarding pulp therapy. The clinician instead should be cognizant of the dental age of the patient, stage of development and position of the permanent successor, and other factors in the decision-making process. Choices **C** and **D**: Teeth with caries involvement that are mobile, have swelling, furcation radiolucency, pain to percussion, and spontaneous pain likely either have advanced inflammation or are necrotic. The pulpotomy procedure is reserved for vital teeth only. Choice **E**: Marginal ridge breakdown is a common issue with severely decayed teeth. This condition alone does not rule out a pulpotomy procedure unless the caries is very extensive and renders the tooth nonrestorable either by extending cervically excessively or by interproximal space loss secondary to the carious process. Choice **F**: Amelogenesis imperfecta is not a contraindication to a pulpotomy procedure. Choice **G**: Carious exposures with normal pulp tissue are typically treated with a pulpotomy procedure.

Answer Key for Section 6

1. **B.** The four processes of motivational interviewing are engaging, focusing, evoking, and planning.

2. **C.** Important tenets of social cognitive theory are the notion of self-efficacy, behavioral modeling, and social reinforcement.

3. **B.** Sustain talk is communication that conveys a desire to maintain the current behavior.

4. **C.** Informed consent requires that the patient be advised of reasons for the procedure and the benefits and risks of the procedure and anticipated outcome, any alternatives and their risks and benefits including no treatment at all, and the costs of the procedure and the alternatives and be given an explanation of the procedure in understandable terms for a layperson (not technical terms).

5. **C, E.** The ethical principles listed in the question that are found in the ADA *Principles of Ethics and Code of Professional Conduct* include beneficence ("do good") and veracity ("truthfulness"). The remaining ethical principles found in the ADA *Principles of Ethics and Code of Professional Conduct* include patient autonomy ("self-governance"), nonmaleficence ("do no harm"), and justice ("fairness").

6. **B, C.** The required elements for a patient to give consent include the patient must voluntarily agree to treatment and the patient must have the opportunity to ask questions. Additional elements required for a patient to give consent include the following: information and consent must be given in a language that the patient understands; the doctor must be available to answer any patient questions; only the patient or the patient's legal guardian can authorize treatment decisions; and all state regulations that outline who must obtain consent from the patient and whether it must be in writing or signed are met.

7. **C.** Risk management is a concept derived from industry wherein one identifies areas possibly exposing one to liability; weighs the risks against the benefits; and controls that exposure by monitoring, ensuring, or eliminating the dangerous activity. Risk management does not include intentionally and knowingly exposing oneself to liability.

8. **A, D, F.** A very important weapon against a possible lawsuit is appropriate and adequate documentation of patient contacts. When making entries in patient records, be sure to include specific facts, document completely the patient visits and contacts, make timely entries, and avoid gaps in time. Never make personal characterizations that criticize patient behavior; instead, be objective and factual in documentation. Entries must be readable, and use of abbreviations and shorthand should be avoided.

9. **C.** Habituation is the decrease in response that occurs as a result of repeated or prolonged exposure to a conditioned stimulus.

10. **A.** A rational response is a cognitive therapy technique in which the patient develops (with or without assistance) a more adaptive thought or statement as a means of coping.

11. **E.** Creating a child-oriented environment (e.g., having toys and books in the waiting room, hanging pictures on the wall or ceiling that a child would find interesting), conveying interest in the child by asking about their interests, and having the parent present in the operatory all are variables that may put child patients more at ease.

12. **B.** Research has demonstrated that behavioral intervention is typically more effective than patient education. A combination of the two is considered the most effective approach to increasing patient compliance.

13. **B.** Clinicians should use caution in providing premature reassurance because trust and rapport may be compromised if the outcomes are inconsistent with what the clinician asserted.

14. **D.** The tongue is the most common place for incident cancers in the oral cavity.

15. **A.** Community water fluoridation is the most cost-effective and economical method to prevent dental caries. However, fluoride is believed to be the least effective on the occlusal surface. Most decay among school-age children occurs on the pits and fissures of the chewing surfaces.

16. **C.** Double-blind designs help prevent the potential for a biased interpretation of a treatment effect that might occur if either the investigator or the subject knows to which group the latter belongs.

17. **D.** The methods section of a scientific article allows the reader to assess the validity of the study and the reliability of the measures. This section provides the reader with specific and detailed information regarding how the study was conducted. Based on this information, the reader should be able to replicate the study.

18. **C.** The variance determines the way individual values are located around the mean. The larger the variance, the more widely the data items are spread about the mean value. Variance is measured in squared units (s^2). The standard deviation is the square root of the variance. The mean is expressed in the same units as the data items, but the variance is expressed in squared units. The standard deviation measures the average deviation from the mean in the same units as the mean.

19. **D.** Parenteral contact is defined as the transmission of pathogenic microorganisms by piercing the skin or mucous membrane (e.g., intravenous, subcutaneous, intramuscular) by an accidental or intentional stick with a needle or other sharp instrument that is contaminated with blood or other body fluid.

20. **E.** Masks that cover the mouth and nose reduce inhalation of potentially infectious aerosol particles. They also protect the mucous membranes of the mouth and nose from direct contamination. Masks should be worn whenever aerosols or spatter may be generated. If a mask is worn longer than 20 minutes in an aerosol environment, the outside surface of the mask becomes a nidus of pathogenic bacteria rather than a barrier. It is recommended that a new mask be worn for each patient and that masks be changed routinely at least once every hour and more often in the presence of heavy aerosol contamination.

21. **D.** Disinfection refers *only* to the inhibition or destruction of pathogens. Spores are not killed during disinfection procedures. By custom, the term *disinfection* is reserved for chemicals applied to inanimate surfaces, and the term *antiseptic* is used for antimicrobial agents that are applied to living tissues.

22. **A.** The spore test is a biologic monitor. The process consists of placing into the autoclave bacterial spores on strips or in envelopes along with a normal instrument load. If the autoclave is working properly, the autoclave reaches the temperature and pressure to kill the spores. Spore testing must be conducted weekly.

23. **E.** A disinfectant should be able to kill *M. tuberculosis*. This is the benchmark organism for disinfectants. It is much harder to kill than most bacteria, viruses, fungi, and protozoa. This resistance is partially due to the waxy cell wall of *Mycobacterium*.

24. **E.** MSDSs are an easy reference for information on hazardous substances. MSDSs must be "readily accessible" to workers exposed to hazardous substances. MSDSs provide information on hazardous materials, substances, and wastes. Chemical manufacturers develop and provide an MSDS for each hazardous product. The distributor is responsible for getting MSDSs to employers. At least one copy of the MSDS should be maintained with each chemical.

25. **B.** Prospective reimbursement is a mechanism in which the dentist is compensated before treatment is provided (i.e., in capitation systems). Managed care is an arrangement in which a third party mediates between providers and patients negotiating reimbursement for certain services and overseeing the treatments delivered.

26. **E.** Fluoridated water is odorless, colorless, and tasteless at the recommended level of fluoride for a community water supply, which ranges from 0.7 to 1.2 parts per million (ppm) of fluoride. At this dosage, it is imperceptible to the human senses.

27. **D.** According to the U.S. Centers for Disease Control, in 2012, more than 210 million people in the United States lived in fluoridated communities.

28. **D.** According to the CDC, in 2010, about 74% of the U.S. population on a public water supply lived in fluoridated communities.

29. **D.** Studies shows that fluoridation prevents tooth decay for people of all ages. It has both a topical and a systemic effect.

30. **D.** The best response is school sealant programs because it is the only choice that is a community-level or population-level prevention program. Choices **A**, **B**, and **E** are individual prevention measures.

31. **E.** Flossing daily is the only choice that is an individual prevention measure, not a community prevention program. Flossing does not prevent tooth decay.

32. **B.** According to the CDC, the recommended level of fluoride for a community water supply is 0.7 to 1.2 ppm of fluoride depending on the mean annual temperature over 5 years. In 2011, the U.S. Department of Health and Human Services proposed decreasing this to 0.7 ppm, but as of July 2013, it had not been implemented. The rationale is that fluid intake of people is the same regardless of yearly air temperature of a community.

33. **D.** Community water fluoridation is the most cost-effective and the most practical preventive measure to prevent tooth decay. Everyone in the community benefits with no individual or group effort needed, at a minimal cost to society and at no cost to an individual. All the other prevention programs listed require staff or individual effort for everyone.

34. **C.** For a child who lives in a nonfluoridated community it is recommended, depending on existing water fluoride levels, to start fluoride dietary supplements from 6 months until 16 years old. For children 3 years old or younger, it is much easier to use fluoride drops because children at that age have difficulty swallowing or chewing tablets.

35. B. Secondary prevention is the elimination or reduction of a disease after it occurs. An amalgam restoration is considered secondary prevention because tooth decay is removed and a restoration is placed.

36. E. All health care providers—dentists, hygienists, nurses, and physicians—are responsible for educating the public on the safety and effectiveness of a public health measure that benefits everyone such as community water fluoridation.

37. C. Sealants seal in and block the caries process before or after it has begun. Sealants prevent incipient caries in pits and fissures from progressing. Sealants are primarily recommended for first and second permanent molars. Sealants are not the best preventive measure for large populations; fluoridation is. Sealants are primarily for children at risk for dental caries. Fluoride mouth rinses have been used in U.S. schools for more than 4 decades.

Answer Key for Section 7

1. B. Wasting diseases of the teeth include erosion (corrosion; may be caused by acidic beverages), abrasion (caused by mechanical wear as with toothbrushing with abrasive dentifrice), attrition (caused by functional contact with opposing teeth), and abfraction (flexure secondary to occlusal loading).

2. D. Wasting diseases of the teeth include erosion (corrosion; may be caused by acidic beverages), abrasion (caused by mechanical wear as with toothbrushing with abrasive dentifrice), attrition (caused by functional contact with opposing teeth), and abfraction (flexure secondary to occlusal loading).

3. A. The periodontal examination includes probing pocket depth (distance from the gingival margin to the base of the pocket) and clinical attachment level (distance from the CEJ to the base of the pocket). Both of these measures are made using a periodontal probe. Gingival recession can be measured as the distance from the CEJ to the free gingival margin. Alveolar bone loss is measured radiographically.

4. C. When the free gingival margin is apical to the CEJ, recession has occurred. Attachment loss is the measure from the CEJ to the base of the periodontal pocket. With the free gingival margin 2 mm apical to the CEJ and the probing pocket depth measurement 6 mm, there has been 8 mm loss of attachment.

5. A. Loss of clinical attachment is the hallmark that distinguishes periodontitis from gingivitis. In both diseases, patients may present with periodontal pocket depths greater than 3 mm. In gingivitis, these are often referred to as "pseudopockets." Gingival recession can occur in a healthy periodontium as a result of factors such as aggressive toothbrushing or orthodontic tooth movement. Bleeding on probing is a hallmark sign of inflammation in the periodontal tissues and can occur in both diseases.

6. D. Supragingival plaque is either tooth-associated or outer layer. Tooth-associated plaque is composed primarily of gram-positive cocci and short rods.

7. C. Saliva is the source of inorganic components (calcium, phosphorus) for supragingival plaque. Gingival crevicular fluid is the source of inorganic components of subgingival plaque.

8. B. *Streptococcus* and *Actinomyces* species are initial colonizers of dental plaque. They are gram-positive, facultative microorganisms.

9. C. Endotoxin or lipopolysaccharide is an important constituent of the gram-negative outer membrane that contributes to initiation of the host inflammatory response.

10. B. Calculus is calcified dental plaque. It is always covered by a layer of uncalcified plaque, which is detrimental to the gingival tissues.

11. B. Supragingival margins are least detrimental to the gingival tissues; subgingival margins are the most detrimental because of the accumulation of dental plaque.

12. C, D, F, G. T cells, B cells, and plasma cells are cells of the acquired immune system. The acquired immune system must "see" a foreign substance to attack it effectively and can confer long-term immunity to the host. Cells of the innate immune system defend the host in a nonspecific manner by responding to foreign substances in a generic way. These cells include neutrophils (polymorphonuclear leukocytes), dendritic cells, monocytes/macrophages, and mast cells.

13. C. Neutrophils are one of the primary defense cells of the innate immune system. T lymphocytes are important activators of the specific (adaptive) immune system. Macrophages are antigen-presenting cells. Plasma cells produce antibodies.

14. B. Matrix metalloproteinases are the most important proteinases involved in the destruction of periodontal tissues.

15. C. Neutrophils are the predominant inflammatory cells in the periodontal pocket and have migrated across the pocket epithelium from the subgingival vascular plexus.

16. C. Preliminary phase therapy is used to treat emergencies and remove hopeless teeth.

17. B. Polymorphisms in the IL-1 genes have been associated with severe chronic periodontitis.

18. D. Single-rooted teeth have a poorer prognosis than multirooted teeth with comparable loss of attachment. Loss of attachment that extends to the apex of the root alters the root/crown ratio and makes the prognosis worse.

19. C. The amount of clinical attachment loss is most important in determining the prognosis. Deep pocket depths and bleeding on probing can be found in both gingivitis and periodontitis. Although the level of alveolar bone is usually consistent with the amount of clinical attachment loss, there are circumstances under which these two measures are not comparable.

20. **B.** Diabetic patients may experience hyperglycemia, which is greater than normal amounts of glucose in the blood. However, this is not the most common problem for diabetic patients undergoing dental treatment. They are more likely to experience hypoglycemia, or low blood glucose concentrations, as a result of inadequate carbohydrate ingestion. Insulin resistance is a physiologic condition in which cells do not respond normally to the actions of insulin. Insulin deficiency is when the pancreas does not produce enough insulin.

21. **C.** Sickle scalers and universal curettes do not have offset angulation of the blade. The working ends of area-specific curettes are offset at a 60-degree angle relative to the terminal shank. The working ends of sickle scalers and universal curettes are not offset—they are at a 90-degree angle relative to the terminal shank.

22. **C.** Patients with active infectious diseases should not be treated with ultrasonic instruments because of the aerosol that is created when using this type of instrument.

23. **B.** During the course of periodontal treatment, a wound (space) is created that becomes an area where cells from multiple tissue types are present in close proximity. Because of their diverse characteristics, different cell types have dissimilar proliferative and migratory capabilities that affect the speed and order of healing. Epithelial cells are typically fastest in their response and migratory capabilities and engage in this process first, resulting in what is often called "healing by long junctional epithelium." Connective tissue cells from the gingival tissue and the PDL cells follow in their migratory abilities, with bone cells being the slowest in these capabilities. Although this process is dependent on the physiologic capabilities of the different cell types in general, it can be influenced by other systemic or local factors. During periodontal treatment, the ultimate goal is the creation of new attachment, which can be achieved only if the PDL cells repopulate the area of lost attachment.

24. **A.** Plaque removal during the initial postoperative visits after periodontal surgery is essential to healing of the periodontal tissues.

25. **D.** Laterally positioned flaps should be performed only when there is adequate bone and adequate width and thickness of attached gingiva on the facial of the donor site.

26. **B.** If the bone is overheated (>47°C) for prolonged periods (>1 minute) during the preparation of the osteotomy, it leads to necrosis of the bone cells and bone tissue, causing bone sequestration or creation of nonmineralized soft scar tissue at the osteotomy site. This type of aberrant bone healing leads to prevention or disruption of the normal process of osseointegration around the dental implant, causing implant failure. During the osteotomy phase, it is critical to use profuse irrigation (cooling), along with gentle moderate-speed drilling and sharp drills, to prevent overheating of the site.

27. **C.** Three-walled defects respond best to regenerative therapy.

28. **C.** The primary goal of guided tissue regeneration is to prevent the migration of epithelial cells into the healing surgical site. When those cells are present on the root surface, healing is by establishment of a long junctional epithelium. By excluding these cells, the membrane allows for stabilization of the clot and regeneration of the periodontium—the deposition of cementum on the root surface and regeneration of alveolar bone and the PDL. Plaque accumulation does occur on the surface of the membrane during this healing process.

29. **C.** Although tooth migration can be a sign of occlusal trauma, tooth mobility is the most common clinical sign.

30. **B.** Most patients who have been treated for periodontitis should be seen at 3-month intervals for supportive periodontal therapy (maintenance).

31. **C.** The minimal space needed between an implant and a natural tooth or between two implants in mesiodistal direction is 2 mm of bone. This dimension provides at least 1 to 1.5 mm of adjacent bone present to allow for proper healing and prevent bone loss around or between implants. If two implants (4 mm each; 8 mm total) are used, 6 mm (2 + 2 + 2) is needed to allow a sufficient amount of mesiodistal bone between tooth #1/implant #1, implant #1/implant #2, and implant #2/tooth #1. The minimum dimensions of the total mesiodistal space needed for placement of two 4-mm implants is 14 mm.

Answer Key for Section 8

1. **C.** Only weak acids and weak bases are greatly affected in their distribution by changes in pH. Weak organic acids dissociate more from protons at higher pH, making a higher percentage of their molecules charged; this traps them in that compartment.

2. **A.** Drug agonists have an intrinsic activity of greater than 0 and less than or equal to 1. Intrinsic activity refers to the maximal effect attainable by the drug. Potency and receptor affinity are not directly related to intrinsic activity. The therapeutic index requires a quantal dose-response curve, in contrast to the other characteristics listed, which require graded concentration-response curves. Drugs with the same intrinsic activity may vary a great deal in their aqueous solubility.

3. **A.** Inhibition of adenylyl cyclase through G_i, resulting from stimulation of α_2-adrenergic receptor, leads to a reduction in intracellular cAMP.

4. **C.** Circulating muscarinic cholinergic receptor agonists stimulate these receptors on endothelial cells, leading to release of nitric oxide and vasodilation.

5. **B.** Carbidopa is used to inhibit dopa decarboxylase. Its usefulness is based on reducing conversion of levodopa to dopamine outside the CNS. Carbidopa does not penetrate the blood-brain barrier and does not interfere with the beneficial effect of levodopa in the brain, but it prevents the adverse effects of dopamine in the periphery.

6. **A.** Bupivacaine has the highest lipid solubility of the drugs listed. Lipid solubility is the major chemical characteristic of the local anesthetic that determines duration of action. Procaine is the only ester given as a choice and is rarely used.

7. **B.** Nitrous oxide oxidizes the cobalt in vitamin B_{12}, resulting in the inhibition of methionine synthase. Nitrous oxide has greater analgesic potency than other inhaled anesthetics (e.g., halothane, isoflurane). Ketamine is not inhaled; rather, it is injected. It also does not inhibit methionine synthase. The same is true for propofol.

8. **C.** α-Adrenergic receptor stimulation accounts for the vasoconstrictor effect of levonordefrin.

9. **A—3, B—5, C—1, D—2, E—4.** Botulinum toxin prevents fusion of the secretory vesicles with the plasma membrane in cholinergic nerves, preventing the release of acetylcholine. Tranylcypromine is a nonselective MAO inhibitor. It increases the concentration of catecholamines and serotonin in the cytoplasmic pool of nerves but indirectly reduces the level of neurotransmitter in the secretory granule. Amphetamine is well known for its sympathetic effect because of release of catecholamines. Physostigmine inhibits acetylcholinesterase, which metabolizes acetylcholine. The enzyme is primarily located on the postjunctional and postsynaptic membranes. Fluoxetine is an antidepressant that inhibits the reuptake of serotonin.

10. **D.** Naloxone is a competitive antagonist at opioid receptors.

11. **C.** COX is a key enzyme in the synthesis of prostaglandins. Prostaglandins, including PGE_2 and $PGF_{2\alpha}$, are important mediators for functions such as pain and are a product of COX. Aspirin inhibits both COX-1 and COX-2.

12. **C.** Oral ketorolac (an NSAID) is used only to continue therapy after a parenteral dose.

13. **E.** Basophils and mast cells release histamine. However, the cell that responds to histamine stimulation at the H_2 receptor is the parietal cell of the stomach. Stimulation of this receptor leads to proton release and a decrease in the pH of the stomach lumen. H_2 histamine receptor blockers are used to reduce stomach acid.

14. **A.** Renin release from the kidney is enhanced by stimulation of the β_1-adrenergic receptors in the juxtaglomerular cells. Among the answer choices, only β blockers reduce renin release. Although ACE inhibitors and angiotensin II receptor blockers act on the renin-angiotensin system, they do not inhibit renin release. These agents tend to increase plasma renin.

15. **C.** α-Adrenoceptor blockers, such as phentolamine, inhibit the vasoconstrictor effect of epinephrine but not the vasodilator effect of epinephrine. The administration of α blockers results in epinephrine reversal. Propranolol would block only the vasodilator effect of epinephrine. Guanethidine and tyramine act largely at prejunctional sites and do not block adrenergic receptors.

16. **B.** Enoxaparin is a low-molecular-weight heparin. It activates antithrombin III and inhibits factor Xa.

17. **D.** The effect of glucocorticosteroids remaining in the mouth after inhalation is to make the oral cavity more susceptible to fungal infection. The mouth should be rinsed with water after inhalation use.

Inhaled methacholine, in contrast to the other drugs listed, is not used therapeutically, but rather is used to diagnose hyperactive airway.

18. **E.** Divalent and trivalent cations, such as those found in oral antacids, chelate tetracyclines and prevent their absorption.

19. **D.** A decrease in glycogen breakdown is a classic effect of insulin. Epinephrine (by acting as an agonist at α_1-adrenergic and β_2-adrenergic receptors), albuterol (by acting as an agonist at β_2-adrenergic receptors), and glucagon (by acting at glucagon receptors) all tend to increase glycogenolysis. Parathyroid hormone has little effect on glycogenolysis.

20. **B.** Nitroglycerin is a nitrovasodilator. It produces nitric oxide, which activates guanylyl cyclase which catalyzes the production of cGMP.

21. **C.** Clavulanic acid has very little antimicrobial activity. Its value in combination with certain penicillins is due to its ability to inhibit certain penicillinases. This inhibition protects the penicillin from bacterial enzyme attack. Transpeptidase is inhibited by β-lactams, such as penicillin. DNA gyrase is inhibited by fluoroquinolones, such as ciprofloxacin.

22. **E.** Transpeptidase is the enzyme that catalyzes the peptide cross-linking of peptidoglycan. Transpeptidase is inhibited by penicillins and cephalosporins.

23. **E.** Trimethoprim, by virtue of its inhibition of bacterial dihydrofolate reductase, acts synergistically with the sulfonamides.

24. **D.** Clindamycin is useful for some oral infections, including infections involving viridans streptococci. *K. pneumoniae* and *P. aeruginosa* are gram-negative rods and not subject to clinical inhibition by clindamycin. Methicillin-resistant staphylococci are insensitive to clindamycin and most traditional antistaphylococcal drugs. *C. albicans* is a yeastlike fungus and is not inhibited by antibacterial drugs such as clindamycin.

25. **E.** The mammalian enzyme form of dihydrofolate reductase is the target for methotrexate. Bleomycin produces strand breaks in DNA. Cisplatin is an alkylating agent. Doxorubicin intercalates with DNA and inhibits topoisomerase. 5-Fluorouracil, after undergoing activation, inhibits thymidylate synthase.

26. **1—C, 2—A, 3—E, 4—D, 5—B.** Glipizide is an oral hypoglycemic drug that causes the release of insulin from the beta cells of the pancreas by closing the ATP-dependent potassium channels. The effect of insulin is mediated by binding to its receptor, followed by several events including the movement of the glucose transporter, GLUT-4, to the plasma membrane, resulting in an increase of glucose uptake into the cell.

27. **A, D, F.** Phentolamine blocks both α_1-adrenergic and α_2-adrenergic receptors. It blocks the vasoconstrictor effects of norepinephrine and epinephrine, both of which cause vasoconstriction by stimulating α-adrenergic receptors. The effect of phentolamine would last long enough to block the vasoconstrictor effect of a subsequent injection of epinephrine. Phentolamine does not block β-adrenergic receptors or sodium channels. It does not block protein synthesis in bacteria and does not have an antimicrobial effect. Phentolamine is used in dentistry to reverse soft tissue anesthesia more quickly after local anesthesia.

28. **A—3, B—5, C—1, D—7, E—2.** Several drugs are approved for the treatment of overactive bladder. These are typically antimuscarinic drugs that block the effect of acetylcholine on the detrusor muscle of the bladder. Solifenacin is a newer drug that happens to be a selective antagonist at the M_3 muscarinic receptor. Stimulation of α_2-adrenergic receptors in the brain and spinal cord reduces sympathetic outflow and leads to sedation, analgesia, and reduced blood pressure. As a result of this mechanism, dexmedetomidine is a useful intravenous sedative. Quetiapine is a newer antipsychotic drug that is able to block both the dopamine D_2 and the 5-HT$_2$ receptors, resulting in fewer adverse effects compared with older antipsychotic drugs. Zaleplon blocks the BZ_1 receptor selectively, whereas a benzodiazepine, such as diazepam, blocks both the BZ_1 and the BZ_2 receptors. Both are located on chloride channels. Gabapentin binds selectively to the $\alpha_2\delta$-1 subunits of the high-voltage calcium channel. Pregabalin has a similar mechanism. These drugs are useful for certain partial seizures and for neuropathic pain and, at least for pregabalin, for fibromyalgia. Codeine is an opioid receptor agonist that has analgesic and antitussive properties. Pilocarpine is a muscarinic receptor agonist that does not act at any of the receptors mentioned and would have an effect on the bladder opposite to that desired for overactive bladder. Carbamazepine is a sodium channel blocker, which is used as an antiepileptic drug and for neuropathic pain such as trigeminal neuralgia.

29. **A—5, B—7, C—1, D—11, E—4, F—9, G—10.** The effect of neostigmine on acetylcholinesterase makes it a useful drug for myasthenia gravis. ACE inhibitors end in "pril" (generic names) and are useful for various cardiovascular indications. By inhibiting dipeptidyl peptidase-4, sitagliptin reduces the breakdown of the incretin, GLP-1. The resulting increase in GLP-1 reduces glucose uptake from the gut, inhibits glucagon release, increases insulin release, and normalizes insulin levels. This mechanism makes sitagliptin a useful drug for type

2 diabetes. Rifampin inhibits DNA-dependent RNA polymerase, making it effective in certain bacterial infections. It is useful in treating tuberculosis in combination with other drugs. The enzyme, 14 α-demethylase, is important in the synthesis of ergosterol and for membrane integrity of many fungi. Inhibition of this enzyme is the antifungal mechanism of the azoles, including fluconazole. DOPA decarboxylase catalyzes the conversion of DOPA to dopamine. By inhibiting this enzyme, carbidopa reduces the conversion of DOPA to dopamine. The reason this inhibition is useful is because it allows more DOPA to enter the CNS where it can be converted to dopamine. Neither dopamine nor carbidopa enters the CNS, so preserving DOPA for CNS conversion to dopamine is effective in treating parkinsonism, and the use of carbidopa means that the dose of DOPA does not have to be large, and the side effects of dopamine are minimized. MAO-B is selective for the metabolism of dopamine. Selegiline increases the level of dopamine in the CNS, making the drug useful for parkinsonism and without as many adverse effects as nonselective MAO inhibitors. Terbinafine inhibits squalene epoxidase (squalene monooxygenase), making it useful for dermatophyte fungal infections. Aliskiren is a direct inhibitor of renin. This drug is useful in treating hypertension. Ciprofloxacin inhibits DNA gyrase and topoisomerase IV, making it useful as an antibacterial drug. Lithium inhibits inositol monophosphate phosphatase. This and other mechanisms mediate an antimanic effect from the drug.

30. **B, D, E.** The drugs that most effectively antagonize pilocarpine are agents that block muscarinic receptors because pilocarpine is a muscarinic receptor agonist. Tolterodine and oxybutynin are used to treat overactive bladder, whereas benztropine is used principally to overcome Parkinson-like (extrapyramidal) adverse effects from antipsychotic drugs. All three drugs are antimuscarinic agents. Rivastigmine increases salivary flow rate because of its inhibition of acetylcholinesterase with resultant muscarinic effects in the salivary glands. Metoprolol is a selective β_1-adrenergic receptor blocker and does not directly affect the secretory flow rate increase from pilocarpine. Epinephrine stimulates α-adrenergic and β-adrenergic receptors and does not directly affect the secretory flow rate increase from pilocarpine.

31. **C, E.** Acyclovir and penciclovir both become initially phosphorylated by thymidine kinase in the herpes simplex virus. The eventual activation of the drugs by host enzymes results in the inhibition of viral DNA polymerase. The drugs are selective for the virus because they are poorly phosphorylated by thymidine kinase in mammalian cells. Their toxicity is low despite their effectiveness against the virus. Ganciclovir is also activated in a similar way; however, its selectivity is lower, and its toxicity precludes its use for herpes simplex virus, although the risk/benefit ratio is acceptable in treating cytomegalovirus. Indinavir is an inhibitor of HIV aspartyl protease and is targeted to HIV. Zidovudine is a nucleotide derivative that inhibits HIV reverse transcriptase, restricting its use to retroviruses. Ribavirin inhibits RNA synthesis and is used to treat respiratory syncytial virus.

32. A—3, B—9, C—1, D—6, E—7, F—4. Bisphosphonates, especially at doses used to treat neoplasms of the bone, have been linked to osteonecrosis of the jaw. Pamidronate is a member of this class of drugs. ACE inhibitors are known commonly to cause a nonproductive cough. This cough is likely due to the increase in bradykinin resulting from inhibition of bradykinin breakdown by ACE. The generic names of ACE inhibitors end in "pril" (e.g., fosinopril). The α-adrenergic receptor blockers, including α_1-selective blockers such as terazosin, are associated with a risk of first dose hypotension because of the high degree of sensitivity to these drugs until the body adapts to them. Diphenhydramine is an H_1 histamine receptor blocker. It also passes through the blood-brain barrier. These two characteristics predict a high probability of sedation when given. The drug is used for its antihistaminic effects, but it is also used to produce sedation. The use of aspirin, and by extension other salicylates, in individuals younger than 20 years old with concurrent or recent viral infections has been linked to Reye's syndrome. This syndrome is characterized by encephalopathy and liver damage and is often fatal. It has not been implicated with use of acetaminophen. Although there have been some anecdotal reports of methemoglobinemia with acetaminophen or lidocaine, these cases are extremely rare. There is a more direct connection with the use of prilocaine because it is metabolized to o-toluidine, which can lead to oxidation of hemoglobin. Neither acetaminophen nor lidocaine is metabolized to o-toluidine. Clopidogrel blocks the $P2Y_{12}$ receptor for ADP in platelets and reduces platelet aggregation. It is not linked to any of the descriptions given here. Bleeding is its most important adverse effect.

Answer Key for Section 9

1. **B.** Irreversible hydrocolloid or alginate is the material of choice to produce diagnostic casts. Its composition is mainly sodium or potassium salts of alginic acid. The salts react chemically with calcium sulfate to produce insoluble calcium alginate.

2. **B.** A closed or insufficient vertical dimension of occlusion is thought to be one predisposing condition for angular cheilitis, which usually is associated with *Candida albicans*. Improperly balanced occlusion and poor contour of the denture base are not predisposing conditions for angular cheilitis.

3. **A.** Paget's disease of bone is a bone disease characterized by bone resorption followed by attempts at bone repair involving proliferation leading to bone deformities. Its etiology is unknown, and it occasionally involves the maxilla and mandible. Papillary hyperplasia is characterized by multiple papillary projections of the epithelium caused by local irritation, poor-fitting denture, poor oral hygiene, and leaving dentures in all day and night.

4. **A.** Maxillary teeth should contact the wet dry lip line when fricative sounds *f*, *v*, and *ph* are made. These sounds help to determine the position of the incisal edges of the maxillary anterior teeth.

5. **C.** Using more monomer than needed causes increased shrinkage. The more monomer used, the less expansion, less heat, and reduced strength produced.

6. **D.** Occlusal adjustment of dentures should be done with the premise of obtaining even occlusal contacts with balanced occlusion to stabilize the dentures during function.

7. **C.** Bone loss is usually seen on the most coronal aspect of the implant in the form of a wedge. There is no periodontal ligament on implants, so there is no feeling of soreness.

8. **C.** Rests are critical for the health of the soft tissues underlying the denture resin basis and the minor and major connectors. Rests should prevent tilting action and should direct forces through the long axis of the abutment tooth. To function as specified, an occlusal rest should have a rounded (semicircular) outline form and be one third the facial lingual width of the tooth, one half the width between cusps, and at least 1.5 mm deep for base metal. The rest floor inclines apically toward the center of the tooth, and the angle formed with the

vertical minor connector should be less than 90 degrees.

9. **D.** This is the best answer because generally it is the dentist's fault and not the technician's. Incorrect opaque may influence the resultant shade. Inadequate vacuum affects the esthetics. If the opaque does not mask well, the metal result is a gray appearance or lower value in the restoration.

10. **C.** Usually, vertical fractures refer pain when biting. In this case, the patient had recent endodontic treatment, but there is no periapical lesion to indicate the pain is due to inadequate root canal therapy. There is no sign that the crown is loose, no premature contact, and no mobility.

11. **C.** The condyles should be in centric relation, which is defined as "the maxillomandibular relationship in which the condyles articulate with the thinnest avascular portion of their respective disks with the condyle-disk complex in the anterior-superior position against the shapes of the articular eminences" (The glossary of prosthodontic terms. *J Prosthetic Dent* 94:21-22, 2005).

12. **D.** Any time there is a question regarding the treatment outcome involving a prosthetic device or the need to produce templates for provisional restorations that reproduce a desired form of teeth, it is recommended that a diagnostic wax-up be generated.

13. **A.** The length, canal enlargement, and a finish line for the post are unimportant if there is no sound remaining coronal tooth structure to get a ferrule of the final restoration.

14. **E.** Bone resorption around dental implants can be caused by inadequate oral hygiene, premature loading, and repeated overloading. If an implant-supported framework does not fit passively, the implant is placed under constant force. If significant compressive forces are placed on the interfacial bone, these can lead to implant failure.

15. **D.** When checking the occlusion of a cast restoration, mylar paper or shim stock is a very accurate method for testing occlusal contacts. The procedure is to check with the mylar paper before placing the restoration in the teeth adjacent to the tooth to be restored and the opposing side. The dentist places the restoration and checks whether the same occlusal contacts are maintained on the tested teeth. When all teeth, including the one being

restored, hold the mylar paper on occluding and even, articulating markings are present, occlusion contacts are correct.

16. **E.** An FDP replacing the first bicuspids improves the prognosis of the second bicuspids when placing an RDP. Implants would also improve the prognosis by not leaving the second bicuspid standing alone and acting as a cantilever when in function with the removable prosthesis.

17. **D.** The surveyor is used for surveying a diagnostic cast and to measure a specific depth of undercut. It also helps to determine the most desirable path of placement for an RDP. It identifies bony areas that may need to be surgically removed because they interfere during insertion of the RDP. It is also used to survey crowns, place intracoronal retainers, machine or mill cast restorations, and survey and block out a master cast before constructing an RDP.

18. **C.** Anterior guidance must be preserved by means of construction of a custom incisal guide table, especially when restorative procedures change the surfaces of anterior teeth that guide the mandible in excursive (lateral, protrusive) movements.

19. **D.** The tooth does not exhibit any pathology to indicate that the radiolucency is derived from the tooth. The mental foramen can appear on the apex, depending on the direction of the x-ray beam.

20. **A.** The minor connector for the mandibular distal extension base should extend posteriorly about two thirds the length of the edentulous ridge; this adds strength to the denture base.

21. **D.** Rigidity is provided by cross-arch stability through the principle of broad distribution of stress. The major connector should not alter dramatically the contours of the supporting structures, and it should contribute to the support of the prosthesis.

22. **B.** Common reasons for an FDP not to fit in one piece are lack of parallelism between the abutments and distortion of the wax pattern during removal from the dies. In any of these cases, the framework may not fit in the prepared abutment teeth and must be sectioned between one of the connectors between the pontic and retainer to fit the two pieces individually, and a solder record must be made to solder the pieces.

23. **A.** The soldering flux used with gold alloys is usually borax glass ($Na_2B_4O_7$) because of its affinity for copper oxides. Flux is applied to a metal surface to remove or prevent oxide formation. With an oxide-free surface, the solder wets the surface freely and spreads over the metal surface.

24. **C.** The rest should be spoon-shaped and is slightly inclined apically from the marginal ridge of the abutment tooth. It should restore the occlusal morphology of the tooth and not interfere with the normal existing occlusion.

25. **A.** Metamerism is the phenomenon where a color match under a lighting condition appears different under a different lighting condition.

26. **B.** The patient's main concern is not to lose the anterior teeth and lose esthetics. Maintaining the vertical dimension is not the main concern when fabricating complete dentures because vertical dimension can be accurately reproduced. Extracting the posterior teeth and maintaining the anterior teeth until the day of delivery of the dentures is the preferred method when placing immediate dentures because the posterior teeth can be set (teeth placed in a wax setup). The vertical dimension and the maxillomandibular relationship (centric relation) can be determined. The anterior teeth are set by means of removing the teeth from the cast and replacing them with the denture teeth in a position that is similar to that of the teeth in the cast or in a improved position if necessary, being careful not to make very drastic changes. Also, extracting the posterior teeth beforehand and allowing a period of about 1 month helps to reduce major changes in the anatomic configuration of the ridges, which provides stable ridges posteriorly for the dentures at the time of delivery. It is better to extract all the teeth and allow healing and construct the dentures. However, in this scenario, the patient would lose all the teeth, and this presents an esthetic issue, which is the main concern of the patient (and generally this is the case with most patients). Esthetics is the main concern, so the anterior teeth should be maintained. In some situations, the anterior teeth might not be worth retaining even for a short time, such as if they have severe mobility or are broken down. In the case presented, there is no indication that the anterior teeth are severely mobile or broken down.

27. **A.** Border molding can be challenging with teeth present because there can be tissue undercuts, and it is more difficult to border mold areas with teeth. The area around anterior teeth is usually a difficult area because of anatomic form. Sequencing the treatment is not the most difficult step because generally the steps are similar whether constructing a conventional denture or immediate denture. Delivery is performed in the same manner as most dentures.

28. **C.** A tooth with an occlusal prematurity is often sore when occluding, and patients usually complain that the tooth occludes before the others. An area of abfraction is generally sensitive to passing an explorer over it and sensitive to concentrating a puff of air on the abfraction. A cracked tooth is difficult to diagnose because often the crack is invisible. Pain generally can be elicited by chewing something hard and during the release of the force

applied to a tooth sleuth. The tooth is sensitive to cold liquids. In some cases, there is discoloration of a cusp if the crack passes through the cusp.

29. **D.** Zirconia crowns can be placed on a preparation with the same reduction required as for a full metal crown. A full metal crown requires less reduction than a metal-ceramic crown. A Zirconia crown can also be used on a tooth that has additional reduction needed for a metal-ceramic crown or an all-ceramic crown, such as lithium disilicate crowns.

30. **D.** Assessment and adjustment of occlusal relationships and axial contours does not have any effect on marginal integrity or how the fixed prosthesis fits between the retainer teeth. Proximal contact is the first step when trying any fixed restoration because a tight proximal contact does not allow the prosthesis to seat completely on the tooth and obtain marginal integrity.

Answer Key for Sample Examination

Endodontics

1. A. Acute apical (periradicular) periodontitis is characterized by *pain*, commonly triggered by chewing or percussion. Acute periradicular periodontitis alone is *not* indicative of irreversible pulpitis. It indicates that apical tissues are irritated, which may be associated with an otherwise vital pulp.

2. C. The most important part of the restored tooth is the tooth itself. No combination of restorative materials can substitute for tooth structure. Posts do not reinforce the tooth, but rather weaken it further by additional removal of dentin and by creating stress that predisposes to root fracture.

3. A. Lingering spontaneous pain is evidence of C-fiber stimulation. Even in degenerating pulps, C fibers may respond to stimulation. The excitability of C fibers is less affected by disruption of blood flow compared with A fibers. C fibers are often able to function in hypoxic conditions (e.g., at the early stage of pulpal necrosis).

4. A. Nasopalatine duct cyst is a circular radiolucent area seen as a marked swelling in the region of the palatine papilla. It is situated mesial to the roots of the central incisors, at the site of the incisive foramen. The pulps of the anterior teeth test vital (whereas a periapical cyst tests nonvital). This is the most common type of maxillary developmental cyst. They often remain limited in size and are asymptomatic; they may become infected and show a tendency to grow extensively.

5. E. A patient's immune response to a periradicular infection varies according to the individual. The size and volume of the pulp, the number and quality of the nerves, and the pulpal vascularity and cellularity all are unique to the individual patient. The different virulence of organisms causing the infection may cause differences in pain experienced and differences in the amount of orthoclastic activity. Sheer numbers of organisms can influence their virulence.

6. B. Any notion of moral decision making assumes that rational agents are involved in making informed and voluntary decisions. In health care decisions, respect for the autonomy of the patient would, in common parlance, mean that the patient has the capacity to act intentionally, with understanding, and without controlling influences that would mitigate against a free and voluntary act. It implies knowledge and understanding of the risks and benefits to treatment. This principle is the basis for the practice of "informed consent" in the physician-patient transaction regarding health care.

7. B. The pulp contains two types of sensory nerve fibers: myelinated (A fibers) and unmyelinated (C fibers). A fibers include A-beta and A-delta, of which A-delta are the majority. A-delta fibers are principally located in the region of the pulp-dentin junction, are associated with a sharp pain, and respond to relatively low-threshold stimuli. C fibers are distributed throughout the pulp, are associated with a throbbing pain sensation, and respond to relatively high-threshold stimuli.

8. A. The paralleling, not right-angle, technique is best for endodontics. The film is placed parallel to the long axis of the tooth, and the beam is placed at a right angle to the film. The technique allows for the most accurate and reproducible representation of tooth size.

9. C. The principles of flap design are as follows: (1) flap design should ensure adequate blood supply, and the base of the flap should be wider than the apex; (2) reflection of the flap should adequately expose the operative field; and (3) flap design should permit atraumatic closure of the wound.

10. D. Studies have shown that 50% of the roots of maxillary lateral teeth were distally dilacerated. Oversight of the distal direction of root dilaceration of upper lateral incisors can be a contributing factor in the failure of endodontic treatment of these teeth.

11. B. EDTA is the chelating solution customarily used in endodontic treatment. Chelators remove inorganic components, leaving the organic tissue elements intact.

12. D. Periodontal disease can have an effect on the pulp through dentinal tubules, lateral canals, or both. Primary periodontal lesions with secondary endodontic involvement differ from primary endodontic lesions with secondary periodontic involvement in their temporal sequence. Primary periodontal problems have a history of extensive periodontal disease.

13. D. The buccal object rule (Clark's rule or "SLOB" rule [*S*ame *L*ingual, *O*pposite *B*uccal]) is used to identify the buccal or lingual location of objects in relation to a reference object. If the image of the object moves mesially when the x-ray tube is moved mesially, the object is located on the lingual. If the image of the object moves distally when the x-ray tube moves mesially, the object is located on the buccal (facial).

14. D. Ledges can sometimes be bypassed; the canal coronal to the ledge must be sufficiently straightened to allow a file to operate effectively. This straightening may be achieved by anticurvature filing (file away from the curve). The dentist precurves the file severely at the tip and uses it to probe gently past the ledge. Otherwise, the dentist cleans to the ledge and fills; the patient is warned of the poorer prognosis.

15. D. Factors affecting the long-term prognosis of teeth after perforation repair include the location of the defect in relation to the crestal bone, the length of the root trunk, the accessibility for repair, the size of the defect, the presence or absence of a periodontal communication to the defect, the time lapse between perforation and repair, the sealing ability of the restorative material, and technical skill. Early recognition and repair improve the prognosis. Smaller perforations (<1 mm) cause less destruction. Subcrestal lesions, especially lesions closer to the apex, have a better prognosis.

16. B. If an instrument is broken at the filling stage, it is not necessary to remove or bypass the instrument because the canal has already been cleaned and shaped. Prognosis depends largely on the extent of undébrided material remaining within the canal. The dentist should attempt to obturate as much of the canal as possible.

17. D. Teeth that have been endodontically treated have lost much of their coronal dentin in the access formation, regardless of the caries state before endodontic treatment. This loss of dentin compromises the internal architecture of the tooth. Less internal tooth structure, combined with the absorption of external forces (usually occlusal) may exceed the strength of dentin and result in fracture. Endodontic treatment and loss of pulp vitality are no longer thought to desiccate the tooth to the point of increasing risk of fracture.

18. C. When a root fractures horizontally, the coronal segment is displaced to a varying degree, but generally the apical segment is not displaced. Because the apical pulpal circulation is not disrupted, pulp necrosis in the apical segment is extremely rare. Pulp necrosis in the coronal segment results because of its displacement; this occurs in only about 25% of cases. Because 75% do not lose vitality, emergency treatment involves repositioning the segments in as close proximity as possible and splinting the teeth for 2 to 4 weeks. After the splinting period is completed, follow-up is as with all dental traumatic injuries, at 3, 6, and 12 months and yearly thereafter.

19. B. Radiographic examination for root fractures is extremely important. Because a root fracture is typically oblique (facial to palatal), one periapical radiograph may easily miss its presence. It is imperative to take at least three angled radiographs (45, 90, and 110 degrees) so that in at least one angulation the radiographic beam passes directly through the fracture line and makes it visible on the radiograph.

20. D. For decades, controversy has surrounded the validity of thermal and electrical tests on traumatized teeth. Only generalized impressions may be gained from these tests after a traumatic injury. They are sensitivity tests for nerve function and do not indicate the presence or absence of blood circulation within the pulp. It is assumed that after traumatic injury, the conduction capability of the nerve endings or sensory receptors is sufficiently deranged to inhibit the nerve impulse from an electrical or thermal stimulus; this makes the traumatized tooth vulnerable to false-negative readings from these tests. Teeth that give a positive response at the initial examination cannot be assumed to be healthy or that they will continue to give a positive response over time. Teeth that yield a negative response or no response cannot be assumed to have necrotic pulps because they may give a positive response at later follow-up visits. It may take 9 months for normal blood flow to return to the coronal pulp of a traumatized, fully formed tooth. As circulation is restored, responsiveness to pulp tests returns.

21. A. The K-file and K-reamer are the oldest instruments for cutting and machining dentin. They are made from a steel wire that is ground to a tapered square or triangular cross section and then twisted to create either a file or a reamer. A file has more flutes per unit length than a reamer. The K-Flex file is a modification of the shape of the K-file, with a non-cutting tip design.

22. B. The indications for a direct pulp cap for a tooth are (1) asymptomatic tooth, (2) with little or no hemorrhaging, (3) small (<1 mm), and (4) well-isolated traumatic pulp exposure. A direct pulp cap acts to stimulate the formation of a reparative *dentin bridge* over the exposure site and to preserve the underlying pulpal tissue. It is especially successful in *immature teeth*. Failure of direct pulp capping is indicated by (1) symptoms of pulpitis at any time and (2) lack of vital pulp response after several weeks. Failures result in pulpal necrosis (continual pulpal insult), calcification of the pulp, or (rarely) internal resorption. Direct pulp capping is primarily used on permanent teeth. It is not used often in primary teeth because of the alkaline pH of calcium hydroxide. It can cause either mild or (often) severe pulp irritation. With severe irritation, the risk of internal resorption is increased. With primary teeth, severe resorption is more common; in permanent teeth, formation of reparative dentin occurs more often.

23. **E.** If an immature tooth is nonvital, the diseased tissue must be removed via pulpectomy. Apexification is the treatment of choice.

24. **A.** Internal bleaching alone causes 3.9% of external cervical root resorption (also referred to as *peripheral inflammatory root resorption*). A barrier (base material) of approximately 4 mm between the root filling material and the internal bleaching material should be present to prevent this resorption.

25. **B.** Sodium perborate is more easily controlled and safer than concentrated hydrogen peroxide solutions and should be the material of choice for internal bleaching.

26. **C.** In newly erupted teeth, the apical root end has not fully formed, allowing for greater blood supply to the tooth. Subsequent pulpal regeneration leads to greater long-term success.

27. **C.** The physical and chemical properties of zinc oxide eugenol are beneficial in preventing pulpal injury and in reducing postoperative tooth sensitivity. Zinc oxide eugenol provides a good biologic seal; also, its antimicrobial properties enable it to suppress bacterial growth, reducing formation of toxic metabolites that might result in pulpal inflammation.

28. **C.** When endodontic treatment is done properly, healing of the periapical lesion usually occurs with osseous regeneration, which is characterized by gradual reduction and resolution of the radiolucency on follow-up radiographs. The rate of bone formation is slow, and complete resolution may take longer than the standard 6-month follow-up, especially with elderly patients. As long as the radiolucency appears to be resolving as opposed to enlarging, an extended reevaluation is in order.

29. **B.** Pulpotomy is normally not recommended in permanent teeth unless root development is incomplete. If incomplete, calcium hydroxide pulpotomy is recommended. This procedure is performed in permanent teeth with immature root development and with healthy pulp tissue. The success is indicated when the root apex, if not completely formed, completes its full development. This procedure is done only on teeth free of symptoms.

30. **B.** Internal resorption is most commonly identified during routine radiographic examination. Histologically, it appears with chronic pulpitis, including chronic inflammatory cells, multinucleated giant cells adjacent to granulation tissue, and necrotic pulp coronal to resorptive defect. Only prompt endodontic therapy can stop the process and prevent further tooth destruction.

31. **C.** The best treatment of symptomatic irreversible pulpitis with a corresponding bony lesion is removal of the source of infection via pulpectomy.

32. **B.** The current recommendation for patients with a recent MI is to postpone dental or surgical treatment for at least 6 months. Risk for a second MI in patients with recent MI if given a general anesthetic is as follows: 0 to 3 months after MI, 31% risk of reinfarction; 3 to 6 months after MI, 15% risk of reinfarction; more than 6 months after MI, 5% risk of reinfarction.* defer elective care for at least 6 months after MI.

33. **D.** Incision and drainage techniques work best for fluctuant abscesses, so as to release purulent exudate. Local anesthesia should be obtained first. An incision should be placed at the most dependent part of the swelling. The incision should be wide enough to facilitate drainage and allow blunt dissection. After irrigation, a drain may be placed to maintain patency of the wound.

34. **C.** Many studies have shown definitively the predominant role of gram-negative obligate anaerobic bacteria in endodontic periapical infections. Earlier studies generally implicated facultative organisms, but improved culturing techniques established the predominance of obligate anaerobes.

35. **C.** "Danger zone" refers to the distal area in the mesial root in mandibular molars. Usually a straight layer of dentin, it becomes a preferable site for strip perforation during instrumentation. "Safety zone" is described as the mesial area of the root, with a thicker layer of dentin, slightly touched by the endodontic instruments.

36. **D.** In an intrusive dental injury, the patient may complain of pain. The patient's tooth is misaligned, or there is no sense of tooth mobility. This type of displacement has the worst prognosis. For intruded primary teeth, teeth should be allowed to reerupt before possible repositioning. For intruded adult teeth, treatment is allow reeruption and then stabilize.

37. **A.** Internal resorption begins on the internal dentin surface and spreads laterally. It may or may not reach the external tooth structure. The process is often asymptomatic and becomes identifiable only after it has progressed enough to be detectable radiographically. The etiology is unknown. Trauma is often, but not always, implicated. Resorption that occurs in inflamed pulps is characterized histologically by dentinoclasts, which are specialized, multinucleated giant cells similar to osteoclasts. Treatment is prompt endodontic therapy. However,

once external perforation has caused a periodontal defect, the tooth is often lost.

38. **A.** Internal bleaching alone causes 3.9% of external cervical root resorption (also referred to as *peripheral inflammatory root resorption*). The presence of a barrier (base material) between the root filling material and the internal bleaching material should be approximately 4 mm to prevent this resorption.

39. **E.** Emergency treatment of localized swelling associated with an endodontic infection is to achieve drainage either through the root canal or by incision and drainage and to remove the source of infection. Administration of antibiotics should be considered with the concomitant presentation of fever and malaise and for diffuse swelling (cellulitis).

40. **A.** The manufacturing process of a K-type instrument (K-file or K-reamer) is grinding a stainless steel wire to a tapered square or triangular cross section.

Operative Dentistry

1. **D.** Altering the organism, its nutrients, and its environment enhances prevention and treatment objectives.

2. **B.** A restored tooth indicates potential past carious activity but not current activity. Plaque presence does not indicate caries presence. Sealants are used for preventive purposes, not caries treatment.

3. **C.** When an alteration (a break in continuity) occurs to the tooth surface from a carious attack, restoration is usually necessary. When a lesion is evident in the dentin with an x-ray, the lesion usually needs a restoration.

4. **D.** When doing an indirect pulp cap, some caries may be left, a liner (probably calcium hydroxide) is usually placed over the excavated area, and the area may be assessed 6 to 8 weeks later. Regardless, the prognosis for indirect pulp caps is better than the prognosis for direct pulp caps.

5. **D.** Smooth surface caries occurs on any of the axial (facial, lingual, mesial, distal) tooth surfaces but not the occlusal surface.

6. **C.** A finishing bur is designed to provide a smoother surface and has more blades than a cutting bur. The increased number of blades results in a smoother cut surface.

7. **E.** The advantages and benefits of rubber dam usage are reflected in all of the items listed. The rubber dam isolation increases access and visibility.

8. **C.** When the rubber dam edge around the tooth is turned gingivally (inverted), it significantly reduces the leakage of moisture occlusally, sealing around the tooth better and resulting in a better isolated operating area.

9. **A.** The first number is the *width of the blade* or primary cutting edge in tenths of a millimeter (0.1 mm). The second number of a 4-number code indicates the *primary cutting edge angle*, measured from a line parallel to the long axis of the instrument handle in clockwise centigrades. The angle is expressed as a percent of 360 degrees. The instrument is positioned so that this number always exceeds 50. If the edge is locally perpendicular to the blade, this number is normally omitted, resulting in a 3-number code. The third number (second number of a 3-number code) indicates the *blade length* in millimeters. The fourth number (third number of a 3-number code) indicates the *blade angle*, relative to the long axis of the handle in clockwise centigrade.

10. **D.** A tooth preparation for a mandibular molar should have a narrow isthmus, should be initiated in the most carious (or distal) pit, and should establish the initial pulpal floor depth of 1.5 to 2 mm. However, it should be oriented parallel to the long axis of the *crown*, which tilts to the lingual. If prepared in the long axis of the tooth, there is greater potential of weakening the lingual cusps.

11. **C.** Retention locks, when needed in class II amalgam preparations, should be placed entirely in dentin, not undermining the adjacent enamel. They are placed 0.2 mm internal to the DEJ, are deeper gingivally (0.4 mm) than occlusally (i.e., they fade out as they extend occlusally), and translate parallel to the DEJ. If the axial wall is deeper than normal, the retention lock is not placed at the axiofacial or axiolingual line angles, but rather is positioned 0.2 mm internal to the DEJ. If placed at the deeper location, it may result in pulp exposure, depending on the location of the axial wall depth.

12. **C.** The guide for axial wall depth for a typical class II preparation that has a gingival margin occlusal to the CEJ is 0.2 to 0.5 mm internal to the dentinoenamel junction—the greater depth is necessary when placing retention locks. However, when there is no enamel proximally, the axial wall needs to be deep enough internally to provide for adequate strength of the amalgam material as well as to have room to place retention locks if needed. This depth is approximately 0.75 mm.

13. **D.** Because of the typical shape of a carious lesion in the cervical area, the resulting restoration is kidney-shaped or crescent-shaped, and the extensions are to the line angles, resulting in the mesial and distal walls diverging externally. The convexity of the tooth in the gingival one third results in the occlusal and gingival walls diverging externally. There are several retention groove designs that are appropriate, including four corner coves, occlusal and gingival line angle grooves, and

circumferential grooves. However, as with any restoration, if there is only a small amount of tooth structure (<1 mm) between the new and existing restoration, it is best to join the two restorations together and prevent the possibility of fracture of the small amount of remaining tooth structure.

14. **B.** When needed for large restorations, retention form usually consists of a gingival groove and incisal cove prepared with a small round bur (No. ¼). The placement of the groove or cove is dependent on the dentinoenamel junction (DEJ), placing the retention 0.2 mm internal to the DEJ entirely in dentin. It is not placed at the axiogingival or axioincisal line angles if those line angles are deeper than ideal; otherwise, the retention form may be too deep or cause a pulpal exposure.

15. **B.** Typically, the class I composite preparation has occlusally converging walls that provide primary retention form. The actual bonding also provides retention form. However, an occlusal bevel is not indicated on class I preparations, and retention grooves are not used.

16. **C.** A successful amalgam restoration requires 90-degree amalgam margins. Amalgam margins less than 90 degrees result in increased potential for fracture of the amalgam. Greater than 90-degree amalgam margins are good for the amalgam, but the corresponding enamel margin is less than 90 degrees and potentially undermined and prone to fracture. Because the amalgam is not bonded to the tooth, it must be retained in the tooth with undercuts, in either the primary or the secondary preparation. An amalgam restoration needs a minimum 1-mm thickness in nonstress areas and 1.5- to 2-mm thickness in areas that may be under load. The preparation must provide this dimension. Except for class V amalgams, the prepared walls generally converge to the exterior. The prepared walls may diverge or converge externally.

17. **B.** A tooth preparation is dictated by the extent of the carious lesion or old restorative material, the creation of appropriate convenience form for access and vision, and the anticipated extensions necessary to provide an appropriate proximal contact relationship. Fracture lines present should normally be included the restoration. However, it is rare that the size of the tooth affects the design of the tooth preparation.

18. **B.** Although the amalgam margin must be 90 degrees, the enamel margin might not be 90 degrees, especially on the occlusal surface. Most walls converge occlusally, but many class V amalgam preparations have walls that diverge externally. No retention form should be placed at the DEJ because the adjacent enamel is undermined and becomes subject to fracture.

19. **D.** A "skirt" is a minicrown preparation around a line angle. It should be prepared by a diamond instrument in the long axis of the tooth crown, extended to the gingival one third, and result in an appropriate amount of tooth removal. It is placed to increase both retention form (having opposing "skirt" vertical walls retentive with each other) and resistance form (enveloping the line angles similar to a barrel hoop around a barrel). It extends the outline form and so may be least appropriate for highly esthetic areas in the mouth.

20. **C.** The primary causes of postoperative sensitivity for amalgam restorations are voids (especially at the margins), poor condensation (that may result in void), or inadequate dentinal sealing. Extension onto the root surface does not result in increased sensitivity.

21. **C.** Tensile and compressive strengths may have relevance for composite materials but not for dentin bonding systems. The success of bonding depends on the various dentin structural factors, tooth factors, polymerization shrinkage, C-factor considerations, and technique sensitivity.

22. **B.** Amalgam carving should result in coincidence with the cavosurface margin and should not result in deep occlusal anatomy because such form may create acute amalgam angles that are subject to fracture. Depending on the condensation rate of the amalgam used, waiting a couple of minutes before initiating carving may allow the amalgam to harden enough so that the carving is easier and overcarving is minimized. When carving the occlusal cavosurface margin, the discoid carver should rest on the adjacent unprepared enamel, which serves as a guide for proper removal of amalgam back to the margin.

23. **A.** Generally, composite can be properly polymerized in 1- to 2-mm increments.

24. **D.** The trituration process mixes the amalgam components, and the reaction results in the alloy particle being coated by mercury and a product being formed.

25. **C.** The half-life of mercury in the body is 55 days.

26. **C.** Proper proximal contacts reduce the potential for food impaction, preserving the health of the underlying soft tissue. A missing proximal contact may result in tooth movement, which would have an adverse effect on the occlusal relationship of the tooth. Having a correct contact does not enhance the retentive properties of the restorative material.

27. **B.** Using the adjacent unprepared enamel at the cavosurface margin to guide the discoid carving instrument when carving away excess amalgam at the occlusal margin is the best way to develop the junction correctly.

28. **A.** Self-etch dentin bonding systems differ from total-etch dentin bonding systems by removing less of the smear layer (they use a less potent acid); creating a weaker bond to enamel, especially nonprepared enamel; and not requiring wet bonding, which may be necessary for some total-etch systems. Although fewer actual materials may be needed with some self-etch systems, they need to be applied in multiple coats, and the time necessary to apply the materials is similar for both systems.

29. **A.** Dentin bonding in laboratory studies may create bond strengths similar to or greater than bond strengths to enamel. However, clinical studies cannot corroborate that the dentin bond is stronger, and the bond may deteriorate over time. Available information is insufficient to predict accurately the bond potential to dentin in every application. However, bonding to enamel is predictable and good. The attempt to simplify the bonding mechanism has resulted in fewer materials being involved and less decision making on the part of the operator—both in an effort to get more predictable results. However, the newer bonding systems have not yet been proven to be better.

30. **D.** Occlusal reduction would not affect the ability to seat a casting. However, temporary cement, heavy proximal contacts, or tooth undercuts could keep the casting from seating completely.

31. **D.** Zinc is added to act as a scavenger for oxygen during the casting process. Copper and palladium increase the hardness and affect the color. Silver has an effect on the color as well.

32. **A.** If a patient has a notched cervical area that is very sensitive or esthetically objectionable, restoration is usually indicated. If the notched area is very deep, adverse pulpal or gingival responses may occur. Although more notched areas are encountered in older patients, a patient's age is not a factor in the need for restoration.

33. **B.** Slots and pins may be used interchangeably. They both provide good secondary retention form. Slots are usually better when box forms or vertical walls exist in the preparation, and pins are usually better when there are few or no vertical walls. The retention is similar for both.

34. **A.** The longer a slot, the better. They should be inside the DEJ and prepared with an inverted cone bur to a depth of 1 mm.

35. **A.** The bond of adhesives to dentin (and enamel) is primarily a mechanical interlocking of the material within the dentin (or enamel). The etching causes some removal of the surface, creating irregularities or spaced collagen fibrils into which the adhesive enters. When polymerized, the adhesive is mechanically locked into the surface.

36. **C.** Although some self-etch bonding systems use milder acid, the primary acid system used for etching tooth structure is phosphoric acid.

37. **D.** Bonding is primarily for sealing the dentin and enhancing the retention of the restorative material in the preparation. Esthetic benefits are a welcome side benefit when using a composite restoration. Thermal insulation is provided by the use of composite compared with amalgam but is not a benefit of the bonding. Bonding does not alter tooth flexure under normal load but may help bond the unprepared tooth structure together better.

38. **B.** Triturating (mixing) the amalgam particle with mercury is intended to result in coating the particles with a surface of mercury and creating the desirable phases in the set amalgam. All of the alloy particle is not dissolved in the mercury, and the size is not significantly reduced.

39. **B.** The only constant contraindication for the use of composite is when the operating area cannot be properly isolated, decreasing the potential success of the bond.

40. **D.** Direct gold and tooth structure have similar linear coefficients of expansion. Amalgam exhibits twice that expansion, whereas composite expansion would be even greater (2.5 times greater than tooth structure).

41. **D.** Self-threaded pins are used by most operators, when pin use is indicated.

42. **D.** All of these factors indicate a cervical lesion should be restored. In addition, if the lesion is large and the pulpal or gingival tissues are in jeopardy, restoration should be considered.

43. **B.** No known alternative low-mercury or no-mercury systems have been developed that provide the same properties or clinical performance as amalgam. The other statements are true.

44. **B.** Composite restorations are more technique-sensitive than amalgam restorations because the bonding process is very specific (requiring exact, correct usage of the various materials and an isolated, noncontaminated field), and the insertion and contouring of composites are more demanding and time-consuming. Composites are not stronger than amalgams and have similar wear resistance compared with amalgams. Composites are indicated for class II restorations.

45. **C.** The restoration of a proximal contact is easier with amalgam than with composite. Amalgam is easier to use and is less technique-sensitive. Either material can be used for class II restorations. Because amalgam restorations require a tooth preparation that has (1) a specified depth (for strength of the amalgam), (2) cavosurface marginal configurations that result in 90-degree amalgam margins, and (3) an undercut form to its walls or secondary

retention form features, they require more tooth structure removal than composite tooth preparations. Composite tooth preparations require (1) removal of the fault, defect, or old material; (2) removal of friable tooth structure; and (3) no specific depths—they are more conservative.

46. **A, D, E.** Eburnated dentin is also known as sclerotic dentin and has darkened from extrinsic staining. It is firm to the touch of an explorer and may be rough but is cleanable. It is seen in patients (usually older) whose oral hygiene and diet in recent years are good.

47. **A.** Resistance form preparation features help the restoration and tooth resist fracturing as a result of occlusal forces. Resistance features that assist in preventing the tooth from fracturing include rounded internal preparation angles.

48. **A.** *Abfraction* is tooth loss in the cervical area caused by biomechanical loading. *Abrasion* is mechanical wear resulting from abnormal forces (e.g., toothbrushing). *Attrition* is normal tooth wear. *Erosion* is wear secondary to chemical presence.

49. **B.** A direct pulp cap is recommended for a mechanical pulp exposure that is noncarious (<1.0 mm). No pulp therapy is required when the remaining dentin thickness is greater than 2.0 mm over vital pulp. Endodontic therapy is recommended for a carious pulp exposure (>1.0 mm) with purulent exudate. An indirect pulp cap is recommended when there is residual questionable dentin near pulp in an asymptomatic tooth.

50. **E.** Collars provide bracing.

51. **D.** The correct order is D, B, C, A, E.

Oral and Maxillofacial Surgery and Pain Control

1. **A.** The surgical guide template is a critical factor for the placement of implant in the esthetic area.

2. **C.** The most difficult impaction to remove is the distoangular tooth because the withdrawal pathway runs into the ramus of the mandible and requires greater surgical intervention.

3. **B.** An impacted tooth is one that fails to erupt into the dental arch within the expected time. Consequently, the third molar in a 13-year-old patient would be classified as unerupted or in the process of erupting.

4. **A.** The primary principle of management of odontogenic infections is to perform surgical drainage and removal of the cause. Abscesses do not resolve on antibiotics alone and may progress even if the patient is on antibiotics.

5. **D.** Any radiolucent lesion that requires biopsy should undergo aspiration before surgical exploration. This procedure may yield material for biopsy and would rule out a vascular lesion (e.g., arteriovenous malformation), which could be dangerous to enter without prior diagnosis.

6. **D.** Criteria for implant success include mean vertical bone loss of less than 0.02 mm annually after the first year of service. In this question, no further treatment is necessary at this time.

7. **B.** The major causes for loss of osseointegrated implants are similar to the causes for loss of natural teeth: poor hygiene, occlusal load, and the resultant inflammatory processes that occur.

8. **D.** Traditionally, 6 months has been the recommended period for integration and subsequent loading of posterior maxillary implants. Today, because of technologic advancements in specified cases, earlier loading may be possible.

9. **C.** Imaging tools used in the evaluation of TMJ pathology include panoramic radiographs, traditional and computer-generated tomograms, magnetic resonance imaging, nuclear imaging, and arthrography.

10. **A.** Distraction osteogenesis is preferred over traditional osteotomies when large skeletal movements are required and the associated soft tissue cannot adapt to the acute changes and stretching that results. Larger movements may be at increased risk of some relapse; this is particularly true in a patient with a cleft palate, where there is significant soft tissue scarring from previous surgeries.

11. **C.** Bilateral sagittal split osteotomy is the most commonly used osteotomy for mandibular advancement.

12. **B.** OSAS may result in mood disorders, daytime fatigue, and personality changes. Aggressive behavior is not considered a sequela of OSAS.

13. **C.** Although less invasive, arthrocentesis and splint therapy are not considered surgical interventions.

14. **C.** The mandibular condyle is the most common location of mandibular fractures. The alveolus, ramus, and coronoid are the least common sites.

15. **D.** Le Fort level fractures are associated with maxillary injuries. Mandibular fractures are classified according to anatomic location, condition of the bone and soft tissue, and muscle pull on the segments.

16. **A.** A proper occlusal relationship is a prerequisite for satisfactory bony reduction. This is most commonly accomplished by the use of intermaxillary fixation, or wiring the jaws closed, during surgery.

17. **A.** Most nerve injuries are transient; however, in an injury that lasts greater than 4 weeks, a surgical evaluation is indicated.

18. **C.** Sites commonly used for reconstruction of the atrophic mandibular ridge are dictated by the deficiency and include chin, hip, ribs, prosthetic materials, and donor bone (human and bovine). Dental

implants are commonly used, not just as a last resort. The use of distraction of ridge augmentation has been reported and is useful in certain applications. The mandibular alveolar ridge is more problematic in terms of resorption and denture retention, which more commonly necessitates reconstructive measures.

19. **A.** A dry socket (alveolar osteitis) occurs on day 3 to 4 after extraction and, except for pain, does not have the classic signs of infection.

20. **B.** Older age, diabetes, and smoking are risk factors for delayed healing.

21. **A.** Ideally, a local anesthetic should be relatively free from producing allergic reactions, and it should be stable in solution and readily undergo biotransformation in the body. It is an absolute requirement that it should be either sterile or capable of being sterilized by heat without deterioration. If proper doses are used and are properly injected, there is a high success rate of obtaining anesthesia, while being able to minimize adverse effects.

22. **B.** All local anesthetics are vasodilators to some degree.

23. **C.** The pK_a of lidocaine is 7.9. It is packaged as a 2% solution both with and without epinephrine and has a rapid onset of action.

24. **B.** Of needles commonly used in dentistry, 25-gauge needles have a much lower incidence of breakage versus any other needle size, whereas 30-gauge needles have the highest incidence of breakage.

25. **B.** A 2% solution is 20 mg/mL; 1.0 mL of a 20 mg/mL solution is 20 mg.

26. **B.** The supine position is correct. This position prevents fainting during or immediately after the injection of local anesthetic. Reclined or semisupine is not back far enough, and Trendelenburg is too far back.

27. **B.** Malamed recommended that one cartridge of local anesthetic be delivered over not less than 1 minute; 1 mL (one half cartridge) should be delivered over not less than ½ minute (30 seconds).

28. **A.** Posterior superior alveolar nerve block is the only injection listed that leads to pulpal anesthesia in the maxilla. Nasopalatine nerve block is a maxillary injection that leads to soft tissue anesthesia of the premaxilla only. Inferior alveolar and long buccal nerve blocks are mandibular injections.

29. **B.** The proper depth of penetration for the posterior superior alveolar nerve is half the length (16 mm) of a long needle or three fourths the length (15 mm) of a short dental needle. Penetration beyond 16 mm has a significantly higher incidence of positive aspiration and hematoma formation.

30. **B.** The greater palatine injection provides soft tissue anesthesia of the hard palate from the junction of the premaxilla to the junction of the hard and soft palate and from the gingival margin to the midline of the palate.

31. **A.** Jastak and Yagiela published data demonstrating that patients with cardiovascular compromise who are well monitored begin to show elevation of vital signs when more than about 40 µg (0.04 mg) of epinephrine is administered in a local anesthetic solution.

32. **C.** Malamed recommended that a maximum of 4.4 mg/kg (2.0 mg/lb) of lidocaine be administered regardless of whether vasoconstrictor is in the formulation. The package insert for lidocaine allows up to 7 mg/kg when lidocaine is packaged with vasoconstrictor.

33. **B.** Inferior alveolar, posterior superior alveolar, and infraorbital injections all lead to pulpal anesthesia when performed properly. The lingual injection leads to soft tissue anesthesia only.

34. **B.** A true anterior superior alveolar nerve block, also called infraorbital nerve block, requires a volume of one half cartridge of local anesthetic solution, or about 1.0 mL.

35. **C.** The local anesthetic drug of choice for administration in children is 2% lidocaine with 1:100,000 epinephrine because it allows the greatest volume to be administered safely. Mepivacaine in either 2% or 3% allows less volume to be safely administered, and bupivacaine is not approved by the U.S. Food and Drug Administration for use in children.

36. **B.** All local anesthetics cause some amount of vasodilation. Agents packaged as plain drugs (i.e., without vasoconstrictor) cause less vasodilation than agents that must be packaged with vasoconstrictor to have efficacy. Of the listed drugs, mepivacaine is the only one packaged in dental cartridges without vasoconstrictor.

37. **D.** The formulation 2% lidocaine contains 36 mg of lidocaine per cartridge. Because 80 mg is the amount of lidocaine that can safely be administered to this child, the number of cartridges that can be administered is 80 mg divided by 36 mg per cartridge, which is roughly two cartridges.

38. **C.** By definition, a low pK_a means a fast onset of action. Hydrophobicity and protein binding directly affect duration of action and potency.

39. **A.** The (long) buccal injection anesthetizes the soft tissues and periosteum buccal to the mandibular molar teeth.

40. **C.** Lipid solubility (hydrophobicity) and protein binding are the most important factors in determining duration of action of a local anesthetic. Bupivacaine has the longest duration of action of the local anesthetics listed and has the highest hydrophobicity; it is bound 95% to protein. The other agents have lower hydrophobic qualities and are bound 75% or less to protein.

41. B. With all intraoral injections of local anesthesia, the intent is to anesthetize a portion of cranial nerve (CN) V. With an improperly placed needle in a mandibular block, it is possible to anesthetize a portion of CN VII inadvertently, and it is possible to anesthetize CN VI inadvertently with certain second-division nerve blocks.

42. D. Articaine has an ester bond and an amide bond. Because esters are biotransformed much more rapidly than amides, articaine has a much shorter half-life than the other local anesthetics.

43 D. Antibiotics used to treat odontogenic infections should be effective against streptococci and oral anaerobes, which are common pathogens in the oral cavity. *S. aureus* is commonly seen in the respiratory tract and on the skin, not on oral mucosa, so choices **B** and **C** are incorrect. Most oral infections such as abscesses are not primarily due to fungal or viral organisms.

44. A, C, D. An asymptomatic full bony impaction in someone older than 35 years of age is usually not surgically removed, if no pathology exists. All the other choices are reasons to remove the impaction.

45. C. Aspiration biopsy or fine-needle biopsy on a soft tissue lesion deep to mucosa should be done first to confirm if the entity is truly cystic, vascular, or solid. However, an attempt to obtain a biopsy specimen of a soft tissue lesion that is vascular in origin (e.g., arteriovenous malformation) can result in hemorrhagic complication. Hard tissue biopsies and full-thickness flaps apply to bone lesions. Incisional and excisional biopsies are used for surface soft tissue lesions.

46. E. The pK_a determines the degree to which a drug is charged. A low pK_a for a local anesthetic favors more of the noncharged species of a drug; this increases the ability of the drug to penetrate to the nerve and increases the rate of onset of anesthesia.

47. A. The nasopalatine nerve block leads to anesthesia of palatal soft tissue from canine to canine, bilaterally (the premaxilla). The mental nerve block is in the mandible. The greater palatine nerve block leads to anesthesia in the palate from the canine distally to the posterior aspect of the hard palate and from the gingival margin to the midline. The anterior superior alveolar nerve block anesthetizes from the midline of the maxilla to the mesiobuccal aspect of the maxillary first molar but does not anesthetize palatal tissue. The posterior superior nerve block anesthetizes from the maxillary third molar anteriorly to the maxillary first molar with the possible exception of the mesiobuccal aspect of the maxillary first molar. This injection does not anesthetize palatal tissue.

Oral Diagnosis

1. D. An acute exudate (pus) at the apex of a tooth follows the path of least resistance (e.g., into surrounding bone, gingiva, or skin). If the offending tooth is not treated and the abscess becomes chronic, a periapical granuloma may result.

2. A. Reduced enamel epithelium that overlies the crown of an unerupted tooth may give rise to a cyst occurring in the same position—by definition, a dentigerous cyst. The stimulus for cystic epithelial proliferation is unknown.

3. A. The key to this question is the description of the cystic lining of thin, parakeratinized epithelium with basal cell palisading, which is typical of odontogenic keratocyst. Tooth vitality, lack of symptoms, and more than one lesion also support the diagnosis.

4. C. Odontogenic keratocysts are notable because of their recurrence rate, their aggressive clinical behavior, and their occasional multiplicity. When multiple, they may be part of the nevoid basal cell carcinoma syndrome.

5. A. Ameloblastic fibro-odontoma is the only lesion listed that is lucent with opaque foci. The patient's age is also characteristic for this lesion. Paget's disease may show a mixed opaque and lucent pattern, but it occurs only in patients older than 50 years.

6. C. *Herpetic whitlow* is a term used for secondary herpes simplex infections that occur around the nail bed. The cause of aphthous ulcers is unknown. Herpangina is caused by coxsackievirus, and herpes zoster is caused by varicella-zoster virus.

7. E. Premature tooth loss is seen in several conditions, especially malignancies and Langerhans' cell disease because of cellular invasion of the periodontal ligament. Sharply marginated bone lesions are characteristic of Langerhans' cell disease (and Paget's disease affecting elderly patients). The eosinophils in a round cell infiltrate suggest Langerhans' cell disease (the round cells would be Langerhans' cells).

8. E. Numb lip is malignancy of the jaw until proved otherwise. About half of patients with numb lip have associated malignancies. The other 50% of patients have acute bone infections or neurologic problems.

9. E. Sclerotic bone margins indicate a long-term, low-grade process because it takes a considerable amount of time for bone to become radiodense. The signs and symptoms listed in choices **A** through **D** are associated with malignancies.

10. A. Peripheral and central giant cell granulomas have very different clinical presentations and behaviors but identical light microscopic features.

11. **D.** Acquired angioedema is a rapidly developing allergic reaction that results in characteristic nonerythematous swelling of lips, face, and neck.

12. **A.** Regional odontodysplasia is often referred to as "ghost teeth" because of the thin layers of dentin and enamel produced. One quadrant of teeth is affected, and the teeth are nonfunctional.

13. **B.** Salivary gland tumors manifest as submucosal masses. The combination of epithelial and connective tissue elements is indicative of pleomorphic adenomas, also termed *mixed tumors*. Oral warts and leukoplakias are surface or epithelial lesions. Peripheral giant cell granulomas are exclusively gingival lesions, and granular cell tumors are composed exclusively of cells with grainy or granular cytoplasm.

14. **E.** Oral cancers (squamous cell carcinomas) manifest typically as indurated nonhealing ulcers. They can also manifest as white patches, red patches, or irregular masses.

15. **E.** Dermoid cyst occurs in the midline floor of the mouth when above the mylohyoid and geniohyoid muscles and in the neck when below the mylohyoid and geniohyoid muscles.

16. **C.** Ectopic (normal tissue, abnormal site) lymphoid tissue is commonly seen in the floor of the mouth as well as in the posterior lateral tongue, soft palate, and tonsillar pillar. It appears as one or more small, dome-shaped yellow nodules.

17. **C.** Schwann's cell is of neural origin and gives rise to several neoplasms, including neurofibroma and schwannoma.

18. **C.** Nasopalatine duct cysts are anterior midmaxillary lesions that occur in the nasopalatine canal. The associated lucency is often heart-shaped because of the superimposition of the nasal spine over the lesion. These cysts do not devitalize teeth.

19. **B.** *Globulomaxillary lesion* is a clinical term used to designate any lucency that occurs between the maxillary lateral incisor and canine.

20. **E.** Peripheral giant cell granuloma is the exception. Although it is red, it occurs only in the gingiva. Choices **A** through **D** are differential diagnoses for red atrophic tongue.

21. **C.** Multiple odontogenic keratocysts are part of nevoid basal cell carcinoma syndrome.

22. **E.** The mean age for ameloblastoma is 40 years. All other lesions listed occur in children and teenagers.

23. **A.** Behçet's syndrome includes lesions in the mouth, eye, and genitals. The other diseases do not affect the genitalia.

24. **B.** Nicotine stomatitis appears as opacification of the palate, with red dots representing inflamed salivary ducts.

25. **C.** X-ray photons (Bremsstrahlung radiation) results from the interaction of high-speed electrons with tungsten nuclei in the target.

26. **C.** X-rays are produced in most dental x-ray machines half the time (i.e., in bursts at the rate of 60 per second, each lasting $\frac{1}{120}$ second) owing to the alternating current supplied to the tube.

27. **A.** Deterministic effects are effects with dose thresholds, requiring at least moderate levels of exposure, where the severity of response is proportional to dose.

28. **E.** "Direct effect" refers to production of free radicals from the ionization of water (choice **C**). These free radicals formed in the radiolysis of water are highly reactive and may alter biologic molecules (choice **D**). The presence of oxygen *increases* the number of free radicals.

29. **D.** The radiosensitivity of cells depends on mitotic future, mitotic activity, and degree of differentiation.

30. **B.** Using a rectangular collimator restricts the area of the patient's face exposed to the size of the receptor, reducing the patient exposure by more than half.

31. **E.** If someone must hold a film and the patient cannot, it should be a family member or friend of the patient, not an x-ray operator in the dental office.

32. **A.** The dispersion of visible light from the crystals in the phosphor layer of the intensifying screen reduces image resolution compared with direct-exposure film.

33. **C.** The base needs to be flexible to go through automatic processors and be put into film mounts. Usually, the base is not completely clear, and it is the emulsion that is sensitive to x-rays.

34. **B.** The film should be parallel to the long axis of the tooth, and the central ray of the beam should be perpendicular to both the film and the tooth. Increasing the vertical angulation foreshortens the image of the tooth.

35. **B.** The central ray should be *perpendicular* to the object.

36. **C.** The smaller the focal spot size, the greater the resolution. Other factors remaining equal, density, contrast, and magnification are unchanged.

37. **A.** Developer reduces silver bromide to solid silver grains.

38. **E.** Exposure time should be reduced. Development parameters should not be changed if they are correct.

39. **B.** Silver halide in the emulsion of an exposed film is converted into grains of metallic silver in the developer.

40. **D.** The "penny test" is a test of darkroom safelighting. A penny is placed on an exposed film (after removing the film from its cover) for 2 minutes, and the film is processed. If the processed film shows a

lighter area on the film corresponding to the penny, the safelighting is too bright and is fogging the film.

41. **E.** Film packets need not be sterilized because the goal is to prevent cross-contamination, not ensure that everything that goes into a patient's mouth is sterile.

42. **A.** The TMJ is much too far from the occlusal plane (the location of occlusal film) to be imaged with this technique. The other choices all are proper indications for using occlusal film.

43. **A, D, E.** Celiac sprue, Behçet's disease, and Crohn's disease all are examples of diseases in which immune system dysfunction is an important factor in their pathogenesis. Aphthous or aphthouslike ulcers may develop in patients with these diseases, but there is no clear link to a dysfunction of the immune system for aphthous ulcers or for the other disorders. Although oral manifestations may be variable, lesions in patients with sarcoidosis, amyloidosis, and neurofibromatosis typically manifest as submucosal nodules and masses.

44. **A, D, E.** These three signs clearly point to primary Sjögren's syndrome. Hairy leukoplakia is associated with Epstein-Barr virus. Aphthous ulcers may be associated with other disorders.

45. **B, C, D.** Filtration increases the mean energy of the x-ray beam because it filters out the low-energy radiation, leaving the higher energy radiation. The filtration reduces low-energy radiation to the patient.

46. **D.** This anatomic position is the usual extent of the maxillary sinus. The zygomatic process of the maxilla usually appears as a U-shaped radiopaque line with the open end pointing upward. A dentigerous cyst is associated with a tooth such as an impacted third molar. An ameloblastoma usually occurs in the molar ramus. Neither a dentigerous cyst nor an ameloblastoma would be expected normally to duplicate the typical location of the maxillary sinus.

47. **C.** Discoid (chronic type) lupus erythematosus does not involve systemic disorders and rarely progresses to the systemic form. Systemic lupus erythematosus often affects the kidney, heart, and joints as well as skin and the oral cavity.

Orthodontics and Pediatric Dentistry

1. **A.** Class I is the most common malocclusion, affecting about 50% of the U.S. population, compared with class II (15%) and class III (about 1%).

2. **C.** Reproductive tissues grow at the same time as the adolescent growth spurt, and the appearance of secondary sexual characteristics can be used to help predict the timing of growth.

3. **B.** Although developmental indicators generally correlate well with each other, using dental age to predict timing of growth is the least reliable of the methods offered.

4. **C.** Fusion of the palate proceeds from anterior to posterior, so any disturbance that occurs during that time stops fusion at that point, leading to an opening posteriorly.

5. **B.** Young children often present with minimal overbite or anterior edge-to-edge relationship. Habits such as thumb-sucking increase the likelihood that less overbite will be present.

6. **B.** Small diastemas between the maxillary incisors of 2 mm or less generally close on their own as more permanent teeth, specifically the canines, erupt. The presence of a midline diastema before canine eruption is referred to as the "ugly duckling" stage.

7. **D.** If the mandibular molar buccal groove is mesial to the mesiobuccal cusp of the maxillary molar, the relationship is described as Angle Class III.

8. **A.** The molars are class II, but the skeletal relationship described by the ANB (the anterior-posterior angular difference between the maxilla and mandible) measurement is normal, so the malocclusion is dental in origin.

9. **B.** All of the choices are possible solutions to correct a deep overbite. Erupting posterior teeth would increase the already excessively long lower face height, whereas intrusion of maxillary incisors would improve the excessive maxillary incisor show at rest.

10. **B.** Heavy forces cause compression of the periodontal ligament with hyalinization.

11. **B.** Root resorption is common during orthodontic treatment, although lesions often repair on the root surface. Mobility of teeth is also common as the periodontal ligament reorganizes and widens during tooth movement. It is uncommon for teeth to become devitalized as a result of orthodontic movement unless they have also been substantially compromised by injury or infection.

12. **A.** Although controversial, it is believed that types of tooth movements that concentrate force in small areas of the PDL are more likely to result in root resorption during orthodontic treatment.

13. **B.** The center of resistance is defined as the point at which force application causes pure translation of a tooth.

14. **C.** Because $M = Fd$, doubling the force would double the moment, or tendency to rotate, tip, or torque.

15. **D.** This is the definition of a couple. A couple results in a rotational tendency or pure moment.

16. **C.** The sum of the forces and moments on an appliance must equal zero. If the incisors intrude, the molars extrude. These two forces form a couple with a moment in one direction. The molars

experience a couple in the opposite direction, which causes them to tip distally.

17. **D.** Class II elastics work in the direction that would be used to correct a class II malocclusion, to pull the mandibular teeth forward and the maxillary teeth distally.

18. **B.** Nickel-titanium archwires can exist in more than one phase: austenitic and martensitic phases. Superelastic behavior of these wires is attributed to the reversible transformation between these two phases.

19. **B.** A second-order bend is placed to provide angulation of a tooth in the mesiodistal direction, also called "tip." A first-order bend is placed in an archwire to position a tooth in the labiolingual direction (in-out bend) or to rotate a tooth as seen in the occlusal plane. A bend to provide angulation in the labiolingual direction is called a *third-order bend* (torquing bend).

20. **B.** Class III elastics are worn from the maxillary first molars to the mandibular canines. The force system created by class III elastics produces mesial movement and extrusion of the maxillary first molars.

21. **D.** This patient, if still growing, may be treated with a growth modification approach using headgear (either cervical or high-pull, not reverse-pull) to correct the class II malocclusion. Because deep overbite is present, a cervical headgear should be used because this type of headgear extrudes the molars, which aids in reducing overbite; however, this was not one of the choices. If the patient is finished growing, the second approach to treat class II malocclusion is class II camouflage, which includes extraction of maxillary first premolars to correct the malocclusion. An intrusion arch along with full fixed appliances should be used to correct the deep bite.

22. **B.** The line of force generated by a cervical headgear causes the maxillary first molar to move distally, usually also tip distally, and to extrude. A high-pull headgear would cause the molar to move distally and intrude.

23. **B.** Primary canines are extracted to encourage alignment of the crowded incisors. However, the incisors align and upright, borrowing space otherwise needed for eruption of the permanent canine. Primary first molars are extracted to encourage eruption of the first premolar so that it may be extracted to make room for the permanent canine to erupt.

24. **B.** There is a high likelihood that a small diastema of 2 mm or less will close on its own over time as the permanent teeth erupt. However, if a child experiences psychological trauma because of esthetic concerns, the diastema can be closed. Parents should be informed of the reason for treatment and

understand that there are some risks of performing orthodontic treatment.

25. **D.** Excessive crowding may influence the decision in favor of canine substitution. However, esthetic concerns may deter a decision to substitute canines for lateral incisors. Patients with a class II interarch relationship requiring maxillary extractions anyway may be better served to substitute canines for laterals rather than extracting healthy first premolars.

26. **C.** Excessive crowding may necessitate extractions. Also, extraction of maxillary premolars may be indicated to camouflage a class II molar relationship. Anterior open bites may be improved by uprighting anterior teeth to increase overbite. Flat lips would not be improved by extraction of permanent teeth, but other considerations may necessitate extraction even in those patients.

27. **A.** Fixed retention requires no patient cooperation to achieve retention. However, fixed retainers are more difficult to clean and cannot be modified to move teeth or control overbite relapse.

28. **D.** Class II correction by surgery requires moving the mandible forward or the maxilla back. In a patient with a deficient mandible, it is preferable to move the mandible forward. Moving the maxilla back significantly is difficult or impossible.

29. **D.** Inferior movement of the maxilla, especially without bone grafting and rigid fixation, has been shown to relapse over time because of vertical occlusal forces generated by the masticatory musculature.

30. **B.** All anterior permanent teeth begin calcification during the first 6 months except for maxillary lateral incisors. The maxillary lateral incisor may be used as a key to timing; if this tooth is affected, the causative event is likely to have occurred at 1 year of age or older.

31. **D.** Localized infection, trauma, and excessive systemic fluoride ingestion may cause hypocalcification. Disturbances in apposition result in incomplete tissue formation. For example, an intrusive injury to a primary incisor may disrupt enamel apposition and result in an area of enamel hypoplasia.

32. **D.** Implants are osseointegrated and behave as ankylosed teeth. As teeth erupt and alveolar bone formation occurs, an osseointegrated implant appears to submerge.

33. **B.** Many mentally challenged individuals can be mainstreamed and treated as any other patient. Because a moderately challenged 6-year-old may function as a preschool child, the normal management techniques are likely applicable. The correct answer for such a question would include some kind of normalization response.

34. A. Studies show that there is a high correlation between maternal anxiety and a child's negative behavior in the dental office. This effect is greatest for children younger than 4 years old.

35. D. Inferior alveolar, lingual, and buccal nerve blocks are required to anesthetize this area adequately when performing deep restorations, pulp therapy, and extractions. Some studies have shown that local infiltration anesthesia for primary molars is effective, but this is primarily reserved for restorative procedures because there is an increased probability for anesthesia failure using local infiltration for pulp therapy and extraction procedures.

36. C. In patients with primary dentition, the mandibular foramen is located lower than the plane of occlusion. Mandibular block injections for these patients are lower than for adult patients.

37. D. Minimum alveolar concentration is a measure of potency. It is the concentration required to produce immobility in 50 vol % of patients responding to surgical incision. A minimum alveolar concentration of 105 vol % indicates that nitrous oxide alone does not produce profound surgical anesthesia at a normal atmospheric pressure.

38. A. The total flow rate is 4 to 6 L/min for most children. The practitioner can check the bag and make adjustments if necessary. The maintenance dose of nitrous oxide during an operative procedure is typically about 30%. In other words, a standard maintenance dose would usually be 4 L of oxygen and 2 L of nitrous oxide. After a lengthy administration, it is wise to reduce the concentration because of tissue saturation and nausea.

39. A. It is difficult to know which treatment is indicated without more information than is presented in the question. The tooth could be mobile because of furcation involvement, internal or external root resorption, exfoliation, or a combination of all of these. A radiograph needs to be taken to obtain more clinical information before any further treatment is rendered.

40. D. Because of the small size of primary molars and small restorations, it is helpful to reduce stresses within the restorative material. It has been demonstrated that rounded internal line angles aid in reducing stress compared with sharp internal line angles. Many of the burs recommended for use in primary molars have a rounded end to help achieve softened internal line angles.

41. A. The treatment decision in this case should be made based on the presence or absence of furcation involvement. Absence of furcation involvement generally indicates a vital pulp. It is necessary to have vital tissue to perform a pulpotomy. Presence of furcation involvement generally indicates

progression to a nonvital pulp. If furcation involvement is present, a pulpectomy would be the treatment of choice in the absence of external or internal root resorption.

42. A. Mineral trioxide aggregate pulpotomies are very promising and generally show higher success rates than formocresol pulpotomies. However, mineral trioxide aggregate is very expensive at the present time and is not used as often as formocresol or ferric sulfate.

43. B. The pulp chambers of primary teeth are proportionately larger compared with the size of the crown; this is significant because there is a higher risk of accidental pulp exposures on primary teeth. In particular, the mesiobuccal pulp horn of the first primary molar is close to the external surface of the tooth.

44. C. Tooth I typically exfoliates before the eruption of tooth #13. One of the "abutments" of the space maintainer would be lost and render the space maintainer ineffective. A palatal holding arch and a Nance holding arch, although bilateral holding arches, would be good options. However, there may be situations where tooth #13 would have an accelerated eruption because of bone loss in the area and where the band-loop space maintainer would be appropriate.

45. D. The only possibility among these choices is the distal shoe space maintainer. Some clinicians find that a removable "kiddie" acrylic partial can also be successful. These "kiddie" partials extend distally to the point where the mesial of the first permanent molar would be. Some clinicians advocate placing a 1-mm-deep labial-lingual groove in the cast on the alveolar ridge on the mesial of the first permanent molar. This groove results in extra acrylic at the tissue-acrylic interface that causes pressure; this may aid in keeping the unerupted first permanent molar in position.

46. B. The systemic fluoride "rule of 6s" states the following: (a) If fluoride level is greater than 0.6 ppm, no supplemental systemic fluoride is indicated. (b) If the patient is younger than 6 months old, no supplemental systemic fluoride is indicated. (c) If the patient is older than 16 years old, no supplemental systemic fluoride is indicated. The statement, "If the patient is less than 12 months old, no supplemental systemic fluoride is indicated" is false.

47. C. Anticipatory guidance is counseling patients and parents regarding the child's home oral health care that is age appropriate and is focused on prevention. Subjects to discuss with parents include oral hygiene, oral development, fluoride, diet and nutrition, oral habits, and trauma and injury prevention.

48. **B.** Most natal and neonatal teeth are primary teeth (90%); very few are supernumerary teeth (10%). Most are mandibular incisors (85%). Extraction of primary teeth should be accomplished only if they are extremely mobile and there is danger of aspiration. Most commonly, natal and neonatal teeth are left in position.

49. **D.** Munchausen syndrome by proxy is a condition in which a person, usually a parent, presents factitious symptoms and illnesses in a child, which may result in extensive testing and hospitalizations. Examples of emotional abuse include denial of affection, isolation, extreme threats, and corruption. A parent who knowingly and willingly does not seek care for a child who has pain, infection, or inadequate function is guilty of neglect.

50. **E.** The location of lesions of primary herpetic gingivostomatitis is on mucous membrane, including tonsils, hard and soft palates, buccal mucosa, tongue, palate, and gingiva. Children with this disease can become very sick and require close supervision and support. They typically have a significant fever and can become dehydrated, and the disease can last 2 weeks. Treatment may consist of (a) topical anesthetics such as 0.5% dyclonine hydrochloride and viscous lidocaine, (b) coating solutions such as diphenhydramine elixir and kaolin-pectin compound, (c) antivirals such as acyclovir, and (d) analgesics such as acetaminophen and ibuprofen.

51. **B.** Localized aggressive periodontitis in the primary dentition, previously known as *localized prepubertal periodontitis*, is most common in the primary molar area and occurs most commonly in African-American children. Treatment includes débridement and antibiotic therapy.

52. **C.** The appropriate splint for an avulsed tooth is a nonrigid splint, which is left in place for about 7 to 14 days. A 0.016 × 0.022 stainless steel orthodontic wire, a 0.018 round stainless steel wire, and a monofilament nylon (20- to 30-lb test) line are considered nonrigid. Long-term rigid splinting of replanted teeth increases risk of replacement root resorption (ankylosis). Rigid splinting is indicated for root fractures and remains in place for 2 to 3 months. A 0.032 to 0.036 stainless steel wire is considered a rigid splint.

53. **D.** If a tooth is incompletely erupted or is being orthodontically treated, the tooth may be normal even if there is little sensitivity to electrical pulp tests. In the absence of other symptoms, treatment is contraindicated.

54. **A.** Rapid root resorption, pulp necrosis, and ankylosis are common sequelae to intruded permanent teeth with mature apices. Treatment includes the following: (a) gradual repositioning orthodontically (2 to 3 weeks), (b) stabilization for 2 to 4 weeks, and (c) calcium hydroxide pulpectomy 2 weeks after injury.

55. **C.** The other three conditions listed may occur as the result of trauma but do not cause loss of vitality. Pulpal hyperemia causes increased intrapulpal pressure and swelling, which may result in an interruption of the pulp's blood supply. Without an adequate blood supply, the pulp becomes necrotic. This process can take time, and symptoms (either radiographic or clinical) may not manifest for weeks or months. Typically, follow-up examination and radiographs are indicated at 1-, 2-, and 6-month intervals following a traumatic incident.

56. **B, A, C, D.** In any comprehensive treatment plan, the most urgent consideration is control of disease processes. In this case, caries control is the most urgent need. Orthodontic movement should be second because alignment of teeth changes bony contours and modifies the occlusion. Final bone recontouring can be performed if orthodontic treatment did not correct previous defects. Definitive prosthetic treatment should be done last so that restorations can be fabricated to fit the final occlusion.

57. **C, E, F.** Most bones of the craniofacial complex form by intramembranous ossification. The bones of the cranial base are endochondral bones separated by synchondroses during development. The three bones of the cranial base are the occipital, sphenoid, and ethmoid bones.

58. **C.** The adolescent growth spurt occurs during puberty and is characterized by an increase in body height. Also, because puberty is the process of sexual maturation, reproductive tissues increase in size during adolescence. In contrast, neural development, characterized primarily by growth of the brain, occurs rapidly in young children and is mostly complete by age 7. Lymphoid tissue, important for development of immunity, increases until puberty, and then these tissues shrink in size until adulthood.

59. **A, D.** Although any of the features listed are possible, the most common presentation of the occlusion in the primary dentition is spacing and decreased overbite. Spacing is an important and desirable characteristic because the permanent incisors and canines will be much larger than their deciduous predecessors. Decreased overbite is common because of sucking habits.

60. **A.** Angle's classification of malocclusion is based on the anterior-posterior position of the buccal groove of the mandibular first molar relative to the mesiobuccal cusp of the maxillary first molar. If the mandibular first molar is distal to this position, the Angle classification is class II. An ANB angle of 2

degrees is the average (or "normal") adult skeletal relationship, so the origin of the class II relationship must be dental and not skeletal.

61. **B.** The other choices all are common or even expected during orthodontic treatment. Root resorption, to some degree, is likely to occur in most patients as a result of orthodontic treatment but usually has no clinical significance. Mobility of teeth and transient occlusal interferences are expected during tooth movement. Devitalization of teeth as a result of orthodontics rarely occurs unless the teeth have been previously traumatized or otherwise compromised.

62. **C.** The rotational tendency or "moment" is equal to the magnitude of the force applied times the perpendicular distance of the line of action of the force away from the center of resistance of the tooth ($M = Fd$). Doubling the force would double the tooth's tendency to rotate.

63. **A, D, F.** The "ugly duckling" stage occurs during the process of eruption of the maxillary canines. As the maxillary canines migrate mesially before they erupt, their crowns put pressure on the roots of the erupted permanent lateral incisors, causing the crowns to tip distally and spaces to appear between the incisor crowns. This is called the "ugly duckling" stage, and although it does not occur in everyone, it is considered a normal stage of development during the mixed dentition. As the canines erupt, their crowns compress the crowns of the incisors together, and any spacing that was present is expected to close without treatment.

64. **B.** Class III elastics are used to correct a class III relationship and are stretched from the maxillary first molar region to the mandibular canine region. The maxillary first molar would be expected to move mesially and extrude.

65. **A, C, D, B.** Serial extraction is a process that is used only when the decision is made early in dental development that there will be a future need to extract permanent premolars to create space for tooth alignment owing to a severe arch length deficiency (severe crowding). When the decision is made to proceed, the primary canines are extracted to allow the permanent incisors, which are usually crowded and rotated in these patients, to align on their own. The primary first molar is extracted to encourage early eruption of the permanent first premolar so that it may be extracted atraumatically.

66. **B.** A midline diastema greater than 2 mm is uncommon during normal development, and it is unlikely to close on its own. The possible presence of a supernumerary tooth (mesiodens) should be ruled out radiographically before any attempt to close the space orthodontically is made.

67. **A.** Intruding maxillary incisors directly reduce the amount of overbite, and this is the best answer. Uprighting incisors would result in an increase of overbite as the teeth become more vertically overlapping. High-pull headgear would intrude maxillary molars and encourage rotation of the mandible closed, increasing overbite. "Using a lip bumper" is a distractor choice that is unrelated to controlling overbite. However, it is possible that use of a lip bumper would encourage flaring of lower incisors that would indirectly cause a reduction of overbite eventually.

68. A—4, B—3, C—2, D—1.

69. **B, D, E.**

70. 1—D, 2—E, 3—B, 4—A, 5—C.

Patient Management

1. **B.** Of the options given, the best response would be to interpret what the patient is trying to communicate and reflect the communication back to her. This approach gently encourages the patient to express openly and discuss the concern with the clinician. It also serves to establish an environment of openness and acceptance.

2. **C.** Of the options given, it is best to acknowledge that the patient is trying to convey information that is important to him or her and establish that there will be a time to talk about those issues, while gently redirecting him or her to the task at hand.

3. **A.** When a number of alternatives are presented and the first on the list is more desirable, there is a tendency for individuals to select the first option and view the successive options as less desirable.

4. **B.** Focusing on long-term goals is not only a poor motivator, but also it is often a pitfall in the effort to change behavior because patients are less motivated when goals seem too big, impossible, or far from their current circumstances.

5. **A.** Although the behavioral contract is not a legal document, it can be a useful approach in solidifying behavioral strategies and goals.

6. **B.** Extinction is the process of identifying all positive reinforcements (in this case, the dentist ceasing work on the child's teeth) that maintain a behavior and ceasing or withholding these.

7. **E.** Both positive and negative events or situations are experienced as stress.

8. **D.** Systematic desensitization is the process of systematically pairing a relaxation response with a hierarchy of feared stimuli.

9. **B.** Muscle tension is associated with the experience of anxiety. Heightened anxiety contributes to lower pain thresholds, or sensitivity to the perception of pain.

10. **E.** All of the strategies listed may be considered appropriate cognitive interventions in pain management.

11. **D.** Classical conditioning (also known as respondent or Pavlovian conditioning) occurs when a neutral stimulus, one that is not associated with a particular response, is paired with an unconditioned stimulus (US), a stimulus that naturally elicits a particular response (UR). After numerous pairings, the neutral stimulus (CS) elicits a conditioned response (CR), which is essentially a weaker form of the UR without the presence of the US.

12. **C.** Providing the patient with information and control over his or her environment is likely to contribute to increased trust over time. Avoiding the issue of trust or providing reassurance that the patient can trust you without evidence is likely to maintain poor trust.

13. **E.** Contrary to their behavior in the waiting room, anxious patients are typically more likely to sit very still, often holding onto the arms of the dental chair, and engage in minimal verbal communication unless encouraged by the clinician.

14. **E.** Diaphragmatic breathing naturally activates the parasympathetic nervous system, producing a relaxation response.

15. **D.** Systematic desensitization is the systematic process of exposing the patient to a hierarchy of increasingly anxiety-provoking stimuli while the patient uses relaxation skills such as diaphragmatic breathing exercises.

16. **B.** Operant conditioning posits that behavior is largely influenced by the consequences associated with the particular behavior.

17. **D.** Research suggests that the most integral component of the treatment of anxiety is exposure to the feared stimulus.

18. **B.** Of the choices, distraction would most likely be the least effective approach—the attention of a very anxious individual cannot typically be easily diverted. In such cases, distraction can have detrimental effects, such as compromising rapport or increasing anxiety by failing to provide a positive coping experience. Providing education and coping strategies—increasing predictability, familiarity, and controllability—are typically more effective strategies in working with anxious patients.

19. **C.** Controllability, familiarity, predictability, and imminence are significant factors that influence the cognitive appraisal of stress.

20. **B.** Graded exposure is the systematic process of exposing the patient to a hierarchy of increasingly anxiety-provoking stimuli.

21. **A.** Asking the child about his or her fears creates an environment in which the child is encouraged to discuss any worries or concerns and to ask questions. This approach also serves to alleviate anxiety, provide an opportunity to correct any misperceptions regarding dentistry, and establish or maintain trust and rapport further.

22. **A.** Perceived stress and distress in one's life has been demonstrated to be a significant predictor (positively correlated) with self-reported health concerns.

23. **A.** Patients who are experiencing stress and anxiety typically feel more comfortable in having greater interpersonal space than they normally would when not experiencing stress and anxiety.

24. **E.** The use of silence can be a useful technique to encourage patient comment following a statement or question posed to the patient.

25. **E.** Individuals respond to stress physiologically, behaviorally, cognitively, and emotionally.

26. **A.** Periodontal disease, measured by the PI, and gingival disease, measured by the GI, are reversible processes. The amount of the debris and calculus, measured by the OHI-S, can decrease as well. Caries is not a reversible process.

27. **E.** The recommended level of fluoride for a community water supply in the United States ranges from 0.7 to 1.2 ppm of fluoride, depending on the mean maximum daily air temperature over a 5-year period. The fluoride level would be lower in a warm climate and would be higher in a cold climate. In the United States, most communities are fluoridated at approximately 1 ppm, which is equivalent to 1.0 mg of fluoride per 1 L of water.

28. **D.** Physicians and dentists can help prevent fluorosis by prescribing dietary fluoride supplements according to the Supplemental Fluoride Dosage Schedule recommended by the American Dental Association Council on Scientific Affairs.

29. **D.** Experimental epidemiology is used primarily in intervention studies. When an etiology for a particular disease has been determined, the researchers try to establish the effectiveness of a particular program of prevention or therapy. Descriptive epidemiology is used to quantify disease status in a community. Analytical epidemiology, also called *observational epidemiology*, is used to determine the etiology of a disease.

30. **D.** In this case, the investigator chooses or defines a sample of subjects who do not yet have the outcome of interest (in this case, cancer). The investigator measures risk factors in each subject (e.g., habits that may predict the subsequent outcome) and follows these subjects with periodic surveys or examinations to detect the outcomes of interest.

31. **C.** In a retrospective cohort study, the investigator chooses a sample of individuals who have the outcome of interest (in this case, squamous cell carcinoma) and looks into the past for possible

variables that may have caused the disease (e.g., chewing tobacco).

32. **E.** The abstract allows the reader to determine whether the study is of interest. The abstract usually appears at the head of the article and is reproduced in the literature database.

33. **C.** In the results section, the researcher describes the specific findings and actual outcomes of the project but does not interpret them. The interpretation and analysis of the results are part of the discussion, where the researcher attempts to explain the results.

34. **E.** The median is the middle of a distribution: half the scores are above the median, and half are below the median. The median is less sensitive to extreme scores than the mean, making it a better measure than the mean for highly skewed distributions. For instance, the median income of a population is usually more informative than the mean income. When there is an even number of numbers, the median is the mean of the two middle numbers. In this case, the median is $(64 + 68)/2 = 66$.

35. **C.** The correlation coefficient (r) quantifies the relationship between variables (x and y). A positive correlation coefficient indicates that the variables increase in the same direction; a negative correlation coefficient indicates that the variables vary in opposite directions. The correlation coefficient ranges from -1 to $+1$.

36. **C.** A false-positive test is a test result that erroneously assigns an individual to a specific diagnostic or reference group.

37. **D.** The average risk of infection for HBV after a needle-stick injury *does not fall* between HCV and HIV. For HBV, the risk of transmission after percutaneous injury is 30%; this figure is 1.8% for HCV and 0.3% for HIV.

38. **A.** Very specific tests are appropriate for confirming the existence of a disease. If the result of a highly specific test is positive, the disease is almost certain. High specificity is required in situations where the consequences of a false-positive diagnosis are serious or unduly alarming (e.g., HIV positivity).

39. **E.** All of these measures help ensure the safety of dental personnel.

40. **D.** Disinfection refers *only* to the inhibition or destruction of pathogens. Spores are not killed during disinfection procedures. By custom, the term *disinfection* is reserved for chemicals applied to inanimate surfaces, and the term *antiseptic* is used for antimicrobial agents that are applied to living tissues.

41. **D.** The proper time and temperature for autoclaving is 250° F (121° C) for 15 to 20 minutes, which yields 15 pounds pressure of steam, or 270° F (134° C) for a minimum of 3 minutes, which yields 30 pounds

pressure of steam. Moist heat destroys bacteria—denaturation of the high-protein–containing bacteria.

42. **E.** A thorough medical history, physical examination, and laboratory tests do not always detect patients who are carriers of infectious diseases. You must assume that all patients are infected with HIV, HBV, or other bloodborne pathogens. Similar infection control procedures must be used for all patients, regardless of their medical history or the type of treatment to be performed.

43. **D.** Alcohol is *not* an accepted disinfectant. Alcohol evaporates too quickly to be an effective disinfectant. The term *disinfection* is reserved for chemicals applied to inanimate surfaces, and the term *antiseptic* is used for antimicrobial agents (e.g., alcohol) that are applied to living tissues.

44. **E.** Mercury can be absorbed through the skin as well as absorbed by inhalation. Safe handling, resulting in part from proper training, helps reduce the risk of exposure.

45. **C.** The CDC recommends, at a minimum to meet nationally recognized drinking water standards, less than 500 CFU/mL of heterotrophic bacteria. In 1995, the American Dental Association addressed the dental water concern by asking manufacturers to provide equipment with the ability to deliver treatment water with less than 200 CFU/mL of unfiltered output from waterlines.

46. **A.** There are five principles in the ADA Principles of Ethics:
    1. *Patient autonomy* ("self-governance"). The dentist has a duty to respect the patient's rights to self-determination and confidentiality.
    2. *Nonmaleficence* ("do no harm"). The dentist has a duty to refrain from harming the patient.
    3. *Beneficence* ("do good"). The dentist has a duty to promote the patient's welfare.
    4. *Justice* ("fairness"). The dentist has a duty to treat people fairly.
    5. *Veracity* ("truthfulness"). The dentist has a duty to communicate truthfully.

47. **E.** Being specific helps to avoid misinterpretation of reports. Being objective provides the basis for accuracy in describing events. Being complete provides the basis for a thorough review of the facts when reviewing the report. Being timely ensures the best opportunity to recall all relevant events.

48. **A.** A preferred provider organization (PPO) is an arrangement between a plan and a group of dentists whereby the providers agree to accept certain payments (usually less than their usual fees) in anticipation of a higher volume of patients. Capitation is a payment mechanism whereby the dentist is paid a fixed amount regardless of the number of

patients seen or services provided. Health maintenance organizations (HMOs) are also called capitation plans because of the payment mechanism they use. An individual practice association (IPA) is a type of plan that combines the risk of capitation with fee-for-service reimbursement.

49. **A.** The Centers for Disease Control and Prevention (CDC) monitors and prevents disease outbreaks, implements disease prevention strategies, and maintains national health statistics. The U.S. Food and Drug Administration (FDA) is responsible for protecting the health of the nation against impure and unsafe foods, drugs, cosmetics, and other potential hazards. The Drug Enforcement Administration (DEA) determines the levels of controlled substances that have abuse potential. The Indian Health Services (IHS) focuses on the goal of raising the health status of Native Americans and Native Alaskans.

50. **A.** The Department of Health and Human Services (DHHS) is the principal agency of the U.S. government for protecting the health of all Americans and providing essential human services. DHHS includes 11 agencies and more than 300 programs. The other agencies listed are part of the DHHS. The National Institutes of Health (NIH) is the world's premier medical research organization. The Health Resources and Services Administration (HRSA) provides access to essential health care services for people with low income, people with no health insurance, and people who live in rural areas or urban neighborhoods where health care is scarce. The Agency for Healthcare Research and Quality (AHRQ) supports research on health care systems, health care quality and cost issues, access to health care, and effectiveness of medical treatments.

51. **A, C, D.** In a case-control study, people with a condition ("cases") are compared with people without the condition ("controls") but who are similar in other characteristics. Hypothesized causal exposures are sought in the past medical records of the participants. The case-control study could establish a temporal relationship between the exposure and disease of interest, such as a history of alcohol drinking before the appearance of oral cancer. Choice **B** applies to a prospective cohort study.

52. **A, B, C, E.** Sampling strategy provides a description of the sampling strategy, the sample size, and the methods for assigning samples to conditions. Measurement strategies and measurement instruments indicate how the variables are measured. Although the variables studied are discussed in the abstract, the introduction, and the conclusion, the actual definitions of the variables are stated in the measurement strategy. Experimental design describes operationally the study design in a step-by-step

sequence. Statistical analytical procedures explain the proposed strategy for quantifying, evaluating, and analyzing the results and is presented along with the actual statistical procedures proposed. The commentary on the results is placed in the discussion section and the summary and conclusion section.

53. **D.** The mean or average is the value obtained by adding all the measurements and dividing by the number of measurements. Choice **A** is equal to choice **C**. The most frequent measurement in a set of data is termed the *mode*. The median is determined by sorting the observations in order of magnitude and finding the middle number.

54. **A.** The χ^2 test measures the association between two categorical variables. The correlation coefficient quantifies the relationship between variables (e.g., x and y). If the r value is +1, there is a perfect correlation, with both values increasing in the same direction. A multiple regression analysis provides a mathematical model of linear relationship between a dependent (i.e., an outcome variable) and two or more independent or predictor variables.

55. **B.** Supplemental fluoride in addition to proper water fluoridation could lead to fluorosis. Fluoride has both a topical and a systemic effect. The U.S. Centers for Disease Control and Prevention (CDC) directive on the level of fluoride in the water is still in effect even though suggestions have been made to reduce it to 0.7 ppm. The CDC reported in 2010 that 74% of the U.S. population have water fluoridation.

56. **B.** Three doses are given to confer immunity: an initial dose, followed by a second dose at 1 month, and a third dose 6 months after the first. Because HBV is highly infectious, all dental personnel should be vaccinated against HBV. The mainstay of postexposure prophylaxis is hepatitis B vaccine, but in certain circumstances hepatitis B immune globulin is recommended in addition to HBV vaccine for added protection.

57. **C.** Blue identifies the health hazard. Red identifies the fire hazard. Yellow identifies the reactivity or stability of a chemical. White identifies the required personal protective equipment (PPE) when using this chemical. The level of risk for each category is indicated by the use of numbers 0 through 4, the higher the number, the greater the danger.

58. **A, B, C, D.**

Periodontics

1. **A.** Wasting diseases of the teeth include erosion (corrosion; may be caused by acidic beverages),

abrasion (caused by mechanical wear as with toothbrushing with abrasive dentifrice), attrition (secondary to functional contact with opposing teeth), and abfraction (flexure secondary to occlusal loading).

2. **A.** Keratinized gingiva extends from the free gingival margin to the mucogingival junction. The attached gingiva extends from the free gingival groove to the mucogingival junction.

3. **C.** Gingivitis is characterized by inflammation of the gingival tissues with no loss of clinical attachment. Periodontitis is characterized by inflammation with loss of clinical attachment.

4. **D.** Because there is no loss of attachment, the diagnosis would not be periodontitis. The clinical description of pain, erythema, blunt papillae, pseudomembrane, and halitosis is consistent with necrotizing ulcerative gingivitis.

5. **C.** Radiographs must be taken in a standardized format at repeated visits to be assessed for small changes in bone density over time, using subtraction radiography. Radiographs are usually standardized by using a bite registration block to relocate the x-ray at the same place and angulation each time.

6. **D.** Maxillary molars usually have three roots (mesiobuccal, distobuccal, and palatal). Furcation involvement can be assessed on these teeth from the facial (bifurcation between the mesiobuccal and distobuccal roots), mesial (bifurcation between the mesiobuccal and palatal roots), and distal (bifurcation between the distobuccal and palatal roots).

7. **A.** Subgingival plaque can be in the cervical area or more apical. In both areas, it can be either tooth-associated or tissue-associated. The apical tooth-associated plaque is composed primarily of gram-negative rods.

8. **C.** Calcium, phosphorus, sodium, and potassium are inorganic components of dental plaque. Polysaccharides, proteins, glycoproteins, and lipids are organic components of dental plaque.

9. **D.** *F. nucleatum* can be found in health and disease. This bacterium is an important bridge between early and late colonizers of the dental plaque biofilm.

10. **C.** Periodontal health is characterized by a microflora dominated by gram-positive, facultative cocci and rods.

11. **B.** *P. gingivalis* has been associated with chronic periodontitis. *A. viscosus* is usually associated with health or gingivitis. *S. mutans* is associated with dental caries. *A. actinomycetemcomitans* has been associated with localized aggressive periodontitis.

12. **D.** Although age, gender, and nutrition may have an impact on periodontal disease, the accumulation of the bacterial plaque biofilm is the primary initiator of the disease.

13. **B.** Inadequate or overhanging margins serve as a nidus for dental plaque accumulation and make plaque removal difficult.

14. **C.** Individuals who smoke cigarettes are more likely to have periodontal disease than nonsmokers. The number of cigarettes smoked and the number of years of smoking affect the severity of disease. Former smokers usually have less disease than current smokers.

15. **D.** The extent and severity of periodontal disease in a patient with well-controlled diabetes are usually no more than the extent and severity of disease in patients without diabetes. Patients with well-controlled diabetes can usually be treated with conventional periodontal therapy.

16. **D.** Oral contraceptives can exacerbate the impact of bacterial plaque on the gingival tissues. However, oral contraceptives cannot cause gingivitis.

17. **D.** Neutrophils are one of the primary defense cells of the innate immune system. T lymphocytes are important activators of the adaptive immune system. Macrophages are antigen-presenting cells. Plasma cells produce antibodies.

18. **D.** Although defects in any of the host defense cells could affect periodontal disease susceptibility, defects in neutrophils have been most frequently described.

19. **D.** The initial, early, and established lesions of gingivitis do not have attachment loss associated with them.

20. **A.** IL-1 is important in the activation of osteoclasts and stimulation of bone loss.

21. **E.** Scaling and root planing are used in all phases of periodontal therapy where there has been loss of attachment through periodontitis.

22. **C.** Although changes in gingival color and consistency and loss of gingival stippling can be indicators of gingival inflammation, bleeding on probing is the most objective clinical indicator.

23. **A.** Marginal gingivitis not complicated by systemic problems or medications usually can be treated successfully with phase 1 therapy, and a patient with this diagnosis would have a good prognosis.

24. **B.** Polishing is used to remove plaque and stains from the teeth. Gingival curettage is used to remove the epithelial lining of a periodontal pocket. Root planing is used to create a smooth root surface through the removal of calculus and rough cementum. Scaling is used to remove plaque, calculus, and stains from the tooth.

25. **A.** Scalers, with their pointed ends and back, are designed for supragingival instrumentation; curettes, with their rounded ends and back, can be

used for both supragingival and subgingival instrumentation.

26. **B.** Scalers have a pointed back; curettes have a rounded back, making them suitable for subgingival instrumentation.

27. **C.** Three incisions are made in the modified Widman flap—internal bevel, crevicular, and interdental. The flap is designed to provide exposure of the tooth roots and alveolar bone. However, the flap is not reflected beyond the mucogingival junction.

28. **A.** Surgical techniques designed to increase the width of attached gingiva include free gingival grafts and apically repositioned flaps.

29. **C.** The Miller classification system for mucogingival defects takes into consideration the degree of recession (whether or not it extends to the mucogingival junction) and presence or absence of bone loss in the interdental area. Both class I and class II defects are characterized by no loss of bone in the interproximal areas. In class I defects, the marginal tissue recession does not extend to the mucogingival junction. In class II defects, recession extends to or beyond the mucogingival junction.

30. **B.** Ostectomy is the removal of supporting alveolar bone. Osteoplasty is the reshaping or recontouring of nonsupporting alveolar bone.

31. **B.** An interdental crater has two bony walls remaining. These walls are usually the facial and lingual walls.

32. **D.** Cells from the periodontal ligament are proposed to allow for regeneration of the periodontal tissues.

33. **D.** Through-and-through (class III) furcation defects are least likely to be treated with bone graft procedures.

34. **B.** When evaluated by light microscopy, there appears to be direct contact at the bone-implant interface.

35. **A.** Chlorhexidine is the most effective antimicrobial agent currently available.

36. **D.** PerioChip is a biodegradable local delivery agent for chlorhexidine.

37. **B.** Epithelial cells migrate approximately 0.5 mm/day. It takes 5 to 14 days after a gingivectomy for surface epithelialization to be complete.

38. **A.** Increased tooth mobility is the most common clinical sign of trauma from occlusion. Increased periodontal ligament width is the most common radiographic sign.

39. **C.** The term *trauma from occlusion* refers to the tissue injury that occurs when occlusal forces exceed the adaptive capacity of the tissues. An occlusion that produces such an injury is called a *traumatic occlusion*. The tooth may become damaged as a result of excessive occlusal forces. The periodontal ligament also may become widened as a result of the force.

40. **C.** Teeth are usually splinted to improve patient comfort during mastication.

41. **C.** Establishment of drainage is the first step in treating an acute periodontal abscess. The patient may then use self-applied mouth rinses and be prescribed antibiotics if there is evidence of systemic involvement (e.g., fever, lymphadenopathy). A flap would be reflected in a subsequent appointment if the abscess did not resolve and became a chronic problem.

42. **B.** Calcium channel blockers, cyclosporine, and phenytoin often result in overgrowth of gingival tissues.

43. **C.** Patient cooperation and effectiveness in removing bacterial plaque is of primary importance in maintaining a healthy periodontium.

44. **D.** Mature dental plaque usually reforms on the teeth within 24 to 48 hours after effective plaque removal.

45. **C.** The Bass technique of brushing is designed to direct the bristles of the brush toward the gingival sulcus.

46. **C.** Under these conditions, doxycycline inhibits metalloproteinases. By inhibiting matrix metalloproteinase (MMP)-8 and MMP-13, collagen breakdown is reduced. Amylase is a normal constituent of saliva. β-Lactamases break down β-lactam antibiotics such as penicillins. Cyclooxygenases are inhibited by nonsteroidal antiinflammatory drugs. 5-Lipoxygenase is important for the formation of leukotrienes. None of the last four mentioned enzymes is significantly affected by doxycycline.

47. **C, B, D, A.** Immediately after suturing to close a periodontal flap, a clot forms that connects the flap to the tooth and alveolar bone. Epithelial cells begin to migrate over the border of the flap 1 to 3 days after surgery. An epithelial attachment consisting of hemidesmosomes and a basal lamina is in place 1 week after surgery. The clot is replaced by granulation tissue. Collagen fibers appear 2 weeks after surgery. Within 1 month, the gingival crevice is lined with epithelium.

48. **C, D.** Only lymphadenopathy and fever indicate a spreading infection.

49. **B.** Furcation involvement can be classified as follows: grade I, incipient; grade II, cul-de-sac with definite horizontal component; grade III, complete bone loss in the furcation; grade IV, complete bone loss in the furcation and recession of the gingival tissues resulting in a furcation opening that is clinically visible.

50. **C.** *Streptococcus* and *Actinomyces* species are early or primary colonizers. *P. gingivalis* and *A. actinomycetemcomitans* are late (secondary) colonizers, as are *Campylobacter* species. *F. nucleatum* serves as a middle or bridging microorganism.

Pharmacology

1. **B.** The brain has especially tight capillary junctions as well as glial cells that result in a blood-brain barrier.

2. **E.** Oxycodone is a scheduled drug, requiring DEA registration on the part of the prescriber.

3. **B.** The characteristic response to a competitive antagonist is a parallel shift to the right of the agonist curve, with the two curves reaching the same maximal effect.

4. **C.** The fourth phase constitutes postmarketing surveillance.

5. **D.** This situation for sweat glands is atypical for the sympathetic nervous system.

6. **A.** Nicotinic receptors are located at the skeletal-neuromuscular junction, in the ganglia, at the junction of the sympathetic nerve to the adrenal gland and the adrenal chromaffin cells, and in the central nervous system.

7. **E.** All other choices are typical of muscarinic cholinergic receptor agonists.

8. **D.** α-Adrenoceptor blockers such as phenoxybenzamine inhibit the vasoconstrictor effect of epinephrine but not the vasodilator effect of epinephrine. The administration of α blockers results in epinephrine reversal. Atropine would have little effect because it does not act at adrenergic receptors. Propranolol would block only the vasodilator effect of epinephrine and the effect of epinephrine on the heart. Guanethidine and tyramine act largely at prejunctional sites and do not block adrenergic receptors.

9. **D.** The nigrostriatal pathway contains dopaminergic neurons, which are important in muscle control. Many antipsychotic drugs block these, leading to the motor adverse effects.

10. **C.** The antimuscarinic action of benztropine tends to reduce the Parkinson-like symptoms and some other motor symptoms caused by haloperidol, a dopamine receptor blocker. Benztropine does not improve the antipsychotic effect of haloperidol. Histamine release appears to play little role in this interaction. Benztropine reduces salivary flow, and xerostomia can easily result from its administration. Benztropine has little effect on renal clearance of haloperidol.

11. **B.** The two benzodiazepine receptor subtypes (targets for drugs such as diazepam) are located on the same chloride channel as the γ-aminobutyric acid A receptor.

12. **C.** Only prilocaine is metabolized to *o*-toluidine.

13. **B.** Halothane sensitizes the heart to epinephrine and other catecholamines.

14. **A.** Inhibiting sodium channels leads to the inhibition of the nerve action potential and inhibition of nerve conduction. Sodium channels are examples of ion channel receptors. Ion channel receptors contain several subunits arranged in a barrel shape. Drugs that bind to the channel can alter conductance to the ion associated with that channel.

15. **D.** Benzocaine lacks the terminus group that procaine, mepivacaine, prilocaine, and lidocaine have. This amine group can become protonated, making these drugs more water-soluble and facilitating an injectable form. Benzocaine must be provided in a cream-based or oil-based preparation allowing just a topical form. Procaine and mepivacaine have poor topical anesthetic properties.

16. **C.** An area of inflammation is an area of low pH. The acid environment would convert more of the drug into the charged form, making it less able to diffuse to the nerve cells. This would reduce the rate of onset and the net anesthetic effect of the drug.

17. **D.** All of the choices are combinations of an opioid and an inhibitor of cyclooxygenase (COX), except two: ibuprofen, naproxen and aspirin, ibuprofen. Ibuprofen and naproxen are both reversible inhibitors of COX and are propionic acid derivatives. Aspirin is a salicylate and is an irreversible inhibitor.

18. **C.** Thromboxane A_2 increases platelet aggregation. Its inhibition is the target of low-dose aspirin, which inhibits cyclooxygenase. Inhibition of this enzyme leads to a reduction in important downstream products, including thromboxane A_2.

19. **C.** The INR value indicates that the patient has received anticoagulant therapy for atrial fibrillation. Aspirin increases the risk of postsurgical bleeding. The combination of increase in prothrombin time, surgery, and the antiplatelet effect of aspirin makes aspirin contraindicated in this situation. The effect of ibuprofen on the platelet is reversible, whereas the effect of aspirin on the platelet is irreversible. Aspirin poses a greater risk than ibuprofen in this situation.

20. **C.** The first three choices are all H_1 histamine receptor blockers. However, fexofenadine is largely excluded from the central nervous system, in contrast to diphenhydramine and hydroxyzine. Albuterol is a β_2-adrenergic receptor agonist. Famotidine is a H_2 histamine receptor antagonist.

21. **B.** The cardiovascular risks may be associated with adverse hematologic effects, but the exact mechanism is not yet known.

22. **A.** All the drugs listed are diuretics. However, only bumetanide acts on the ascending limb of the loop of Henle. It is called a "loop" and "high-ceiling" diuretic because of its site of action in the nephron and maximal effect, respectively.

23. **D.** The long Q–T interval observed as a result of certain drugs or as a hereditary condition makes the patient more susceptible to this condition.

24. **C.** Lisinopril, by virtue of the fact that it inhibits angiotensin-converting enzyme (also called peptidyl dipeptidase), inhibits the breakdown of bradykinin.

25. **D.** Diazepam, epinephrine, and insulin act at ion channel receptors, G-protein–linked receptors, and tyrosine kinase–linked receptors, respectively. These three receptor types are cell surface receptors. Thyroid hormone and steroid hormones or drugs, such as prednisone, act on nuclear receptors, accounting for much of their action. The action of heparin is to stimulate antithrombin III in the plasma. Its action is extracellular.

26. **A.** All of the choices are oral hypoglycemic agents. Only acarbose inhibits α-glucosidase.

27. **D.** Spironolactone, a potassium-sparing diuretic useful in treating edema and heart failure, is a competitive antagonist at the aldosterone receptor.

28. **B.** Aldosterone and fludrocortisone are selective mineralocorticosteroids. Hydrocortisone has significant mineralocorticoid and glucocorticoid activity. Dexamethasone has very little mineralocorticoid activity.

29. **B.** Glucocorticoids characteristically stimulate gluconeogenesis and lipolysis. Insulin has the opposite effects. The other hormones listed have minor or negligible effects.

30. **C.** Renal tubular acidosis, aminoaciduria, and hyperphosphaturia are some of the manifestations of proximal tubule damage in Fanconi's syndrome.

31. **D.** Of the choices given, only vancomycin is effective against many methicillin-resistant staphylococci. Various penicillins, macrolides, and clindamycin are ineffective.

32. **C.** Because it lacks a cell wall, *M. pneumoniae* is not sensitive to cell wall inhibitors such as penicillin V. The macrolides (e.g., clarithromycin) are ribosomal protein synthesis inhibitors that are effective against *M. pneumoniae*. Viridans streptococcus, *S. pneumoniae*, and *S. pyogenes* are gram-positive cocci. *L. buccalis* is a gram-negative oral bacillus.

33. **A.** The short elimination half-time for penicillin V is due to rapid excretion of penicillin in the urine. About 90% of this renal excretion is a result of active tubular transport, a rapid and efficient process. (Very little metabolism of penicillin occurs.)

34. **E.** Amoxicillin, clarithromycin, and clindamycin are effective against some anaerobes, but their spectrum is not limited to anaerobic bacteria. Aminoglycosides are effective only against aerobes. The action of metronidazole requires a reduced environment. Its antibacterial spectrum is limited to anaerobes. Metronidazole is also effective against many parasites.

35. **B, D.** Nonspecific esterase in the plasma can metabolize various esters. Articaine and acetylcholine have ester bonds that are susceptible to these enzymes. Bethanechol and carbachol are designed to be resistant to hydrolysis by acetylcholinesterase and plasma esterases. Pilocarpine is an alkaloid that is not significantly affected by these enzymes.

36. **A—4; B—5; C—2; D—3; E—1.** Glibenclamide is a newer sulfonylurea-type drug that increases insulin secretion by closing adenosine triphosphate–sensitive potassium channels in the cell membranes of β cells. Activating AMP kinase has an effect of regulating energy production, leading to the effects indicated above. An increase in glucagonlike peptide leads to stimulation of insulin release, inhibition of glucagon release, and reduced food intake.

37. **A, E.** Inhibitors of the α2/δ-1 protein subunit of high-voltage–activated calcium channels have selective antiepileptic effects and have been found to be useful in treating neuropathic pain. Phenobarbital enhances chloride channel activity. Carbamazepine is a sodium channel blocker, and ethosuximide is an inhibitor of T-type calcium channels.

38. **D, E.** The half-lives are as follows: chlordiazepoxide, 5 to 30 hours; diazepam, 30 to 60 hours; lorazepam, 10 to 18 hours; midazolam, 2 to 5 hours; triazolam, 1 to 2 hours.

39. **B, E.** Cleavage of the aromatic ring rarely, if ever, occurs in the metabolism of local anesthetics. Lidocaine does not possess an ester bond to be metabolized.

40. **C, D, E.** Flumazenil blocks both types of benzodiazepine receptors associated with γ-aminobutyric acid A ($GABA_A$) channels, blocking the effects of diazepam, zaleplon, and zolpidem, the latter two being selective for the Bz_1 receptor. Baclofen stimulates $GABA_B$ receptors, and buspirone is a partial agonist at serotonin 5-hydroxytryptamine 1A receptors.

Prosthodontics

1. **A.** The incisive papilla provides a guide for the anterior-posterior position of the maxillary anterior teeth. The labial surfaces of the central incisors are usually 8 to 10 mm in front of the papilla. This distance varies depending of the amount of resorption of the residual ridge, the size of the teeth, and the labiolingual thickness of the alveolar process.

2. **E.** All of the statements are correct. VDR is a physiologic rest position; it is the position of the mandible when the muscles are in their minimum state of tonicity, which occurs when a patient is relaxed with the trunk upright and the head unsupported.

In this position, the interocclusal distance is usually 2 to 4 mm when observed at the first premolar area.

3. **C.** Stability is resistance to movement toward the residual ridge. The function of the posterior palatal seal is to improve retention, not stability. Stability is determined by the size, height, or shape of the ridge.

4. **A.** "Failure of an occlusal rest rarely results from a structural defect in the metal and rarely if ever is caused by distortion. Therefore the blame for such failure must often be assumed by the dentist for not having provided sufficient space for the rest during mouth preparations" (Carr AB, et al: *McCracken's Removable Partial Prosthodontics*, ed 11. St Louis, Mosby, 2005).

5. **D.** To preserve the mounting relationship in the articulator of the maxillary cast (face-bow record) after processing a denture, an occlusal index of the maxillary denture is made after occlusal adjustments and before decasting the denture. This procedure has nothing to do with the mandible's relationship to the maxilla.

6. **D.** Angular cheilosis is described as inflamed and cracked corners of the mouth that can become infected with bacterial and fungal organisms. It is commonly seen in patients with dentures with diminished vertical dimension of occlusion. It is best treated with antifungal creams and correcting the vertical dimension of occlusion.

7. **A.** When performing an occlusal adjustment, the goal is to make centric relation and maximum intercuspation to coincide. None of the other choices allows one to mount the casts reliably in centric relation or allows one to perform this procedure accurately.

8. **B.** The main purpose is to capture the influence of the mylohyoid muscle. The extent of this flange is determined by the elevation of the floor of the mouth when the patient wets the lips with the tip of tongue. Pursing the lips forms the extension of the buccal vestibule. The buccal vestibule is influenced by the buccinator muscle, which extends from the modiolus anteriorly to the pterygomandibular raphe posteriorly and has its lower fibers attached to the buccal shelf and the external oblique ridge.

9. **B.** The function of the direct retainer is to retain the removable partial denture by means of the abutments. Stabilization is provided by the minor connector. Support is provided by the rest. The indirect retainers improve the efficiency of the direct retainers. Direct retainers do not add strength to the major connector.

10. **D.** Tooth mobility is prevented or diminished during function by the reciprocating clasp. The reciprocating clasp should contact the tooth on or above the height of contour of the tooth, allowing for insertion and removal with passive force. Displacement of the RPD toward the tissue, causing tissue recession, is a function of the lack of occlusal rests.

11. **D.** This meets the definition of centric relation and the normal anatomic relationships of the temporomandibular discs to the condyles. Centric relation is a clinically repeatable mandibular position primarily defined by the temporomandibular joints, not the teeth.

12. **A.** The retromolar pad should always be covered for support of the mandibular denture base. The retromolar pads and the buccal shelf are considered primary areas of support for a mandibular distal extension RPD or complete denture.

13. **B.** Anatomic landmarks to be used as guides in arranging the anterior teeth are the incisive papilla, midsagittal suture, and ala of the nose (canine lines). The incisive papilla is a good guide for the anterior-posterior positioning of the maxillary anterior teeth. The labial surfaces of the central incisors are usually 8 to 10 mm in front of the papillae. This distance varies depending on the size of the teeth and the labiolingual thickness of the alveolar process, so it is not an absolute relationship.

14. **A.** The vibrating line is located by finding the pterygomaxillary (hamular) notches and continues to the median line of the anterior part of the soft palate slightly anterior to the foveae palatinae. A V-shaped groove 1 to 1.5 mm deep and 1.5 mm broad at its base is carved into the cast at the vibrating line. The narrow and sharp bead sinks easily into the soft tissue to provide a seal against air being forced under the denture. Stability is resistance to movement toward the residual ridge. The post dam improves retention, not stability. It is carved shallow in the midpalatal suture area. Stability is determined by the size, height, or shape of the ridge.

15. **D.** The ala-tragus line posteriorly and the interpupillary line anteriorly are used as guides to align the occlusal plane for complete dentures. The Camper's line is also known as the ala-tragus line.

16. **A.** Teeth come together every time a patient swallows. This can dislodge dentures secondary to breaking the denture seal.

17. **B.** Epulis fissurata is a reactive growth to an overextended or ill-fitting denture flange. It is best removed surgically. Papillary hyperplasia is found in the palatal vault. It is caused by local irritation, poor-fitting dentures, poor oral hygiene, or leaving dentures in 24 hours a day. Candidiasis is associated with papillary hyperplasia. Fibrous tuberosity is commonly seen with large tuberosities.

18. **C.** "Failure of an occlusal rest rarely results from a structural defect in the metal and rarely if ever is caused by accidental distortion. Therefore the blame for such failure must often be assumed by the dentist for not having provided sufficient space for the rest during mouth preparations" (Carr AB, et al: *McCracken's Removable Partial Prosthodontics*, ed 11. St Louis, Mosby, 2005).

19. **B.** Resin-modified glass ionomers combine some of the advantages of glass-ionomer cements, such as fluoride release and adhesion, but provide higher strength and low solubility. These materials are less susceptible to early moisture exposure than glass-ionomer cements, but they exhibit increased thermal expansion because of the addition of resin.

20. **A.** The width of an anterior tooth is usually identified by the mesiofacial and distofacial position of the line angles, the shape of the surface contour, and light reflection between these line angles. The contralateral tooth features should be duplicated closely in the pontic, and the space discrepancy can be compensated by modifying the shape of the proximal areas.

21. **C.** The carboxylate groups in the polymer molecule chelate to calcium.

22. **B.** Gold alloys are heavier for a given volume. Gold alloys are softer. Base metals are cast at higher temperatures, leading to greater shrinkage.

23. **B.** Polysulfide has the highest tear strength of all elastomeric impression materials.

24. **B.** *Chroma* is the saturation or intensity of the color or shade. *Value* is the relative lightness or darkness of a color. *Opalescence* is the light effect of a translucent material.

25. **B.** Noble metals are gold, platinum, and palladium. Silver is not considered noble; it is reactive but improves castability. Noble alloys (old term was *semiprecious metal*) have a noble metal content greater than or equal to 25%. To be classified as noble, palladium-copper, palladium-gold, and palladium-cobalt alloys have no stipulation for gold. High noble alloys have a high content of gold (>60%).

26. **D.** All these reasons are correct. The provisional is placed to protect the tooth and preserve healthy tissues if proper contours and marginal integrity are present. This is an excellent time to evaluate and give feedback to the patient on how well he or she is brushing and flossing.

27. **C.** Compomer cements (also known as *resin-modified glass ionomer cements*) have low solubility, low adhesion, and low microleakage. They are not recommended to be used with all-ceramic restorations because they have been associated with fracture, which is probably due to water absorption and expansion.

28. **D.** An important factor that affects the metal-ceramic bond is the surface treatment of the alloy before firing porcelain. Air-abrasion of the cast alloy is typically performed before the oxidation step to help remove surface contaminants that remain from devesting and to help clean the casting and provide microscopic surface irregularities for mechanical retention of the ceramic. The oxidation step for the alloy can be performed in air or by using the reduced atmospheric pressure (approximately 0.1 atm) available in dental porcelain furnaces.

29. **D.** The casting alloy and luting agent have been shown to have a minimal effect on the retention of a crown. The geometry of the preparation, parallelism between the walls (taper), and surface texture of the preparation have an effect on the retention of a crown.

30. **B.** The arcon articulator is capable of duplicating a wide range of mandibular movements but is generally set to follow the patient's border movements. The terminal hinge axis is located, and a pantograph is used to record the mandibular movements. These mandibular movement tracings or recordings are used to set the articulator.

31. **A.** If there is an existing pulp chamber and remaining sound tooth structure, there is no need to place a post. Placement of a post tends to require taking additional tooth structure, which weakens a tooth.

32. **E.** A tooth moves within the limits of its periodontal ligament during function. The relative immobility of the osseointegrated implant compared with the functional mobility of a natural tooth can create stresses at the neck of the implant up to two times the implied load on the prosthesis. Potential problems when connecting an implant with a tooth include (1) breakdown of the osseointegration, (2) cement failure on the natural abutment, (3) screw or abutment loosening, and (4) failure of the implant prosthetic component. Fracture in the connector area is rarely seen in this situation.

33. **C.** The minor connector must have sufficient bulk to be rigid so that it transfers functional stresses effectively to the abutment or supporting teeth and tissues. It should be located in the interdental embrasure where it does not disturb the tongue and should be thickest in the lingual surface, tapering toward the contact area but not located on a convex surface.

34. **E.** The posterior and anterior factors, position in the mouth, and side shift influence the occlusal anatomy of a restoration.

35. **E.** The contact of the framework with parallel tooth surfaces acting as guide planes provides a positive path of placement and removal for the RPD. In addition, guide planes can provide retention by

limiting the movement of the framework. The rest on the RPD prevents vertical or cervical movement.

36. **C.** The clasps are meant to be flexible to engage in undercut. The rest of the components of the RPD should be rigid.

37. **A.** Circumferential cast clasps are more rigid than combination clasps or wrought wire clasps. Because there is good stability of the prosthesis when the tooth is supported, there is no need for the added flexibility in a normal situation.

38. **E.** The impression should be rinsed and disinfected with glutaraldehyde or iodophor and should be poured within 15 minutes from the time the impression was removed from the mouth.

39. **B.** Isolation is the most important factor because it prevents bacterial contamination, increasing the success of the pulp cap procedure.

40. **E.** On a tooth-supported RPD with a circumferential cast clasp assembly, there should be more than 180 degrees of encirclement by the clasp in the greatest circumference of the tooth (that passes from diverging axial surfaces to converging axial surfaces). Mesial and distal rests anterior and posterior to the edentulous areas, respectively, are generally used.

41. **A.** Nonrigid connectors are used when it is not possible to prepare two abutments for a fixed partial denture (FPD) with a common path of placement or to segment a large or complex FPD into shorter components. Nonrigid connectors can be prefabricated plastic patterns (female or keyway portion and male or key portion) that are embedded in the waxed crown and pontic patterns or custom-milled in the cast crown. The second part is custom-fitted to the milled retainer and cast.

42. **C.** The recommended space or distance between the border of the framework and the marginal gingiva should be at least 6 mm.

43. **B.** The minor connectors are the components that serve as the part of the removable partial denture that connect the major connector and other components, such as the clasp assembly, indirect retainers, occlusal rests, or cingulum rests.

44. **D.** The Munsell Color System, which is the basis of shade guides such as Vita Lumin, is divided into three dimensions: *hue* is the shade or color of an object, *chroma* is the saturation or intensity of the color or shade, and *value* is the relative lightness or darkness of a color.

45. **D.** Opaque porcelain is used for masking the oxide layer of the metal and provides the porcelain-metal bond. The minimum thickness of the opaque is about 0.1 mm.

46. **B.** *Chroma* is the saturation or intensity of the color or shade. *Value* is the relative lightness or darkness of a color. *Metamerism* is the phenomenon in which a color match under a lighting condition appears different under a different lighting condition. *Fluorescence* is the physical property in which an object emits visible light when exposed to ultraviolet light.

47. **B, C, D.** Silver is not considered noble. It is reactive. It improves castability but can cause porcelain "greening."

48. **B.** The base paste in polyether impression material contains a polyether polymer. Polydimethylsiloxane is the main base component of condensation silicone. Polysulfide polymer is found in polysulfide impression material. None of these is a reversible impression material.

49. **A, B, C, D.** Electrosurgery is contraindicated under all of the conditions listed.

50. **A, D.** Retentive clasps need to be occlusal to the survey line because they approach the tooth from the occlusal. The I bar and T bar engage the undercuts of teeth by way of a gingival approach.

Index

Page numbers followed by "f" indicate figures, "t" indicate tables, and "b" indicate boxes.

A

ABC model, 240
Abfraction, 260
  treatment, 46
Abrasion, 252
  treatment, 46
Abscesses, 284
Absorption (drugs), 292-293
Abstract/vague communication, usage, 237
Abused tissues, management, 351-352
Abutment teeth
  alignment, 343
  torqueing force, reduction, 355
Acarbose, 327
Accelerator, type, 359
Accidental traumatic lesions, 255
Acetaminophen, 315
  effects, 315-316
  metabolic pathways, 315f
  preference, 316
Acetylcholine (ACh), biosynthetic pathway, 296
Acid-base drug properties, 292
Acid etching, 212
Acknowledging, usage, 236
Acquired immunodeficiency syndrome (AIDS), oral complications, 113b
Acrylic partial denture, 201
Acrylic resins, 356
  porosity, 356
  shrinkage, 356
  usage, 344
Actinic cheilitis (solar cheilitis), 117
Actinomyces odontolyticus, 260
Actinomycosis, 113
Activating hand instruments, 273
Activator, 175
Active retainers, 181
Acute acetaminophen toxicity, 315
Acute apical abscess, 4
  differentiation, 4
  presenting signs/symptoms, 4
Acute aspirin toxicity, 315
Acute candidiasis, 114f
Acute gingival diseases, 283-285
Acute herpetic gingivostomatitis, 204, 283
Acute necrotizing ulcerative gingivitis, 205
  treatment, 283
Acute osteomyelitis, 129
Acute pericoronitis, 283
Acute radiation syndrome, 136
Addition silicone (vinyl polysiloxane), 359
A-delta fibers, 2
Adenoid cystic carcinoma, 122
Adenomatoid odontogenic tumor, 126
Adenosine, 319
Adenosine diphosphate (ADP) receptor, 290
Adhesive techniques, uses, 66
Adjunctive endodontic treatment, 28-30
Adjunctive therapeutic approaches, 281f
Administration for Children and Families (ACF), 235
Admixed amalgam, 66

Adrenal corticosteroids, 327-328
Adrenal medulla, hormone secretion, 296
Adrenergic agonists, 296-298
  cardiovascular effects, 297f
  uses, 298t
Adrenergic neuron blockers, 298-299
Adrenergic receptor blockers, 298-299, 298t
Adults
  children, physiologic differences, 194
  coronal caries, 218
  psychological considerations, 181
  risk-based interventions, 39t
  treatment, 181-182
    periodontal aspects, 182
Adverse reactions, examples, 192
Aerosols, usage, 229
Affordable Care Act (ACA), 235-236
Agency for Healthcare Research and Quality (AHRQ), 236
Aggregatibacter actinomycetemcomitans, 257, 259
Aggressive horizontal brushing technique, 260
Aggressive periodontitis, 205, 256, 258, 283-284
  systemic neutrophil abnormalities, association, 263t
Agonists, graded dose-response curves, 291f
Airborne particles, environmental contaminants, 232-233
Air-driven particle abrasion equipment, 49
Akers clasp, 355
Albers-Schönberg disease (osteopetrosis), 131
Aligners, 175
All-ceramic crowns, 362
All-ceramic restorations, 362
All-ceramic systems, comparison, 362t
Allograft, 83, 277
  materials, 277
Alpha-adrenergic receptor blockers (alpha blockers), 298, 321
  adverse effects, 298
  dental implications, 299
Alpha-hydroxylation, 305
Alpha particles, 132
Aluminum chloride/aluminum sulfate, 359
Aluwax, 344
Alveolar bone, periodontal disease measure usage, 253
Alveolar concentration, minimum, 194
Alveolar crest, radiographic anatomy, 144
Alveolar process fractures, 82
Alveolar ridge preservation, 83
Alveoloplasty, 349
Alveolus, grafting, 83
Alveoplasty, 82
Amalgam
  blues, 43
  carving, 64-65
  insertion, 63-64
  knives, usage, 65f
  scrap, collection/disposal problems, 66
  tattoo, 111

Amalgam restorations, 62-66
  cavosurface margin, 58
  clinical examination, 43-44
  convenience form, 59
  finishing, 65
  outline form, 57-58
  primary resistance form, 58-59
  primary retention form, 58
  repair, 65
  requirements, 63
  resistance form, 58-59
  restorative technique, 63-65
  safety, 66
  tooth preparation, 56-59
  usage, 62
Amalgam tooth preparation
  external/internal walls, 52f
  retention, 59f
Amantadine, 308
Ameloblastic carcinoma, 126
Ameloblastic fibroma, 127
Ameloblastic fibro-odontoma, 127
Ameloblastoma, 10, 125-126, 125f
Amelogenesis imperfecta, 131, 131f, 189
Amides, 308
  bond, hydrolysis, 309
Amiloride, 322
Aminoglycosides, 333
Amino terminus, dealkylation, 309
Amiodarone, 318
Amoxicillin, 281, 332
Amphetamine/dextroamphetamine, 192
Amylin analogue, 327
Amyloidosis, occurrence, 123
Anaerobic bacteria, role, 94t
Analgesics, 313-317
Analysis of variance (ANOVA) test, 228
Analytical epidemiology, 223-224
Analytical statistics, 226
Anatomic contours, problems, 44
Anatomic radiolucencies, 10
Anchorage, 171-172
  cortical anchorage, 172
  implants, 172
  reinforced anchorage, 172
  stationary anchorage, 172
Anesthetics, 308-313
  amounts, calculation, 310
  properties, 294t
Aneurysmal bone cyst, 128
Angiotensin-converting enzyme (ACE) inhibitors, 290, 322
  adverse effects, 321
  dual function, 320f
  usefulness, 321
Angiotensin II receptor antagonists, 321
Angle classification, 155-156, 160
Angle class III malocclusions, 155
Angle class II malocclusions, 155
Angle-formers, 48
Angular cheilitis, 351
Angular defects, 276
Angular osseous defect, 149